Clinical Blood Gases

Assessment and Intervention

Clinical Blood Gases

Assessment and Intervention

Second Edition

William J. Malley, MS, RRT, CPFT
Administrative Director, Respiratory Services
The Western Pennsylvania Hospital
Program Director, School of Respiratory Care
Indiana University of Pennsylvania/The Western Pennsylvania Hospital
Pittsburgh, Pennsylvania

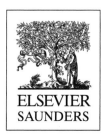

ELSEVIER
SAUNDERS

ELSEVIER
SAUNDERS

11830 Westline Industrial Drive
St. Louis, Missouri 63146

CLINICAL BLOOD GASES: ASSESSMENT
AND INTERVENTION, SECOND EDITION
Copyright © 2005, Elsevier (USA). All rights reserved.

NOTICE

Pharmacology is an ever-changing field. Standard safety precautions must be followed, but as new research and clinical experience broaden our knowledge, changes in treatment and drug therapy may become necessary or appropriate. Readers are advised to check the most current product information provided by the manufacturer of each drug to be administered to verify the recommended dose, the method and duration of administration, and contraindications. It is the responsibility of the licensed prescriber, relying on experience and knowledge of the patient, to determine dosages and the best treatment for each individual patient. Neither the Publisher nor the author assumes any liability for any injury and/or damage to persons or property arising from this publication.

Previous edition copyrighted 1990.

ISBN-13: 978-0-7216-8422-2
ISBN-10: 0-7216-8422-X

Managing Editor: Mindy Hutchinson
Senior Developmental Editor: Melissa K. Boyle
Publishing Services Manager: Melissa Lastarria
Project Manager: Joy Moore
Designer: Amy Buxton

Printed in the United States of America

Last digit is the print number: 9   8   7

To my dad (rest in peace),
    For his inspiration, spirit, and wit.

To my mom,
    For her understanding and love.

To my wife, Margie,
    For her infinite endurance and love.

Reviewers

ALLEN W. BARBARO, MS, RRT
Program Director, Respiratory Care
St. Luke's College
Sioux City, Iowa

SUSAN BLONSHINE, BS, RRT, RPFT,
  FAARC, AE-C
Director, TechEd Consultants
Mason, Michigan
Technical Director, Pediatric Pulmonary
  Function Laboratory
Michigan State University
East Lansing, Michigan

LINDA K. EVANS, RN, MSN
Instructor of Clinical Nursing
Sinclair School of Nursing
University of Missouri
Columbia, Missouri

CATHERINE M. FOSS, BS, RRT, RPFT
Clinical Research Coordinator, Pulmonary
  and Critical Care
Duke University Medical Center
Durham, North Carolina
AARC Diagnostic Specialty Section Chair

LAVERNE YOUSEY, RRT, MSTE
Chair, Allied Health Department
Program Director, R.C. Program
Professor of Respiratory Care
University of Akron
Akron, Ohio

Preface

More than a decade has passed since the first edition of *Clinical Blood Gases*, yet the need for clinicians with a comprehensive understanding of blood gas analysis and interpretation persists. Overall, I suspect we do fewer blood gases today than we did then primarily as a result of cost-containment initiatives and the ubiquitous availability of pulse oximetry. Nevertheless, even today, arterial blood gases remain the undisputable gold standard in the critical assessment of oxygenation, acid-base balance, and ventilation.

It could be argued that because of the decreased incidence of blood gas sampling, blood gas analysis has become of lesser importance. Indeed, the opposite is the case. Acquisition of arterial blood gases seems to be reserved for more critical situations, specifically in those patients where vital life functions are in question. In many cases, electrolytes or other analytes are measured concurrently with blood gases to provide a more comprehensive glimpse into disease or emergent needs.

It has been my observation that with fewer blood gases being drawn, many clinicians fail to maintain interpretative competence or, worse yet, never achieve it. Thus, when a patient crisis exists and a definitive analysis of oxygenation, acid-base, and/or ventilation is essential, no one may be available or sufficiently experienced to respond. Therefore now, as perhaps never before, clinicians who are expert in the nuances of this assessment are vital. This text is written to ensure that blood gas experts are never extinct. This second edition is also designed for the critical thinker and life-long student of oxygenation, acid-base balance, ventilation, and related pathophysiology.

Because of the widespread acceptance of the first edition, the book is organized in much the same manner with a few key exceptions. Classification, or naming, of blood gases (referred to as *interpretation* by some) has been relocated to Chapter 2 (Chapter 7 in the first edition) because the skill needed to be able to categorize blood gases must be mastered in the early phase of clinical practice. In an effort to be more consistent with common clinical practice and exams, I have also abandoned the use of the terms *acidemia* and *alkalemia* in classifications. Since one must have an acidosis to cause an *acidemia*, I have simply used the term acidosis in blood gas classification. Also, the chapter on technical accuracy (Chapter 8 in the first edition) has been relocated to Chapter 5 so that all technical issues are covered in Unit 2.

In addition to overall updates regarding technology and clinical application, probably the most significant enhancement to the text as a teaching tool is the addition of two "On-Call Cases" within each chapter. These cases involve critical thinking and application and deal specifically with important content contained within each chapter. On-Call Cases are germane to the particular content of a specific chapter which differentiates them from the more comprehensive cases in Chapter 16. Detailed discussion regarding the On-Call Cases is provided in the Answers section near the end of the book. Case questions are designed in a consistent manner to encourage analytical problem-solving skills and specific action.

Another new feature, "NBRC Challenge," offers five multiple-choice questions at the end of each chapter. These questions were cross-referenced to the National Board for Respiratory Care (NBRC) examination matrices in effect at the time of development of the book. Various questions may be based on any of the various exams used for Certified or Registered Respiratory Therapist credentialing. Although the NBRC matrix is continuously evolving and specific references to the matrices may change, the goal of these multiple-choice questions is critical thinking with particular reference to actual job functions, experiences, and responsibilities. The slight change in the subtitle to *Clinical Blood Gases: Assessment and Intervention* highlights the clinical decision-making focus of the text.

Like the first edition, the second edition of *Clinical Blood Gases* remains the most comprehensive, current, and easy-to-read reference for clinical issues pertaining to acid-base balance, oxygenation, blood gases, and noninvasive blood gas measurements. Furthermore, it again provides a lavish supply of clear illustrations and tables to organize thinking and visualize concepts.

Clinical Blood Gases remains unique in its role as a medical textbook. It is not only a reference book but also a clearly organized, comprehensive, interactive educational vehicle. It is my hope that, like the first edition, it will be enthusiastically received by respiratory therapists, physicians, nurses, and other health-related professionals. Most importantly, I hope it will be a rich source of information and understanding that will, in turn, ultimately enhance patient care.

William J. Malley, MS, RRT, CPFT

Please feel free to forward any unusual cases, questions, or correspondence to William Malley at bmalley@icubed.com.

Acknowledgments

Very few textbooks of this magnitude are written by a single author. I believe the value and advantage of a single author is a continuity of writing style, organization, focus, and approach. The potential disadvantage of the single-author approach is the critical need for peer review and multiple viewpoints. I have been fortunate to be surrounded by outstanding colleagues and a rich source of reviewers through Elsevier.

My first source of review includes the outstanding faculty at the Indiana University of Pennsylvania/The Western Pennsylvania Hospital baccalaureate respiratory therapy program. The extensive clinical and professional knowledge of Kathy Kinderman, Jeff Heck, Jack Albert, Catherine Myers, and Jackie Heisler is always readily accessible. Whenever I feel uncertainty, I look to their remarkable clinical expertise and guidance.

Another valuable reference for me is Bud Jozwiak, director of the excellent laboratories at The Western Pennsylvania Hospital. Bud is an invaluable resource for accurate laboratory and technical information. He's always readily available to provide direction, information, and counsel. Robin Nitkulinec, Manager of Respiratory Services, Charlie Morgan, Supervisor of Pulmonary Diagnostics, and Paul Fiehler, MD, Medical Director, are likewise always available to provide valuable expertise.

I am also a recipient of the tremendous resources and commitment to excellence from Elsevier. Elsevier is relentless in their pursuit of accuracy and quality. Melissa Boyle, Senior Developmental Editor, and Mindy Hutchinson, Managing Editor, have provided me with a rich source of expert reviewers and feedback in times of uncertainty. They have also gently provided me with the needed encouragement and support to complete this project in the midst of our harried careers, families, and lives. They were patient but helped me stay the course. Joy Moore, Production Project Manager, and Janine White, Production Editor, were also a pleasure to work with.

The advantage and resources of a first-class publisher is clearly evident to me. Without the resourceful and cordial negotiations of Andrew Allen, Publishing Director, I suspect this second edition would never have reached fruition. He provided creativity, open communication, patience, and support throughout.

Most importantly, friends, family, and co-workers who I see every day need a special thanks. My secretary, Georgeann Meyers, Clinical Director Kathy Kinderman, and faculty are always there to provide help, support, and understanding in my daily work environment. Finally, my wife, Margie, who has endured the most, has provided the ultimate positive support to complete a project of this magnitude.

Contents

Introduction to Blood Gases

Blood gas and pH analysis has more immediacy and potential impact on patient care than any other laboratory determination.

National Committee for Clinical Laboratory Standards[690]

There is no substitute for PO$_2$, PCO$_2$, and pH when you are really in the dark about oxygenation status, acid-base, or ventilatory status.

Woody Kagler, M.D.[105]

Outline

INTRODUCTION

The *arterial blood gas report* is the cornerstone in the diagnosis and management of clinical oxygenation and acid-base disturbances. An abnormal blood gas report may be the first clue to an acid-base or oxygenation problem: It may indicate the onset or culmination of cardiopulmonary crisis and may serve as a gauge with regard to the appropriateness or effectiveness of therapy. Thus, the arterial blood gas report plays a pivotal role in the overall care of cardiopulmonary disease. Using the arterial blood gas report as a reference point, this text explores the diagnosis, assessment, and intervention of clinical acid-base and oxygenation problems.

Over the past decade, the incidence of arterial blood gas sampling has decreased primarily for cost-containment reasons. Clinicians, casually and increasingly, rely on pulse oximetry as a complete substitute for arterial blood gas data. Although pulse oximetry is extremely valuable and provides us with real-time information, it provides only one small piece in oxygenation assessment. Furthermore, it has been shown that many junior physicians and nurses do not fully understand this technology and make serious errors in its interpretation.[167]

More importantly, pulse oximetry provides absolutely no information regarding ventilation and acid-base balance. In one study, more than 50% of surgical patients who had arterial blood gases drawn manifested alkalemia at some point during their hospital stay.[106] With only pulse oximetry, these acid-base abnormalities may easily go unnoticed and untreated. In contrast to pulse oximetry, there are myriad reasons for arterial blood gas analysis. According to Clinical Guidelines published by the American Association for Respiratory Care (AARC), indications also include assessment of the adequacy of ventilation, acid-base evaluation, diagnostic evaluation, quantification of response to therapy, and monitoring of severity and progression of disease.[15]

Several studies have shown that by avoiding the use of blood gases, we may be delaying or preventing detection of serious oxygenation and acid-base disturbances.[108–111] The real incremental cost of an arterial blood gas report is minuscule. The neglected and unquantifiable cost of overlooked clues in the diagnosis of life-threatening disturbances (i.e., acid-base, ventilation, and oxygenation) is immeasurable. Arterial blood gases remain the gold standard in comprehensive emergency and critical care assessment. Their value must be weighed against the potential for real, substantial cost savings and patient harm.

NORMAL BLOOD GAS VALUES

Indices

Table 1-1 shows the various indices that are typically reported when an arterial blood gas is acquired. Collectively, these indices give us valuable information about the important triad of patient oxygenation, ventilation, and acid-base balance.

Oxygenation

Arterial blood gases remain the indisputable gold standard for evaluation of arterial oxygenation.

Dean Hess, Ph.D., RRT, FAARC[168]

There are two indices shown in Table 1-1 (i.e., PaO_2 and SaO_2) that basically reflect the amount of O_2 present in the blood. Oxygen is carried

in the blood in two forms, dissolved O_2 and combined O_2. The PaO_2 is the partial pressure of O_2 *dissolved* in arterial blood, whereas the SaO_2 is the oxygen saturation of arterial hemoglobin (an indicator of *combined* O_2).

Technically, the partial pressure of oxygen (denoted PO_2) is defined as the pressure of O_2 in both a gas phase and a solution in equilibrium.[6] In contrast, oxygen saturation is the amount of oxyhemoglobin in a solution expressed as a fraction (%) of the total amount of hemoglobin able to bind oxygen.[6] It is noteworthy that abnormal (inactive) forms of hemoglobin (dyshemoglobins) are not considered in this calculation.[241]

The PaO_2 is directly measured and is the most sensitive indicator of oxygenation directly measured. The PaO_2 should be a focal point of every blood gas interpretation. The SaO_2 is a calculated value and a less sensitive indicator. There are times when a calculated SaO_2 may be misleading (e.g., burn patients) so it is sometimes not included with the routine blood gas report. Calculated SaO_2 should not be used for further clinical calculations such as shunt fraction because it may introduce significant error.[241] SaO_2 can actually be measured directly with co-oximetry (as opposed to calculated) in cases when this value is essential. Clinical and technical issues related to co-oximetry are discussed in Chapters 11 and 15.

Ventilation

The single best way to evaluate the adequacy of ventilation is via the $PaCO_2$ of an arterial blood gas. One cannot make a definitive evaluation of whether an individual is hypoventilating or hyperventilating by observation alone. Ventilatory status is best assessed via arterial blood gases.

Acid-Base Balance

The arterial pH is the single best indicator of global and blood acid-base status. In addition to providing definitive information about ventilation, the $PaCO_2$ also allows us to evaluate the respiratory component of acid-base balance. Thus, we can determine if a given acid-base problem is of respiratory system origin.

The remaining indices shown in Table 1-1 ($[HCO_3]$ and $[BE]$) are "non-respiratory"

Table 1-1. NORMAL ARTERIAL BLOOD GAS VALUES

pH	7.35–7.45
$PaCO_2$	35–45 mm Hg
[BE]	0 ± 2 mEq/L
PaO_2	80–100 mm Hg
$[HCO_3]$	24 ± 2 mEq/L
SaO_2	97%–98%

acid-base indices. Non-respiratory indices are commonly referred to as *metabolic indices*. Metabolic indices will be abnormal when the patient has a so-called metabolic (non-respiratory) acid-base disturbance. Actually, the term *metabolic* is sometimes misleading because the patient often does not have a problem with metabolism per se, nevertheless, it is well ingrained in the acid-base lexicon and will be used in this text.

Although it is common practice, it is really unnecessary to include both [BE] and plasma [HCO_3] on a report. This practice originates from the *Great Transatlantic Debate*[4,5] between the Boston and Copenhagen schools of thought regarding acid-base diagnosis and treatment.

The Boston school has always advocated the use and application of plasma [HCO_3] as the most appropriate metabolic index. This index is calculated by most blood gas machines via the application of the well-known Henderson-Hasselbalch equation. The plasma [HCO_3] is also historically involved in the development of blood gas analysis because it was the first metabolic index to be routinely reported. Understanding of plasma [HCO_3] is also essential because it is the metabolic index most often used in respiratory care credentialling examinations.

The Copenhagen school, on the other hand, advocates the use of the [BE] as the primary metabolic indicator, purporting its superiority both diagnostically and therapeutically. The index of choice is really a matter of personal preference because the patient can be treated appropriately with use of either index. The level of understanding of the particular index being used has greater importance, because both indices may be misleading if their particular nuances are not well understood.

Historically, a variety of other metabolic indices have been reported (e.g., standard bicarbonate, total body buffer base, and CO_2 combining power[2,3]), but none of these indices is currently well accepted. Furthermore, they provide us with no additional information necessary for optimum care of patients. They may, however, serve as a source of confusion and are probably best omitted from the blood gas report.

Normal Ranges

The various quantities shown in Table 1-1 are referred to collectively as arterial blood gases (ABGs). The values indicated in Table 1-1 are normal ranges for adults. Normal ranges are defined by the criterion that 95% of the normal population have values that fall within this range. Normal values for any laboratory measurement are established through measurements made on individuals assumed to have normal health. The average value is calculated as well as the dispersion of values around the average, which is described by a statistical term called the *standard deviation*.

A large number of measurements made on any normal population generally yields a distribution pattern similar to the one shown in Figure 1-1. The most frequent value observed would be identical to the arithmetic mean. As values deviate more and more from the mean, they occur less and less frequently. The curve represented in Figure 1-1 is referred to as the *normal* (or gaussian) *distribution*. In the normal distribution, 68% of the population has values that fall within 1 standard deviation and 95% of the values measured in the population fall within 2 standard deviations. Finally, 99.73% of measurements fall within 3 standard deviations.

Normal laboratory values are generally considered to be within ±2 standard deviations

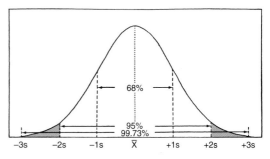

Figure 1-1. **Normal distribution of laboratory values.** Of the normal population, 68% have measurements that fall within 1 standard deviation from the mean ($\bar{x}$). Ninety-five percent of the population values fall within 2 standard deviations, and 99.73% fall within 3 standard deviations. Normal laboratory values are considered to be ±2 standard deviations from the mean.

from the mean because these values represent the vast majority of the population. The distribution pattern underlying the establishment of normal values is important to understand because 5% of the normal population has values that fall outside the normal range. Nevertheless, it is highly unlikely that an abnormal value reported in this population will deviate greatly from the normal range.

Interestingly, there are data that suggest that the mean normal pH is closer to 7.38 than 7.40.[3] Nevertheless, there is little support or reason to change the accepted normal range because the difference is minimal and the range of 7.35 to 7.45 is well ingrained.

Regarding the normal blood gas values shown in Table 1-1, one study showed significantly lower values for arterial carbon dioxide tension ($PaCO_2$) in young women compared to values in young men.[7] Mean arterial PCO_2 in the female group was 33 mm Hg. Lower arterial PCO_2 in women compared with men is also consistent with some earlier findings.[8] Indeed, values of 30 to 46 mm Hg may more accurately characterize the normal range for the entire population, which is calculated from seven published studies.[9] While keeping these issues in mind, the *accepted* normal range of 35 to 45 mm Hg is used in this text for standardization and to avoid confusion.

Normal values for [BE] and [HCO_3] may likewise be slightly (i.e., 1 to 2 mEq/L) lower in women than in men.[7] Nevertheless, here again, a single accepted normal range of 24 ± 2 mEq/L for [HCO_3] and 0 ± 2 mEq/L for [BE] is used because the difference is slight and has little clinical significance.

The mean partial pressure of oxygen dissolved in arterial blood (PaO_2) in a normal young male is 97 mm Hg at sea level.[10] Normal oxygen saturation of arterial hemoglobin (SaO_2) is 97.5%. Both PaO_2 and SaO_2 values tend to decrease with aging.

Oxygenation values may also differ slightly with body position; they are typically higher in the sitting position than in the supine (lying on the back) position particularly in the obese or elderly. Finally, altitude and the percentage of O_2 inspired also affect PaO_2. The effects of these variables on PaO_2 are discussed in Chapter 3. In this text, room air (21% oxygen)

and sea level (760 mm Hg) are presumed unless otherwise noted.

The normal PaO_2 in the supine position for an adult 40 to 75 years old can be calculated specifically by the formula $PaO_2 = 109 - (0.43 \times age)$.[242] A PaO_2 within ± 8 mm Hg of the predicted value is considered to be normal. Because the *minimum* normal PaO_2 at 40 years of age in the supine position is 80 mm Hg, most tables show the normal PaO_2 range as being approximately 80 to 100 mm Hg. Technically, however, a PaO_2 of 80 mm Hg in a 20-year-old individual is not normal.

Arterial PO_2 is approximately 5 mm Hg higher in the sitting position than in the supine position and the mean normal value at a given age can be calculated more precisely by the formula $PaO_2 = 109 - (0.27 \times age)$.[11] In general, the difference in PaO_2 associated with positional change is minimal in young adults but magnified in the elderly.

In clinical practice, it is not usually practical or expedient to calculate PaO_2 based on these formulas. An approximate rule of thumb is sometimes useful to estimate the *minimum* normal PaO_2 in adults of different ages. Minimum normal PaO_2 should exceed 90 mm Hg if the patient is younger than 45 years old. Above the age of 45, PaO_2 generally decreases with age; however, low minimum normal PaO_2 should exceed 75 mm Hg regardless of age.[242] Interestingly, PaO_2 seems to progressively decrease between the ages of 45 to 75, then actually increases slightly and levels off beyond age 75.[242] This is contrary to earlier beliefs.

Units of Measurement

It is essential to have a clear understanding of the particular units in which any laboratory value is being measured. The pH value is dimension-less, and SaO_2 is measured as a percentage. The [HCO_3] and [BE] are usually reported in milliequivalents per liter (mEq/L). Nevertheless, because mEq/L is equal to millimoles per liter (mM/L) in ions with a univalent charge (e.g., HCO_3^-, Na^+), mM/L may also be used as the units for these values.

The PaO_2 and $PaCO_2$ are measured in millimeters of mercury (mm Hg), a unit of pressure. The unit *torr* is synonymous with (mm Hg) and either may be substituted interchangeably.

The International System of Units (SI) has attempted to standardize the reporting of all scientific data and has made recommendations with regard to the most appropriate units that should be used.

The recommended SI unit for pressure is the pascal (Pa). Because this unit is too small for clinical use, the kilopascal (kPa) has been recommended for use in blood gases (1 kPa = 1000 Pa). The conversion factor from mm Hg to kPa is 0.133. Thus, the normal range of PaO_2 (i.e., 80 to 100 mm Hg) becomes 10.6 to 13.3 kPa, and the normal $PaCO_2$ (i.e., 35 to 45 mm Hg) becomes 4.6 to 6.0 kPa. The clinician may see PaO_2 and $PaCO_2$ reported in SI units in some foreign literature, but the awkwardness of the decimal units has hampered general acceptance and there has been a general retreat from SI units in American journals and laboratories.[13] Likewise, clinicians continue to use mm Hg or torr when they report pressure measurements in blood gas analysis. A chart of pressure conversion factors between mm Hg, kPa, and cm H_2O is shown in Table 1-2.

ARTERIAL VERSUS VENOUS BLOOD

Blood vessels that carry blood away from the heart are classified anatomically as arteries, whereas vessels that return blood to the heart are called veins. Arterial blood in the systemic circulation (Fig. 1-2) provides more information than systemic venous blood with regard to ventilation and oxygenation assessment. Arterial blood is a uniform substance presented to all organs for their metabolic needs.

An important concern in oxygenation assessment is the adequacy of O_2 delivery to all

Table 1-2. PRESSURE UNIT CONVERSION FACTORS

cm H_2O	mm Hg	kPa
1.0	0.736	0.098
1.359	1.0	0.133
10.197	7.501	1.0

From Burke, J.F.: Surgical Physiology. Philadelphia, W.B. Saunders, 1984.

human cells. To assess delivery, one must analyze arterial blood en route *to* the cells. The PO_2 of peripheral venous blood, on its journey back to the heart *from* the cells, provides little information concerning O_2 delivery.

Arterial blood also provides direct information with regard to lung function and the adequacy of CO_2 excretion. When $PaCO_2$ levels are excessive, the ventilatory system has failed to perform one of its primary functions—namely, CO_2 regulation in the blood. The *venous* PCO_2 level, on the other hand, is primarily a result of local metabolic rate and perfusion. Either an increase in local metabolism or a decrease in local perfusion elevates venous PCO_2. Thus, venous PCO_2 varies in different areas of the body and provides little useful information regarding the adequacy of pulmonary ventilation.

Finally, arterial blood is superior to peripheral venous blood in both acid-base and oxygenation assessment because it reflects *overall* blood or body conditions. *Arterial blood gases are uniform regardless of the specific artery from which the sample was drawn.* This is true because arterial blood, after being well mixed in the heart, does not change appreciably in O_2 or CO_2 composition until it reaches the systemic capillaries. The systemic capillaries are the small vessels between arteries and veins within which gas exchange takes place between blood and body tissues. In general, samples of blood gases taken from any artery should have identical blood gas values.

Peripheral venous blood, on the other hand, reflects only localized conditions. The O_2 and CO_2 levels in a given peripheral vein depend on the metabolic rate and perfusion of the tissue traversed earlier. Because local metabolism may vary widely, venous blood gas samples acquired simultaneously from different peripheral veins likewise vary substantially. The different PvO_2 levels in various peripheral veins are discussed later in Chapter 7 and are shown in Table 7-1.

Although less accurate than arterial samples, venous samples from a well-perfused patient may provide a gross indication of acid-base balance,[5] electrolyte levels, or abnormal hemoglobins.[241] Likewise venous blood pH appears to correlate well with arterial blood in patients

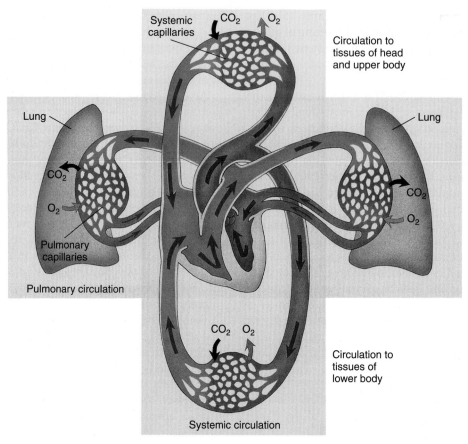

Figure 1-2.   Pulmonary and systemic circulation. Blood from the pulmonary circulation flows back to the left heart after gas exchange in the lungs. Oxygenated blood flows from the left heart to the systemic circulation.

with uremic acidosis and diabetic ketoacidosis.[112] One should also realize that any difference between arterial and venous blood will be exaggerated when the general or local circulation is impaired.[107] Thus, measurement of arterial blood gases is the gold standard in the diagnosis and clinical management of oxygenation and acid-base disturbances.

TECHNIQUE

The collection of arterial blood is not only technically difficult but can be painful and hazardous to the patient. Therefore, it is essential that individuals performing arterial puncture be familiar with the proper techniques, with the dangers of the procedure, and with necessary precautions.

National Committee for Clinical Laboratory Standards[107]

Compared with the acquisition of venous blood, arterial sampling is technically more difficult and has greater potential for serious complication. The higher arterial pressure can make bleeding complications more profuse. Furthermore, large clot formation or prolonged spasm in an artery could cut off vital supply of O_2 to the tissue. Arterial blood gas samples are also very vulnerable to improper handling technique because of their high gas content. Arterial blood is one of the most sensitive specimens sent for clinical laboratory analysis.[107]

Despite these drawbacks, after appropriate training, arterial blood sampling may be accomplished simply, safely, accurately, and expediently by respiratory therapists, laboratory technologists, nurses, or physicians. The following section involves pre-analytical considerations when preparing to draw an arterial blood sample; this is followed by a description of a technique of arterial puncture and specimen collection.

Preparation and Pre-analytical Considerations

Status of Patients and Control of Infection

Before attempting to perform an arterial puncture, the clinician should always be aware of the patient's primary diagnoses and current status. A brief review of the chart, inspection of the patient, and observation for respiratory care modalities (e.g., O_2 therapy, mechanical ventilation) are essential. This initial evaluation may alert the clinician to a potential complication or suggest that the sample should be drawn at a later time. When the sample is to be drawn by a non-physician, the first step is to verify that a written order is documented in the patient's chart. The chart should then be evaluated for factors (e.g., medications) that might suggest the need for special precautionary measures.

Anticoagulants/Bleeding Disorders

Pharmacologic therapy should be reviewed to ascertain whether the patient is undergoing anticoagulant or thrombolytic therapy. Commonly prescribed anticoagulants include heparin, warfarin (Coumadin), and dipyridamole. The mild anticoagulant effect of aspirin may be of lesser importance.[15] Anticoagulant therapy is associated with an increased likelihood of bleeding complication after puncture, and additional preventive measures should be taken. Consideration may be given to scheduling the arterial puncture approximately 30 minutes before the next scheduled dose of anticoagulant, if feasible.[16]

Thrombolytics (e.g., streptokinase, tissue plasminogen activator) differ from anticoagulants in that they are administered to break down (lyse) blood clots rather than simply to prevent clotting. Nevertheless, excessive bleeding after arterial puncture may also occur when these drugs are being administered.[15]

When evaluating the patient's history and progress notes, the clinician should be especially alert for documentation of blood coagulation disorders (coagulopathy). Hemophilia, a genetic disorder found in men, is characterized by a prolonged blood clotting time and, therefore, a predisposition to bleeding complications. Similarly, a low platelet count or a prolonged bleeding time on laboratory reports should also be noted. Identification of any coagulation disorder should activate implementation of special bleeding precautions.

Infection Control

The clinician should always be cognizant that infectious diseases may be transmitted by contact with blood. The disease foremost on our minds in this regard is the acquired immunodeficiency syndrome (AIDS). AIDS is caused by the human immunodeficiency virus (HIV), formerly known as the human T-lymphotropic virus type III–lymphadenopathy-associated virus. This viral disease has essentially no cure as yet and may be contracted through intimate contact with the body secretions of an infected individual.

The body secretions that contain the greatest amount of the virus are blood, semen, and vaginal secretions.[17] The virus may be transmitted by sexual contact, percutaneous (through the skin) exposure, absorption through mucous membranes (e.g., mouth, eyes), and through non-intact mucous membranes or skin (e.g., cuts, open wounds).[17] The risk that healthcare workers may acquire the disease is related to the potential for percutaneous exposure or mucous membrane contact with contaminated body secretions.

A major problem in controlling the spread of this disease is the fact that individuals infected with the virus are asymptomatic early in the disease while at the same time they are contagious. Thus, all blood samples must be treated as though infectious and handled with standard precautions.[107] Standard precautions are new guidelines that include the major features of universal fluid precautions and body substance isolation procedures.[107] Standard precautions are more comprehensive than universal precautions, which only account for bloodborne pathogens. Standard precautions address the transmission of all bloodborne pathogens.[107] Both standard precautions and universal precautions are available through the Centers for Disease Control.

Other infectious disorders that may be acquired through blood contact include viral hepatitis, syphilis, Jakob-Creutzfeldt disease, and septicemia. Viral hepatitis is a generalized inflammation of the liver caused by hepatitis virus A, B, or C. Hepatitis vaccination, which prevents hepatitis B on a long-term basis, is available and healthcare workers who routinely perform arterial puncture should receive it. There is also an injection available to prevent hepatitis A in the short term; however, no protection is available for hepatitis C. Syphilis is a chronic infectious venereal disease that may also be transmitted through the blood. Jakob-Creutzfeldt disease is a rare, fatal neurologic disorder that is transmitted by a virus. Septicemia is a systemic infection in which pathogens are present in the blood.

In the past, samples obtained from individuals with any of the above disorders were marked as *precaution samples*, and special procedures were implemented to minimize the risk of infection to the healthcare worker. Today, however, *all* blood samples should be handled as if they are infected, because most individuals who have HIV are not diagnosed and are asymptomatic.

Standard precautions require diligent handwashing and use of gloves when the hands are likely to come into contact with body secretions (e.g., during arterial blood gas sampling[14]). The Centers for Disease Control also recommends the use of masks and protective eyewear (to avoid contact with mucous membranes) if a procedure is likely to generate droplets of blood and aprons or gowns if blood is likely to be splashed during a procedure.[19]

Handwashing is critical between examinations of patients and immediately after any direct contact with blood. Gloves should always be worn when acquiring an arterial blood sample, and the gloves should be changed before contact with each new patient. Remember, however, that gloves are an adjunct to, but not a substitute for, handwashing.

Furthermore, needles must be handled carefully to prevent accidental puncture. Needle sticks are the most frequent source of transmission of bloodborne diseases in healthcare workers.[19,20] Needles should not be purposely bent or broken by hand, removed from syringes, or manipulated by hand in any way. Specimen sampling devices in which the needle retracts

after use or use of some other device to assure that inadvertent puncture cannot occur is essential. After use, needles should be placed in puncture-resistant containers that are located as close as is practical to the area where they are being used.

Patient Identification and Assessment

Identification of the correct patient is extremely important. NCCLS document H3—*Procedure for the Collection of Diagnostic Blood Specimens by Venipuncture*—describes this in more detail.[691]

Likewise, the patient and the clinical indication for the sample should be assessed before acquisition. Knowledge of current vital signs and a general awareness of the patient's background and psychological status may also contribute to acquisition of the sample smoothly and efficiently. The more information the clinician has with regard to a particular patient, the more prepared he or she is to care for that patient most effectively. Notwithstanding, the review of the chart is most often brief in clinical practice due to time constraints and the need for efficiency.

Steady State

When oxygen therapy or mechanical ventilation is used, a period of time is required before the complete effect of the therapy is reflected in the arterial blood specimen. Similarly, the same principle is true when therapy is changed or discontinued and following exercise. Because blood gases are often the major criteria on which major therapeutic decisions are made regarding oxygenation and acid-base disturbances, it is crucial that the blood gas results provide us with an accurate and current reflection of the patient's status.

During this period of adjustment to a change in therapy, blood gas values are in a *dynamic, changing state*. In time, the entire cardiopulmonary system reaches a new equilibrium or *steady state*. Blood gas values remain relatively constant from this point on, and the complete impact of the therapy is reflected in the arterial blood.

Arterial blood samples must always be drawn only when the patient is in a steady state. The actual time required for the attainment of a steady state differs slightly with the patient's pulmonary status. In patients free of overt pulmonary disease, a steady state is likely achieved in as few as 1 to 3 minutes[1,21] and almost certainly within 10 minutes.[22,23]

In patients with chronic airway obstruction, up to 24 minutes after a change in therapy may be necessary.[24] In clinical practice, a 20- to 30-minute waiting period is usually recommended before sampling arterial blood after a change in oxygen therapy or ventilation.[1,15,25] As described previously, however, only 3 to 10 minutes is necessary to achieve steady-state conditions in the *absence* of pulmonary disease.

Ideally, a patient who is breathing spontaneously should also be at rest for at least 5 minutes before sample acquisition.[14] Likewise, temporary fluctuations in therapy also compromise steady-state conditions, which may occur if the patient removes his or her oxygen mask or must be suctioned for excessive pulmonary secretions. The clinician drawing the sample is responsible for ensuring that the patient is in a steady state before arterial puncture. When a sample is thought to represent non–steady-state conditions, a repeat puncture with related pain, risks, and cost is probably necessary. Worse yet, if the non–steady state goes unnoticed, incorrect or inappropriate therapy may be prescribed. Thus, before arterial puncture, the patient must be carefully assessed to ensure steady-state conditions.

Samples drawn to assess response to exercise require special considerations. They are best drawn at peak exercise, however, samples drawn within 15 seconds of termination of exercise are acceptable.[15] Outside this time range, samples may yield false-negative results for hypoxemia.[15]

Mild to moderate pain may accompany arterial puncture.[26] The clinician should be aware that pain and anxiety associated with arterial sampling may in itself cause changes in ventilation that, in turn, alter blood gas results. Thus, the patient should be approached calmly with a quiet voice and reassurance to promote physical and mental comfort[14]; and the sample should be obtained as quickly as possible. Some suggest the use of numbing agents before the actual puncture[26] and this issue is discussed later in this chapter.

Spontaneous Variability of PaO₂

The clinician should also appreciate that some studies have shown considerable spontaneous variability in PaO_2 in apparently stable patients.[169] This variability may be as much as 10% and may be due to patient or machine issues.[168] The important point here is that changes in PaO_2 of as much as ±8 mm Hg should be viewed with skepticism because they are commonly a result of spontaneous variability.

Documenting Current Status

Many times, the individual who interprets and acts upon the blood gas report is not the same individual who drew the sample. Therefore, it is important that sufficient information regarding the patient's status at the time of the sample be documented. Sound decisions can be made only in the proper context of circumstances at the time of sampling.

Specific information regarding identification of the sample and the date and time of acquisition is essential on the requisition slip. This information must include the patient's full name and hospital or emergency room number. The blood vessel source should also be noted (i.e., arterial, venous, or mixed venous). Potential technical issues that may impact the quality of the sample should be noted as well. These might include issues such as improper storage of the sample or transportation delays. Other desirable information includes the location of the patient, working diagnosis, clinical indication, name of the physician requesting the sample, the initials of the individual who obtained the sample, and the sample site.[14]

The patient's temperature and respiratory rate should likewise be recorded. The position of the patient (e.g., supine, sitting) at the time of sampling and the activity of the patient (e.g., comatose, convulsing) may also provide valuable information when the data are interpreted. Hemoglobin concentration may be useful in assessing oxygenation status or calculating [BE]. Notations of fluid infusions and location may likewise be useful in some cases. The type and flow rate of O_2 therapy should be checked and recorded. When positive airway pressure (e.g., Continuous Positive Airway Pressure [CPAP] or Biphasic Positive

Airway Pressure [BIPAP]) is being applied, the inspiratory and expiratory pressures being delivered should be observed and recorded.

In the case of the patient receiving mechanical ventilation, a host of other variables should be documented. The type of ventilator and mode of ventilation should be recorded. The respiratory rate setting on the machine as well as the actual respiratory rate of the patient should be determined and included on the report. When applicable, the positive end-expiratory pressure (PEEP) level or BIPAP levels should be observed on the pressure manometer of the machine and recorded. Finally, the fraction of inspired oxygen (FIO_2) and exhaled tidal volume (VT) should be *measured* and recorded. All of this information may be important for interpreting blood gas results. In plotting the future course of treatment, it is essential to know clearly what has transpired.

Materials

Equipment needed for an arterial puncture includes a plastic syringe, anticoagulant, alcohol swabs, tape, and sterile gauze pads. A local anesthetic and sterile towel are optional. If the sample will not be run within 30 minutes or is being used to evaluate the $P(A-a)O_2$ gradient, a glass syringe and an iced transport container are also necessary. Many institutions now use commercially available arterial blood gas kits that eliminate the need to gather all of these materials.

Syringe

The basic components of a hypodermic needle and syringe are shown in Figure 1-3. The typical syringe is a 1-, 3-, or 5-mL self-filling, disposable, plastic syringe that comes pre-filled with dry heparin anticoagulant. A 20- to 25-gauge, short-beveled needle with a clear hub is usually recommended for arterial sampling in the adult.[14,16] Smaller (i.e., higher gauge) needles may not be desirable in adults because they may obscure the visual pulsation of blood characteristic of entering an artery. The volume of the syringe should be equal to the volume of blood to be sampled. The length of the needles range from $5/8$ to $1\frac{1}{2}$ in.; the longest needles are used for brachial or femoral artery sampling.[14]

In children or neonates, a 25-gauge syringe is preferable to minimize vessel trauma and bleeding.[16] Similarly, a small (high-gauge) syringe

---

ON CALL | CASE 1-1 *ABGs and Critical Thinking*

You are the only person available to care for this patient. You must assess the patient/situation and act accordingly.

A 70-year-old female in Denver arrives in the emergency room complaining of shortness of breath. She is placed on 2 Lpm of oxygen via nasal cannula. A few minutes later, a therapist arrives and draws an arterial blood gas.

ARTERIAL BLOOD GASES

pH	7.42
$PaCO_2$	34 mm Hg
PaO_2	62 mm Hg
$[HCO_3]$	21 mEq/L

ASSESSMENT

Abnormalities: List abnormal data and other noteworthy information.
The physician requests an additional sample 45 minutes later on room air. The patient is immediately placed on room air and the following results are obtained in 45 minutes.

ARTERIAL BLOOD GASES

pH	7.45
$PaCO_2$	32 mm Hg
PaO_2	60 mm Hg
$[HCO_3]$	20 mEq/L

ASSESSMENT

Abnormalities: List abnormal data and other noteworthy information.
Explanation: List possible diseases, pathology, or other circumstances that may have lead to this patient's condition.
Evaluation: Suggest additional data which would be useful in helping understand the situation or in making a diagnosis.

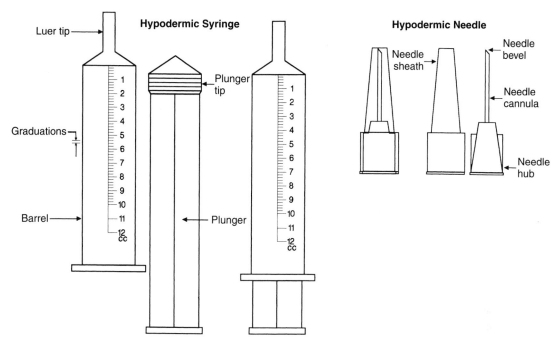

Figure 1-3.   Basic components of hypodermic needle and syringe.

may be best for arterial puncture in the patient receiving anticoagulant therapy to minimize actual vessel damage and bleeding, despite the disadvantage of masked pulsation.[16]

Either glass or plastic syringes are acceptable for specimen collection, however, there may be substantial diffusion of room air through plastic syringes particularly when they are iced.[34] PaO_2 is most affected by diffusion in plastic syringes when the PaO_2 is high or when hemoglobin in the sample is low.[1] When it is important to get a precise PaO_2 from a specimen (e.g., $P(A-a)O_2$, very high leukocyte or platelet count), a glass syringe should be used[34,65,116] and the sample analyzed quickly (i.e., within 5 to 10 minutes).[1,65,107]

Currently, quality plastic syringes with or without pre-filled heparin are available that fill spontaneously upon entry into the artery and in most cases provide acceptable results.[14] Other syringe designs allow blood to fill the syringe under its own pressure and allow filling to a predetermined volume. For example, some new syringe designs allow for filling to a predetermined volume while the blood pushes air out a vent that closes when the syringe is filled.[1]

In addition, newer syringes are often designed more safely to prevent accidental needle punctures in healthcare professionals (e.g., needle guides and retractable needles; Fig. 1-4). Some interesting points are noted in the Box 1-1.

Anticoagulant

Blood is activated to form clots after leaving the body. If allowed to proceed, this clot formation (coagulation) within the specimen would interfere with the acquisition or analysis of blood samples. Even microscopic clotting can adversely affect a blood gas analyzer. Most new blood gas syringes are pre-filled with a dry anticoagulant. Occasionally, however, in emergency situations, a *liquid* anticoagulant must be added to a standard syringe before drawing a blood gas sample. When adding liquid anticoagulant, it is important that the volume or type of anticoagulant does not alter the acid-base and oxygenation values being measured.

Type of Anticoagulant

Lithium heparin is the anticoagulant of choice in arterial blood gas sampling.[1] Lyophilized (dry) heparin is usually included in prepackaged

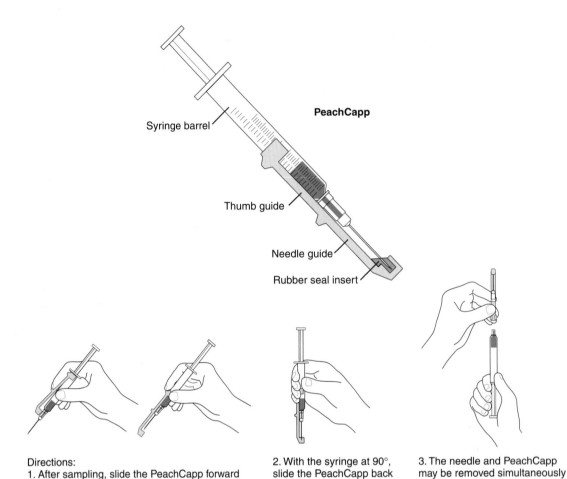

PeachCapp

Syringe barrel

Thumb guide

Needle guide

Rubber seal insert

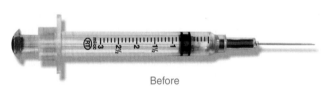

Directions:
1. After sampling, slide the PeachCapp forward until the Needle Guide clears the needle.

2. With the syringe at 90°, slide the PeachCapp back to embed the needle.

3. The needle and PeachCapp may be removed simultaneously by twisting the needle at its hub and sliding it forward.

A

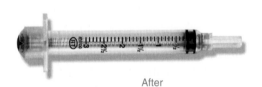

Before

After

VanishPoint Retractable Needle Syringe:
When the plunger handle is fully depressed, a spring mechanism automatically retracts the needle directly from the patient into the barrel of the syringe. This virtually eliminates any risk of accidental contaminated needle stick injury to the healthcare worker.

B

Figure 1-4.   **Safe syringe designs.** The Peachtree syringe design by Marquest Medical products (**A**) and the syringe designed by Retractable Technologies (**B**) are examples of syringes designed to prevent accidental needle punctures in healthcare workers. (Note: The Peachtree Syringe by Marquest Medical is no longer being produced or manufactured.)

Box 1-1	Needle Safety

In the United States in the year 2000:
The nation used more than 500 million needles.
There were 600,000 inadvertent needle punctures.
There were 30 needle stick injuries per year for each 100 hospital beds.
Only 15% of hospitals used safer needle designs because their cost was up to four times greater.

Reference: Neergard, L. (The Associated Press): Hospitals urged to use safer needles to reduce injuries, Pittsburgh Post Gazette, November 23, 1999, p A-14.

blood gas syringes. When liquid heparin must be added, it should be sodium heparin (1000 IU/mL). Also, when samples will be drawn to measure electrolytes as well as blood gases, *balanced heparin* should be used. Balanced heparin is physiologically balanced for the electrolytes being measured (e.g., Ca^{2+}, K^+, Cl^-, Na^+) and therefore should minimize any distortion of electrolyte concentrations in the sample.

All heparin salts have some potential to cause the formation of small fibrils in the sample which, in turn, may interfere with some equipment. Lithium heparin, because of the quantity of lithium used, is least likely to cause these problems.[27] As a rule, heparin salts (lithium, sodium) in 1000 IU/mL are the only acceptable anticoagulants for blood gas analysis. Higher concentrations of heparin (e.g., 10,000 U/mL) may alter pH and ionized calcium of the sample.

Volume of Anticoagulant

Only 0.05 mL of 1000 U/mL liquid heparin is required to anticoagulate 1 mL of blood. Because the deadspace volume of a standard 5-mL syringe with a 1-inch, 22-gauge needle is 0.2 mL, filling the syringe deadspace with heparin provides sufficient volume to anticoagulate a 4-mL blood sample.[1]

When *liquid* heparin is used, the syringe is heparinized by drawing a small amount into the syringe then distributing it throughout by working the plunger in and out several times. Because the objective is only to coat the inner walls of the syringe, the plunger is completely, albeit gently, pushed in, and any excess of heparin is expelled.[28] This procedure leaves heparin only in the syringe deadspace (needle and hub). The use of minimal liquid heparin is important because an excess of heparin is known to alter blood gas values.[1] Most new blood gas syringes

come prepackaged with dry lyophilized heparin and thus obviate syringe preparation with liquid heparin.

Transport

Because blood is living tissue, O_2 is consumed and CO_2 is produced as the blood sample sets in the syringe. The speed and significance of these changes depend on the metabolic rate.

Plastic syringes containing blood for blood gas and/or electrolyte analysis should be maintained at *room temperature* and analyzed within *30 minutes*.[34,107,116] The reader should note that this is in contrast to previous practice when all samples were iced (see discussion below). When an elevated leukocyte or platelet count is present, however, blood samples should be placed in ice and analyzed immediately or within 5 minutes.[107,116]

It was earlier practice to place all samples immediately in an ice water bath to minimize metabolism. More recently, however, it has been shown that icing samples in plastic syringes is unnecessary unless blood is being used for special studies (e.g., $P(A-a)O_2$ analysis) or more than a 30-minute delay is anticipated before analysis.[34,107]

When icing is necessary, the ice container should be large enough to allow for immersion of the syringe barrel. A mixture of ice and water in the container may facilitate more uniform cooling and an immediate decrease in metabolic function. The ice or ice/water should be capable of maintaining the blood sample at a temperature of 1° to 5° C.[14]

Alcohol, Gauze and Tape

Asepsis is the absence of disease-producing microorganisms. The aseptic technique is the use of methods that minimize the risk of infection to the patient. Most importantly, the clinician should always wear aseptic gloves for the protection of both practitioner and patient. An alcohol swab or a similar antiseptic agent is used to clean and disinfect the skin before puncture. A 2×2 in. sterile gauze pad should be available so that manual pressure can be applied aseptically to the puncture site after the needle is withdrawn. Pressure dressings are not an acceptable substitute.[14] Nosocomial (i.e., hospital-acquired) infection is a potentially serious complication of arterial puncture that can be avoided mainly through the use of proper handwashing and aseptic technique.

Local Anesthetic

Administration of a local anesthetic to the sample site to alleviate anxiety and pain is sometimes recommended.[26] Administration of a local anesthetic may relieve discomfort and minimize the risk of vasoconstriction.[1] It is theoretically plausible that the pain or anxiety associated with arterial puncture may cause hyperventilation and alteration of blood gas values, although this has not been clearly demonstrated.[29] Many clinicians do not advocate the use of local anesthesia and think that the additional cost, time, discomfort, and potential for complications are not justified.[1,30,31]

This controversy persists, however, and one recent study reported that the injection of local anesthetic before puncture significantly decreased the amount of pain felt and did not make the procedure either more difficult or more time-consuming.[26] This study concluded that local anesthesia is indeed indicated with routine arterial puncture.[26] Notwithstanding, the National Committee for Clinical Laboratory Standards (NCCLS) states that local anesthetic with arterial puncture is optional.[1]

If a local anesthetic is to be used, a 25-gauge or 26-gauge hypodermic needle and a local anesthetic (e.g., 1.0% lidocaine without epinephrine) is also needed. A few drops of anesthetic is injected just under the skin and in the tissues surrounding the vessel. The patient can then be calmed by showing him or her that a needle prick cannot be felt in this area. It should be noted, however, that lidocaine without epinephrine may cause prolonged bleeding in patients receiving anticoagulant therapy.[1]

Puncture Technique

A general procedure for performing an arterial puncture is described later in this chapter. Local preferences and conditions determine the actual technique used by a specific individual or laboratory.

Explanation

The patient should always fully understand the reason for a particular diagnostic test as well as the procedure that will be followed. The individual should realize that arterial blood is useful for evaluating his or her breathing, blood oxygenation, and acid-base status. The individual should be seated or lying in bed comfortably for at least 5 minutes before the procedure.[107] Also keep in mind that longer than 5 minutes may be necessary for outpatients to achieve a steady state.[107] The patient should be encouraged to relax and should understand that some discomfort may be felt. All individuals drawing blood gases should work hard to develop communication skills that promote a calm, reassuring environment.

Selection of Site

Because blood gas values are identical in all arteries, the specific artery chosen for the acquisition of the sample is based on accessibility, safety, departmental policy, and the patient's comfort. Box 1-2 lists the primary physiologic criteria that determine site selection. The three vessels most commonly punctured for blood gases in the adult are the radial, brachial, and femoral arteries (Fig. 1-5). Other arteries that may be used include the axillary, ulnar, dorsalis pedis, and superficial temporal arteries.[32] The carotid artery should be avoided because of the potential for cerebral air embolism or damage to neighboring vital structures. Arterial puncture should also be avoided through skin

---

Box 1-2	Physiologic Criteria for ABG Site Selection

1. Collateral blood flow
2. Accessibility and size of artery
3. Proximity of nerves, veins, supporting structures

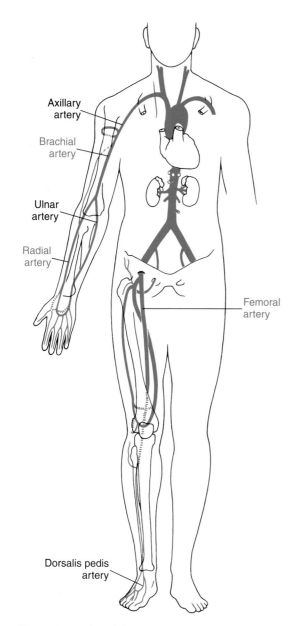

Figure 1-5. **Arterial puncture sites.** The three preferred arteries for arterial puncture are the radial artery, the brachial artery, and the femoral artery.

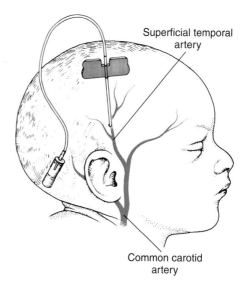

Figure 1-6. **Puncture of superficial temporal artery.** The superficial temporal artery may be punctured in the newborn by using a 25-gauge butterfly scalp vein needle.

temporal artery is usually used.[14] Alternatively, in the newborn, the umbilical arteries are easily accessible for sampling without puncture. The umbilical arteries are patent during the first 24 to 48 hours after birth but these arteries constrict rapidly if they are not kept open by catheterization (insertion of a catheter into the arteries for sampling).

The *ideal* vessel for arterial puncture would be large and superficial and would thus be an easy target for puncture. Also, the vessel would not lie extremely close to large veins or nerves that might predispose to inadvertent venous puncture or significant pain or complication in association with the procedure. Most important, other arteries that could maintain perfusion to distal tissue if an obstruction occurred in the punctured artery (i.e., collateral circulation) should be available in the general area.

Complications of Arterial Puncture

A potentially serious, albeit uncommon, complication of arterial puncture is *thrombosis*. Thrombosis involves the formation of an abnormal adherent clot (thrombus) on the inner wall of the vessel. The thrombus grows

lesions and through (or distal to) a surgical shunt (e.g., dialysis).[15]

In the infant, the radial and scalp (temporal) vessels are often recommended. The location of the superficial temporal artery (which may be even wider than the radial artery) is shown in Figure 1-6. One of the two main branches of the

gradually with subsequent diminution or cessation of blood flow. Thrombi are generally more serious in arteries than veins due to lesser collateral circulation. Thrombus is most likely when a needle or cannula is left in a small artery for an extended time.

The possibility of hemorrhage secondary to the high arterial pressure is also of considerable concern, particularly in the case of patients who receive anticoagulant therapy or who have known blood coagulation disorders. Hematoma, the leakage of blood into the tissues, is not uncommon, especially in the elderly, who may lack sufficient elastic tissue to seal the puncture site. The probability of hematoma or external bleeding will vary directly with the diameter of the needle. Hematoma is also more likely in patients receiving anticoagulant therapy or individuals with serious coagulopathies such as patients with end-stage hepatic disease or cancer.[107]

Arteriospasm (transient constriction of the artery) may occur as a reflex secondary to pain or anxiety and make it difficult or impossible to obtain a sample. Other complications include pain, air emboli, infection, and peripheral nerve damage. Occasionally, vasovagal (vascular and vagal) responses occur; these responses consist of precordial (region over the heart and stomach) distress, anxiety, feeling of impending death, nausea, and respiratory difficulty.[33] A vasovagal reaction may also result in loss of consciousness. The practitioner should be alert to signs and symptoms that suggest a vasovagal reaction (e.g., sweating, hypotension, bradycardia). In the event of a vasovagal reaction, the patient should lie down or if sitting, lower their head and arms and loosen light clothing.[107]

Although it has yet to be reported, anaphylaxis, a severe allergic reaction, may accompany the administration of a local anesthetic. In general, the overall incidence of complication with arterial puncture is low.[32] Arterial puncture is a safe, simple procedure[35,36] that can be done by qualified respiratory care practitioners and other healthcare personnel.

Common Sample Sites

Radial Artery. The vessel of choice for puncture in the adult is the radial artery (Figs. 1-7 to 1-9), which lies on the thumb side of the forearm.[10,32,35] The radial artery, although

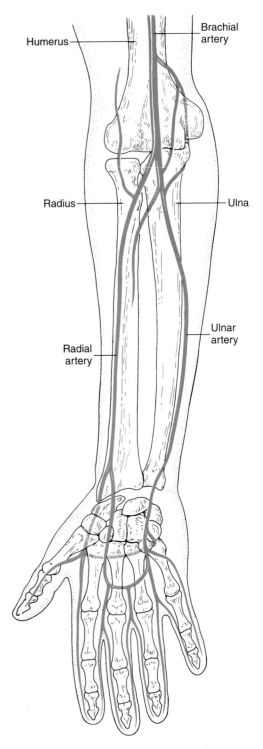

Figure 1-7. **Major arteries of the right lower arm.**

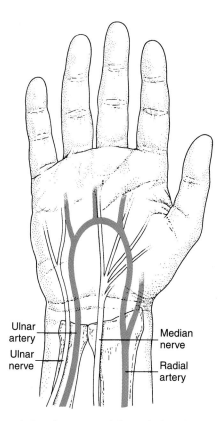

relatively small, is very accessible. The arm is convenient and the vessel is superficial and easy to stabilize and palpate. The vessel is also easily compressed over the wrist ligaments and the incidence of hematoma is low.[107] The radial nerve and vein are not particularly close to the artery and, most importantly, collateral circulation is usually excellent. Conversely, the ulnar artery is smaller, deeper, and lies close to the ulnar nerve.

Although complications from arterial puncture are rare, the non-dominant hand should be considered whenever possible.[41,697] This is particularly true when brachial puncture is necessary.[41] Punctures should also be avoided near the site of a surgical scar because this may predispose to a risk for injury, especially nerve injury.[107] Selection of the non-dominant hand is still controversial, however, and not considered standard of practice by some authorities. Some clinicians think that the site most comfortable for the clinician and with the best pulse is optimal. This approach may increase the likelihood of optimal technique and successful sampling and decrease the potential for complication.

Pulsations from the radial artery are readily palpable approximately 1 inch from the wrist

Figure 1-8.   Anatomy of the right hand and wrist. Pulsations from the radial artery are palpable approximately 1 inch from the crease of the wrist. The radial nerve runs underneath the radius.

Figure 1-9.   Superficial dissection of radial area. Actual proximity of radial artery (*A*) to median nerve (*B*) in cadaver is shown.

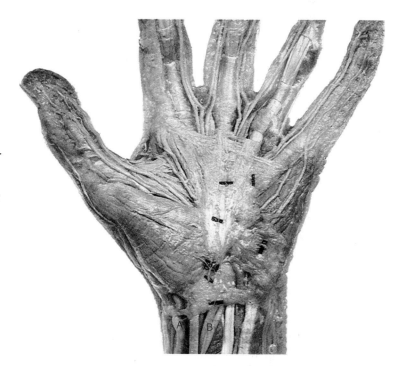

where the artery passes above the radius bone (see Figs. 1-7 to 1-9). The radial nerve is avoided at this location because its course runs below the radius (Fig. 1-10). Notwithstanding, radial artery puncture may still be painful if the puncture is deep and/or the bone covering (periosteum) is pierced.

Before performing an arterial puncture in the radial artery, however, the presence of adequate collateral circulation *must* be ensured. The vessel of collateral circulation to the hand, in the event of damage or obstruction to the radial artery, is the ulnar artery. The ulnar artery is capable of providing adequate perfusion to the hand; however, in 3% to 5% of the population, ulnar perfusion may be either absent or minimal. The incidence of abnormalities appears to increase with age from 2% in the first decade of life to nearly 7% after the ninth decade.[115] In the absence of adequate collateral circulation (ulnar circulation), radial artery puncture is not recommended.

A technique used to determine the adequacy of ulnar circulation is the *Allen test*, or more correctly, the *modified Allen test*. Technically, the Allen test was first described as a method of confirming radial artery occlusion[38]; nevertheless, the basic principles involved can be used to evaluate the adequacy of ulnar collateral circulation. Alternatively, ulnar circulation can be assessed with a Doppler ultrasonic flow indicator.[14]

The procedure for performing the modified Allen test is shown in Figure 1-11. First, the patient is instructed to clench the fist, thus forcing blood from the hand. If the patient is unable to actively clench the fist, it can be closed tightly by the clinician; however, if this is necessary, the results may be less conclusive.[10] By using his or her fingers, the clinician then applies external pressure to both the radial and ulnar arteries to obstruct blood flow to the hand (see Fig. 1-11,*A*). Relaxation (not full extension) of the hand at this point will result in blanching of the palm and fingers (see Fig. 1-11,*B*). Care should be taken to ensure that the patient does not hyperextend his or her wrist because this may substantially affect the test results.[113,118]

Subsequent release of obstructive pressure on the ulnar artery should result in flushing of the hand (see Fig. 1-11,C) within 5 to 15 seconds provided that ulnar artery blood flow

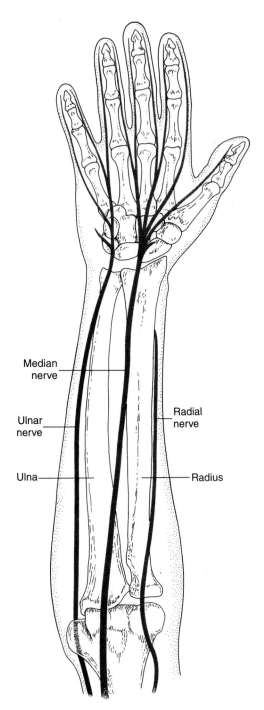

Figure 1-10.   **Major nerves of the right forearm.** The radial nerve passes underneath the radius bone and should not be punctured inadvertently. The course of the median nerve closely parallels the course of the brachial artery.

Median nerve

Ulnar nerve

Radial nerve

Ulna

Radius

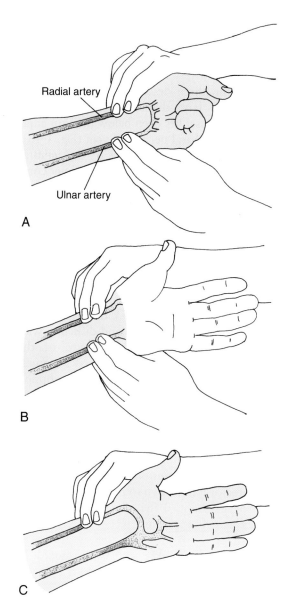

Radial artery

Ulnar artery

A

B

C

Figure 1-11. **Modified Allen test. A,** Blood supply to the hand is depleted. **B,** The hand is relaxed and blanches. **C,** Pressure is released from the ulnar artery. Return of color to the hand within 5 to 15 seconds indicates adequate collateral circulation via the ulnar artery (positive response to the Allen test).

is adequate.[10,14,39,40,107] This normal response is considered to be a positive response to the Allen test. Failure of the hand to flush in the specified time, which represents a negative response to the Allen test, indicates that ulnar

circulation may be compromised and that radial artery puncture should be avoided. Because it is sometimes confusing to state whether the results are positive or negative, it is probably best to record test results as normal or abnormal.

The value and need for use of the Allen test has been challenged,[113,114] and in some institutions it is no longer routinely used.[114] Opponents state that the prevalence of palmar arch arterial insufficiency is low, the patient must be cooperative to clench the fist, results are subjective, and it may not be a valid predictor of negative outcome. Interestingly, many patients may spontaneously hyperextend their wrists, which may delay reperfusion time two- to threefold.[113]

Despite these objections, the modified Allen test is still recommended in this text as a gross screening test. The test is simple, brief, and noninvasive. It may alert the clinician to a potential problem or suggest using the opposite arm for arterial puncture.

Brachial Artery. When the radial arteries are unsuitable for puncture, the brachial arteries should be considered. The brachial artery is the major artery of the upper arm that bifurcates (divides) into the radial and ulnar arteries just below the elbow (see Fig. 1-7). It is a large vessel that can be palpated a short distance above the bend of the elbow on the internal surface of the arm where it passes over the humerus. The patient's arm should be extended completely, and the wrist should be rotated until the strongest pulse is obtained just above the skin crease. Due to minimal vessel support by firm fascia or bone, the vessel may be somewhat difficult to palpate and more susceptible to hematoma. The artery should then be traced 2 to 3 cm up the arm with another finger.

In Figure 1-12, it can readily be seen that the course of the median nerve is parallel to the course of the brachial artery. Puncture of the median nerve with associated pain may occur while brachial puncture is being attempted. More importantly, trauma to the median nerve with subsequent permanent nerve damage has been reported in several cases.[41-43] As stated previously, when pulses are equal, the artery on the non-dominant side should be selected for puncture because, if an injury occurs, the

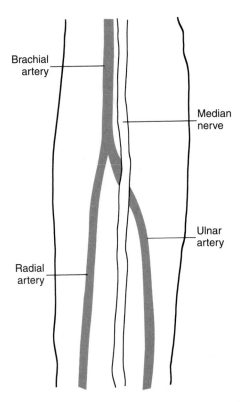

Figure 1-12. **Major arteries of the forearm and the median nerve.** The large median nerve runs close and parallel to the brachial artery.

patient will be less incapacitated.[41,44,697] Interesting legal issues are shown in Box 1-3.

Venous puncture may also occur inadvertently due to the presence of significant large veins in this area. The brachial artery is usually considered the site of second choice in adults because of the proximity of parallel nerves and veins. The brachial artery is not often punctured in children and especially infants due to difficulty in palpation and the absence of collateral circulation.[107]

Femoral Artery. The femoral artery can be palpated just below the inguinal ligament in the patient lying flat with the legs extended. The femoral artery is, however, the least desirable of the three described puncture sites.[31] Although its large diameter makes it an easy target, the vessel lies deep below the skin adjacent to the femoral nerve and vein (Fig. 1-13).

Most important, puncture of the femoral artery has been associated with serious complications. Large quantities of blood may seep from this vessel and may go unnoticed because of its deep, inconspicuous location. Moreover, atherosclerotic plaques are common in this area; they may dislodge and lead to distal artery occlusion. Patency of the femoral artery is vital because collateral circulation is almost nonexistent. In addition, this site may be associated with an increased risk of infection due to pubic hair in this region and difficulty with aseptic technique. Thus, puncture of the femoral artery is generally reserved for emergencies; nevertheless, it may be the only option for the hypotensive patient who has poor peripheral pulses.

Radial Puncture

The general technique used in radial artery puncture is now described. The patient should be seated or lying down to minimize the risk of a vasovagal faint.[31] The patient's wrist should be extended approximately to 30 degrees by placing a rolled towel below the wrist (Fig. 1-14).[14,31] Severe extension should be avoided because it may obliterate a palpable pulse.

The clinician should begin by washing the hands and then by donning gloves. A definite pulse should be palpated by gently pressing the index and middle fingers over the artery. A puncture should not be performed if a palpable

---

Box 1-3	Legal Issues

A California police officer lost use of his right hand following a blood gas procedure:
The technique of re-directing the syringe was alleged to have caused the damage.
An expert plaintiff witness testified that redirecting the syringe constituted a "Singer Sewing Machine technique."
The jury awarded the plaintiff $200,000.

Reference: DeWitt, A. L.: Routine ABGs can carry big risk too. Advance for Respiratory Care Practitioners, August 12, 1996, p 4.

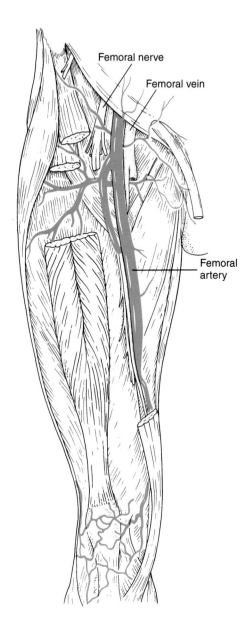

Figure 1-13. **The femoral artery.** The femoral artery lies close to the femoral nerve and vein.

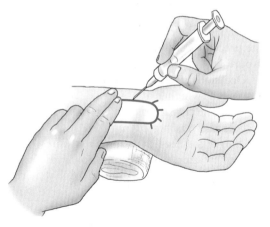

Figure 1-14. **Radial puncture.** The wrist is extended to approximately 30 degrees with the palm upward. The puncture is made at a 45-degree angle opposite the blood flow with the bevel facing upward.

pulse cannot be distinguished. After identification of the pulse, the puncture site should be prepared with 70% isopropyl alcohol swabs.

If the syringe has not been heparinized previously, this procedure should be done by using the method described previously. The radial artery should again be palpated with one hand while holding the heparinized syringe much like a pencil or dart with the opposite hand. While maintaining a palpable pulse, the needle is then inserted 5 to 10 mm distal to the index finger palpating the artery and opposite the blood flow at a 45-degree angle or less with the bevel turned upward (see Fig. 1-14).[10,14,16,46] The near-parallel insertion minimizes vessel wall trauma and provides a longer intraluminal pathway.[31] A 45-degree angle of insertion should be used when performing a brachial puncture and femoral puncture should be done with an angle nearly perpendicular to the skin surface.[14,107]

The needle should be advanced slowly because rapid insertion may force it completely through the vessel. If the needle is advanced too far, an acceptable technique is to withdraw it slowly until blood flow into the syringe commences. Similarly, redirection of the syringe should be done gently if the initial attempt fails to result in entry to the artery. Redirection should not be done while the needle lies deep within the tissue, because the result may be excessive tearing of underlying tissue. The needle should instead be withdrawn almost to the skin surface before redirecting it.

One must be very cautious, however, to avoid contamination of the arterial sample with even a small amount of venous blood. The result could be significantly lower arterial PO_2

values than those actually present in the arterial blood. If an arteriovenous mixture is suspected, the procedure should be repeated to ensure that a pure arterial sample is taken.

Occasionally, there is some question with regard to whether the sample is arterial or venous. The characteristics of an arterial sample include the *flashing pulsation* as blood enters the hub of the needle, and the *auto-filling* of the syringe by arterial pressure without withdrawal effort. In the hypotensive patient, or if a needle smaller than 23-gauge is used,[107] some withdrawal effort (gentle slow pull) may be necessary, but failure to see the flash pulsation should arouse suspicion of venous puncture. Excessive suction should not be applied because it may alter the blood gas results. When using a glass syringe, gentle pressure should also be maintained on the end of the plunger to prevent it from falling out.

After a sufficient sample of blood has been obtained, the needle is quickly withdrawn and a dry, sterile gauze is placed immediately over the puncture site. Digital pressure should normally be applied to the site for a minimum of 3 to 5 minutes.[14,107] This time should be increased slightly after femoral puncture. Immediately after the pressure is released, the site should be inspected for bleeding[14,107]; if any bleeding, oozing, or seepage of blood is present, pressure should be continued until bleeding ceases. A longer compression time (e.g., 15 to 20 minutes) is necessary for patients who are taking anticoagulant therapy or who have bleeding disorders.[16]

When bleeding is of particular concern, one may also leave a pressure bandage on the site for a short period after departure from the bedside. However, *pressure dressings are not a substitute for compression* and they may provide a false sense of security or lead to careless technique regarding manual compression. Also, pressure dressings should be avoided in patients with atherosclerosis because they may depress local circulation and promote thrombus formation. Other safeguards sometimes suggested include checking for a pulse downstream from the puncture site[46] and rechecking the puncture site 5 minutes after releasing pressure to ensure that a hematoma has not formed.[31]

Sample Handling

Needle sticks are the most frequent source of transmission of blood-borne diseases in health care workers.[19,20]

It is important to prevent interface of the blood with air because this may alter blood gas values. After the needle is withdrawn from the skin, it is quickly sealed by removing the needle and capping the syringe in an airtight fashion or following the manufacturer's recommendations. The syringe may be gently tapped while in the upright position to force visible air bubbles to the surface where they can be expelled.

One must be especially careful to avoid inadvertent needle self-puncture. Needle sticks are the most frequent source of transmission of bloodborne diseases in healthcare workers.[19,20] Needles used for blood sampling should be resheathed only with a technique that uses a one-hand device or by careful insertion into a cork or similar device that prevents the sharp point from being accessible.[15,107] Syringes with attached needles should be disposed in puncture-resistant disposal containers. These containers must have a lid and should be made of rigid material. The container must also be marked clearly as a biohazard.[104,107]

The sample should be mixed with the anticoagulant by rolling the syringe between the hands and by inverting the sample several times. Each of these mixing techniques should be done for approximately 5 seconds.

As a general rule, samples should be maintained at room temperature and analyzed within 30 minutes.[107,116] Recent evidence has shown that all blood gas samples are relatively stable for 30 minutes and that there is no need to keep arterial blood in ice if the sample is run within this time.[34,107,116] This is an important finding because icing samples may also artificially alter electrolyte concentrations.

In general, procedures for puncture of other arteries are very similar to those used for radial puncture with minor exceptions. When performing brachial artery puncture, a longer needle is used because the artery lies deep within the tissues especially in obese individuals. It is also more difficult to compress the brachial

ON CALL | CASE 1-2 *ABGs and Critical Thinking*

You are the only person available to care for this patient. You must assess the patient/situation and act accordingly.

A 33-year-old male police officer presents to the emergency department with shortness of breath. The clinician performs a right brachial puncture for an arterial blood gas. During the puncture, the officer experiences involuntary finger movement and pain. The officer returns to the emergency department the next day complaining of numbness, weakness, and difficulty moving his right hand.

ARTERIAL BLOOD GASES

SaO$_2$ 97%
pH   7.42

PaCO$_2$ 33 mm Hg
PaO$_2$ 97 mm Hg
[HCO$_3$]   24 mEq/L

ASSESSMENT

Abnormalities: List abnormal data and other noteworthy information or inappropriate actions.
Explanation: List possible diseases, pathology, or other circumstances that may have lead to this patient's condition.

artery and this must be done for at least 5 minutes. Finally, when puncture of the femoral artery is necessary, the angle of puncture should be more perpendicular to the skin surface.[107]

ARTERIAL CANNULATION

During an acute hypotensive (fall in blood pressure) crisis, two important avenues of patient monitoring may be inaccessible or inaccurate: arterial blood samples may be almost impossible to obtain, and indirect measurement of arterial blood pressure may be misleading.

The insertion of an indwelling arterial catheter will ensure the availability of accurate monitoring information. In addition, an indwelling catheter allows for continuous monitoring, which is preferable to periodic, intermittent measurements. The insertion of a catheter into an artery for blood gas and pressure monitoring is called *arterial cannulation.*

Although the insertion of an arterial line has traditionally been done only by physicians, recent literature suggests that it can be done safely and effectively by respiratory therapists.[45,70] It is important to provide special training and protocols for insertion. With these caveats, it appears that arterial lines can be inserted around the clock in a cost-effective manner by non-physician healthcare professionals without increased complications.[45,70]

The radial artery is usually the vessel of choice for arterial cannulation.[14,47] Nevertheless, larger arteries may be preferred when the risk of thrombosis is high or when the expected duration of cannulation is greater than 7 days.[48,49] Big arteries offer the additional advantages of easier palpation and more accurate blood pressure readings.[49] The large arteries of choice are the femoral and axillary vessels, which have been associated with a low incidence of minor complication and almost no tissue ischemia.[49] Most intensive care units currently attempt to remove arterial cannulas within 72 hours.

Complications

Any invasive procedure such as arterial cannulation may be associated with complications. The potential benefits of invasive monitoring must always be weighed carefully against concomitant risks.

Major complications include hemorrhage and severe vascular occlusion secondary to intraluminal clot formation. On rare occasions, gangrene has necessitated the amputation of a finger or a hand.[50] When coolness of the extremity is observed immediately after insertion of the catheter, the catheter should be removed quickly because tissue damage requiring amputation may occur in less than 2 hours.[48] Careful attention to technique should avoid serious problems. Major complications occur in less than 1% of cases.[47] In fact, severe damage due to vascular occlusion is estimated to occur in less than 1% of patients.[47]

Minor complications include pain, arteriospasm, and localized internal bleeding (i.e., hematoma). Temporary loss of sensation via the median nerve may also occur.[51] Transient occlusion of the radial artery after cannulation is fairly common. Twenty percent to 30% of patients manifest partial or complete radial artery occlusion after cannulation[52–54]; however, there appears to be no clinical tissue damage resulting from the occlusion.[52,53]

The incidence of occlusion appears to be related to the size of the catheter, and a small catheter may decrease the incidence of this complication.[39,53] Radial artery occlusion occurs more commonly in women than in men,[52,53] perhaps because of the smaller vessel size. Furthermore, the occurrence of occlusion appears to be related to the period of cannulation.[54] Radial artery cannulation time should not exceed 6 hours in the absence of clear clinical indication.

Use of a low-flow continuous irrigation system that incorporates a pressurized bag with heparin solution also helps to minimize the risk of thrombus formation and dislodgment. The system shown in Figure 1-15 is an example of a pressurized arterial monitoring system. Flush systems should deliver 1 to 3 mL/hr to ensure patency.[107] The pressurized bag is typically filled with 1000 U of heparin. Administration of heparin may, however, result in thrombocytopenia (decreased platelets) with subsequent hemorrhage or thromboembolism. Heparin should be discontinued if these events occur or the platelet level falls below 100,000/mm[3].[107]

The arterial line is set up to continuously monitor arterial blood pressure. A pressure *transducer* converts mechanical pressure to electrical energy and displays it digitally or graphically on an oscilloscope. The *intraflow flush assembly* allows for a continuous, slow flow of heparin through the system to prevent clot formation. Stopcocks A and B are used primarily for assembly and calibration of the system. Stopcock C is where arterial blood samples are acquired. The procedure for acquiring blood via this stopcock is described in the section on arterial line sampling later in this chapter.

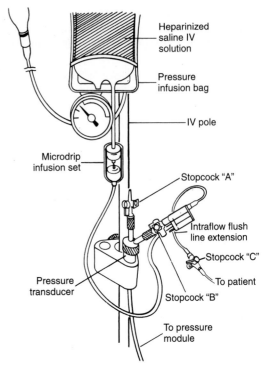

Figure 1-15.   Pressurized arterial line system. Components of a pressurized arterial monitoring system.

Before the development of these systems, arterial lines were kept patent through intermittent high-volume irrigation with heparin solution. Thus, a heparin solution was injected periodically into the system to purge the lines and to avoid clots. This technique is less effective and should be avoided.

Infection is also a potential complication of cannulation. In one prospective study of critically ill patients, 18% developed local infection and 5% developed septicemia.[55] In a study of healthy individuals, only a 4% infection rate was observed.[56] Some physicians contend that the incidence of infection with arterial lines is no greater than that seen with venous cannulation.[10] Generally, the severity of infections seems to be related to the period of cannulation with the most severe infections arising when catheters remain in place for longer than 4 days.[55]

Also, a wise practice is to remove and culture indwelling catheters in the presence of unexplained sepsis. Infections can be minimized by aseptic preparation and application of an antibiotic ointment to the site after cannulation.[14]

Although arterial cannulation is not without risk, it is a valuable method of monitoring critically ill patients. The valuable nature of the data obtained may justify the risk involved especially if the need for serial blood gases is anticipated.

Catheter Insertion

The extremity to be cannulated should be placed securely on a board. The use of local anesthesia is optional but recommended for arterial line insertion.[107] Several techniques can be used for catheter insertion depending on the equipment available and local preferences. The catheter may be inserted (1) over the needle, (2) through the needle, or (3) through a plastic catheter.[14]

When inserting the catheter *over* a needle, the catheter should be advanced slowly. The catheter should *never* be pulled back over the needle after it has been advanced, nor should the needle be advanced again after it has been withdrawn.[14] If resistance is encountered, the needle and catheter should be removed.

If problems are encountered while inserting the catheter *through* a needle, the needle and catheter should always be removed simultaneously to avoid damage to the catheter. While adhering to aseptic technique throughout, the catheter should be secured after it has been inserted the desired distance.

Arterial Line Sampling

Integral to traditional arterial line systems is a three-way stopcock, which is shown in Figure 1-16. Three ports stem from the stopcock: the patient port, a sample port, and a port

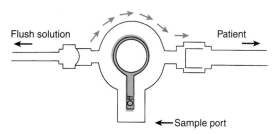

Figure 1-17. **Normal resting position of three-way stopcock.** In the normal resting position, the sample port is closed. The passage between the heparin solution and the patient remains patent.

that leads to a pressurized bag of heparin solution. The lever on the top of the stopcock can be rotated 360 degrees around in a circle. When the lever is not aligned directly with any of the respective ports (see Fig. 1-16), flow through all of the ports will be obstructed.

When the lever is aligned directly with one of the ports, only flow through that port will be obstructed. Fluid can flow readily through the remaining two lines. Figure 1-17 shows the normal resting stopcock position of an arterial line. The pressurized heparin solution is being forced slowly and continuously through the system. This small amount of heparin will keep the lines free and open while not impairing the body's ability to form clots.

When a sample is to be drawn, an empty syringe is attached to the sample port. The stopcock is positioned such that flow to the bag is obstructed while the patient and sample ports remain open (Fig. 1-18). Fluid from within the arterial line is then aspirated into a syringe (i.e., clearance syringe). The volume of fluid

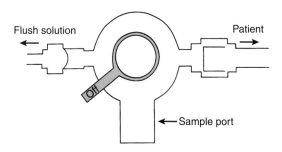

Figure 1-16. **Three-way stopcock.** Flow is obstructed through all ports in the stopcock because the lever is not directly aligned with any of the ports.

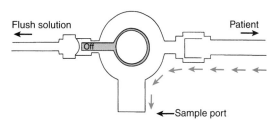

Figure 1-18. **Sampling position of three-way stopcock.** A syringe is attached to the sample port of the three-way stopcock. The stopcock is turned off to the heparin solution, and fluid is withdrawn.

withdrawn will vary with the system used but must be sufficient to ensure blood has reached the syringe. Then, an additional small amount should be withdrawn to prevent any blood dilution.[14] Typically, a volume of flush-blood six times the volume of the catheter and connections is withdrawn.[107] This will ensure that unheparinized arterial blood is present immediately on the patient side of the stopcock.

The stopcock is then repositioned so that all ports are obstructed (see Fig. 1-16). The syringe used to clear the sampling line is discarded, and a new heparinized sample syringe is attached to the sample port. The stopcock is again turned off to the bag, and the patient's blood sample is withdrawn into the syringe. The stopcock is then returned to the obstructed position and the syringe is removed and prepared for transportation.

To cleanse the lines, the stopcock is again turned off to the sample port and heparin is flushed manually through the system. This action forces the blood in the line back to the patient. The stopcock is also turned off briefly to the patient, and heparin is allowed to flow out of the sample port, thus removing any blood residue (Fig. 1-19). A good arterial waveform should be present when the flushing procedure has been completed. Finally, the patient is left with the stopcock in the resting position. Either a cap or a syringe should be placed over the sample port to avoid contamination.

Blood-Conserving Arterial Line Systems

Patients in critical care settings often lose large quantities of blood via phlebotomy (blood

removal) as various diagnostic tests are performed. Critical care patients are also more vulnerable than other patient populations to the adverse affects of blood loss because of frequent coexisting anemia. The mean volume of blood loss per day is often 40 to 50 mL of blood[57,58] in critical care patients; and may be as high as 377 mL/day in patients in some cardiothoracic surgical intensive care units.[59] This problem is especially important in preterm infants who have small total blood volume.[117]

In addition, patients with arterial lines have been shown to commonly have twofold to threefold increased blood loss related to phlebotomy than other critical care patients.[57,60] It is certainly plausible that the ease of blood-drawing from an arterial line makes blood sampling more casual and frequent.

Furthermore, as much as 24% to 30% of daily total blood drawn from traditional arterial lines is for the purpose of clearing the line and is then discarded.[57,59] Newer blood-conserving arterial line systems have been developed that provide a simple and effective method for reducing blood loss secondary to line clearing.[61]

ARTERIAL LINE/BLOOD GAS CONTROVERSY

In the current era of cost containment in healthcare and particularly critical care units, the value and number of laboratory tests being performed have come under great scrutiny. Much of this attention is appropriate because laboratory costs comprise approximately 25% of total hospital costs[62,63] and critical care units alone account for as much as 28% of total hospital costs.[64]

Notwithstanding, although it is relatively easy to quantitate costs of these tests, it is much more difficult to measure the value of laboratory tests performed on critically ill individuals. A *routine* test in a critically ill individual may help us confirm that they are not in a crisis or provide a small first clue to a potentially fatal event or condition (e.g., arrhythmia, electrolyte disturbance). Appropriate use of these tests will remain a matter of controversy, science, and art. We must do all we can to save

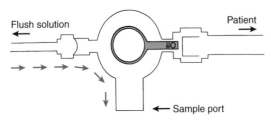

Figure 1-19.   **Flush position of three-way stopcock.** If the heparinized bag to the sample port is opened briefly, solution can flow out of the sample port and rinse away all blood.

money but we must not forget that healthcare is the business of saving lives.

CAPILLARY SAMPLING

Sampling of *arterialized* capillary blood may be used as an alternative to arterial blood gas sampling in infants. Arterialized capillary samples may provide useful information regarding $PaCO_2$ and pH; however, they are of little value in estimating arterial oxygenation.[66] A brief review of the theory and principles of this technique is warranted.

Theory

Capillary blood can be arterialized by warming the skin and thereby increasing and accelerating the flow of blood through the capillary. Thus, theoretically, blood gas values in the capillary approach arterial values. When peripheral perfusion in the patient is normal, arterialized capillary pH and PCO_2 will correlate well with $PaCO_2$ and arterial pH.[67-69] Indeed, even arterialized capillary PO_2 will correlate well with PaO_2 provided PaO_2 is less than 60 mm Hg and peripheral perfusion is good. Higher PaO_2 values do not correlate well with arterialized capillary PO_2 values even with good perfusion.[68,69] Typically, PO_2 values of capillary samples will be considerably lower.

Technique

In infants, the capillary bed most often used for sampling is the heel. Nevertheless, the earlobe or the tip of a finger (or toe) may also be used. Punctures should not be performed over the central area of the foot, the posterior curvature of the heel, or through a previous puncture site.[107] Box 1-4 lists potential contraindications to performance of this procedure.

The site should be heated carefully to a temperature no higher than 42° C.[65,107] This temperature can increase blood flow sevenfold.[107] Warming can be accomplished with warm compresses, a waterbath, a heat lamp, or commercially available hot-packs. Inadequate warming of the site will result in a poor correlation between arterial and capillary values.[66,107]

The skin should be cleaned with an antiseptic solution such as alcohol. A puncture no

Box 1-4	Contraindications to Capillary Blood Sampling

1. Posterior curvature of heel because device may puncture the bone
2. Callus heel of patient who has begun walking
3. Finger samples in neonates to avoid nerve damage
4. Inflamed, swollen, or edematous tissue
5. Cyanotic or poorly perfused tissue
6. Localized infection
7. Previous puncture sites

Reference: Capillary blood gas sampling for neonatal and pediatric patients. AARC Clinical Practice Guideline, Respir. Care, 39:1180–1183, 1994.

more than 2.0 mm deep should then be made on the lateral aspects of the plantar surface (Fig. 1-20).[107] The first drop of blood should be wiped away, and the sample should freely flow into a 75- to 100-μL, heparinized capillary tube. Squeezing the blood into the capillary tube is unacceptable and may alter the values obtained.[66] An alcohol sponge or suitable substitute should be pressed gently against the sample site to stop the flow of blood.

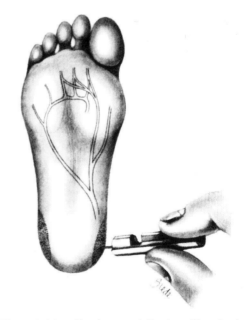

Figure 1-20. Site for arterialized capillary heel sample. Heel puncture for arterialized capillary sample should be done on the lateral aspects of the plantar surface.

The end of the capillary tube where the sample was obtained should be sealed immediately. A metal flea (small piece of metal) is usually then carefully placed in the other end of the capillary tube before it is sealed. A magnet is then applied to the metal flea from the outside of the capillary tube. The magnet is moved backward and forward along the capillary tube for approximately 10 seconds to thoroughly mix the blood and heparin. The sample is then analyzed as soon as possible.

AARC CLINICAL PRACTICE GUIDELINES

The AARC has established Clinical Practice Guidelines for a variety of respiratory therapy modalities and diagnostic tests. Table 1-3 highlights some of the key points of those Clinical Practice Guidelines related to arterial blood gas and capillary sampling. Please refer to the actual guidelines for more comprehensive information on each of these procedures.[15,65,66]

Table 1-3.   AMERICAN ASSOCIATION FOR RESPIRATORY CARE CLINICAL PRACTICE GUIDELINES: NUTS AND BOLTS

Sampling for Arterial Blood Gas Analysis	In-vitro pH and Blood Gas Analysis and Hemoximetry	Capillary Blood Gas Sampling for Neonatal and Pediatric Patients
Anaerobic arterial blood acquired from percutaneous puncture or indwelling catheter	Anaerobic arterial or mixed venous blood from percutaneous puncture or indwelling catheter	Free flowing capillary blood sample from incision with lancet or similar device
To assess:	To assess:	To assess:
1) Acid-base status	1) Acid-base status	1) Acid-base status
2) Ventilation	2) Ventilation	2) Ventilation
3) Oxygenation	3) Oxygenation	
	4) Dyshemoglobin saturations	
Hazards:	Hazards:	Hazards:
1) Hematoma	1) Infection of specimen handler	1) Infection
2) Arteriospasm		2) Burns
3) Emboli		3) Hematoma
4) Anaesthetic reaction		4) Bone calcification
5) Hemorrhage		5) Nerve damage
6) Vascular trauma		6) Bruising
7) Vascular occlusion		7) Pain
8) Vasovagal reaction		8) Bleeding
9) Pain		
10) Infection		
11) Nerve damage		
Key points:	Key points:	Key points:
1) Ensure steady state (20–30 min)	1) 8-hr QC	1) Not good indicator PaO_2
2) Analyze promptly <15 min not iced <1 hr if iced	2) Proficiency testing program	2) Don't squeeze sample out
3) Perform Allen test		3) Ensure proper site warming
4) Heparinize (1000 U/mL)		4) Incision <2.5 mm deep
5) Universal precautions		5) Avoid procedure on infants <24 hr old

References: Sampling for arterial blood gas analysis. AARC Clinical Practice Guideline, Respir. Care, 37:913–917, 1992; Blood gas analysis and hemoximetry: 2001 Revision and Update. AARC Clinical Practice Guideline, Respir. Care, 45:498–501, 2001; Capillary blood gas sampling for neonatal and pediatric patients. AARC Clinical Practice Guideline, Respir. Care, 39:1180–1183, 1994.

EXERCISES

Exercise 1-1   Blood Gas Values

Fill in the blanks or select the best answer.

1. State the normal adult ranges and appropriate units for the following blood gas measurements:
   pH
   $PaCO_2$
   [BE]
   PaO_2
   [HCO_3]
   SaO_2

2. State the two blood gas indices that quantitate the oxygen available in the arterial blood.

3. State the two metabolic indices commonly reported with arterial blood gases.

4. Both [HCO_3] and [BE] are necessary to interpret arterial blood gas results (True/False).

5. What percentage of the total population will have blood gas values that fall within the normal range?

6. Women tend to have (lower/identical/higher) $PaCO_2$ than men.

7. Calculate the specific normal PaO_2 in the supine position in patients of the following ages:
   58 years
   72 years

8. Normal SaO_2 in a young patient in his or her twenties is approximately _____ %.

9. Normal PaO_2 in the sitting position is approximately _____ mm Hg higher than in the supine position in middle-age adults.

10. If the patient is younger than 45 years of age, minimum normal PaO_2 should exceed _____ mm Hg. If older than 45 years of age, PaO_2 decreases with age; however, it should never be less than _____ mm Hg.

11. The International System of Units recommends (mm Hg/kPa) units for blood gas measurements.

12. One hundred mm Hg = _____ kPa.

13. The normal range is usually considered to be within (1/2/3) standard deviations from the mean of the population.

14. One kPa = _____ mm Hg.

15. A PaO_2 of 60 mm Hg = _____ kPa.

16. PaO_2 tends to (decrease/level off) after age 75.

Exercise 1-2   Arterial versus Venous Blood

Fill in the blanks or select the best answer.

1. Define the following terms: arteries and veins.

2. The best type of blood to use in assessing tissue oxygen delivery is (arterial/peripheral venous).

3. The adequacy of CO_2 excretion via the lungs is best assessed by (arterial/venous) blood.

4. Peripheral venous blood provides information primarily about (localized tissue/overall body) conditions.

5. Venous blood samples in the well-perfused patient may fairly accurately reflect (arterial pH/$PaCO_2$/PaO_2).

Exercise 1-3   Preparation for Arterial Sampling

Fill in the blanks or select the best answer.

1. List at least three examples of specific drugs that may interfere with normal coagulation.

2. A genetic disease seen in men that is characterized by an increased clotting time is _____.

3. Establishment of equilibrium throughout the cardiopulmonary system following application of oxygen therapy may be called establishment of a _____.

4. In clinical practice, blood samples are not usually drawn for approximately _____ minutes after a change in ventilator setting or oxygen therapy.

5. When blood samples are drawn during mechanical ventilation, the tidal volume and FIO_2 (should/should not) be measured at the time of sampling.

6. A _____-gauge needle is usually used for arterial puncture in the normal adult.

7. A _____-gauge needle may be most appropriate in children or neonates to minimize vessel trauma during arterial puncture.

8. When a sample is iced, the PaO_2 will be altered due to diffusion in (glass/plastic) syringes.

9. State the recommended anticoagulant to be used for arterial puncture.

10. Sodium or lithium heparin in a concentration of (1000/10,000) U/mL is the anticoagulant of choice.

11. The amount of sodium heparin (1000 U/mL) needed to anticoagulate 1 mL of blood is _____ mL.

12. Metabolism within a blood sample withdrawn from the body will (cease/continue).

13. The use of methods to minimize the risk of infection to the patient is called _____ technique.

14. A hospital-acquired infection is called a _____ infection.

15. Use of a local anesthetic for arterial puncture is (required/optional).

Exercise 1-4   **Arterial Blood Sampling**

Fill in the blanks or select the best answer.

1. List the three recommended vessels for arterial puncture in order of preference.

2. State two alternative arteries that may be punctured in unusual situations.

3. List four potential complications of arterial puncture.

4. Precordial distress, anxiety, nausea, and a feeling of impending doom are part of a clinical picture known as a _____ response.

5. Testing for the adequacy of collateral circulation via the ulnar artery is performed via the _____ test.

6. In performing the modified Allen test, the patient's hand should flush within _____ seconds after release of digital pressure on the ulnar artery.

7. The course of the _____ nerve closely parallels the course of the brachial artery.

8. The most serious complications of arterial puncture have been associated with the _____ artery.

9. The wrist should be extended about _____ degrees for radial puncture.

10. During puncture of the radial artery, the angle of insertion should be _____ degrees or less.

11. State the two signs that indicate acquisition of an arterial sample.

12. Normally, digital pressure should be applied to the puncture site for a minimum of _____ minutes after the syringe has been withdrawn.

13. List the two primary indications for arterial cannulation.

14. When the lever of a three-way stopcock is aligned with one of the ports, that port will be (open/closed).

15. Some advocate selection of the _____ hand or arm for arterial blood sampling.

16. When doing a heel stick, blood (should/should not) be squeezed into the capillary tube.

Exercise 1-5   **Internet Work**

1. State the number of clinical practice guidelines that have been established through the American Association for Respiratory Care (AARC) and list those related to blood gas sampling (www.AARC.org).

2. List at least two *contraindications* cited in the AARC Clinical Practice Guidelines related to "Sampling for Arterial Blood Gas Analysis" (www.AARC.org).

NBRC Challenge 1

Please select the best answer for the following multiple choice questions.

1. The modified Allen test:
   - I. is used to evaluate the presence of collateral circulation.
   - II. is useful in evaluating the radial artery site for arterial puncture.
   - III. should be done preceding all venipunctures.
   - A) I only
   - B) II only
   - C) I, II only
   - D) I, III only
   - E) I, II, and III
   - (CRT EXAM – NBRC MATRIX I,C,1,c)

2. A bluish-colored sample with low PaO_2 and high $PaCO_2$ and of venous origin would be most likely when doing an arterial puncture at the _____ site.
   - A) radial
   - B) brachial
   - C) femoral
   - D) dorsalis pedis
   - E) temporal
   - (CRT EXAM – NBRC MATRIX I,B,9,c)

3. When there are concerns regarding the adequacy of ventilation, acid-base balance, and oxygenation, a(n) _____ would provide the most comprehensive information.
   - A) $P(A-a)O_2$ evaluation
   - B) $C(a-\bar{v})O_2$ evaluation
   - C) pulmonary function study
   - D) arterial blood gas
   - E) flow-volume loop measurement
   - (CRT EXAM – NBRC MATRIX I,A,1,d)

4. What clinical recommendation would be made for a 70-year-old man breathing room air with a PaO_2 of 70 mm Hg?
   - A) Pulmonary function studies
   - B) Chest radiography
   - C) Sleep studies
   - D) Cardiac enzyme studies
   - E) No action necessary
   - (CRT EXAM – NBRC MATRIX I,B,9,c)

5. What is the most likely explanation of the following ABG in a young female?

PaO_2	95 mm Hg
$PaCO_2$	33 mm Hg
pH	7.43
$[HCO_3]$	25 mEq/L

   - A) COPD
   - B) Acute pneumonia
   - C) Neuromuscular disorder
   - D) Severe anxiety response
   - E) Normal
   - (CRT EXAM – NBRC MATRIX I,B,10,c)

Chapter 2

Blood Gas Classification

Of all the concepts employed in the diagnosis and treatment of respiratory disorders, few are more important or less well understood than those of blood gas interpretation.

Robert R. Demers[170]

In interpreting blood gas data, the creative therapist considers not only the present values but attempts to understand what came before and predict what might come afterwards.

Stephen M. Ayres[171]

Outline

INTRODUCTION

The techniques used in the acquisition of arterial blood have been discussed. In this chapter, the first step in the clinical application of arterial blood gases, *arterial blood gas classification*, is explored.

As described previously, the arterial blood gas report is the basis and cornerstone in the assessment and management of clinical oxygenation, ventilation, and acid-base disturbances. The initial objective in clinical management of these areas is to classify the blood gas information into one of several possible *general* categories,

for example, "Partially Compensated Metabolic Acidosis with Mild Hypoxemia."

Sometimes this "naming" of the blood gas is referred to as *blood gas interpretation*. Notwithstanding, simply stating that a patient has a metabolic acidosis without understanding the nature of the acid-base disturbance is taking a very narrow view of "interpretation" and does not facilitate optimal patient treatment. Therefore, in this text, "interpretation" is considered in a much broader context to include detailed analysis and evaluation of the blood gas in conjunction with other patient clinical and laboratory information. This requires critical (diagnostic and therapeutic) thinking and is, indeed, our goal in the clinical management of acid-base balance, ventilation, and oxygenation.

To accomplish these important tasks, the *first* important step in interpretation is "blood gas classification." Even the novice clinician dealing with critical care patients must learn immediately how to "classify an ABG" correctly and expeditiously. Likewise, even the novice must be able to quickly identify critical values and life-threatening situations. These objectives are the aim of this chapter.

SYSTEMATIC APPROACH

The vital nature of blood gas information requires a careful, thoughtful approach. The variety of data that may be reported (e.g., [HCO_3], SaO_2, PaO_2, [BE]) is a potential source of confusion for the novice. Therefore, it is important to process the data on a blood gas report in an orderly, systematic, and thorough manner. A step-by-step approach ensures reproducible results and helps to avoid confusion and omissions.

Although acid-base balance, ventilation, and oxygenation status can often present interrelated problems and issues, individual and separate evaluations of these areas sometimes help to focus and clarify thinking. Although the sequence is somewhat arbitrary, in the classification system presented here, acid-base classification (which also includes ventilation evaluation) is presented first and is followed by classification of blood oxygen levels.

ACID-BASE STATUS

There are three steps in this simple ABC approach to acid-base classification; these steps are shown in Box 2-1. First, Acid-base status (overall body conditions) is assessed by classifying the arterial pH. The arterial pH is the single best index of composite acid-base status in the body.

Second, the Basic primary problem(s) (general type of acid-base disturbance) present is

Box 2-1	ABCs of Blood Gas Classification

Acid-base status
Basic primary problem(s)
Compensation assessment

characterized as either respiratory, metabolic, or both. In this step, we attempt to identify the primary general abnormality that is (are) tending to pull the pH away from normal.

Next, Compensation is assessed. The body's normal response to a single, primary, acid-base disturbance is to alter the acid-base component not primarily affected (respiratory [$PaCO_2$] or metabolic ([HCO_3]) in the opposite direction of the primary problem. This secondary acid-base change is referred to as *compensation*. Because this is an expected occurrence in normal individuals, each blood gas should be evaluated and classified according to the presence and extent of acid-base compensation.

Regarding the sequence of specific indices to be analyzed on a blood gas report, it is recommended that the pH be evaluated first as an index of overall Acid-base balance (Box 2-2). The $PaCO_2$ (respiratory status) is evaluated next followed by [HCO_3] (metabolic) evaluation. Assessment of both of these indices is necessary to complete both step 2 (Basic primary problem determination) and step 3 (Compensation assessment).

As we will see later in this chapter, the clinician should then analyze the PaO_2 (oxygenation classification) and consider it in respect to the FIO_2 (i.e., the concentration of oxygen being inspired) and lung oxygen exchange efficiency. Again, Box 2-2 summarizes the sequence of indices to be evaluated.

Box 2-2	Sequence of ABG Evaluation

pH
$PaCO_2$
[HCO_3]
PaO_2

pH Assessment

Clinical Significance

The pH reported on an arterial blood gas sample is the single best index of overall acid-base status in the body. It is a composite reflection of the net interaction of all acids, bases, buffers, and compensatory mechanisms. It is the logical starting point in comprehensive acid-base assessment. Furthermore, if the pH is severely disturbed and the patient is in a life-threatening situation, this can be identified immediately.

The arterial pH is measured in the blood plasma and reflects quantitatively the hydrogen ion activity in this extracellular fluid compartment. Although the extracellular pH is not identical to the important intracellular pH, alterations in the two values tend to move in similar directions and correlate closely. Thus, the pH on a blood gas report is a good indicator of overall acid-base conditions.

Clinical Manifestations of Abnormal pH

Seemingly slight alterations in blood pH may have profound, life-threatening effects on body chemistry. This is likely due to the small size of the hydrogen ion and the vast number of chemical reactions it may impact. Clinically, it is useful to be aware of the typical manifestations associated with a particular pH disturbance.

Low arterial pH has a generalized depressive effect on the human nervous system (Fig. 2-1).[173] Symptoms may include drowsiness and lethargy. Regardless of the precipitating cause, a very low pH (i.e., pH <7.10) is often associated with coma. A pH of less than 6.80 for any extended period is generally considered to be incompatible with life.

A high blood pH, on the other hand, has a general tendency to excite the central nervous system. Irritability or tetany may be manifest. When the heart muscle becomes more irritable, serious arrhythmias (abnormal beats) may result. When pH remains very high, convulsions may occur. A pH greater than 7.80 is generally considered to be incompatible with life. The clinician should always take note of the patient's symptoms to substantiate, refute, or clarify laboratory findings and disease.

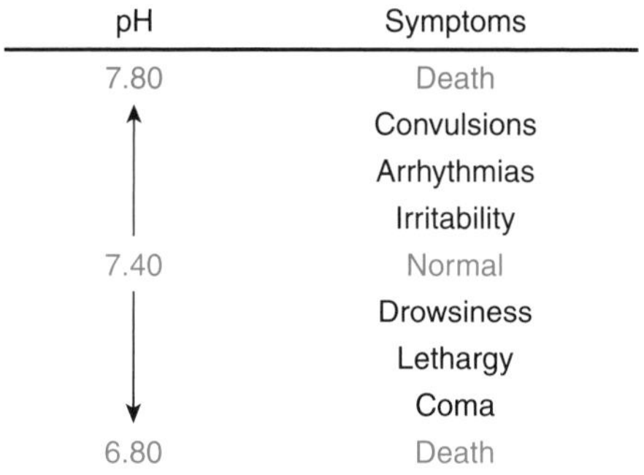

Classification of pH

Normal pH

Normal arterial pH is 7.35 to 7.45. The finding of a normal pH, however, does not preclude further evaluation of acid-base status. Compensation may normalize pH and mask primary acid-base problems that should be identified.

Abnormal pH

A pH of less than 7.35 in the arterial blood is abnormal and is called *acidemia (-emia* is the suffix for a condition in the blood*)*. Likewise, a pH in the arterial blood greater than 7.45 is also abnormal and is called *alkalemia*.

A condition that tends to cause acidemia is called an *acidosis*; therefore, all patients with acidemia must also have a primary acidosis. Similarly, a condition that tends to cause alkalemia is called an *alkalosis*; therefore, all patients with alkalemia must also have a primary alkalosis. For this reason, it is customary to simply call a low arterial blood pH acidosis and a high blood pH alkalosis (Table 2-1).

pH	Symptoms
7.80	Death
	Convulsions
	Arrhythmias
	Irritability
7.40	Normal
	Drowsiness
	Lethargy
	Coma
6.80	Death

Figure 2-1.   **Clinical symptoms associated with abnormal pH.**

Table 2-1.   pH CLASSIFICATION

Classification	pH
Normal	7.35–7.45
Acidosis	<7.35
Alkalosis	>7.45

BASIC (PRIMARY) ACID-BASE DISTURBANCE(S)

It has become standard diagnostic practice to characterize acid-base pathologic conditions into one of two general categories: respiratory and/or metabolic problems. This basic pathologic condition, sometimes referred to as a primary acid-base disturbance, is the root cause or problem that has led to (or has an inclination or tendency to lead to) overall acid-base disruption.

To determine the primary problem, the clinician should first evaluate (or classify) the respiratory status using the $PaCO_2$. This is followed by evaluation of the metabolic (i.e., non-respiratory) acid-base status using either the plasma bicarbonate concentration $[HCO_3]$ or the base excess concentration $[BE]$. By understanding how these two indices may alter pH, the primary problem or problems can be easily identified as described subsequently.

Respiratory Acid-Base Status

Evaluation or classification of the respiratory component of acid-base balance is a logical starting point in "basic primary problem" determination because the respiratory system is the major organ system responsible for acid excretion and the moment-to-moment regulation of pH.

Regarding acid-base balance, the specific role of the lungs is to excrete carbonic acid at exactly the same rate at which it is being produced by the tissues as a result of carbon dioxide production via metabolism. Therefore, if the lungs are properly excreting carbonic acid, blood leaving the lungs (i.e., arterial blood) should have a constant, normal level of carbonic acid.

Measurement of the carbonic acid levels in the blood leaving the lungs would thus provide us with an index of lung effectiveness in acid-base balance (i.e., carbonic acid excretion). High carbonic acid levels in the arterial blood would indicate that the lungs are failing to adequately excrete this acid. Conversely, low carbonic acid levels in the blood would indicate excessive excretion and depletion of the body stores. Because arterial blood is a mixture of all the blood that has just left the lungs, it is ideal for this assessment.

The technical problem with this approach to respiratory acid-base assessment is that carbonic acid levels in the blood are *very* low, and measurement of carbonic acid levels is not technically feasible. Fortunately, however, *there is a direct linear relationship between arterial carbonic acid levels and* $PaCO_2$. Thus, when $PaCO_2$ is increased, it is indicative of increased carbonic acid in the blood, which tends to decrease pH (acidosis).

Logically, the converse is also true. A decreased $PaCO_2$ indicates below-normal levels of carbonic acid in the arterial blood, which tends to elevate pH (i.e., alkalosis). In summary, *the adequacy of carbonic acid excretion (respiratory acid-base function) can be assessed simply by evaluating* $PaCO_2$.

$PaCO_2$ Classification

A normal level of carbonic acid in the arterial blood corresponds to a $PaCO_2$ level of 35 to 45 mm Hg, which is shown in Table 2-2. Indeed, $PaCO_2$ can be used simply to evaluate and classify the respiratory acid-base status.

Respiratory Acidosis

An increased $PaCO_2$ level in the blood may also be termed *hypercarbia* or *hypercapnia*. These are simply terms that indicate that the amount of carbon dioxide present in the blood exceeds normal. From an acid-base standpoint, hypercapnia means that there is an accumulation of carbonic acid in the blood. The accumulation of acid in the blood is a measurable condition that tends to cause acidemia and therefore fits the criteria to be called a *respiratory acidosis*.

Respiratory Alkalosis

Conversely, a below-normal level of CO_2 in the blood is called *hypocarbia* or *hypocapnia*.

Table 2-2.   CLASSIFICATION OF RESPIRATORY ACID-BASE COMPONENT

Classification	$PaCO_2$ (mm Hg)
Normal respiratory component	35–45
Respiratory acidosis	>45
Respiratory alkalosis	<35

Regarding acid-base status, a low $PaCO_2$ level indicates a depletion in blood carbonic acid levels. Therefore, a $PaCO_2$ level less than 35 mm Hg may be termed a *respiratory alkalosis*.

Inverse Relationship (PaCO₂–pH)

To classify arterial blood gases correctly, it is crucial to understand that *the relationship between $PaCO_2$ and pH is* **inverse**. In other words, when $PaCO_2$ is high (i.e., respiratory acidosis), pH will tend to decrease due to the accumulation of carbonic acid. Conversely, when $PaCO_2$ is low (i.e., respiratory alkalosis), pH will tend to increase due to the depletion of carbonic acid stores in the blood.

A very common classification error for the novice is to see an abnormal pH and $PaCO_2$ and assume the pH has changed because of the $PaCO_2$, despite the fact that the change in pH and $PaCO_2$ is not inverse.

For example, if pH is 7.20 (acidosis) and $PaCO_2$ is 20 mm Hg (respiratory alkalosis), both of these values are abnormal; however, the change in pH *cannot* be due to the respiratory condition (i.e., this is not a primary respiratory acid-base problem) but must be due to some non-respiratory condition (i.e., metabolic acidosis).

If indeed the abnormal $PaCO_2$ had caused an abnormal pH, the pH would be high (alkalosis) because the relationship must be inverse to assume cause and effect. Therefore, in this example, it is clear that the change in pH *must* be due to some other (non-respiratory) cause. To reiterate this important principle; *if the change in pH is due to a respiratory condition, the relationship between pH and $PaCO_2$ must be inverse.*

Metabolic Acid-Base Status

All the numerous conditions that may potentially alter pH have been grouped into two major categories to facilitate differential diagnosis. Blood gas acid-base evaluation involves classification of the data based on these two components. Respiratory disturbances include all those conditions that alter $PaCO_2$ levels in the blood. Metabolic disturbances, on the other hand, are defined by exclusion. Any acid-base disturbance that is not respiratory in origin is called a *metabolic disturbance*.

In some cases, the adjective *metabolic* may actually be misleading because many non-respiratory acid-base disturbances (e.g., vomiting) do not involve changes in "metabolism." In fact, some authors have suggested that the adjective *metabolic* should be replaced with the adjective *non-respiratory*.[174] Nevertheless, the term *metabolic* is well ingrained in clinical medicine and is used throughout this text.

The $PaCO_2$ is a specific, reliable, accurate, and simple indicator of respiratory acid-base disturbance. No single metabolic acid-base index perfectly fits this description. In some cases, metabolic indices will deviate artifactually from their normal ranges owing to reasons unrelated to primary acid-base disorders. Nevertheless, a change in the numerical value of a metabolic index is most commonly due to a metabolic acid-base disturbance and the novice should assume this to be the case. In later chapters, exceptions to this rule will be discussed.

[HCO₃] Classification

Although various different metabolic indices have been advocated through the years, the plasma bicarbonate concentration [HCO_3] (sometimes referred to as the *actual bicarbonate*) is probably the most widely used index and is seen on many clinical, professional, credentialling examinations. Initial blood gas classification examples in this text will include only the [HCO_3] as a metabolic index to avoid confusion. Also, as mentioned previously, there are some uncommon situations when bicarbonate values may be misleading (discussed in Chapter 5). It is best for the novice to assume the bicarbonate is always a clear and concise indicator of metabolic status. Logically, one should first learn the general rules of classification and later address unusual exceptions.

Normal Metabolic Status

Bicarbonate represents the most important base in the blood plasma. The normal value for plasma bicarbonate in the arterial blood is 24 ± 2 mEq/L, which is shown in Table 2-3.

Metabolic Acidosis

The numeric value of bicarbonate decreases in response to either an accumulation of blood

Table 2-3. CLASSIFICATION OF METABOLIC
            ACID-BASE COMPONENT

Classification	[HCO_3]*	[BE]*
Normal metabolic component	24 ± 2	0 ± 2
Metabolic acidosis	<22	<−2
Metabolic alkalosis	>26	>+2

*Base excess and bicarbonate in mEq/L.

fixed acids or to a loss of blood base. This occurs due to blood acid-base buffering, which is discussed in a later chapter. Therefore, a decreased bicarbonate concentration indicates a non-respiratory condition that tends to cause acidemia (i.e., metabolic acidosis). Quantitatively, as shown in Table 2-3, a metabolic acidosis can be defined as a [HCO_3] less than 22 mEq/L.

Metabolic Alkalosis

Conversely, the numeric value of bicarbonate increases in response to increased blood base or to a fall in fixed acid levels. Thus, bicarbonate values higher than normal indicate metabolic alkalosis. Numerically, as shown in Table 2-3, metabolic alkalosis can be defined as a [HCO_3] greater than 26 mEq/L.

Direct Relationship ([HCO_3]–pH)

Unlike the inverse relationship between $PaCO_2$ and pH, the relationship between [HCO_3] and pH is direct. In other words, a low [HCO_3] (e.g., 18 mEq/L termed a *metabolic acidosis*) tends to cause a low pH. Likewise, an increased [HCO_3] (e.g., 30 mEq/L termed a *metabolic alkalosis*) tends to increase pH.

Here again, if one is to assume cause and effect (i.e., a primary acid-base problem), the relationship between the metabolic index and pH must make sense. For example, if pH is 7.60 and the [HCO_3] is 18 mEq/L, this *cannot* be a metabolic acid-base problem because there is not a direct relationship (i.e., pH is above normal whereas [HCO_3] is below normal). *Understanding the effect of $PaCO_2$ and [HCO_3] change on pH are critical to correct blood gas classification.*

Identification of Primary Acid-Base Disturbances

As previously described, the pH should be evaluated first to get an overall view of acid-base status. Then, the $PaCO_2$ and [HCO_3] should be evaluated. If all three parameters (pH, $PaCO_2$, [HCO_3]) are in their normal ranges (Example 2-1), the classification is simply *Normal Acid-Base Status* and therefore no primary acid-base problem is present.

Example 2-1
Classification of Primary Blood Gas Problems
pH 7.38 (normal):

$PaCO_2$	Effect on pH	[HCO_3]	Effect on pH
38 mm Hg	—	23 mEq/L	—

When pH is outside the normal range, one must determine the basic (primary) acid-base disturbance. The key to successful classification is to identify whether the primary problem is respiratory ($PaCO_2$ is abnormal and inverse direction to pH change) or metabolic ([HCO_3] is abnormal and change is in the same direction as pH).

Table 2-4 highlights these key relationships, which must be memorized to identify the primary acid-base problem. Figure 2-2 illustrates the paths by which one can identify primary acid-base disturbances in patients with acidosis or alkalosis. In some less common cases, both respiratory and metabolic components may be pulling pH in the same direction. When there are two primary acid-base problems both pulling pH in the same direction, the problem is said to be "Mixed" or "Combined."

In Example 2-2, the primary problem is clearly metabolic because [HCO_3] is decreased (normal 24 ± 2 mEq/L) along with a decreased

Table 2-4. EFFECT OF $PaCO_2$ AND [HCO_3]
            CHANGE ON pH

Index	Effect on pH
$PaCO_2 \uparrow$	pH $\downarrow$
$PaCO_2 \downarrow$	pH $\uparrow$
[HCO_3] $\uparrow$	pH $\uparrow$
[HCO_3] $\downarrow$	pH $\downarrow$

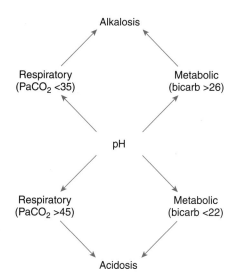

Figure 2-2. **The two potential categories/origins of acidosis or alkalosis.** The related blood gas values associated with each possible cause are also noted.

pH (direct relationship). $PaCO_2$ is within the normal range so this cannot be a primary respiratory acid-base problem. This would be termed a *metabolic acidosis*.

Example 2-2
Classification of Primary Blood Gas Problems
pH 7.28↓:

$PaCO_2$	Effect on pH	[HCO_3]	Effect on pH
37 mm Hg	—	17 mEq/L	↓

In contrast, Example 2-3 shows a *respiratory alkalosis* because the $PaCO_2$ is decreased and the pH is increased. The inverse relationship shows cause and effect indicative of a primary acid-base problem. The [HCO_3] is within the normal range so a primary metabolic problem cannot be present.

Example 2-3
Classification of Primary Blood Gas Problems
pH 7.55↑:

$PaCO_2$	Effect on pH	[HCO_3]	Effect on pH
25 mm Hg	↑	23 mEq/L	—

Example 2-4 shows a *respiratory and a metabolic acidosis*. This blood gas actually

demonstrates two primary problems both pulling the pH in the same direction (lower). Again, $PaCO_2$ is increased (which tends to lower pH because the relationship is inverse) and [HCO_3] is decreased (which tends to lower pH because the relationship is direct). Thus, $PaCO_2$ indicates a respiratory acidosis and [HCO_3] indicates a metabolic acidosis. This may also be classified as a *mixed or combined acidosis*.

A blood gas such as that in Example 2-4 may accompany cardiac arrest. The respiratory acidosis results from decreased ventilation, whereas the metabolic acidosis is a result of anaerobic (without oxygen) metabolism and lactic acid accumulation. Although somewhat inter-related, two primary and separate basic acid-base problems coexist.

Example 2-4
Classification of Primary Blood Gas Problems
pH 7.10↓:

$PaCO_2$	Effect on pH	[HCO_3]	Effect on pH
64 mm Hg	↓	19 mEq/L	↓

Example 2-5 is one of the most common types of blood gases seen and also one of the most commonly misclassified, particularly by the novice. As previously stated, many inexperienced clinicians, after looking at pH and $PaCO_2$, incorrectly classify this as simply respiratory alkalosis. The logic is that pH and $PaCO_2$ are both abnormal; so the abnormal respiratory condition must be the cause of the overall pH acid-base disturbance. The error in this logic is failing to remember the relationship between $PaCO_2$ and pH as shown in Table 2-4. *Whenever the individual has a primary respiratory acid-base disturbance, the relationship between $PaCO_2$ and pH must be inverse.*

This basic primary acid-base disturbance in this blood gas is a metabolic acidosis because a low [HCO_3] tends to lower pH and indeed that explains the abnormally low pH. The low $PaCO_2$ (respiratory alkalosis that tends to increase pH) is actually due to the normal compensatory response of the body, which is described later in this chapter. In summary, when determining primary problems, the key is to understand the relationships in Table 2-4.

Example 2-5

Classification of Primary Blood Gas Problems

pH 7.20↓:

PaCO$_2$	Effect on pH	[HCO$_3$]	Effect on pH
20 mm Hg	↑	17 mEq/L	↓

Base Excess [BE] Assessment

An alternative metabolic index with fairly widespread popularity is the *base excess* [BE]. It is noteworthy for the novice in arterial blood gas classification that the base excess and plasma bicarbonate both provide the clinician with the *same* general clinical information regarding acid-base balance. There is, in fact, no need to evaluate both of these indices.

For the novice, it is recommended that, given a particular blood gas, only one of the metabolic indices should be classified to avoid confusion. Some unusual situations are discussed later in Chapter 5, when the two indices may not completely agree with each other.

If both indices are reported at your institution, the index most commonly used in your particular institution or region should be used for classification. Beginning exercises in this text will use bicarbonate as the metabolic acid-base index. In later examples, the base excess or both metabolic indices (i.e., [HCO$_3$] and [BE]) values may be given.

From a numerical standpoint, the [BE] is easier to understand than bicarbonate since the normal value for base excess is 0 ± 2 mEq/L. A base excess in the negative range (metabolic acidosis) is sometimes called a base deficit. Nevertheless, even in the presence of a "base deficit," this index is still usually referred to as the base excess.

Obviously, if you are using [BE] as the metabolic index, the same rules apply. An elevated [BE] (e.g., +5 mEq/L) would increase pH and would be termed a *metabolic alkalosis* (see Table 2-3). A lower [BE] (e.g., −5 mEq/L) tends to lower pH and would be termed a *metabolic acidosis*.

COMPENSATION ASSESSMENT

Compensation is defined as return of an abnormal pH toward normal by the component (i.e., respiratory or metabolic) that was not primarily affected. For example, when an abnormal respiratory acidosis (i.e., primary pathologic respiratory acidosis) occurs, the body (specifically the kidneys) responds by developing a compensatory increase in blood base (i.e., secondary metabolic alkalosis). The compensatory response helps protect pH and prevents large, abrupt, dangerous swings in pH. Conversely, in the presence of an abnormal (primary) metabolic acidosis, the respiratory system reduces blood PaCO$_2$ levels (i.e., secondary respiratory alkalosis) in an attempt to bring the pH toward normal.

Uncompensated Acid-Base Problems

When one of the acid-base components (i.e., respiratory or metabolic) is abnormal and the other is within the normal range, the abnormal condition is said to be *uncompensated* (e.g., *uncompensated respiratory acidosis*). The absence of compensation may be seen in respiratory acid-base problems that have developed rapidly or when the body is unable to compensate due to disease or some other reason.

Uncompensated respiratory acid-base problems generally indicate that the problem is of recent origin (i.e., acute) and that the kidneys have not had a sufficient time to manifest measurable compensation. Renal compensation is a relatively slow process in that it takes the kidneys considerable time (i.e., 48 to 72 hours) to achieve maximal compensation. As a general rule, it is unusual and, indeed, signals another patient problem when an acid-base disturbance remains uncompensated for a long time.

Total classification of acid-base status in Example 2-6 would be *uncompensated respiratory acidosis*. The patient has respiratory acidosis as described in the previous section because PaCO$_2$ and pH are inverse. Regarding compensation, the respiratory acidosis is uncompensated because no increase in [HCO$_3$] (no secondary metabolic alkalosis) above the normal range is seen.

Example 2-6

Classification of Primary Blood Gas Problems

pH 7.20↓:

PaCO$_2$	Effect on pH	[HCO$_3$]	Effect on pH
68 mm Hg	↓	25 mEq/L	—

Example 2-7 would similarly represent an *uncompensated metabolic alkalosis*. After Compensation assessment for Example 2-2 shown previously, acid-base classification would be *uncompensated metabolic acidosis* rather than simply metabolic acidosis. Example 2-3 would likewise be termed *uncompensated respiratory alkalosis*. In all of these examples, the acid-base component not primarily affected has remained within the normal **range** and therefore no compensation is evident.

Example 2-7
Classification of Primary Blood Gas Problems
pH 7.51↑:

PaCO$_2$	Effect on pH	[HCO$_3$]	Effect on pH
42 mm Hg	—	32 mEq/L	↑

Example 2-8 shows the presence of multiple (combined) acid-base disturbances, specifically a *mixed respiratory and metabolic alkalosis*. Example 2-8 should not be classified as **uncompensated mixed respiratory and metabolic alkalosis**. In the presence of a mixed (combined) acid-base disturbance, it is not necessary to classify this blood gas as being "uncompensated" because this would be redundant. By definition, it is impossible to have compensation for a mixed or combined acid-base disturbance; therefore, no mention of compensation should be in the classification.

Example 2-8
Classification of Primary Blood Gas Problems
pH 7.62↑:

PaCO$_2$	Effect on pH	[HCO$_3$]	Effect on pH
30 mm Hg	↑	30 mEq/L	↑

Partially Compensated Acid-Base Problems

It is typical to see some compensation in individuals with primary acid-base disturbances. In fact, whenever the respiratory and metabolic components are in opposite directions (e.g., acidosis and alkalosis), we routinely assume that compensation is present. Examples 2-9 through 2-11 and, previously, Example 2-5, all show respiratory and metabolic components pulling pH in opposite directions (note arrows indicating opposite effects on pH) and suggesting compensation.

The clinician should understand that what appears to be simple compensation actually could reflect a more complex, dual (i.e., mixed) acid-base problem. Patients may have two *primary*, abnormal acid-base conditions that each pull the pH in a different direction and the blood gas would appear, at first glance, to be consistent with compensation. This is actually not a particularly rare phenomenon and a more detailed discussion of how to recognize mixed disturbances is described in Chapter 14.

Notwithstanding, on initial inspection and classification, *whenever the respiratory and metabolic conditions are in opposite directions* (e.g., respiratory alkalosis and metabolic acidosis), *compensation should be assumed*. A typical blood gas picture in compensation is shown in Example 2-9. Compensation is presumed because the patient has both a respiratory acidosis (i.e., PaCO$_2$ = 68 mm Hg) and a metabolic alkalosis [HCO$_3$] = 32 mEq/L). Because the pH is still clearly below the normal range (acidosis), it would make sense to assume that the primary problem is a respiratory acidosis and that the metabolic alkalosis is a secondary disturbance as a result of compensation.

When compensation is evident but the pH remains outside the normal range, the primary acid-base disturbance is said to be "partially compensated." Hence, Example 2-9 is classified as a *partially compensated respiratory acidosis*. Example 2-10 would be *partially compensated respiratory alkalosis*. Example 2-11 would be a *partially compensated metabolic alkalosis*. Again, one of the most commonly seen (and misclassified) acid-base conditions is the *partially compensated metabolic acidosis* shown earlier in Example 2-5.

Example 2-9
Classification of Primary Blood Gas Problems
pH 7.30↓:

PaCO$_2$	Effect on pH	[HCO$_3$]	Effect on pH
68 mm Hg	↓	32 mEq/L	↑

Example 2-10
Classification of Primary Blood Gas Problems
pH 7.58↑:

PaCO$_2$	Effect on pH	[HCO$_3$]	Effect on pH
17 mm Hg	↑	16 mEq/L	↓

Example 2-11
Classification of Primary Blood Gas Problems
pH 7.49↑:

$PaCO_2$	Effect on pH	$[HCO_3]$	Effect on pH
50 mm Hg	↓	37 mEq/L	↑

Completely Compensated Acid-Base Problems

Determination of the primary problem is obvious when the pH is outside the normal range because compensation has not yet achieved complete pH correction of the primary problem. Notwithstanding, when the respiratory and metabolic components are in opposite directions and *the pH is in the normal range*, the answer to this question is less clear. This point is shown in Example 2-12. Is the metabolic alkalosis compensating for a primary respiratory acidosis or is the respiratory acidosis compensating for a primary metabolic alkalosis?

Example 2-12
Classification of Primary Blood Gas Problems
pH 7.37↑:

$PaCO_2$	Effect on pH	$[HCO_3]$	Effect on pH
50 mm Hg	↓	28 mEq/L	↑

The answer is that this blood gas *most likely* represents an individual with a *compensated respiratory acidosis*. Sometimes these blood gases are also called "completely compensated" because the pH is in the normal range but this is somewhat redundant and therefore not used in this text.

Primary respiratory acidosis is the most likely acid-base situation in Example 2-12 because it is generally accepted that the body does not *overcompensate* for a primary acid-base disturbance. In other words, when the pH reaches the normal **range**, compensatory mechanisms abate.

The most likely sequence of events is shown in Figure 2-3. An individual with a normal pH (Fig. 2-3,*A*) develops an acute respiratory acidosis (Fig. 2-3,*B*). After maximal renal compensation, however, the pH is brought back to the **lower** portion of the normal range (Fig. 2-3,*C*). When the pH reaches the normal range, compensatory mechanisms tend to abate. The fact that the final pH is on the lower portion of the

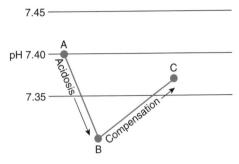

Figure 2-3. **Compensation for a primary acidosis.** *A*, A normal pH of 7.4 is shown. *B*, The individual develops an acidosis that could be either respiratory or metabolic. *C*, After complete compensation, the pH rests on the lower portion of the normal range.

normal pH range strongly suggests that the initial disturbance had pulled the pH down (i.e., it was an acidosis).

Example 2-13
Classification of Primary Blood Gas Problems
pH 7.42↑:

$PaCO_2$	Effect on pH	$[HCO_3]$	Effect on pH
50 mm Hg	↓	30 mEq/L	↑

Conversely, the blood gas shown in Example 2-13 suggests that the primary acid-base problem is a metabolic alkalosis and that the hypercarbia observed is compensatory. In other words, it would be classified as a *compensated metabolic alkalosis*. Figure 2-4 shows the likely sequence of events in this case.

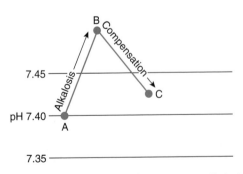

Figure 2-4. **Compensation for a primary alkalosis.** *A*, A normal pH of 7.40 is shown. *B*, The individual develops an alkalosis that could be either respiratory or metabolic. *C*, After complete compensation, the pH rests on the upper portion of the normal range.

Table 2-5. Determination of the Primary Problem

pH	
>7.40	Alkalosis is primary; acidosis is compensatory
<7.40	Acidosis is primary; alkalosis is compensatory

Table 2-6. Classification of Degree of Compensation

pH	Degree of Compensation
<7.35	Partial
>7.45	Partial
7.35–7.45	Complete

An individual with a normal pH (Fig. 2-4, *A*) develops an alkalemia (Fig. 2-4, *B*). After compensation, the pH is returned to the upper portion of the normal range (Fig. 2-4, *C*).

Thus, when the primary problem is not readily apparent, the clinician should assess what side of 7.40 that the pH is on. Table 2-5 shows how the most likely primary problem can be determined when the pH is in the normal range. Similarly, Figure 2-5 illustrates how one can determine the likely primary problem

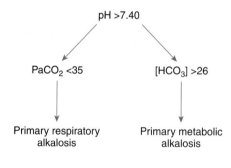

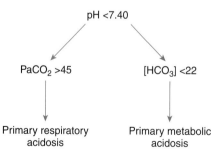

Figure 2-5. **Primary problem determination in complete compensation.** When the pH exceeds 7.40, the patient has a primary alkalosis. If the $PaCO_2$ is less than 35 mm Hg, there is a primary respiratory alkalosis. Similarly, if the $[HCO_3]$ exceeds 26 mEq/L, the patient has a primary metabolic alkalosis. The same approach can be used when complete compensation is present and pH is less than 7.40.

when a blood gas appears to be completely compensated. Partial versus complete compensation can likewise be differentiated by the pH as shown in Table 2-6.

It should be understood that this method for classification of the primary problem when pH is in the normal range is not foolproof. For example, a patient with a compensated metabolic acidosis may hyperventilate in response to an arterial puncture. This, in turn, may push the pH to the alkaline side of 7.40. The numbers in this situation would incorrectly suggest a primary alkalosis.

When compensation is suspected and pH is in the normal range, the clinical history and serial blood gases are more important in making the primary acid-base diagnosis than is the specific pH. More sophisticated tools (e.g., acid-base maps; see Chapter 14) are also very helpful in this regard. Nevertheless, for the student learning basic blood gas classification, it is useful to use the pH method for determining the *probable* primary problem and arriving at an initial classification. This allows the novice to organize concepts into a meaningful, consistent framework.

It is also noteworthy that, physiologically, it is actually unusual to see "complete" compensation. The maximal compensatory response in most cases is associated only with a 50% to 75% return of pH to normal.[172] Thus, most clinical acid-base blood gases will be classified as being partially compensated despite maximal acid-base response by the body.

For the sake of completeness regarding classification, it is also possible for a patient to have two opposing acid-base conditions (e.g., respiratory acidosis and metabolic alkalosis) while having a pH of exactly 7.40. In this case, it is impossible to identify a single primary problem based on the data alone. Thus, this blood gas should be classified as simply a *respiratory acidosis and metabolic alkalosis*, which implies that either condition may be primary or secondary disturbances. Again, the accuracy of this assumption requires further investigation as discussed in subsequent chapters.

ACID-BASE CLASSIFICATION VERSUS INTERPRETATION

By integrating the information acquired in the preceding steps, a complete acid-base classification can now be formulated for any blood gas. The term *classification* is used here to mean stating the overall acid-base status along with carefully selected *general* descriptive adjectives.

The clinician should also realize that an acid-base classification based on only an arterial blood gas is not a definitive acid-base diagnosis. Similarly, a term such as *metabolic acidosis* is not definitive. Rather, it serves as a general categorical classification that may help to direct the clinician to a more definitive acid-base diagnosis (e.g., hypoxia and lactic acidosis). Notwithstanding, acid-base classification based on the arterial blood gas is a good diagnostic starting point.

OXYGENATION STATUS

After acid-base classification, the patient's oxygenation status should be evaluated. The routine classification of oxygenation via the arterial blood gas report is essentially an evaluation of the PaO_2 and its relationship to FIO_2. The SaO_2 may provide valuable information about oxygenation in many clinical circumstances; however, it is not *directly* measured with blood gases or routinely classified. The clinical role of SaO_2 and other factors in oxygenation are discussed in subsequent chapters.

PaO_2 Classification

As shown in Table 2-7, there are three possible general outcomes in adult PaO_2 classification: normoxemia, hyperoxemia, or hypoxemia. Newborns generally have a lower PaO_2 as described in Chapter 1.

Normoxemia

The normal range for adult PaO_2 on room air at sea level is 80 to 100 mm Hg, which is

Table 2-7.   Classification of PaO_2 in the Adult

Classification	PaO_2 (mm Hg)
Hyperoxemia	>100
Normoxemia	80–100
Mild Hypoxemia	60–79
Moderate Hypoxemia	45–59
Severe Hypoxemia	<45

shown in Table 2-7. A PaO_2 value within the normal range is called *normoxemia*. In clinical practice, many clinicians do not use the term *normoxemia* but state simply that (blood gas) oxygenation is normal or PaO_2 is normal.

Hyperoxemia

A PaO_2 level exceeding normal limits (i.e., >100 mm Hg) may be called *hyperoxemia*. Hyperoxemia can occur as a result of hyperventilation or administration of oxygen therapy (Fig. 2-6). PaO_2s are generally less than 130 mm Hg when the cause is hyperventilation but may be much higher (e.g., 400 mm Hg) with the administration of high oxygen concentrations. In most clinical situations, significant hyperoxemia is undesirable and may lead to untoward consequences. Although there are exceptions, as a general rule, one should try to avoid hyperoxemia.

Hypoxemia

A PaO_2 level less than 80 mm Hg is called *hypoxemia*.[10,175] Hypoxemia is very common in hospitalized patients and may be a cause for

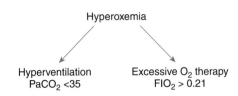

Figure 2-6.   Causes of hyperoxemia. There are only two potential causes of hyperoxemia. Hyperventilation while breathing room air may cause mild hyperoxemia up to about 130 mm Hg. Most often, hyperoxemia is due to oxygen therapy and increased inspired oxygen concentration.

serious concern. One should remember however, that PaO_2 decreases as a normal consequence of aging and mild hypoxemia is expected in the elderly. One can approximate the impact of aging on PaO_2 with the following formula. Assuming a normal PaO_2 of 100 mm Hg at 10 years old, PaO_2 decreases approximately 5 mm Hg for every 10 years thereafter. Notwithstanding, PaO_2 should not be less than 75 mm Hg at any age.[242]

Hypoxic Potential

One must keep in mind that evaluation of blood gas PaO_2 is only an evaluation of how much oxygen is dissolved in arterial blood. A more important clinical question regarding oxygenation is evaluation for the presence of hypoxia. *Hypoxia* is a generalized state of inadequate oxygen to the tissues or cells of the body. Hypoxia is a very serious condition which, if uncorrected, can lead to death of the organism.

Complete hypoxic evaluation is a very important and much more complex process that is described later in this text. Nevertheless, simple classification of the PaO_2 is a good first step in oxygenation assessment, which can be done with only the use of the blood gas information. Simply stated, hypoxemia *may* lead to hypoxia. Furthermore, the likelihood of hypoxia (i.e., cellular oxygen deprivation) depends on the severity of the hypoxemia. For this reason, it is customary to specify the degree of hypoxemia when classifying an arterial blood gas. The degree of hypoxemia can be classified as being mild, moderate, or severe depending on the propensity of the PaO_2 to result in hypoxia (Fig. 2-7).

Mild Hypoxemia

The presence of hypoxemia does not necessarily mean that oxygen levels in the blood are insufficient to meet cellular needs. Mild hypoxemia (i.e., PaO_2 value of 60 to 80 mm Hg), which is shown in Table 2-7, is generally well tolerated, and tissue hypoxia is rare. The SaO_2 value remains at 90% even when the PaO_2 value falls to 60 mm Hg. *The presence of mild hypoxemia, although not normal, is unlikely to result in hypoxia in the absence of other oxygenation disturbances.*

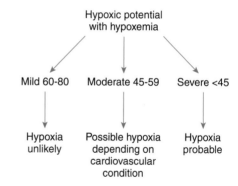

Figure 2-7. Hypoxic potential with hypoxemia. The potential for hypoxia is directly related to the degree of hypoxemia. With mild hypoxemia, hypoxia is unlikely because SaO_2 remains above 90%. With moderate hypoxemia, hypoxia may be present if the body's compensatory mechanisms (especially cardiac output) are unable to maintain tissue oxygenation. With severe hypoxemia, it is highly likely that the patient will have concurrent hypoxia. Severe hypoxemia and hypoxia represent a critical situation that must be addressed.

Moderate Hypoxemia

Moderate hypoxemia leads to a more substantive decrease in blood oxygenation and typically requires an increased cardiac output to maintain tissue oxygen delivery. In the individual with a normal cardiovascular system, tissue oxygenation is usually maintained despite moderate hypoxemia. In the presence of cardiovascular disease, however, the individual may not be capable of delivering sufficient oxygen to the tissues and hypoxia may ensue. Thus, *moderate hypoxemia may or may not result in hypoxia depending on the integrity of the patient's cardiovascular system.* Moderate hypoxemia is usually corrected to decrease cardiovascular work and preclude the development of hypoxia.

Severe Hypoxemia

When hypoxemia is severe, it is unlikely that tissue oxygenation can be maintained even with a normal cardiovascular system. Therefore, *the patient with severe hypoxemia should be presumed to be in a state of hypoxia. Severe hypoxemia requires immediate attention and action (e.g., oxygen administration)!* Patients should never be left in a state of severe hypoxemia.

Efficiency of Oxygen Uptake

Normal FIO$_2$–PaO$_2$ Relationship

The adult PaO$_2$ classification system is based on the assumption that patients are breathing room air (FIO$_2$ of 0.21). When a patient is receiving oxygen therapy, the PaO$_2$ value may be in the normal range or higher despite the presence of substantial pulmonary dysfunction. A PaO$_2$ value of 80 mm Hg may be called normoxemia and it does indicate a sufficient amount of dissolved oxygen in the blood, nevertheless, it is indicative of pulmonary dysfunction if the patient is breathing a high concentration of oxygen (e.g., an FIO$_2$ of 0.8, 80% oxygen). Oxygen uptake in the lungs is very inefficient.

In normal individuals, the PaO$_2$ value is approximately four to five times higher than the percentage of oxygen being inspired. Thus, normal PaO$_2$ on room air ($\approx$20% O$_2$) is approximately 80 to 100 mm Hg (e.g., 5 $\times$ 20 = 100). Normal PaO$_2$ on 40% O$_2$ is approximately 160 to 200 mm Hg (e.g., 40 $\times$ 5 = 200). Normal PaO$_2$ on 70% O$_2$ is approximately 280 to 350 mm Hg (e.g., 70 $\times$ 5 = 350) and so forth.

PaO$_2$/%FIO$_2$ (Oxygenation Ratio)

If one takes the PaO$_2$ and divides it by the percentage of inspired oxygen (i.e., PaO$_2$/%FIO$_2$), an efficiency rating of pulmonary oxygen exchange can be calculated. The normal oxygenation ratio is approximately 5 (100/20 = 5). The lower the oxygenation ratio, the less efficient oxygen uptake in the lungs is and the more severe is the pulmonary impairment. Values in the range of 4 to 5 are clinically normal.

Ratios in the range of 2 to 3.9 indicate moderate pulmonary dysfunction (Table 2-8).

Table 2-8. OXYGENATION RATIO (PaO$_2$/%FIO$_2$)

Pulmonary Status	Oxygenation Ratio (PaO$_2$/%FIO$_2$)
Normal	4.0–5.0
Moderate pulmonary dysfunction	2.0–3.9
Substantial pulmonary dysfunction	<2.0

Ratios less than 2 suggest substantial pulmonary dysfunction. Generally, the lower the ratio, the higher the shunt component in the lungs.

It is not customary to state the FIO$_2$ as part of the blood gas classification. Nevertheless, at the very least, the clinician should always take note of the FIO$_2$ when classifying a blood gas to get some idea as to the normalcy of pulmonary gas exchange.

COMPLETE BLOOD GAS CLASSIFICATION

Acid-base and oxygenation status have been described separately as an introduction to the classification of blood gases. In clinical practice, blood gas classification refers to the combined assessment of both acid-base and oxygenation status. Conventionally, acid-base status is stated first followed by classification of the oxygenation status. Complete blood gas classification of Example 2-14 below would thus be *partially compensated metabolic acidosis with moderate hypoxemia.* The clinician should note that the patient is breathing room air.

Example 2-14

(Room Air Blood Gases)

pH	7.22
PaCO$_2$	22 mm Hg
[HCO$_3$]	9 mEq/L
PaO$_2$	51 mm Hg

It is especially important for the novice in blood gas classification to complete the exercises at the end of this chapter to ensure mastery of the important clinical skill of basic blood gas classification. More sophisticated approaches to acid-base and oxygenation assessment are provided in later chapters.

ALTERNATIVE TERMINOLOGY

Ventilatory Failure

The clinician should be aware that alternative terminology is used sometimes to classify these same data from an arterial blood gas report. Shapiro introduced the term *ventilatory failure* to characterize a PaCO$_2$ greater than 50 mm Hg.[10]

ON CALL | CASE 2-1 *ABGs and Critical Thinking*

You are the only person available to care for this patient. You must assess the patient/situation and act accordingly.

A 27-year-old woman arrives in the emergency department comatose, with a very slow respiratory rate.

ARTERIAL BLOOD GASES

SaO_2	89%
pH	7.24
$PaCO_2$	69 mm Hg
PaO_2	69 mm Hg
$[HCO_3]$	26 mEq/L

ASSESSMENT

Abnormalities: List abnormal data and other noteworthy information. Classify ABG.

Explanation: List possible diseases, pathology, or other situations which may have lead to this patient's condition.

Evaluation: Suggest additional data which would be useful in helping understand the situation or in making a diagnosis.

INTERVENTION

Importance: Prioritize concern(s) of treatment in order of urgency and/or seriousness as you see the overall situation.

The term *ventilatory failure* is based on the concept that ventilation has failed to excrete CO_2 at the same rate that it is being produced; thus, the process of alveolar ventilation has failed. The advantage of this terminology is that it draws attention to the fact that $PaCO_2$ is essentially a product of CO_2 production and alveolar ventilation. Thus, the presence of ventilatory failure suggests the potential need for ventilation (compared with oxygenation) therapy.

The process of ventilation, however, is not an end in itself. Rather, its importance is based on the impact that ventilation has on the broader concerns of acid-base balance and oxygenation. For this reason and because of the continued widespread use of acid-base focused terminology, this alternative terminology is not routinely used for basic blood gas classification in this text.

Nevertheless, the overall concept of ventilatory failure is useful, and the reader should be aware of it. The clinician should understand that ventilatory failure is synonymous with respiratory acidosis.

Temporal Adjectives

The term *temporal* means of or pertaining to time. The fact that the renal compensatory response to respiratory acid-base disturbances is a time-dependent process has prompted the use of temporal related adjectives to classify blood gases. It is well known that maximal renal compensation for primary respiratory disturbances may take up to or beyond 72 hours. Knowledge of this fact often allows us to determine whether a particular respiratory acid-base problem is of recent origin.

Usefulness

In particular, an *acute* respiratory problem can often be recognized by the conspicuous absence of renal compensation. Similarly, a *chronic* respiratory problem is likely to manifest substantial or complete compensation. This information may be very important in trying to evaluate if an individual in the emergency room has chronic pulmonary disease and may hypoventilate or become apneic following oxygen therapy.

Table 2-9 shows the temporal adjectives that correlate with absent or complete compensation. Again, remember that complete

Table 2-9. TEMPORAL ADJECTIVES FOR PRIMARY RESPIRATORY ACID-BASE PROBLEMS

Temporal Adjective	Degree of Compensation
Acute	Uncompensated
Chronic	Completely compensated

ON CALL | CASE 2-2 *ABGs and Critical Thinking*

You are the only person available to care for this patient. You must assess the patient/situation and act accordingly.

A 68-year-old man is admitted with a history of heavy smoking, a barrel chest, shortness of breath, and excessive sputum production.

Explanation: List possible diseases, pathology, or other situations which may have led to this patient's condition.

Evaluation: Suggest additional data which would be useful in helping understand the situation or in making a diagnosis.

ARTERIAL BLOOD GASES

SaO$_2$	78%
pH	7.32
PaCO$_2$	68 mm Hg
PaO$_2$	48 mm Hg
[HCO$_3$]	32 mEq/L

INTERVENTION

Importance: Prioritize concern(s) of treatment in order of urgency and/or seriousness as you see the overall situation.

ASSESSMENT

Abnormalities: List abnormal data and other noteworthy information. Classify ABG.

---

compensation for any respiratory acid-base disturbance is uncommon. Thus, chronic problems may present as partially compensated disturbances.

Caveats

Several caveats or cautions should be realized regarding the use of temporal adjectives. First, what appears to be compensation may in fact be a *primary* acid-base problem in the opposing direction. The duration of a particular acid-base disturbance is best assessed by carefully reviewing the history and physical examination.

Second, this terminology is appropriate only for *primary respiratory acid-base problems.* The temporal nature of primary metabolic problems cannot be assessed by the degree of compensation present. Substantial respiratory compensation for metabolic acid-base problems occurs immediately (i.e., certainly within an hour). Therefore, the degree of compensation in primary metabolic disorders does not provide any useful information regarding the duration of the primary acid-base disorder.

EXERCISES

Exercise 2-1 **pH Assessment**

Fill in the blanks or select the best answer.

1. The single best indicator of acid-base status in the body is the (PaCO$_2$, [HCO$_3$], [BE], pH).

2. The pH of arterial blood is measured in (intracellular/extracellular) fluid.

3. The pH in the arterial blood reflects (overall/local) acid-base conditions in the body.

4. The pH range generally considered compatible with life is _____ to _____.

5. A low arterial pH tends to have an overall (depressive/stimulatory) effect on the nervous system.

6. Convulsions may be seen with severe (acidemia/alkalemia).

7. A normal pH (does/does not) ensure that all acid-base components are completely normal.

8. Technically, (acidosis/acidemia) is a below-normal pH in the blood.

9. Because all patients with acidemia must have a causative acidosis, it is common clinical practice to refer to a low blood pH as simply _____.

10. State the three steps (ABCs) in classification of acid-base status from a blood gas report.

11. List the four blood gas values to be assessed and the appropriate sequence of assessment.

12. Classify the following arterial blood pH measurements:
    a. 7.34   d. 7.45   g. 7.62
    b. 7.20   e. 7.32   h. 7.45
    c. 7.60   f. 7.48   i. 7.46

Exercise 2-2   Respiratory Acid-Base Status

Fill in the blanks or select the best answer.

1. Regarding acid homeostasis, the specific role of the lungs is to excrete _____ acid at exactly the same rate at which it is being produced by the tissues.

2. There is a direct, linear relationship between arterial carbonic acid levels and _____.

3. An increased $PaCO_2$ level in the blood is called (hypercarbia/hypocarbia).

4. Classify the following $PaCO_2$ values as either a respiratory acidosis, normal $PaCO_2$, or respiratory alkalosis.
   a. 30   b. 42   c. 35   d. 20   e. 55

5. State whether the presence of the following $PaCO_2$ values will tend to increase or decrease pH.
   a. 80   b. 58   c. 32   d. 75   e. 15

Exercise 2-3   Metabolic Acid-Base Status

Fill in the blanks or select the best answer.

1. Any acid-base disturbance that is not respiratory in origin is called a _____ disturbance.

2. Some authors have suggested that the term *metabolic* should be replaced with _____.

3. The plasma bicarbonate is also sometimes referred to as the _____ bicarbonate.

4. The normal value for plasma bicarbonate in the arterial blood is _____ mEq/L.

5. Classify the metabolic acid-base status as metabolic acidosis, metabolic alkalosis, or normal [HCO_3] given the following values for plasma bicarbonate.
   a. 25 mEq/L   b. 30 mEq/L   c. 18 mEq/L

6. Determine which way the following [HCO_3] values tend to move pH (increase or decrease).
   a. 20 mEq/L   b. 28 mEq/L   c. 15 mEq/L

7. The two most commonly used metabolic indices in the basic classification of blood gases are the _____ and the _____.

8. The normal value for base excess is _____ mEq/L.

9. A base excess in the negative range is sometimes called a _____ _____.

10. Given the following values for base excess, classify metabolic status.
   a. −5 mEq/L   d. −20 mEq/L
   b. +5 mEq/L   e. −1 mEq/L
   c. +12 mEq/L   f. +20 mEq/L

Exercise 2-4 Compensation Assessment

Fill in the blanks or select the best answer.

1. Return of an abnormal pH toward normal by the component that is not primarily affected is called _____.

2. The organ system responsible for compensation for metabolic acid-base problems is the _____ system.

3. The organ system responsible for compensation for respiratory acid-base problems is the _____ system.

4. The body responds to metabolic acidosis with (hypercarbia/hypocarbia).

5. Uncompensated respiratory acid-base problems usually indicate that the problem is (acute/chronic).

6. Most clinical blood gases with severe primary problems manifest (partial/complete) compensation.

7. To determine whether or not a blood gas is completely compensated, one must evaluate the (pH/$PaCO_2$).

8. A pH of 7.30, with a $PaCO_2$ value of 30 mm Hg and a [HCO_3] of 14 mEq/L, is classified as a (completely/partially) compensated metabolic acidosis.

9. In the patient with a long-standing hypercapnia, one would expect to see a(n) (increased/decreased) bicarbonate.

10. Determine the probable primary problem given the following (completely compensated) acid-base data:

	pH	$PaCO_2$	[HCO_3]
a.	7.36	50	28
b.	7.38	48	28
c.	7.44	30	20
d.	7.42	51	30
e.	7.36	30	18

Exercise 2-5   Acid-Base Classification

Write the complete acid-base classification for the following:

	Set A				Set B		
	pH	**PaCO$_2$**	**[HCO$_3$]**		**pH**	**PaCO$_2$**	**[HCO$_3$]**
1.	7.28	60	26	1.	7.38	54	31
2.	7.50	40	30	2.	7.25	80	33
3.	7.62	28	28	3.	7.52	23	18
4.	7.22	50	20	4.	7.44	37	24
5.	7.52	28	23	5.	7.32	32	16
6.	7.52	42	33	6.	7.32	36	17
7.	7.60	30	29	7.	7.51	15	12
8.	7.10	40	12	8.	7.49	44	34
9.	7.20	36	13	9.	7.48	64	49
10.	7.34	50	25	10.	7.25	48	20

Exercise 2-6   Alternative Terminology

Fill in the blanks or select the best answer.

1. A PaCO$_2$ in excess of 50 mm Hg is sometimes referred to as ventilatory (insufficiency/ failure).

2. The term _____ means of or pertaining to time.

3. A/an (acute/chronic) respiratory problem can often be recognized by the conspicuous absence of renal compensation.

4. Temporal adjectives can be used for primary (respiratory/metabolic/respiratory and metabolic) acid-base problems.

5. Classify the following blood gases using temporal adjectives where possible.

	pH	PaCO$_2$	[HCO$_3$]
a.	7.35	58	30
b.	7.28	58	25
c.	7.60	26	25
d.	7.28	40	18
e.	7.55	28	25
f.	7.57	36	35

Exercise 2-7 Oxygenation Assessment

Fill in the blanks or select the best answer.

1. The routine classification of the pulmonary component of oxygenation using an arterial blood gas is essentially an evaluation of the (SaO_2/PaO_2).

2. The normal range of adult PaO_2 in the clinic is _____ to _____ mm Hg.

3. A PaO_2 value within the normal range is called _____.

4. A PaO_2 value less than 80 mm Hg is called _____.

5. In this text, the term *hypoxemia* refers to a low oxygen (content/partial pressure).

6. A PaO_2 value exceeding normal limits (i.e., >100 mm Hg) is termed _____.

7. In general, (lower/higher) PaO_2 values are seen in the newborn.

8. Mild hypoxemia (is/is not) usually associated with hypoxia.

9. SaO_2 is approximately _____% at a PaO_2 of 60 mm Hg.

10. The presence of hypoxia in moderate hypoxemia depends on the integrity of the (pulmonary/cardiovascular) system.

11. The patient with severe hypoxemia (should/should not) be presumed to be in a state of hypoxia.

12. In normal individuals, PaO_2 values are approximately _____ times higher than the percentage of oxygen being inspired.

Exercise 2-8 PaO₂ Classification

Classify the following adult PaO_2 values as mild, moderate, or severe hypoxemia.

Adult	PaO₂ (mm Hg)
1.	160
2.	31
3.	56
4.	43
5.	59
6.	415
7.	75
8.	260
9.	92
10.	80

Exercise 2-9 Complete Blood Gas Classification

Classify both the complete acid-base status and the oxygen status of the following adult blood gases:

	pH	PaCO$_2$	[HCO$_3$]	PaO$_2$
1.	7.58	20	19	63
2.	7.44	52	33	28
3.	7.21	66	25	47
4.	7.44	31	20	111
5.	7.60	28	27	59
6.	7.50	50	37	75
7.	7.41	42	24	229
8.	7.52	41	33	45
9.	7.46	44	30	87
10.	7.44	35	23	97

Exercise 2-10 Complete Blood Gas Classification using [BE] as Metabolic Index

Classify both the complete acid-base status and the oxygen status of the following adult blood gases:

	pH	PaCO$_2$	[BE]	PaO$_2$
1.	7.32	30	−10	58
2.	7.52	34	+4	32
3.	7.32	38	−6	145
4.	7.40	30	−5	90
5.	7.20	50	−9	60
6.	7.20	80	+2	90
7.	7.55	25	+1	72
8.	7.34	30	−9	41
9.	7.37	56	+5	57
10.	7.40	38	−2	350

Exercise 2-11   Complete Blood Gas Classification Additional Examples

Classify both the complete acid-base status and the oxygen status of the following adult blood gases:

	Set A						Set B			
	pH	PaCO$_2$	[HCO$_3$]	PaO$_2$			pH	PaCO$_2$	[HCO$_3$]	PaO$_2$
1.	7.10	60	18	53		1.	7.53	27	22	83
2.	7.60	26	25	42		2.	7.32	69	34	28
3.	7.40	36	22	183		3.	7.18	56	20	53
4.	7.30	30	14	90		4.	7.46	33	23	151
5.	7.20	72	26	63		5.	7.20	28	11	59
6.	7.32	70	35	82		6.	7.14	60	20	75
7.	7.59	30	28	32		7.	7.41	42	25	229
8.	7.37	30	18	41		8.	7.52	41	34	45
9.	7.41	56	34	87		9.	7.64	32	34	87
10.	7.39	58	33	350		10.	7.33	54	28	97

Exercise 2-12   Internet Work

1. Search the Internet for arterial blood gas interpretation and list at least two sites that you found useful.

2. State the major problems associated with using the Internet to research and learn about various medical topics. How might you minimize these problems?

NBRC Challenge 2

Please select the best answer for the following multiple choice questions.

1. Given: pH   7.16
           $PaCO_2$ 68 mm Hg
           $[HCO_3]$ 23 mEq/L
           PaO_2 62 mm Hg

   Which of the following would be the most likely treatment for a patient presenting with this blood gas?
   A) Mechanical ventilation
   B) Continuous Positive Airway Pressure (CPAP)
   C) Oxygen via nasal cannula
   D) Oxygen via mask
   E) Leave patient as is
   (CRT EXAM – NBRC MATRIX III,C,1)

2. A patient in the emergency room appears short of breath. The following blood gas is obtained:
   pH   7.15
   $PaCO_2$ 17 mm Hg
   $[HCO_3]$ 5 mEq/L
   PaO_2 110 mm Hg

   What is the likely explanation for the shortness of breath?
   A) Hypoxemia
   B) COPD
   C) Compensation for severe metabolic acidosis
   D) Primary hyperventilation
   E) Paradoxical oxygen response
   (CRT EXAM – NBRC MATRIX I,B,10,c)

3. An elderly patient presents to the emergency room with the following blood gas.
   pH   7.36
   $PaCO_2$ 58 mm Hg
   $[HCO_3]$ 31 mEq/L
   PaO_2 62 mm Hg

   A likely diagnosis for this patient is:
   A) drug overdose.

B) primary metabolic acidosis.
C) primary metabolic alkalosis.
D) pulmonary embolus.
E) COPD.
(CRT EXAM – NBRC MATRIX I,C,2,c)

4. A patient presents to the emergency room with the following blood gas:
   pH   7.50
   $PaCO_2$ 29 mm Hg
   $[HCO_3]$ 22 mEq/L
   PaO_2 42 mm Hg

   The patient should be treated immediately with:
   A) mechanical ventilation.
   B) low flow oxygen.
   C) oxygen via mask.
   D) sedatives.
   E) respiratory stimulants.
   (CRT EXAM – NBRC MATRIX III,C,1)

5. A blood gas is drawn from a patient on a general floor.
   pH   7.16
   $PaCO_2$ 55 mm Hg
   $[HCO_3]$ 18 mEq/L
   PaO_2 42 mm Hg

   Based on the results, the patient appears to have:
   I. primary respiratory acidosis.
   II. primary metabolic acidosis.
   III. primary metabolic alkalosis.
   IV. tissue hypoxia.

   A) I and II only
   B) I and III only
   C) I, II, and IV
   D) II, III, and IV
   E) I, II, III, and IV
   (CRT EXAM – NBRC MATRIX I,C,1,c)

Technical Issues in Blood Gas Analysis

Chapter 3

Blood Gas Sampling Errors

In blood gas and pH analysis, an incorrect result can often be worse for the patient than no result at all.
National Committee for Clinical Laboratory Standards[1]

Outline

INTRODUCTION

Improper sampling technique or blood specimen handling may introduce marked error into the blood gas measurements.[10,72] Blood gas values are not particularly stable, and they may undergo significant alteration by apparently minor sampling flaws. The incidence of sampling error increases when inexperienced clinicians are responsible for obtaining the blood.[72,73] Given the vital nature of decisions depending on blood gas values, proper education with regard to potential sampling errors is essential. Blood gas sampling technique must be given careful attention.

BASIC PHYSICS OF GASES

Molecular Behavior

The basic principles of gas behavior are reviewed as a prerequisite to understanding potential blood sampling errors. Gases consist of minute molecules in rapid, continuous, random motion, which is sometimes referred to as *Brownian movement*. The *kinetic energy* (energy of motion) of these molecules will generate a force as the molecules collide with each other and bounce from one surface to another. The force per unit area generated by a gas is called *pressure*.

Pressure, in turn, can be measured by a device called a *manometer*. Water molecules may also be present in a gas phase and likewise generate pressure. The force per unit area generated by the water molecules in a gas is called *water vapor pressure*.

Air is a mixture of gases that usually includes water vapor. The air surrounding the earth is called the *atmosphere*. The total pressure exerted by all gases in the atmosphere is called *atmospheric pressure*. Atmospheric pressure at sea level is approximately 760 mm Hg; therefore, this pressure is often referred to as 1 *atmosphere*. The unit *torr* is synonymous with millimeters of mercury; therefore, these units may be used interchangeably.

Gravity tends to attract molecules to the center of the earth. Therefore, atmospheric pressure is higher than 760 mm Hg below sea level, whereas above sea level it is lower than 760 mm Hg. Atmospheric pressure can be measured by a specific type of manometer called a *barometer*.

Because air is a mixture of gases, many different types of gas molecules are present within it. Each individual gas in the mixture is likewise responsible for a portion of the total (i.e., atmospheric) pressure. The specific pressure exerted by a single gas is called its *partial pressure* (P) or tension. The specific gas that is being referred to is denoted by including its chemical formula. For example, the symbol for the partial pressure of carbon dioxide is PCO_2. The symbol for water vapor pressure is PH_2O.

Dalton's law states that the *sum* of the partial pressures in a mixture of gases is equal to the total pressure. Thus, atmospheric pressure is equal to the sum of all the partial pressures of gases that are present in the air.

Fractional Concentration

It is important to understand the distinction between partial pressure of a gas and fractional concentration of a gas. Fractional concentration of a gas in a dry gas phase (F) is the percentage of total gas molecules occupied by a particular gas *excluding* water vapor molecules. Fractional concentration is expressed as a decimal; for example, 21% O_2 is equivalent to an FO_2 of 0.21. In a container filled with only O_2 and water vapor, the fractional concentration of O_2 is 100% ($FO_2 = 1.0$),

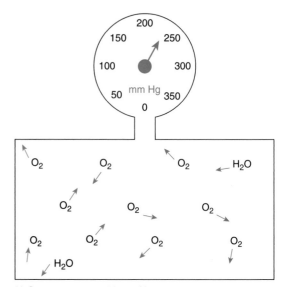

H$_2$O vapor pressure 40 mm Hg
Temperature 20° C

Figure 3-1. **Fractional concentration and partial pressure of a gas in a closed container.** The fractional concentration of O_2 in the dry gas phase is 100% ($FO_2 = 1.0$). The total pressure on the manometer is 240 mm Hg. The partial pressure of O_2 can be calculated:
(total pressure – water vapor pressure) × F = P
(240 – 40 mm Hg) × 1.0 = 200 mm Hg.

which is shown in Figure 3-1. The true concentration of O_2 would be less than 100% because some molecules in the container are H_2O rather than O_2; nevertheless, the percentage of O_2 in the *dry* gas phase (i.e., excluding PH_2O) is 100%.

Partial Pressure

The partial pressure of oxygen (PO_2) in Figure 3-1 could be determined by the application of Dalton's law; the sum of the partial pressures equals the total pressure. Because there are only two gases in the container, the sum of their partial pressures must be equal to 240 mm Hg. Because PH_2O is given as 40 mm Hg, the balance of pressure must be due to O_2. Thus, in this example, the PO_2 is 200 mm Hg. The formula used to calculate the partial pressure of a gas is (see Fig. 3-1):

(total pressure – water vapor pressure) × the fractional concentration of that gas.

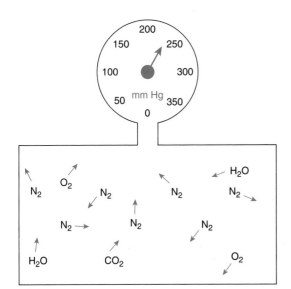

H$_2$O vapor pressure 40 mm Hg
Temperature 20° C

Figure 3-2. **Fractional concentration and partial pressure of a gas in a mixture of gases.** The total number of molecules in the container excluding water vapor is 10. Because two of the 10 non–water molecules are O$_2$, the FO$_2$ is 0.2. The PO$_2$ can be calculated:
(total pressure − water vapor pressure) × F = P
(240 − 40 mm Hg) × 0.2 = 40 mm Hg.

A similar container with an identical PH$_2$O and the same total pressure is shown in Figure 3-2. However, only two of the ten non–water molecules in this mixture of gases are O$_2$ molecules. Thus, the fractional concentration of oxygen (FO$_2$) in this mixture is 0.2 (20% O$_2$). The partial pressure of O$_2$ in this mixture of gases can be calculated by:

(total pressure − water vapor pressure) × 0.2.

Symbols

The symbol FIO$_2$ is used to refer to the percentage of *inspired oxygen*. It is customary to use capital letters as symbols to indicate gas measurements related to the *lung* or its function (e.g., I, inspired; E, expired; A, alveolar; T, tidal). Alveoli are the tiny air sacs within the lungs in which gas exchange with the blood takes place. Tidal refers to the movement of gas into and out of the lungs during normal (tidal) ventilation.

Lowercase symbols, on the other hand, are usually reserved for measurements made in the *blood* (e.g., a, arterial; v, venous; c, capillary). A bar (—) over the symbol is used to represent the mean or average. For example, P$\bar{v}$O$_2$ designates the average PO$_2$ in the veins. P$\bar{v}$O$_2$ can be measured in the pulmonary artery. In this blood vessel, all venous blood that has returned to the heart from throughout the body has been thoroughly mixed.

Composition of Atmospheric and Alveolar Air

The major gases present in dry atmospheric air with their respective partial pressures and percentages are shown in Table 3-1. It can be seen that the normal FIO$_2$ while breathing room air is 0.21 and that the normal PIO$_2$ is approximately 158 mm Hg. Partial pressures shown are based on a total atmospheric pressure of

Table 3-1. COMPOSITION OF AIR AT SEA LEVEL

Compound	Dry Air		Alveolar Air	
	Partial Pressure (mm Hg)	Percent	Partial Pressure (mm Hg)	Percent
Nitrogen	590.0	78.09	569	74.8
Oxygen	158.0	20.95	104	13.7
Carbon dioxide	0.2	0.03	40	5.3
Argon, neon, etc.	7.8	0.93	(<1)	(<0.1)
Water vapor	—	—	47	6.2
	760	100	760	100

From Ziment, I.: Respiratory Pharmacology and Therapeutics. Philadelphia, W. B. Saunders, 1978.

760 mm Hg present at sea level. For simplicity, Table 3-1 shows no water vapor pressure in the atmospheric air. In reality, the air that we breathe contains some water vapor pressure, and the normal partial pressure of inspired oxygen in *humidified* air is only approximately 148 mm Hg.

The partial pressures and percentages of these gases in alveolar air are also shown in Table 3-1. Two major processes are responsible for changing the quality of the air in the alveoli compared with inspired air: humidification and external respiration.

Humidification

The water vapor pressure actually present in air at any particular time is a function of the temperature and relative humidity. The warmer the air, the more humidity it is capable of holding. The relative humidity (RH) is a ratio of humidity actually present in the air (absolute humidity) compared with the maximum amount of humidity that air at that temperature could hold (i.e., potential humidity). Relative humidity is expressed as a percentage.

A relative humidity of 100% means that the air is holding the maximum amount of molecular water possible at that temperature (i.e., actual humidity = potential humidity). Air with a relative humidity of 100% is *saturated*. Table 3-2 shows the water vapor pressures that would be present in air that is saturated at various temperatures. The fact that warm air can hold more moisture than cold air is readily apparent.

Air that is completely saturated at body temperature (i.e., 37° C) has a PH_2O of 47 mm Hg. Fully saturated room air (i.e., 20° C), on the other hand, has a PH_2O of only 17 mm Hg. Obviously, if gas is not fully saturated at a particular temperature, water vapor pressure is less than that shown in Table 3-2. Air is heated to body temperature (37° C) and is completely humidified (100% RH) as it travels through the upper airway on its way to the lungs. Therefore, it is safe to assume that PH_2O in the alveoli is approximately 47 mm Hg. Thus, alveolar air has a higher water vapor pressure than atmospheric air. The total pressure in the alveolus is the same as atmospheric pressure.

Table 3-2. EFFECT OF TEMPERATURE ON WATER VAPOR PRESSURE (100% RELATIVE HUMIDITY)

Temperature (°C)	Vapor Pressure (mm Hg)	Temperature (°C)	Vapor Pressure (mm Hg)
0	4.6	39	52.0
5	6.5	40	54.9
10	9.1	41	57.9
14	11.9	42	61.0
16	13.5	43	64.3
18	15.3	44	67.8
20	17.4	46	75.1
22	19.6	48	83.2
24	22.2	50	92.0
26	25.0	55	117.5
28	28.1	60	148.9
30	31.5	65	187.1
31	33.4	70	233.3
32	35.3	75	288.8
33	37.4	80	354.9
34	39.5	85	433.2
35	41.8	90	525.5
36	44.2	95	633.7
37	46.6	100	760.0
38	49.3		

From Guyton, A. C.: Textbook of Medical Physiology, 9th ed. Philadelphia, W. B. Saunders, 1996.

Thus, the partial pressures of other gases must decrease as a result of the increased PH_2O.

External Respiration

External respiration is the exchange of O_2 and CO_2 between the alveoli and the blood. Oxygen, of course, diffuses from the alveoli into the blood, whereas CO_2 is diffusing from the blood into the alveoli. Therefore, it is not surprising that alveolar PO_2 is lower than atmospheric PO_2 because of the loss of O_2 from the alveolus to the blood. Likewise, one would expect that alveolar PCO_2 would be higher than atmospheric PCO_2 owing to the influx of CO_2 into the alveolus. Table 3-1 simply confirms this exchange.

Finally, it should be noted that alveolar PN_2 and the partial pressure of trace gases are lower in the alveoli. These changes, however, are passive results owing to external respiration and humidification.

Body Temperature and Pressure Saturated

Clinical measurements of gases are made under standardized conditions for comparison of values and reproducibility of results. Blood gases are measured at body temperature and pressure saturated (BTPS). The BTPS notation refers to normal standardized conditions within the body (i.e., temperature 37° C, ambient pressure, and PH_2O of 47 mm Hg).

Temperature, Pressure, and Volume

An introduction or review of gas behavior would be incomplete without some mention of the basic gas laws; in particular, the laws that describe the interdependent relationships between volume, pressure, and temperature are briefly described.

Gay-Lussac's law states that if volume and mass remain fixed, the pressure exerted by a gas varies directly with the absolute temperature of the gas.[74] Absolute temperature is measured in

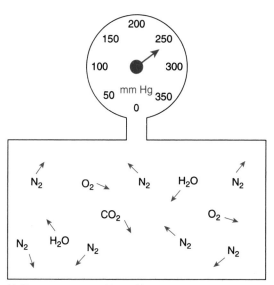

H₂O vapor pressure 40 mm Hg
Temperature 38° C

Figure 3-3. **Effects of increasing temperature of gas in a closed container.** If the temperature of a closed container is increased, the speed and energy of the enclosed molecules will also increase and will thus raise the pressure. The concentration of the molecules remains constant while partial pressure increases.

Kelvin degrees and 0° Celsius is equivalent to 273° Kelvin (K). The total pressure in Figure 3-2 is 240 mm Hg, and the gas is at a temperature of 20° C (293° K). If the temperature of the gas increased to 38° C (311° K), which is shown in Figure 3-3, Brownian movement and kinetic energy of the gas would increase and the total pressure within the container would increase. As show in Figure 3-3, the new pressure is 255 mm Hg.

Similarly, the partial pressures of other gases within the container also increase. Partial pressure must be distinguished from fractional concentration, which would not change. The partial pressure of O_2 in Figure 3-3 can be calculated as described earlier:

$$PO_2 = (\text{total pressure} - PH_2O) \times \text{fractional concentration}$$

$$PO_2 = (255 \text{ mm Hg} - 40 \text{ mm Hg}) \times 0.2$$

$$PO_2 = 43 \text{ mm Hg}$$

The gas laws pertaining to changes in volume are less important with regard to blood gases but are included here for completeness. *Boyle's law* states that if absolute temperature and mass remain unchanged, volume varies inversely with pressure. Similarly, *Charles' law* states that if pressure and mass are unchanged, volume varies directly with changes in absolute temperature.

Gases in Liquids

Gases dissolve freely in liquids. The particular gas may or may not react chemically with the liquid, depending on the chemical nature of each substance. Nevertheless, all gases remain in a free gaseous phase to some extent within the liquid. The dissolution of gases in liquids is a physical, not a chemical, process. Gases within liquids exert pressure in much the same manner as described in pure gaseous environments.

Henry's law states that when a gas is exposed to a liquid, the partial pressure of the gas in the liquid phase equilibrates with the partial pressure of the gas in the gaseous phase. Thus, if O_2 in the air is exposed to blood or water, there is an exchange of O_2 molecules between the liquid and gaseous phases until the respective partial pressures are equal. The progressive equilibration of the partial pressure of O_2

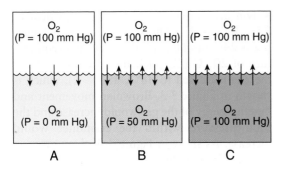

Figure 3-4. **Equilibration of partial pressures between liquid and gas phases.** Solution of oxygen in water. **A,** When the oxygen first comes into contact with pure water. **B,** After the dissolved oxygen is half way to equilibrium with the gaseous oxygen. **C,** After equilibrium has been established.

between the gaseous and the liquid phases is shown in Figure 3-4.

Change in Altitude

The barometric pressure is lower as altitude increases. Air at a high altitude still has a 21% O_2 concentration; however, the partial pressure of O_2 is much lower. The effect of high altitude on barometric pressure and PO_2 is shown in Table 3-3.

At the summit of Mount Everest, which has the highest altitude on earth, the PO_2 is approximately 42 mm Hg.[75] Again, the FIO_2 remains at 0.21 but the PO_2 decreases tremendously. Thus, the normal PaO_2 at a high altitude (e.g., Denver) is obviously much lower than the normal PaO_2 at sea level.

Table 3-3. EFFECTS OF HIGH ALTITUDE ON BAROMETRIC PRESSURE PO_2

Altitude (ft)	Barometric Pressure (mm Hg)	PO_2 in Air (mm Hg)
0	760	159
10,000	523	110
20,000	349	73
30,000	226	47
40,000	141	29
50,000	87	18

From Guyton, A. C.: Basic Human Physiology, Normal Function and Mechanisms of Disease, 2nd ed. Philadelphia, W. B. Saunders, 1977.

Box 3-1	Potential Sampling Errors

Air in the blood sample
Venous sampling or admixture
Excessive or improper anticoagulant
Rate of metabolism
Temperature disparities between patient
  and machine

POTENTIAL SAMPLING ERRORS

Five common types of arterial blood sampling error are discussed: air in the blood sample, inadvertent venous sampling or admixture, anticoagulant effects, changes due to metabolism, and alterations in temperature (Box 3-1). The significance of each type of error and also the mechanism of these changes are explored.

Proper labeling of the sample is also paramount. If the specimen is to be submerged in water or ice, the label must remain legible. Incorrect matching of laboratory results with the patient is unacceptable.

Air in the Blood Sample
Effects of Air Contamination

Clinical studies have shown that the major effect of an air bubble in a blood gas sample is a change in PaO_2.[76-79] According to Henry's law, when a blood specimen with a PaO_2 of less than 158 mm Hg is interfaced with an air bubble, the PaO_2 of the blood sample spuriously increases. This action occurs because the partial pressure of O_2 in the air at sea level is approximately 158 mm Hg. The magnitude of the increase depends partly on the duration of exposure, whereas the volume of the air bubble, although important, seems to make less difference.[77] Other factors that may determine the ultimate effect of air contamination include the temperature of the sample and the degree of agitation (Fig. 3-5).

Furthermore, the change is greatest when the patient's actual PaO_2 exceeds 100 mm Hg.[79] This change can be explained by the chemical relationship between O_2 and hemoglobin that is discussed in Chapter 7 under the oxyhemoglobin dissociation curve.

In certain clinical situations (e.g., in the operating room where high concentrations of inspired O_2 are often used), the initial PaO_2 of

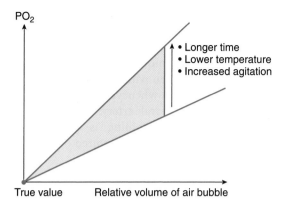

PO$_2$

• Longer time
• Lower temperature
• Increased agitation

True value   Relative volume of air bubble

Figure 3-5. **Effect of air contamination on PaO$_2$.** Air bubbles may seriously influence PO$_2$, even when very small (1% of sample volume). The effect depends on many factors, e.g., size of air bubble relative to sample volume, initial oxygen status of sample, and storage conditions (time, temperature, agitation).

the blood sample may exceed 158 mm Hg. In this event, O$_2$ tends to migrate from the blood phase to the bubble and results in measurement of an erroneously low PaO$_2$ in the blood sample being analyzed.[76]

As shown in Table 3-1, the PCO$_2$ in room air is essentially zero. Thus, one would expect blood PCO$_2$ levels to decrease if blood were exposed to an air bubble. This effect does occur, but is less marked than the change in PO$_2$. The different blood solubility coefficients of O$_2$ and CO$_2$ probably explain the disparity in response. Finally, the pH increases when arterial blood is exposed to an air bubble as a direct consequence of the decrease in PaCO$_2$.

Clinical Guidelines

Mixing or agitating a sample contaminated with an air bubble tends to escalate the error (see Fig. 3-5). Also, because the duration of exposure to an air bubble is a factor in the degree of error, all air bubbles should be expelled *immediately*. Results are reasonably stable when blood samples are not prematurely mixed and when foreign air bubbles are expelled within 2 minutes.[77]

When froth is observed in a blood gas sample, the likelihood of significant error is great. Froth represents many minute air bubbles

with great surface area exposed to blood. Furthermore, froth is essentially impossible to expel. *All samples with visually apparent froth should be discarded.*

Finally, serious error is likely if air is allowed to remain in the sample or is introduced into the blood gas machine when the actual measurements are being made. Electrodes used in blood gas machines register incorrect results when they are in contact with an air bubble.

Summary

The presence of air in an arterial blood gas sample is unacceptable and may introduce notable error. The PaO$_2$ tends to migrate toward 158 mm Hg; PaCO$_2$ tends to fall, and pH may increase if the decrease in PCO$_2$ is substantial. The most important change is the alteration in PaO$_2$, which is particularly marked when initial PaO$_2$ is greater than 100 mm Hg. This can be explained by the oxyhemoglobin dissociation curve, which is explained in Chapter 7.

The expulsion of air bubbles within 2 minutes and the delay in mixing the sample until air bubbles have been expelled helps to prevent contamination of the sample from the air. The clinician must also take care not to introduce air into the blood gas machine. Thus, every effort must be made to ensure the acquisition of the sample under *anaerobic* (i.e., in the absence of free O$_2$) conditions.

New blood gas syringes have been designed which have special vent mechanisms. These vents allow the syringe to be filled to a preselected volume while air is pushed out and the vent is closed.[1] Use of these syringes precludes air contamination of the sample.

When laboratory samples are unacceptable, this should always be documented in the laboratory along with the reason. In addition, corrective measures to ensure this error will not be repeated should also be noted. This is true for all sample errors or inaccurate readings.

Venous Sampling or Admixture
Venous Samples

Inadvertent venous puncture is a potential source of error in blood gas sampling, particularly in the hypotensive (low blood pressure) patient and when femoral artery puncture is attempted. As discussed previously, failure to observe the characteristics of an arterial sample (i.e., a flash of blood on entry into the vessel, pulsations during syringe filling, and auto-filling of the syringe) should arouse suspicion of this type of error. Peripheral venous blood has little value in oxygenation assessment. Furthermore, therapeutic decisions based on venous blood that is assumed to be arterial may be grossly inappropriate.

Venous Admixture

A less recognized, albeit important, technical error is contamination of the arterial sample with a small amount of venous or capillary blood during an attempt at arterial puncture. Entry into a vein may occur easily during an attempt to puncture the femoral artery because the large femoral vein lies close and posterior to the artery. Overshooting any artery with subsequent withdrawal may result in the entry of some venous blood into the syringe. Moreover, femoral venous anomalies, in which the vein may lie anterior to the artery, are fairly common and predispose to this type of error.

The addition of one-tenth part of venous blood to an arterial sample could produce as much as a 25% decrease in measured PaO_2.[80] For example, mixture of 0.5 mL of venous blood having a PO_2 of 31 mm Hg (not unusual for a skeletal muscle vein[81]) with 4.5 mL of arterial blood having a PO_2 of 86 mm Hg would lead to a mixture having a PO_2 of 56 mm Hg (Table 3-4).[80] Certainly, the clinical treatment of a patient with a PaO_2 of 56 mm Hg is considerably different from that of a patient with a PaO_2 of 86 mm Hg.

Precautions

Some precautions could decrease the likelihood of venous sampling or contamination.

Table 3-4.   VENOUS CONTAMINATION OF AN ARTERIAL SAMPLE

Blood	Volume (mL)	PO₂ (mm Hg)
Arterial	4.5	86
Venous	0.5	31
Mixed	5.0	56

From Doty, D. B., and Moseley, R. V.: Reliable sampling of arterial blood. Surg. Gynecol. Obstet., 130:701, 1970.

The use of short-beveled needles minimizes the surface area available for aspiration and thus decreases the potential for venous admixture. The puncture technique of overshooting the blood vessel and then withdrawing the syringe should be avoided whenever possible. Most important, the femoral artery, where venous contamination or sampling is particularly likely to occur, should be punctured only when absolutely necessary.

Recognition of Venous Error

Venous contamination error should be suspected whenever the patient's clinical status and picture is remarkably better than the blood gas data suggest. The patient with serious acid-base or oxygenation impairment is rarely asymptomatic. When the laboratory data are not congruent with the patient's appearance, it is most likely that the laboratory data are incorrect.

Occasionally, there is some question with regard to whether a particular blood sample is arterial or venous in origin. Although hypoxemia (low PO_2) and hypercarbia (high blood PCO_2) suggest that the sample is venous, one cannot be certain of this on the basis of blood gas numbers alone. It is not uncommon to find arterial hypoxemia and hypercarbia in critically ill patients.

The technology of pulse oximetry is discussed in Chapter 15. Pulse oximetry is a noninvasive technology used to monitor O_2 saturation of arterial blood. When pulse oximetry is being used, it may serve as a crosscheck of saturation measured via arterial blood gases. For example, a saturation of 90% via pulse oximetry and a blood gas saturation of 78% strongly suggest that the blood gas sample may not be arterial. This crosscheck may be useful when the origin of blood gases (i.e., arterial versus venous) is in doubt.

Mixed versus Peripheral Venous Blood

Mixed venous blood from the pulmonary artery typically approximates the blood gas values shown in Table 3-5. A sample of mixed venous blood may be taken only from a catheter in the patient's pulmonary artery. The values shown in Table 3-5 are normal for *mixed* venous blood, which is an average of all venous blood returning to the heart. Occasionally, some

Table 3-5.   NORMAL MIXED VENOUS GASES

Parameters	Values
pH	7.38
$P\bar{v}CO_2$	48 mm Hg
$P\bar{v}O_2$	40 mm Hg
$S\bar{v}O_2$	75%

healthcare personnel presume that *all* venous blood has these same values—this assumption is incorrect.

Peripheral venous blood from different organs and tissues has different PvO_2 values depending on various factors, including local metabolism, perfusion, and tissue function. For example, the PO_2 of venous blood exiting skeletal muscles may be near 34 mm Hg, whereas the PO_2 of blood leaving the skin is approximately 60 mm Hg.[81] Because venous blood inadvertently sampled while attempting an arterial puncture is peripheral venous blood, it is impossible to predict exactly how the blood gas values will change. Lower PO_2 values and higher PCO_2 values should be expected. However, a sample cannot be judged to be venous solely because the values nearly approximate normal mixed venous values.

Verification

One method that has been suggested to determine whether a sample is arterial or venous is to repeat the sample while simultaneously drawing a known venous sample from the same anatomic area for comparison. The discomfort, expense, and potential for complication appear to make this a poor option. Alternatively, a carefully acquired new sample taken by an experienced therapist or clinician usually provides a satisfactory answer to the question of sample accuracy. If repeated samples become necessary, perhaps an arterial line is indicated to ensure that all samples are arterial.

Anticoagulant Effects

Anticoagulation of the blood gas sample is essential to prevent clotting of the specimen. Nevertheless, introduction of an anticoagulant to the sample may in itself cause a technical error. The type, concentration, and volume of

ON CALL | CASE 3-1 *ABGs and Critical Thinking*

You are the only person available to care for this patient. You must assess the patient/situation and act accordingly.
A 52-year-old man is treated in the emergency department for suspected pneumonia. An arterial blood gas sample is drawn on room air. The sample appears a little frothy and is bright red.

ARTERIAL BLOOD GASES

pH	7.50
$PaCO_2$	29 mm Hg
PaO_2	153 mm Hg
$[HCO_3]$	22 mEq/L

ASSESSMENT

Abnormalities: List abnormal data and other noteworthy information.

anticoagulant must be carefully controlled. Most new blood gas kits come with syringes that have been pre-filled with the appropriate type and amount of anticoagulant.

Nature of Anticoagulant

Lithium heparin is the current recommended anticoagulant for blood gas and/or electrolyte sampling.[1] Sodium heparin (1000 U/mL) is still sometimes used, although it has a slightly higher potential to cause the formation of very small fibrils in the sample and will likely increase [Na] by approximately 3 mEq/L if Na is also being measured.[82,241] Heparin, however, is expensive, and the supply fluctuates in some parts of the world. Therefore, the use of alternative anticoagulants has been explored.[72] Most other anticoagulants are unsuitable for blood gas samples; however, Heller-Paul oxalate and citrate have been identified as being potential substitutes that may be cheaper and acceptable.[72] Further studies are necessary before these agents can be recommended for routine use.

The concentration of sodium heparin recommended is 1000 U/mL. The pH of this solution closely approximates the normal pH of arterial blood. Stronger concentrations of heparin and other anticoagulants have pH values that differ

Table 3-6. pH OF ANTICOAGULANT
SOLUTIONS

Anticoagulant	pH
Citrate	7.65
Heparin (1000 U/mL)	7.33
Heparin (5000 U/mL)	7.10
Oxalate	6.94
Heparin (25,000 U/mL)	6.53
EDTA	4.73

Adapted from Goodwin, N. M., and Schreiber, M. T.:
Effects of anticoagulants on acid-base and blood gas
estimations. Crit. Care Med., 7:473, 1979.

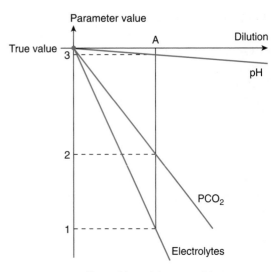

Figure 3-6. **Effect of liquid heparin dilution on blood gases and electrolytes.** Diluting the blood sample (to point *A*) may significantly decrease electrolyte values (*1*) and pCO_2 values (*2*). There is almost no change in pH values (*3*).

significantly from arterial blood and are more likely to contaminate blood pH (Table 3-6) and electrolyte readings.

Dilution Error

The normal technique for manually heparinizing a syringe has been described previously. The clinician must be careful not to add unnecessary heparin volume because it may substantially alter blood gas results. Inexperienced clinicians sometimes add extra heparin in stress situations to ensure anticoagulation.[72] This error can be avoided through proper education and training.

Blood Gas Change with Excessive Dilution

Liquid heparin is essentially a weak acid equilibrated with room air. Therefore, the effects of heparin on an arterial blood sample are very similar to those that would occur if the sample were exposed to an air bubble. Unlike air contamination, however, the major blood gas error associated with excessive heparin in the sample is a drop in the $PaCO_2$ (Fig. 3-6). Apparently, $PaCO_2$ is affected more than PaO_2 because of the different solubility coefficients of the two gases in the liquid phase. As shown in Figure 3-6, electrolyte measurements are also significantly altered when simple sodium heparin is used.

A decrease in $PaCO_2$, in turn, tends to increase pH. Surprisingly, however, the actual pH may slightly fall (see Fig. 3-6), presumably because the low CO_2 effect is offset by the low pH and bicarbonate concentration of the heparin solution.[28,72,73,83] When dilution is

extreme, the pH, bicarbonate, and base excess concentrations may fall more appreciably.[84] The PaO_2 is usually relatively unchanged in response to heparin dilution. If the initial PaO_2 is very high, however, heparin dilution may result in a notable decrease.[85]

Clinical Significance

In some cases, even normal syringe heparinization technique has been purported to significantly lower $PaCO_2$ and bicarbonate values.[28,86] Similarly, hematocrit and hemoglobin values measured from heparinized arterial samples have been falsely low owing to the dilution effect.[72] Dilution correction factors are available to correct for these errors.

New syringe designs with minimal deadspace and the use of dry (lyophilized) crystalline heparin have increased accuracy and virtually eliminated the need for concern regarding sample dilution.[85,86,241] The concern that dried heparin may increase technical error through an air bubble effect does not appear to be justified.[85] The only blood gas concern with dry heparin is that it may not dissolve adequately or quickly which may, in turn, lead to clot formation.[241]

In laboratories still using standard 5-mL or 10-mL syringes, the sample volumes for adults should always exceed 2 mL.[16] For additional accuracy, correction factors are available for PCO_2 and bicarbonate level.[5] As a general rule, each 1% dilution results in a 1% decline in PCO_2. The primary concern in the clinical setting is the use of a standard technique that allows for an accurate comparison of serial measurements.[83]

Neonatal Considerations

Neonatal blood gas samples are often drawn into 1-mL tuberculin syringes. Thus, they are particularly vulnerable to the dilution effects of heparin because of the small sample volume. Whereas an adult's sample may be diluted only 6%, a neonatal sample may be diluted up to 40%.[72] Although the blood gas machine may be capable of providing results with a mere 0.2-mL neonatal sample,[83] this volume may not be sufficiently large to preclude significant heparin dilution.

Error in arterial PCO_2 may be 14% to 15% if a 0.2-mL blood sample is introduced into a 1-mL tuberculin syringe with deadspace heparin.[83] Therefore, neonatal sample volumes should exceed 0.6 mL to minimize dilution effects. Notwithstanding, larger samples should be avoided in neonates because blood volume depletion and anemia may occur with repeated sampling.[87]

Metabolism

Qualitative Effects of Metabolism

Metabolism continues within blood cells in the syringe after the blood has been drawn from the patient. These metabolic processes consume O_2, produce CO_2, and thus tend to alter blood gas values. Likewise, the accumulation of CO_2 in the sample lowers pH. The speed and magnitude of these changes depend, in large part, on the temperature of the sample. Generally, the extent of blood gas alterations due to metabolism is proportional directly to the temperature of the sample.

Quantitative Effects of Metabolism

Table 3-7 shows the magnitude of blood gas changes that would occur if a sample were maintained at 37° C (body temperature). In 1 hour, arterial PCO_2 would increase by approximately 5 mm Hg and pH would decrease

Table 3-7. Effects of Metabolism on Blood Gases at 37° C

Measurement	Direction	Magnitude/Hr
pH	Decrease	0.05
$PaCO_2$	Increase	5 mm Hg
PaO_2	Decrease	150 mm Hg[*]
		20 mm Hg[†]

[*]Initial PaO_2 >250 mm Hg.
[†]Initial PaO_2 <150 mm Hg.

approximately 0.05 units.[10,88] The magnitude of the drop in arterial PO_2 would depend mainly on the initial PO_2 level.

Very high initial PO_2 values (e.g., PaO_2 > 300 mm Hg) tend to decrease precipitously, perhaps by as much as 150 mm Hg per hour. Conversely, lower initial PaO_2 values (e.g., 100 mm Hg) tend to decrease only approximately 20 mm Hg per hour. Furthermore, PaO_2 values less than 60 mm Hg fall much less than this. The large discrepancy between initial high and low PaO_2 groups can be explained by the oxyhemoglobin dissociation curve and O_2 transport (see Chapter 7).

At room temperature (20° to 24° C), metabolism is slowed to approximately 50% of levels at 37° C.[88] Thus, the changes quantified in Table 3-7 may take 2 hours instead of 1 hour to occur. Placing the sample in iced water (almost at 4° C) slows metabolism to approximately 10% of levels at 37° C.[88] Thus, in iced samples, the quantitative changes indicated in Table 3-7 may take up to 10 hours. Placing blood gas samples in refrigerators is not an adequate substitute for placing samples in ice, and this practice should be avoided.[77]

Plastic versus Glass Syringes and Icing

It has long been known that blood gases (i.e., oxygen, carbon dioxide) could diffuse more readily (thereby tending to equilibrate with ambient gases) through plastic syringes than glass syringes. Notwithstanding, however, this increased permeability through plastic syringes has been thought to be clinically insignificant. Therefore, with the advent of plastic syringes that filled freely without friction, and with increased attention to cost containment, it is common to use plastic syringes for blood gas acquisition.

Surprisingly, it has been found that PaO_2 and $PaCO_2$ in *iced samples within plastic syringes* may actually change over time in opposite directions to what would be expected by metabolism.[34] In other words, PaO_2 increased and $PaCO_2$ decreased in iced samples within plastic syringes. This can only be explained by the increase in solubility coefficients caused by cooling within the sample. The change in solubility tends to lower partial pressures within the blood and enhances diffusion of ambient gases through the plastic syringe with the sample.

When blood is cooled to 4° C, the solubility of oxygen in blood nearly doubles.[34] In addition, the oxyhemoglobin curve is shifted to the left and increased dissolved oxygen is combined with hemoglobin. These two factors result in a decreased PaO_2 within the iced blood sample. The increased diffusion gradient between ambient air ($PO_2 \sim 155$ mm Hg) and the sample allows additional oxygen to diffuse from the ambient gas to within the plastic syringe.

Subsequently, when the blood is re-warmed within the blood gas machine, oxygen is released from within the blood to the gaseous phase. The oxygen is released from hemoglobin due to the right shift of the oxyhemoglobin curve and is also released into physical solution due to the decreased solubility coefficient at the higher temperature. In summary, the ambient oxygen that had diffused into the sample due to cooling now results in a falsely *elevated* PaO_2.

Surprisingly, *blood gases drawn in plastic syringes remain more stable within the first 30 minutes at room temperature as compared to iced samples.*[34] Therefore, *if plastic syringes are used and samples will be run within 30 minutes, they need not be iced.*

On the contrary, samples that are not likely to be run within 30 minutes or known to have increased oxygen consumption (e.g., leukocytosis or thrombocytosis), *should be iced immediately and a glass syringe should be used for sampling.* This same procedure should be used when high PaO_2s are expected (as in the operating room) or when determining the $P(A\text{-}a)O_2$ gradient.

Clinical Guidelines

In clinical practice, all *room temperature* blood gas samples should be analyzed within 30 minutes to avoid the introduction of significant error.[1,34,77,79] Iced samples remain generally stable for 2 hours or more if the initial PaO_2 is less than 150 mm Hg.[14,34,65] Arterial PCO_2 and pH are especially stable in iced samples. Error in these measurements is minimal even 2 to 4 hours after the time when the sample is placed in ice.[77–79,88] The decrease in PaO_2 in the iced sample, however, may be substantial after only 30 minutes when the initial PaO_2 is high.[79] The change factors shown in Table 3-7 may also be used to approximate blood gas values if the sample cannot be iced or analyzed within 30 minutes.[88]

Leukocyte Larceny

The metabolic activity responsible for blood gas changes occurs predominantly in *leukocytes* (white blood cells), *platelets*, and *reticulocytes* (immature red blood cells).[34,75] Normal, mature *erythrocytes* (red blood cells) are not responsible for significant metabolism and blood gas change because 90% of their metabolism is anaerobic. Immature leukocytes, when present, consume even more O_2 than that noted for normal leukocytes.[89] The effect of reticulocytes on oxygen depletion is usually slight due to their small concentration.

The term *leukocyte larceny* was coined by Fox to describe the rapid decrease in PaO_2 that was observed in blood samples with high leukocyte counts (leukocytosis).[89] In one case, a patient with leukemia and a leukocyte count of 276,000 cells/mm[3] blood (normal leukocyte count is 6000 to 10,000 cells/mm[3]) showed a decline in PaO_2 from 130 to 58 mm Hg in 2 minutes.[89] The phenomenon of leukocyte larceny was unveiled after several patients with leukemia presented with unexplained hypoxemia. The term *pseudohypoxemia* has also been used to describe the spuriously decreased PaO_2.[100]

In an extraordinary case, a 57-year-old man with leukemia and a leukocyte count of 450,000 cells/mm[3] had a PaO_2 of 0 in four repeated blood samples from an arterial line.[90] Apparently, all the O_2 in the blood sample was consumed by the rapid metabolism of the numerous immature leukocytes. Much of this

ON CALL | CASE 3-2 *ABGs and Critical Thinking*

You are the only person available to care for this patient. You must assess the patient/situation and act accordingly.

An arterial puncture is drawn on a 44-year-old woman who is notably cyanotic and diaphoretic. She is on a nasal cannula at 2 L/min. An experienced technician noted that he observed a flash of blood upon entry into the artery and the syringe auto-filled. The results of the blood gas and vital signs are shown.

VITAL SIGNS

B/P	145/96 mm Hg
RR	30/min
HR	116/min
Temp	39° C
S_pO_2	77%

ARTERIAL BLOOD GASES

SaO_2	75%
pH	7.53
$PaCO_2$	28 mm Hg
PaO_2	40 mm Hg
$[HCO_3]$	26 mEq/L

A physician is notified of the blood gas results by telephone. After reviewing the results, the physician responds "These must be venous gases…normal venous PO_2 is 40 mm Hg." What is your response?

ASSESSMENT

Abnormalities: List abnormal data and other noteworthy information.

---

consumption of O_2 undoubtedly occurred after the blood sample left the patient's body; however, the actual PaO_2 in the patient's blood may also have been very low.

The quantitative blood gas changes secondary to metabolism shown in Table 3-7 are based on normal blood conditions and cell counts. In severe leukocytosis (e.g., leukemia) or thrombocytosis, blood gas values change much more quickly.[89,91] Therefore, samples from patients with these disorders should be drawn in glass syringes, then iced and analyzed immediately.

Alterations in Temperature

As stated previously, blood gas values should be measured under standardized BTPS conditions because they are affected by temperature changes. To ensure that blood gas values are actually measured at 37° C, blood samples are warmed through a water bath or similar mechanism that is integral to the analyzer. Obviously, failure to heat the sample to precisely 37° C leads to incorrect results.

Quantitative Effects of Alterations in Temperature

The direct physical relationship between temperature and pressure results in higher arterial PO_2 and PCO_2 readings at higher temperatures (Fig. 3-7). Although normal adult arterial PO_2 is approximately 100 mm Hg

at 37° C, this reading would almost double at 47° C.[92] A more modest increase in temperature from 37° to 39° C would increase arterial PO_2 less markedly, from 100 to 110 mm Hg.[93]

An increase in temperature would similarly increase arterial PCO_2 values. Arterial blood

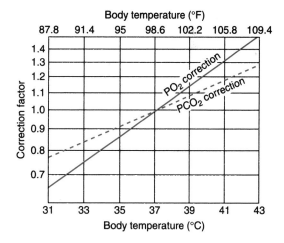

Figure 3-7. **Blood gas temperature correction nomogram.** Nomogram for correction of PO_2 and PCO_2 from temperature of blood gas analyzer (37° C) to patient's body temperature. Read PO_2 or PCO_2 correction factor at patient's body temperature and multiply by measured PO_2 or PCO_2. (Correction for PO_2 from Severinghaus; for PCO_2 from Kelam and Nunn.)

Table 3-8. EFFECTS OF TEMPERATURE ON
NORMAL BLOOD GASES

Temperature (°C)	PO_2	PCO_2	pH
37	80	40	7.40
39	90	44	7.37
30	54	30	7.50

From Walton, J. R., and Shapiro, B. A.: Value and
application of temperature compensated blood gas data
(Response to question). Respir. Care, 25:260, 1980.

with normal PCO_2 (40 mm Hg) at 37° C would
show a PCO_2 level of 62 mm Hg at 47° C.[92]
A slight rise in temperature from 37° to 39° C
would increase PCO_2 from 40 to 44 mm Hg.[93]
Arterial PCO_2 increases approximately 5% per
degree Celsius rise.[88] An increase in arterial
PCO_2 also leads to a decrease in pH. The
pH generally decreases 0.03 unit for every 2° C
increase in temperature.[88]

Just as an increase in temperature leads
to higher gas partial pressures, a decrease in
temperature lowers gas pressure readings.
An arterial PO_2 of 100 mm Hg at 37° C would
be 50 mm Hg at 27° C.[94] A clinically acceptable arterial PO_2 of 60 mm Hg at 37° C would
read 37 mm Hg at 30° C.[94] Similarly, the partial pressure of CO_2 decreases from 40 mm Hg
at 37° C to 30 mm Hg at 30° C, and the pH
simultaneously increases from 7.40 to 7.50.[93,95]

The effects of both cooling and warming on
normal blood gas values are compared in
Table 3-8.

Correction of Temperature of Blood Gases

Figure 3-7 can be used to approximate measured PO_2 and PCO_2 for the patient's temperature, and another nomogram is available to
correct for pH[90]; however, their use is controversial.[88,93–96] NCCLS advocates the use of
specific formulas (see reference 241) if blood
gases are to be temperature corrected. In addition, if temperature-adjusted values are
reported, BTPS values must be simultaneously
reported to allow the clinician to make knowledgeable clinical decisions.[241]

*The problem with temperature corrected
values is that **normal** blood gases at these
various temperatures are unknown.* The
nomogram in Figure 3-4 corrects for only the

physical relationship between temperature and
pressure. They fail to account for the metabolic
and cardiovascular changes that accompany a
change in a patient's temperature.[93] For example, an increase in body temperature of 1° C
increases the O_2 requirements by 10%.[2] What
PaO_2 value is required to meet this demand?

Thus, although one can correct blood gas
values for the direct physical effects of temperature on partial pressure very easily, the ***target
blood gas values*** for therapy are unclear.

Notwithstanding the aforementioned, many
laboratories continue to report temperature-
corrected values,[95] most likely because many
automated blood gas machines can readily
make these corrections. In my opinion, this
exercise does not provide us with more meaningful information on which to base treatment
decisions. For example, the corrected data may
lead to a false sense of security in the febrile
patient if the PaO_2 is in the acceptable range
of 80 to 100 mm Hg because of the higher
temperature.[96]

In conclusion, temperature correction of
blood gas data for clinical application is not
currently recommended.[93,95,97–99] The correction of temperature may be important in
research or academic exercises, but it is probably not useful in clinical application of blood
gases. Blood gases should be interpreted at
37° C—a temperature at which there is a sense
of normalcy and appropriateness.[93–97,99] It is
especially important that if temperature-
adjusted results are reported, the report should
be clearly labeled as such, and results at BTPS
should also be reported.[65,241]

Machine Temperature Error

The blood gas machine must also be monitored carefully to ensure that blood is actually
being warmed to 37° C. The absence of temperature control can lead to grossly inaccurate
reports (see Fig. 3-7). Older machines used
water baths to heat samples to BTPS. In these
cases, the water bath temperature needed to be
frequently monitored. Newer machines use different techniques. Regardless of the technique,
the temperature should be maintained within
±0.1° of 37° C.[241] The manufacturer's literature should be reviewed to understand limitations with each machine.

Table 3-9. Summary Preanalytical Errors Nuts and Bolts

Sampling Error	Effect	Clinical Implications
Air in syringe or icing plastic syringes	↑ PaO_2	* expel air bubbles immediately
	↓ $PaCO_2$	* do not agitate syringe
	↑ pH	* discard samples with froth
Venous sample or contamination	↓ PaO_2	* avoid femoral artery
	↑ $PaCO_2$	* use short-beveled needle
	↓ pH	* watch for flash and auto-filling
Anticoagulant type or concentration	↑ PaO_2	* use 1/1000 U/mL
	↓ $PaCO_2$	* lithium heparin best
	↑↓ pH	* minimize amount liquid heparin
Metabolic effects	↓ PaO_2	* ice samples not run in 30 min
	↑ $PaCO_2$	* use glass syringe if concerned
	↓ pH	* run samples as soon as possible

References: 14, 15, and 65. (See list at end of text.)

Summary of Sampling Errors

Table 3-9 provides a summary of the effects of blood gas preanalytical error on sample results. Key clinical considerations are likewise noted for each of the types of sampling errors.

MEASUREMENT OF BLOOD GASES AND ELECTROLYTES FROM A SINGLE SAMPLE

It is becoming increasingly popular to measure both blood gases and electrolytes from a single sample of arterial blood. This makes good sense from the standpoint of blood conservation, timeliness, and diagnostic value. Many blood gas machines now provide the ability to measure routine blood gas parameters, electrolytes (i.e., sodium, potassium, chloride, and ionized calcium), and other blood values (i.e., glucose, hematocrit, hemoglobin, lactate) from a single sample. Thus, when blood gas samples are obtained, potential technical errors associated with the measurement of these other analytes must also be understood.

There are several potential errors that may occur if routinely handled blood gas samples are also used to measure electrolytes. In general, these errors are most often due to anticoagulants or transporting/icing the sample.

Anticoagulant Errors

The use of simple liquid sodium or liquid lithium heparin as an anticoagulant will lower electrolyte values (see Fig. 3-6) especially ionized calcium.[1] Liquid anticoagulants reduce ionized calcium in three ways: solution dilution, calcium binding, and calcium distortion.[102] The higher the concentration of the heparin, the more calcium binding will occur.[241] Dry (lyophilized) heparin does not dilute the blood significantly but requires sufficient time and mixing for dissolution and proper anticoagulation.[103,241]

The electrolyte measurement problems associated with liquid anticoagulants have been minimized by the use of *dry balanced heparin*.[1] Balanced heparin is a preparation that includes physiologic amounts of calcium and other electrolytes to mitigate electrolyte error; however, it does not completely eliminate calcium distortion.[102] Even when using dry balanced heparin with 50 IU heparin pledgets, sample volume should still exceed 0.6 mL and the syringe should be at least half-filled to avoid potential dilution errors.[153–154] Other forms of commercially available heparin include calcium-titrated or low sodium-titrated heparin.

Other non-heparin anticoagulants have also been evaluated for use in this regard such as the selective thrombin inhibitor, D-phenylalanyl-L-prolyl-L-arginine chloromethyl ketone, also known as PPACK.[101] PPACK has been shown to be an ideal bias-free anticoagulant.[101] A drawback of PPACK is its expense but this would likely change if it was manufactured in larger quantities.

Transporting/Icing Samples

Intracellular potassium is approximately 23 times higher in concentration as compared to the extracellular space. Therefore, anything that disturbs the stability of blood samples (e.g., pneumatic tube systems, centrifuging, or icing) has a tendency to cause hemolysis and spuriously increased potassium measurements. Falsely increased potassium measurements may be seen in fasting individuals or after prolonged setting of a sample. In contrast, ionized calcium tends to decrease with hemolysis because intracellular Ca is about one-thousandth of blood ionized calcium.

Placing blood samples in ice water may also lead to blood trauma, hemolysis, and changes in electrolyte measurements. As described previously, hemolysis will result in an increased potassium[14] concentration and decreased ionized calcium. These changes may also occur if blood is vigorously mixed or if the heel is squeezed while acquiring a capillary sample.[104] Potassium measurements may also increase slightly following exercise or when measured at noon or evening.[241] Ionized calcium will decrease in the presence of alkalosis.

In summary, samples to be used for both blood gas and electrolyte analysis should be handled carefully and not iced. Un-iced samples will remain relatively stable if analyzed within 30 minutes.[34] Failure to measure within this time will also lead to falsely increased lactate measurements. As always, manufacturer recommendations should be carefully reviewed and adhered to because each machine may have unique considerations.

EXERCISES

Exercise 3-1   Basic Physics of Gases

Fill in the blanks or select the best answer.

1. The constant random motion of gas molecules is called _____.

2. Define pressure.

3. The force exerted by molecules of *water* in the air is called _____.

4. Atmospheric pressure may be measured with an instrument called a _____.

5. Atmospheric pressure at sea level is _____.

6. Atmospheric pressure is (increased/decreased) above sea level.

7. State Dalton's law.

8. The energy of motion of gas molecules is called _____ energy.

9. The fractional concentration of a gas in a mixture of gases (will/will not) change with changes in humidity and water vapor pressure.

10. The fractional concentration of a gas (will/will not) change at different altitudes.

11. State what the symbol FIO_2 stands for.

12. Calculate the partial pressure of gases given the following:

	Total Pressure	Fractional Concentration	Water Vapor Pressure
a.	760 mm Hg	0.21	47 mm Hg
b.	700 mm Hg	0.21	47 mm Hg
c.	700 mm Hg	0.50	20 mm Hg
d.	800 mm Hg	0.30	27 mm Hg
e.	500 mm Hg	1.00	17 mm Hg

13. State Gay-Lussac's law.

14. Define BTPS conditions at sea level.

15. At sea level, atmospheric air saturated with humidity at body temperature exerts a partial pressure of oxygen of _____ mm Hg.

16. State Henry's law regarding the partial pressure of gases in liquids.

17. State whether pressure, temperature, or volume is constant in the following gas laws: Charles' law, Boyle's law, Gay-Lussac's law.

18. The blood gas symbol for arterial is (a/A); symbols related to measurements made on the blood are usually (lowercase/capital) letters.

19. The two major processes responsible for the difference between atmospheric and alveolar air are _____ and _____.

20. Relative humidity is a measure of _____ humidity divided by _____ humidity.

Exercise 3-2 Air in Blood Gas Samples

Fill in the blanks or select the best answer.

1. Blood gas values in arterial samples (are/are not) very stable.

2. Generally, the most pronounced blood gas change associated with exposure of the sample to a large air bubble is:
   a. decreased $PaCO_2$
   b. change in pH
   c. change in PaO_2

3. Drawing a blood gas sample under anaerobic conditions means that the sample (is/is not) exposed to air.

4. Which of the following two factors seems to have the greatest impact on the effects of air bubbles on blood gas samples?
   a. Duration of exposure
   b. Size of air bubble

5. An air bubble affects PaO_2 most if the initial PaO_2 of the sample is (greater than/less than) 100 mm Hg.

6. Given the initial PaO_2 values that follow, determine whether the measured PaO_2 increases or decreases when a large air bubble is introduced into the sample.
   a. 40 mm Hg
   b. 100 mm Hg
   c. 250 mm Hg
   d. 80 mm Hg
   e. 180 mm Hg

7. A blood gas sample containing froth (is/is not) acceptable.

8. Blood gas samples remain relatively stable if air bubbles are discarded within _____ minutes.

9. An air bubble always tends to (increase/decrease) blood PCO_2.

10. An air bubble always tends to (increase/decrease) blood pH.

Exercise 3-3   Venous Sampling or Admixture

Fill in the blanks or select the best answer.

1. Mixture of a small amount of venous blood with an arterial sample (will/will not) significantly alter the blood gas values obtained.

2. Blood gas samples thought to contain some venous blood should be (discarded/run quickly).

3. (Short/Long) beveled needles minimize the risk of venous contamination of an arterial blood sample.

4. A blood sample showing a PaO_2 of 40 mm Hg and $PaCO_2$ of 48 mm Hg (means/does not necessarily mean) that the sample is venous.

5. The PO_2 in all veins (is/is not) identical.

6. Mixed venous blood can be obtained only from a (peripheral vein/pulmonary artery).

7. List the normal blood gas values for mixed venous blood.
   $P\bar{v}O_2$ $P\bar{v}CO_2$ $S\bar{v}O_2$

8. Inadvertent venous sampling is particularly likely when attempting to puncture the (brachial/femoral) artery.

Exercise 3-4   Blood Gas Anticoagulation

Fill in the blanks or select the best answer.

1. The recommended anticoagulant for blood gas sampling is _____, although _____ heparin is sometimes still used.

2. The concentration of sodium heparin used for blood gas anticoagulation is _____ U/mL.

3. The major blood gas change associated with excessive volume of heparin is _____.

4. The pH of arterial blood (is/is not) usually significantly altered by the use of excessive heparin.

5. The major effect of heparin on blood gas values is usually via a (chemical/dilution) effect.

6. Hematocrit and hemoglobin measured from a heparinized arterial sample may be falsely (low/high).

7. Blood gas sample volumes in adults should usually exceed _____ mL.

8. As a general rule, a 1% heparin dilution lowers $PaCO_2$ by _____%.

9. What two innovations in blood gas sampling have almost eliminated errors owing to heparin dilution?

Exercise 3-5 Blood Gas Error Due to Metabolism

Fill in the blanks or select the best answer.

1. Metabolism (does/does not) continue in blood after it has left the body.

2. Indicate the effects of metabolism on the following parameters:
   PaO_2
   $PaCO_2$
   pH

3. Normally, in 1 hour at body temperature, PCO_2 increases approximately _____ mm Hg and pH decreases _____.

4. (High/low) initial PaO_2 values tend to drop rapidly owing to metabolism.

5. At room temperature, blood gas changes owing to metabolism occur approximately _____ as fast as they occur at body temperature.

6. Placing a blood gas sample in ice will slow metabolism to approximately _____% of the metabolic rate at body temperature.

7. Non-iced blood gas samples should be run within _____ minutes to avoid significant error.

8. The PO_2 change in an iced blood gas sample may be significant in _____ minutes when the initial PaO_2 exceeds 150 mm Hg.

9. Refrigerating blood gas samples (is/is not) an adequate substitute for placing the sample in ice.

10. The three types of cells primarily responsible for aerobic metabolic activity in blood gas samples are _____, _____ and _____.

11. The rapid fall in PaO_2 that may occur because of leukocytosis is called _____.

12. Iced samples remain stable for _____ hours or more if the initial PaO_2 is less than 150 mm Hg.

13. An elevated leukocyte count is called _____.

14. Immature leukocytes consume (more/less) O_2 than mature leukocytes.

Exercise 3-6 Temperature Effects on Blood Gases

Fill in the blanks or select the best answer.

1. Measurement of blood gases at 39° C would lead to falsely (high/low) PaO_2 and $PaCO_2$ values in blood sampled from an afebrile patient.

2. Arterial PCO_2 increases approximately _____% per degree Celsius temperature increase.

3. The pH generally decreases approximately _____ units/2° C increase in temperature.

4. An increase in body temperature of 1° C increases O_2 requirements by _____%.

5. Although controversial, most clinicians believe blood gas data should (be/not be) corrected to the actual patient's temperature conditions.

Exercise 3-7 Summary of Potential Sampling Errors

Complete the phrases denoted by the acronym AVERT, which is a mnemonic for five common blood gas sampling errors.

A

V

E

R

T

Exercise 3-8 Blood Gas/Electrolyte Specimens

Fill in the blanks or select the best answer.

1. Liquid anticoagulants used for blood gas sampling (will/will not) affect electrolyte results.

2. Heparin with electrolytes added to normal physiologic levels is called _____ heparin.

3. The key consideration when using lyophilized heparin is appropriate (mixing/icing) of the sample.

4. The selective prothrombin inhibitor _____ has been advocated as an ideal anticoagulant for blood gas/electrolyte specimens.

5. Placing blood specimens in ice may (lower, elevate) potassium measurements.

Exercise 3-9 Internet Work

1. Using any search engine, search for the following on the Internet:
   "medscape"
   "PubMed"
   "Medline"

2. Perform a search at one of these sites on the subject of blood gases. How many items were found in your query? What years did you search? Can you view the abstracts of these articles at the site used? If possible, pick two abstracts and describe their conclusions.

NBRC Challenge 3

Please select the best answer for the following multiple-choice questions.

1. One must be especially cautious in interpreting _____ in a patient with leukemia.
   A) PaO_2
   B) pH
   C) $PaCO_2$
   D) $[HCO_3]$
   E) [BE]
   (CRT EXAM – NBRC MATRIX I,C,2,c)

2. The effects of excessive liquid sodium heparin on a blood gas sample are:
   I. related to the partial pressures of the gases in the liquid.
   II. related to the pH of the liquid heparin.
   III. related to the buffer systems in the heparin.
   A) I only
   B) II only
   C) III only
   D) I, II, only
   E) I, II, and III only
   (CRT EXAM – NBRC MATRIX I,C,1,c)

3. Which of the following suggest a blood gas sample may be venous?
   I. Observation of a flash of blood as the syringe begins filling
   II. Bluish coloration of the blood sample
   III. Failure of syringe to auto-fill
   IV. Brownish coloration of blood
   A) I, II only
   B) II, III only
   C) II, IV only
   D) I, II, and III only
   E) I, III, and IV only
   (RRT EXAM – NBRC MATRIX I,C,1,e)

4. Temperature correction of blood gases:
   I. clearly provides the optimal way to guide clinical decision-making.
   II. is only indicated when patient temperature exceeds 40° C.
   III. is easily accomplished with most blood gas machines.
   A) I only
   B) II only
   C) III only
   D) I, III, only
   E) I, II, and III only
   (CRT EXAM – NBRC MATRIX I,C,1,c)

5. Placing a blood sample in an ice-water solution will interfere with analysis of blood:
   A) pH.
   B) hematocrit.
   C) hemoglobin.
   D) electrolytes.
   E) $[HCO_3]$.
   (RRT EXAM – NBRC MATRIX 1,C,2,e)

4

Blood Gas Electrodes and Quality Assurance

Regarding bench blood gas analysis . . .

. . . we have identified a need to restate principles and knowledge which used to be better known to the clinician before the elements of the apparatus disappeared from view in the interests of sophistication, automation, and design.

Alistair A. Spence[119]

Outline

BLOOD GAS ELECTRODES

Basic Electrical Principles

Traditionally, the analysis of blood gas values has been accomplished via electrochemical devices commonly referred to as *electrodes*. The description and function of these specific electrodes is presented later in this chapter. All traditional electrodes used in blood gas analysis measure changes in either electrical current or voltage and equate these changes with chemical measurements. Thus, a brief discussion of basic terms and principles in dynamic electricity is a logical starting point. More recently, new techniques such as optodes, have been used to determine blood gas values. These devices and techniques will be explored near the end of the chapter.

Electricity is a form of energy resulting from the flow of electrons through a substance that is called a *conductor*. An energy source such as a battery or generator is necessary to provide the power for this electrical flow. The energy source may be thought of as an "electron pump" that has two connections or poles. One pole has an excess of stored electrons and is therefore negatively charged. This negative pole is called the *cathode*. Conversely, the remaining pole has a relative shortage of electrons and has a net positive charge. The pole that is positively charged is called the *anode*.

To accomplish work, the electrons flow away from the negative pole, through a conductor, and toward the positive pole. As the electrons flow through the conductor, they can accomplish work such as creating light or producing heat. Electrons always flow from the negative pole to the positive pole.

Voltage

The force responsible for pumping these electrons is called the *electromotive force* or *potential*.[120] The greater the difference in electron concentration between the two poles, the greater is the electromotive force. The unit of measurement for electromotive force is the *volt*. Voltage refers to electromotive potential, and actual electron flow does not occur unless a conductor bridges the positive and negative poles. A *potentiometer* is an instrument that measures an unknown voltage by comparing it with a known reference voltage.[122]

Current

The actual flow of electrons through a conductor is called electrical *current*, and the term for the unit of measurement is the *ampere* or *amp*. Different types of conductors conduct current to various degrees. Good conductors have low *electrical resistance*, whereas poor conductors have high resistance. Long, thin wires are examples of conductors with relatively high resistance. The unit of electrical resistance is the *ohm*.

Ohm's Law

Ohm's law states that the electromotive force is equal to the current times the resistance.

$$\text{Electromotive force} = \text{current} \times \text{resistance}$$

In measurable terms

$$\text{Voltage} = \text{amp} \times \text{ohm}$$

It follows that a 220-volt force will deliver a higher current through a particular wire than a 110-volt force. A fuse or circuit breaker is designed to prevent the danger of fire and to protect electronic circuitry from excessive electron flow that may destroy it.

Consumption of electric power is measured usually in watts. One thousand watts is equal to 1 kilowatt (kW). Actual consumption of power is calculated by the formula

$$\text{Watts} = \text{volt} \times \text{amp}$$

Terminology

As mentioned in the introduction, most blood gas values that are measured directly are analyzed through electrodes. Thus, specific individual *electrodes* measure PO_2, pH, and PCO_2.

Electrochemical Cell Systems

In chemistry, an electrode is defined technically as an electric conductor or terminal through which electricity enters or leaves a medium such as an electrolyte solution.[122] By using this terminology, an *electrochemical cell* is an apparatus that consists of two electrodes placed in an electrolyte solution.[121,122] Similarly, an *electrochemical cell system* is an apparatus that incorporates one or more electrochemical cells to measure a specific chemical species.

Thus, from a chemical standpoint, all the traditional analytical devices used in blood gas analysis should be referred to as electrochemical cell systems. Similarly, within each measuring device there would be at least two electrodes. Nevertheless, clinically, these entire electrochemical cell systems are referred to almost invariably as simply "blood gas electrodes."[123] Therefore, this clinical terminology is used in the text in an effort to promote consistency and avoid confusion in a commonly misunderstood subject. The entire measurement device is referred to as an *electrode* (e.g., PO_2 electrode, pH electrode, PCO_2 electrode), and the term *electrode* is reserved solely for this use.

Half-Cells

Within all blood gas electrodes are *electrode terminals* (sites that chemists would refer to as electrodes). An electrode terminal is a solid site where electrons enter or leave a liquid medium. Electrode terminals may consist of

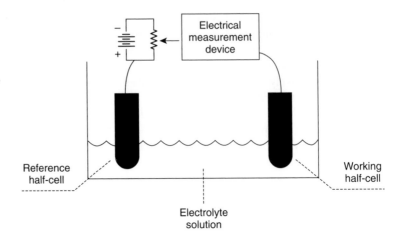

Figure 4-1. **Generic electrode.** The basic components of an electrode (electrochemical cell system) include a battery, an electrical measuring device, a working half-cell, and a reference half-cell.

metal or glass. A single electrode terminal in contact with an electrolyte solution may also be called a *half-cell*. All electrodes require at least two half-cells to function.

There are two types of half-cells: working half-cells and reference half-cells. The working or measuring half-cell is placed at the site where the actual chemical analysis, work, or electrochemical change takes place.[121,123] The reference half-cell is the standard against which the electrochemical change is compared and measured (Fig. 4-1).

A reference half-cell typically consists of a solid metal and a solution of its salt (e.g., silver and silver chloride, mercury and mercurous chloride) attached to an electronic circuit. When the metal is in contact with its salt solution, a constant electrical potential or voltage is produced.[121]

Structure and Function

The structure and function of the three primary blood gas electrodes (PO_2, pH, and PCO_2) will be explained.

PO_2 Electrode

Basic Components

The PO_2 electrode incorporates a battery and an ammeter as the electrical components of the electrode (Fig. 4-2).[123] Wall electricity may be used in place of a battery. The electrode terminal in the *working half-cell* is usually made of *platinum*. The electrode terminal in the *reference half-cell* is made of *silver/silver chloride*. The platinum is negatively charged and serves as a

cathode in the electrical system, whereas the silver is positively charged and serves as the anode.

If blood is then placed directly in contact with the two electrode terminals, the PO_2 of the blood sample can be measured as described in the following section.

Electrochemical Reaction

To initiate the flow of electrical current and the measurement of oxygen, the battery supplies the platinum cathode with a voltage of approximately 700 millivolts (mV).[124] This voltage attracts oxygen molecules to the cathode where they react with water. The ensuing chemical reaction consumes four electrons and produces some hydroxyl ions (see Fig. 4-2). The consumed electrons, in turn, are replaced rapidly in the electrolyte solution as silver and chloride react at the anode.

The net result of these reactions is a flow of electrical current throughout the entire circuit, which is shown in Figure 4-2. The current generated will be in direct proportion to the amount of dissolved oxygen (PO_2) present at the cathode (Fig. 4-3). An *ammeter* is a device used to measure the flow of electrical current.

Polarography

The direct relationship between PO_2 and electrical current is true only when a specific voltage is applied initially to the cathode.[123] The proper voltage to use is determined by analyzing a polarogram, which is a graph that shows the relationship between voltage and current at

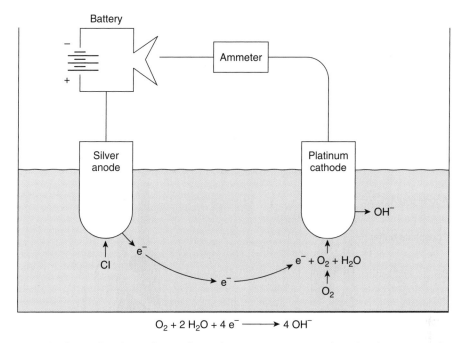

Figure 4-2. **Basic electrochemistry of PO_2 electrode.** Oxygen is attracted to the platinum working half-cell and reacts chemically with water. This reaction consumes electrons that are replaced in solution by the reaction at the silver anode. The entire process results in the generation of electrical current in proportion to the amount of oxygen present in the fluid.

a constant PO_2 (Fig. 4-4). The electrode must operate on the plateau of the polarogram to preserve the relationship between the PO_2 and the current. Thus, PO_2 analysis via the oxygen electrode is often referred to as a *polarographic technique* of gas analysis.[123]

Clark Electrode

The electrode shown in Figure 4-2 is not practical for the clinical measurement of blood PO_2 because protein from the blood deposits on the cathode and alters its electrical characteristics. Clark introduced a clinical version of this electrode in 1953. An illustration of a modern Clark electrode is shown in Figure 4-5.

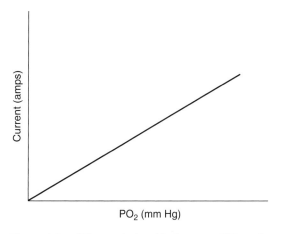

Figure 4-3. **Direct relationship between PO_2 and current.**

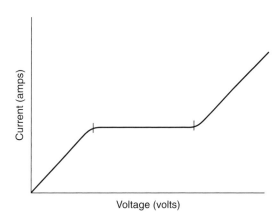

Figure 4-4. **Polarogram.**

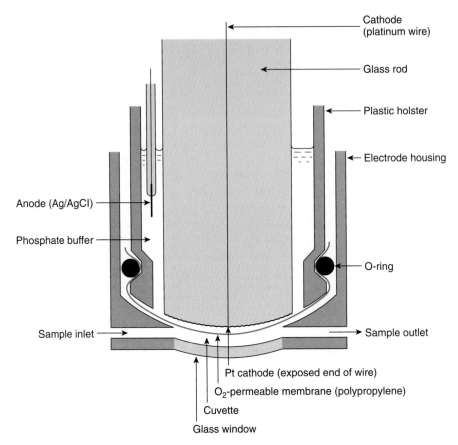

Figure 4-5. **Schematic illustration of a Clark electrode.** A polypropylene membrane separates the platinum cathode from the blood.

In the Clark electrode, blood is separated from the electrode terminals by use of a special membrane, which is permeable to oxygen and is a good electrical insulator. Oxygen from the blood can diffuse easily through the membrane into the electrolyte solution in which the reaction with water can take place. The terminals in the electrode are not bathed directly in blood; they are bathed instead in a phosphate buffer solution, and potassium chloride is added.[121]

Most PO_2 electrodes use polypropylene membranes; however, Mylar, Teflon, and polyethylene all have similar properties and may be used.[123] The membrane is usually secured on the electrode with a rubber O-ring (see Fig. 4-5). In addition, the actual blood sample remains in a chamber known as a cuvette where it is warmed quickly to 37° C and is protected from contamination by the air.

pH Electrode

Electrode Function

The pH electrode differs greatly from the PO_2 electrode in both structure and function. Functionally, the pH electrode measures changes in voltage rather than actual electrical current. Specifically, pH is measured by the *potentiometric method* by which an unknown voltage is measured by comparison with a known voltage and is then converted to pH.[123]

To accomplish this, the pH electrode requires four electrode terminals instead of just two, such as in the case of the PO_2 electrode. A *reference solution* of known pH is placed between two of the terminals to have reference voltage to compare the unknown voltage against. A single unique pH-sensitive glass electrode terminal serves as a common electrode terminal for both the reference solution and the solution of unknown pH (Fig. 4-6).

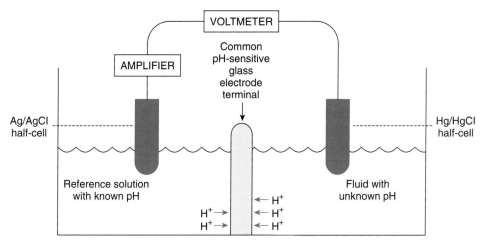

Figure 4-6. **A pH electrode.**

This specially manufactured pH-sensitive glass allows hydrogen ions to diffuse into it in proportion to the hydrogen ion concentration of the fluid to which it is exposed. Because of the different solutions on either side of the glass, a net electrical potential (voltage) develops between the two fluids and is quantitated at the voltmeter.

The relationship between voltage and pH at a particular temperature is described by the modified Nernst equation.[10] In general, for each pH unit difference between the known and unknown solutions, a difference of 61.5 mV develops. A special voltmeter converts voltage to pH units based on the Nernst equation and visually displays the pH.

Actual electron flow (current) secondary to the voltage differences between the two sides is prevented by use of an amplifier between the voltmeter and the reference solution. This amplifier has high electrical resistance that prohibits significant electrical current and this allows for measurement of small voltage differences.[125]

Physical Components

The physical components of a model pH electrode are shown in Figure 4-7. This system can be divided physically into two major components. One component has the pH-sensitive glass at the tip and a silver/silver chloride half-cell inside it. Because this component is the site at which the actual blood comes in contact with the outer surface of the pH-sensitive glass,

it may be referred to as the working half-cell. Thus, the mercury/mercurous chloride (Hg/Hg_2Cl_2) component can be called the reference half-cell.

Although not recommended here, the pH-sensitive glass component is often referred to as the "working or measuring electrode," and the other component is called the "reference electrode." In addition to the confusion surrounding the term *electrode*, these terms are

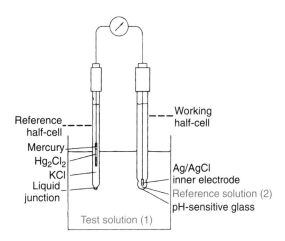

Figure 4-7. **Basic components of the pH electrode.** The reference calomel half-cell is on the left. The KCl diffuses slowly out to form a liquid junction with the test solution. The potential difference between the test solution *(1)* and the reference solution *(2)* is read on a voltmeter calibrated in pH units.

even more misleading because the "measuring electrode" contains the "reference solution." Furthermore, the silver or silver chloride per se is not a working half-cell.

The reference half-cell shown in Figure 4-7 includes an electrode terminal made of mercury coated with mercurous chloride. The term *calomel* is often used for this type of electrode terminal. The calomel electrode terminal interfaces with a platinum wire that transmits the change in voltage to the voltmeter.

The calomel electrode terminal is slightly sensitive and would be damaged if it were in direct contact with blood. Therefore, it is separated from blood samples by creating a salt or contact bridge. The salt bridge is typically a potassium chloride (KCl) solution that is separated from the blood by a thin membrane. The calomel electrode terminal is used because it functions best with KCl. The salt bridge may also be called the *liquid junction*.

Sanz Electrode

Although blood could be sampled in a pH electrode similar to the one shown in Figure 4-7, this particular configuration presents several problems. This system would require a large blood sample volume. Furthermore, the blood would not be at body temperature and would be exposed to air.

The modern, compact, pH electrode (Sanz electrode) facilitates pH measurement at 37° C with a small blood sample and is accomplished by drawing the blood sample into a pH-sensitive glass capillary tube. A membrane at the end of the capillary tube then connects the blood sample to a large reservoir liquid junction and the calomel half-cell.

PCO₂ Electrode

Electrode Function

The PCO_2 electrode (shown in Figure 4-8) is a modified version of the pH. In the PCO_2 electrode, however, blood does not come in direct contact with the pH-sensitive glass. Rather, blood comes in contact with a CO_2 permeable membrane. The membrane may be made of silicone rubber, Teflon, or a similar substance that is readily permeable to CO_2.

On the other side of the membrane is a bicarbonate solution that is in direct contact with the pH-sensitive glass. The bicarbonate solution is also in contact with a silver/silver chloride (Ag/AgCl) electrode terminal. Thus, the PCO_2 electrode actually has two Ag/AgCl electrode terminals within it. No salt bridge is

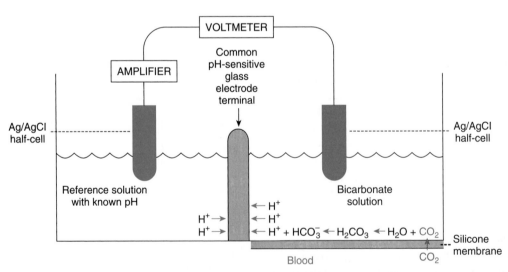

Figure 4-8. **PCO₂ electrode.** The CO_2 from the blood diffuses through the silicone membrane into the bicarbonate solution. The hydrolysis reaction occurs in the bicarbonate solution and results in the production of hydrogen ions in proportion to the amount of dissolved CO_2 present. The difference in voltage is then converted to PCO_2 units and is indicated on the voltmeter. Note also that both metallic half-cells in the PCO_2 electrode are Ag/AgCl.

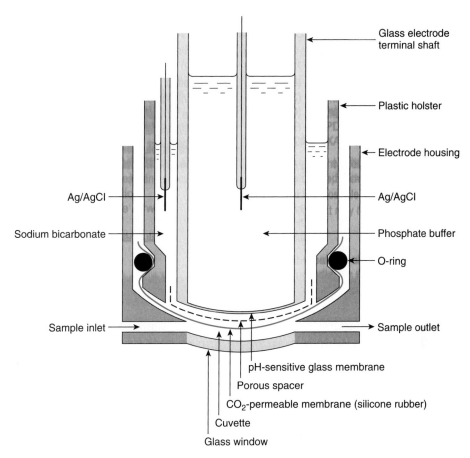

Figure 4-9. Severinghaus PCO_2 electrode.

necessary because blood is not in direct contact with the electrode terminals.

As shown in Figure 4-8, a chemical reaction occurs within the bicarbonate solution as CO_2 diffuses in. This reaction, which is known as the hydrolysis reaction, results in the production of hydrogen ions and a pH change of the bicarbonate solution. The pH change is in direct proportion to the PCO_2. Thus, the corresponding voltage change can be converted into PCO_2 units and reflected on the voltmeter.

Severinghaus Electrode

The clinical PCO_2 electrode is also known as the Severinghaus electrode. An illustration of the structure of a Severinghaus electrode is shown in Figure 4-9. Only a very thin layer of bicarbonate solution is exposed to the blood sample.

Accuracy of Electrodes

A relatively high degree of precision can be expected in the analysis of arterial blood gases today.[10] The approximate accuracy of blood gas electrodes is shown in Table 4-1.[10,123,126–129]

The pH is repeatedly the most reliable and accurate measurement. The PCO_2 variation in historical studies and reports was in the range of 1 to 5 mm Hg.[123,126–130] Today, the variation in PCO_2 should be less than 1 mm Hg.

Table 4-1. ACCURACY OF BLOOD GAS ELECTRODES

Parameters	Values
PO_2	±3 mm Hg
PCO_2	±1 mm Hg
pH	±0.01 units

ON CALL | CASE 4-1 *ABGs and Critical Thinking*

You are the only person available to care for this patient. You must assess the patient/situation and act accordingly.

A 51-year-old man with severe thrombocytosis has a blood gas drawn. He is also on a pulse oximeter, which is reading 95%.

ARTERIAL BLOOD GASES

SaO_2	85%
pH	7.36
$PaCO_2$	37 mm Hg
PaO_2	51 mm Hg
$[HCO_3]$	25 mEq/L

ASSESSMENT

Abnormalities: List abnormal data and other noteworthy information.

Explanation: List possible diseases, pathology, or other situations which may have lead to this patient's condition or these laboratory values.

Evaluation: Suggest additional data that would be useful in helping understand the situation or in making a diagnosis.

Older PO_2 electrodes were the least accurate with reports of as high as 20% inaccuracy, especially at high PO_2 values.[10,131] Variation in PO_2 had been reported to be in the range of 3 to 20 mm Hg at normal PO_2.[126-129] These inaccuracies in the PO_2 electrode were due at least in part to the production of hydrogen peroxide at the cathode site. Furthermore, gases such as carbon dioxide, halothane, and nitrous oxide may cause small changes in current in the system.[123]

Newer designs in PO_2 electrodes, however, continue to make this electrode more accurate. Currently, PaO_2 results should be expected to be accurate to nearly 3 mm Hg at 80 mm Hg.[10]

TOTAL QUALITY MANAGEMENT

Current quality management in the laboratory is much more sophisticated and clinically oriented than in the past. Quality methods and techniques are focused on insuring that the *quality of tests performed in the laboratory allow our clinicians to practice good medicine*.[362] We are becoming increasingly concerned with exactly how the laboratory results impact clinical decision-making. Are they being used for diagnosis, monitoring, or identifying critical levels? This is a much broader concept and goal than simply ensuring that test numbers fall within specific predefined limits.

Thus, many issues and concerns that were previously ignored in laboratory quality management are now becoming increasingly important.

Depending on the particular test, we may be very concerned with accuracy, turn-around time, cost, simplicity, sample size, etc. All these various attributes of a particular test are referred to as *performance characteristics*.[362] Performance characteristics, in turn, can be subdivided into practicability characteristics (e.g., sample size, speed of analysis) and reliability characteristics (e.g., precision, bias).

Ideally, quality specifications would be available for every performance characteristic.[362] Quality specifications are the heart of a quality management system as shown in Figure 4-10. Note that in Figure 4-10, quality management encompasses quality assurance, quality improvement, and quality control. A detailed discussion of laboratory quality management is beyond the scope of this text. Excellent resources are available from the National

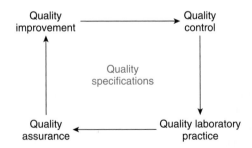

Figure 4-10. **The central role of quality specifications in quality management.**

Committee of Clinical Laboratory Standards [NCCLS], the American Association for Respiratory Care, and books[362] related to this topic. Nevertheless, some of the routine components in quality management within the blood gas laboratory will be briefly discussed.

QUALITY ASSURANCE

Quality assurance is a systematic process used to monitor, document, and regulate the accuracy and reliability of a procedure or laboratory measurement. Errors in blood gases may occur before, during, or after actual analysis of the sample. An error that occurs before or after actual analysis (e.g., an error due to improper sample or data handling) is called a nonanalytical error. On the other hand, an error that occurs during the actual analysis of the sample (e.g., error due to performance of electrode or technician) is called an analytical error.[10,123]

Nonanalytical Error

Preanalytical Error

As described in Chapter 3, an error may be easily introduced into blood gas data during arterial puncture or sample handling. The sample may be inappropriately drawn or transported. Blood gas results could be attributed inadvertently to the wrong patient. A patient's status or therapy may be incorrectly assessed or recorded. Preanalytical error is likely to be the greatest source of incorrect blood gas data. If left unnoticed, this error may have serious consequences on the treatment of the patient.

A comprehensive quality assurance program must include clearly defined departmental procedures and protocols for sample acquisition and handling. In addition, monitoring of the program must ensure and document that department protocol and procedures are being followed.

Postanalytical Error

Recording of results after analysis may be associated with an error in transcription. In particular, the use of telephone reports may easily lead to serious reporting error due to a breakdown in verbal communication.[132] Telephone reporting is done typically in the critical care setting and in regard to critically ill individuals. These individuals cannot afford the potential consequences of incorrect information. The incidence of this type of error may be reduced if the individuals who receive these data are knowledgeable of normal clinical ranges for blood gases.[132] It is also very important that the individuals receiving the data read it back to confirm accuracy. Finally, knowledge of potentially life-threatening values for these parameters also helps to prevent a serious error being made. Ideally, results are directly printed out from the machine at a remote location, and the potential for human error is eliminated.

In summary, blood gas results must be interpreted in light of the potential for both preanalytical or postanalytical error. Unexpected blood gas results should arouse suspicion. Blood gases should be repeated immediately, preferably on another instrument if: (1) they are inconsistent with the patient picture, (2) they are internally inconsistent (see Chapter 5), (3) they are at the extremes of the expected range.[241]

A comprehensive quality assurance program must address the total spectrum of blood gas analysis to include preanalytical and postanalytical error.

Analytical Error

Analytical error includes any error that occurs during the actual analysis of the blood gases. Most often, analytical error is related to the apparatus rather than to the individual and to the equipment rather than to the technique.

An example of human analytical error, however, is failure on the part of the technician to properly mix the sample before it is introduced into the electrode. Failure to mix an iced sample may increase the pH of the sample by as much as 0.11 units.[123]

Also, the technician should not record blood gas values immediately after injecting the sample into the electrode. An adequate exposure time is necessary to achieve sample stabilization at body temperature, ambient pressure, saturated, and to ensure complete electrode response. Most samples achieve equilibrium within 1 to 3 minutes. Two or three times longer may be necessary, however, if PCO_2 is extremely low or if PO_2 is extremely high in the sample.[125,133]

Another source of error is *inherent biologic variation*.[362] The difference between individuals is called *between-subject* or *inter-individual* biologic variation. There are two general types of biologic variation. The difference in a given individual is called *within-subject* or *intra-individual* variation. Intra-individual variation may occur during daily, monthly, or yearly cycles or during the aging process.

Nevertheless, as stated earlier, most analytical error is due to the equipment itself. Various methods must be used by the laboratory technicians to ensure that the electrodes function appropriately. These methods include preventive maintenance and frequent calibration. Quality control will be discussed in the following section.

Preventive Maintenance

Proper maintenance and cleaning of blood gas electrodes is essential. The systems must be kept free of contaminants, and the membranes must be carefully maintained. Most importantly, the technician must be aware of and comply with individual manufacturer specifications and recommendations for each specific instrument.

Calibration

Calibration is a procedure done on blood gas electrodes before analyzing blood samples to establish the accuracy of readings in the anticipated range. *Standards* are gases or buffer solutions with precise, specific blood gas values that are used to set the machine to read linearly over the physiologic range. Gases used for calibration should be extremely accurate and should be traceable to National Institute of Standards and Technology (NIST) certification. Due to the many different protocols, designs, and recommendations of various manufacturers, no specific guidelines can be provided for routine calibration. Operators must adhere to specific manufacturer's recommendations.[241]

The PO_2 electrode is the least accurate of the three blood gas electrodes. The wide clinical range of PO_2 (0 to 600 mm Hg) makes it difficult for the electrode to have a linear response throughout. When high PO_2 is anticipated (i.e., >200 mm Hg), the system should be calibrated to 100% O_2.

An additional problem with the PO_2 electrode is that the PO_2 reading is lower if a gas is introduced into the electrode than if a liquid is introduced into the electrode. This discrepancy has been referred to as the *fluid-gas difference*,[123] the *blood-gas factor*,[10,123] or the *stirring effect*.[125] A rough correction factor for the fluid-gas difference is $1.04 \times PO_2$ of the gas sample.[123]

QUALITY CONTROL

Quality control, concerning blood gas electrodes, refers to the periodic checking of an instrument's performance to ensure calibration, stability, and reliability. Statistical methods are used to evaluate the accuracy and precision of blood gas measurements. Quality control is probably the most controllable aspect of quality assurance. The two major types of quality control systems are internal quality control and external quality control.

Internal Quality Control

Internal quality control programs are designed to ensure that the instruments (i.e., electrodes) within a laboratory perform with precision. They involve routine procedures and protocols designed to detect inconsistencies in performance. Internal quality control is required by most external regulatory or accreditation agencies (e.g., Joint Commission for the Accreditation of Healthcare Organizations [JCAHO], College of American Pathologists [CAP], Clinical Laboratories Improvement Amendments [CLIA]).

External Quality Control

External quality control, also known as proficiency testing, is a system by which laboratories can compare the accuracy of their results with the results obtained from other laboratories. External quality control involves the distribution of identical samples from a central distribution site to participating laboratories. The central distribution site is a noncommercial, independent agency or professional association.

Each laboratory then runs the sample and reports the results to the distribution center. Results reported from one laboratory are then compared with results obtained from other laboratories. Based on these data, individual discrepancies can be identified and evaluated.

A few countries, such as the United States, have identified performance standards that laboratories must meet to maintain accreditation. The US CLIA 88 report documents total error allowable for analysis of certain analytes. This form of regulation is known as an *external quality assessment scheme*.

Finally, laboratories may perform bias studies within their laboratory if they utilize multiple machines. With this technique, the same sample is run on different machines as an additional indicator of control and variability. It is recommended that these types of studies be routinely performed and recorded to detect potential quality concerns within the department.

Statistics

Some fundamental statistics must be understood to evaluate the accuracy and precision of electrodes and thus monitor quality control. There are three pertinent statistical indices: the mean ($\bar{x}$), standard deviation (SD), and coefficient of variation (CV).

Mean

The mean is a fundamental statistic that is calculated by dividing the sum of all the numbers in a group by the number of numeric entries. In lay terms, the mean is known as the *average*. Mathematical calculation of the mean is shown in Equation 4-1.

Equation 4-1

$$\bar{x} = \sum \frac{(X_1 + X_2 + X_3 + \cdots + X_n)}{n}$$

$\bar{x}$ = mean

Σ = sum of

n = number of measurements

Standard Deviation

When considering results of laboratory tests, it is important to understand the difference between the average or *mean* and the *normal range*. The mean is a single number that best characterizes the group. The normal range gives a high and low value within which 95% of the normal population fall when subjected to a particular test.

The normal range is shown well by the bell-shaped curve described in Chapter 1 (see Fig. 1-1). The degree of dispersion (i.e., scattering of values from the average) in a group of numbers can be quantitated by calculating the SD. The SD is therefore a measure of variance around the mean. The formula for calculation of the SD is shown in Equation 4-2.

Equation 4-2

$$SD = \sqrt{\sum \frac{(x - \bar{x})^2}{n - 1}}$$

$\bar{x}$ = mean

x = each measurement

Σ = sum of

n = number of measurements

For each measurement in a series of measurements, the deviation from the mean is calculated ($x - \bar{x}$). Each numeric deviation is then squared ($x - \bar{x}$)^2. Next, the mean of the squared deviations is calculated. Finally, the square root of this value is taken (see Equation 4-2). Note that "n − 1" in Equation 4-2 is used in the denominator in place of "n" and is related to the role that these measures play in statistical inference.[134]

It can be seen how the SD is a measure of the homogeneity or dispersion of the values. A low SD (i.e., minimal dispersion) indicates that the values are generally homogeneous. The SD of $PaCO_2$ in the normal population is approximately 2.5 mm Hg, whereas the SD of PaO_2 is close to 5 mm Hg. Thus, the normal range (±2 SD) of $PaCO_2$ (35 to 45 mm Hg) is more narrow (homogeneous) than the normal range for PaO_2 (80 to 100 mm Hg).

Coefficient of Variation

When comparing the degree of variation (i.e., dispersion) in two groups of measurements with sharply different means, the CV is a more appropriate statistic than the SD. Calculation of the CV is shown in Equation 4-3.

Equation 4-3

$$CV = \frac{SD}{\bar{x}} \times 100$$

CV = coefficient of variation

SD = standard deviation

$\bar{x}$ = mean

Principles and Materials

Controls

To perform internal quality control, samples with known blood gas values must be run periodically to ensure that the machine is operating correctly. These samples in which the true blood gas values are known are referred to as *control samples* or controls. Like any group or population, controls have their own range of normal limits based on ±2 SDs from the mean. Thus, control limits (control normals) can be established based on this information.

The mean and SD are typically given by the manufacturer for commercial controls. Nevertheless, a local mean and SD may also be determined by running more than 20 control samples through a machine over time. This procedure provides a better local standard but may introduce error if the machines are not well calibrated initially.

Controls are available with high, low, and normal values. It has been recommended that at least two levels of controls be run within every 8-hour shift.[10] Furthermore, all three levels of controls should be run in every 24-hour day. Because very high PaO_2s may be seen in some blood gases (e.g., operating room, recovery room), it is often recommended that a fourth high level PaO_2 be run periodically.

Control Limits

Figure 4-11 illustrates how a quality control chart is based on sample control limits. Actual control limits may be set at ±2 or 3 SDs depending on the type of test and on the significance of an abnormal finding. A chart is then developed with horizontal lines drawn in at the mean and the upper and lower selected control limits. Results that fall between the two control lines are "*in control.*" A measurement that is right on the line is also considered to be in control.

Levey-Jennings Control Charts

Description

The results obtained from control sample measurements are run and progressively plotted on a control chart (Fig. 4-12). The control chart shows measured results on the y-axis versus time of measurement (run number) on the x-axis.

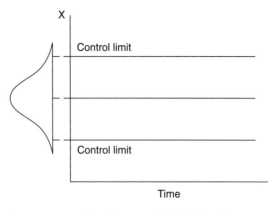

Figure 4-11. **Quality control limits.** Quality control limits are based on the normal distribution curve. They are set at 2 or 3 SDs from the mean. Values falling outside the upper and lower limits indicate that the machine is not *in control*.

This type of quality control chart was introduced into clinical chemistry in the 1950s by Levey and Jennings and is still referred to as a Levey-Jennings chart.

A performance record is a less sophisticated form of documentation that shows the date and time when controls were run and designates whether results were in acceptable limits.

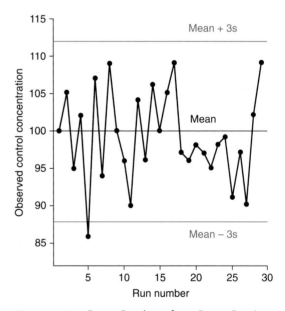

Figure 4-12. **Levey-Jennings chart.** Levey-Jennings control chart with control limits set as the $\bar{x} \pm 3$ SD. Concentration is plotted on the y-axis versus time (run number) on the x-axis.

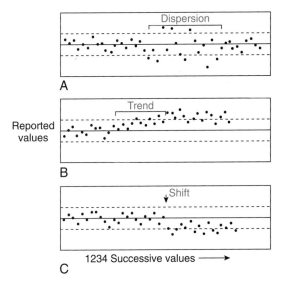

A

B

Reported values

C

1234 Successive values ⟶

Figure 4-13.   **Error patterns in quality control.** Examples of three common changes in quality control data. **A,** *Dispersion* is seen when there is an increased frequency of both high and low outliers. **B,** A progressive drift of the reported values from the previous mean value is called a *trend.* **C,** A *shift* occurs when there is an abrupt change from the established mean value.

Levey-Jennings charts, on the other hand, produce graphic outcomes that may indicate a particular problem or concern.

Error Patterns

Random Error. Random error is characterized by an isolated result outside of control limits, which is shown in Figure 4-12 (run no. 5). A single random error has minor significance and should be disregarded. When random error increases in frequency, however, the machine and techniques should be evaluated carefully. A pattern of frequent random error is shown in Figure 4-13,*A* and is sometimes referred to as *dispersion.*

Systematic Error. Systematic error or bias, on the other hand, is recurrent measurable deviation away from the mean. *Trending* is an example of systematic error in which progressive controls either increase or decrease. An example of a trend is shown in Figure 4-13,*B*. Trending may be caused by an aging electrode, an aging mercury battery, or protein contamination of the electrode.

Shifting is another form of systematic error that is characterized by a relatively abrupt change in measurement outcome followed by clustering or plateauing in a particular area. Shifting is shown in Figure 4-13,*C*. A shift may result from bubbles beneath the membrane, change in temperature, or contamination of calibration standards.[135]

Accuracy versus Precision

The various types of errors that have been described are either problems with accuracy of the measuring device or precision of the measuring device. *Accuracy* is a measure of how closely the measured results reflect the true or actual value (Fig. 4-14). If a PO_2 electrode consistently measures PO_2 10 mm Hg lower than PO_2 actually is, it is inaccurate. Problems related to accuracy are usually characterized by systematic error.

Precision, on the other hand, is an index of dispersion of repeated measurements. If, after repeated measurements, one electrode measured

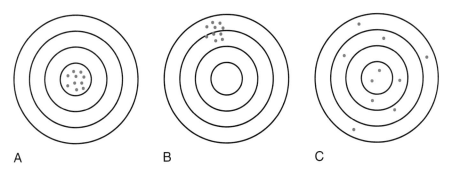

A   B   C

Figure 4-14.   **Accuracy versus precision.** Analytical accuracy and precision are illustrated by the ability to "hit" a known target. **A,** Very good accuracy and precision. **B,** Poor accuracy but good precision. **C,** Occasional accuracy but poor precision.

PO$_2$ to within ±5 mm Hg, whereas another electrode measured PO$_2$ to within ±10 mm Hg, the one with the lesser dispersion would be more precise.

The analogy of shooting at a target has been made to compare the difference between accuracy and precision.[130] The closeness of a particular hit to the bull's-eye represents accuracy, whereas the pattern of hits indicates precision (see Fig. 4-14). Levey-Jennings charts can likewise reflect problems with accuracy or precision (Fig. 4-15) based on the patterns of results obtained.

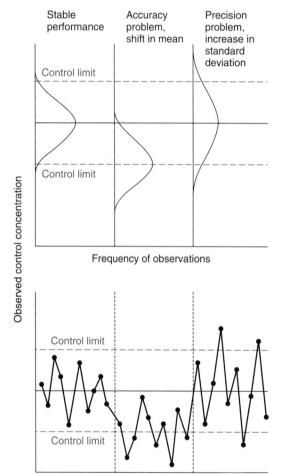

Figure 4-15.   **Problems with accuracy versus precision.** Conceptual basis of control charts. Frequency distributions of control observations for different error conditions (**top**). Display of control values versus time on a control chart (**bottom**).

Troubleshooting

Troubleshooting guides are often available from equipment manufacturers to help the technician detect the problem when the electrodes are not in control. Electrodes are generally considered to be in control when they are accurate to within 2 SDs of known sample values. Most of the new automated machines have sophisticated electronic and computer circuitry that provides periodic self-calibration and troubleshooting.

An example of an old electrode troubleshooting guide is shown in Table 4-2.

Westgard Rules

Westgard and co-workers have defined specific criteria and related actions that should follow when values are found to be out-of-control (Table 4-3).[628] A single measurement outside two standard deviations would warrant *careful observation* (Fig. 4-16,*A*); however, repeated measurements outside the norms or in the same direction requires *corrective action* regarding the sensor.

A random error of greater than 3 standard deviations requires action (see Fig. 4-16,*B*). Similarly, two consecutive measurements more than 4 standard deviations apart (see Fig. 4-16,*D*) would likewise signal the initiation of corrective measures. Finally, systematic errors as shown in Figure 4-16, *C, E,* and *F,* also indicate the need for immediate action.

Electrode Drift

Another indication of electrode integrity is the degree of electrode drift. Electrode drift is the change in the measured values as the sample rests in the electrode. Normally, electrode drift should not exceed 1% to 2% within 5 minutes. The pH electrode drifts slightly to the basic side if buffer solutions are allowed to remain in it. Nevertheless, this drift should not exceed 0.02 units/hour.[123] Electrode drift is minimized in current blood gas systems because single point calibrations are typically performed automatically at least every 30 minutes.[10]

Types of Controls

The ideal quality control material would be almost identical to blood in composition and physicochemical behavior. A variety of control materials have been used to test instrument performance.[130,136]

Table 4-2. ELECTRODE TROUBLESHOOTING GUIDES

Possible Cause	Corrective Action
	pH ELECTRODE
	Calibration
1. Drift or incorrect calibration.	Recalibrate.
2. Calibration buffers are contaminated.	Use fresh solution and recalibrate instrument.
	Sample Handling
1. Improper handling of controls.	Introduce a new control sample.
	a. Ensure that sample has been at room temperature for 24 hours before use.
	b. Shake 10 seconds to equilibrate the gas/liquid phase.
	c. Break open control sample and use within 1 minute.
2. Insufficient aspiration of sample.	Introduce a new sample.
	a. Check for proper suction if automatic aspiration is used.
	b. Replace pump tubing, if necessary.
	c. Check seals around sample chamber.
3. Air bubble entrapment in pH measuring electrode capillary.	Introduce new sample, avoiding bubble.
4. Contamination or carry-over from a previous sample.	Flush system thoroughly, as manufacturer directs, followed by a rinse.
	Electrodes
1. Protein buildup on pH glass electrode.	a. Clean electrode as recommended by manufacturer.
	b. If necessary, soak electrode overnight as manufacturer directs.
2. Concentration of KCl in salt bridge is incorrect (reference electrode).	a. Add some crystals of KCl to reference electrode if saturation is required by manufacturer.
	b. If 4 molar concentration is required, replace 4 molar solution on a *daily* basis.
	c. If KCl tablet is used, replace once a month as manufacturer directs.
	d. If 20% KCl is used, replace as manufacturer directs.
3. Dehydrated glass membrane.	See manufacturer's instructions for rehydration of electrode.
4. Air bubble entrapped in salt bridge of reference electrode.	Tilt repeatedly to dislodge and remove air bubble.
5. KCl—insufficient amount, old or caking.	Replace with fresh KCl solution according to manufacturer's directions.
6. Electrode temperature not at 37° C.	a. Check level of water bath.
	b. Check thermometer for break in mercury column; replace if necessary.
	c. Set instrument temperature to 37° C.
	d. Allow sufficient time for instrument to *fully* equilibrate to 37° C before use.
	e. Check water lines leading to pH bath for crimping or air blockage.
	f. Check circulation of water by pump.
7. Defective glass electrode due to aging or defect (hairline crack or scratches).	Replace glass electrode.
8. Defective pH membrane.	Replace pH membrane.

From bioMérieux, Inc., Durham, NC

Continued

Table 4-2.   ELECTRODE TROUBLESHOOTING GUIDES—*cont'd.*

Possible Cause	Corrective Action
Electrical	
1. Electrical leaks, loose connectors in pH meter.	Contact manufacturer for service.
2. Open circuit.	Check all lines to ensure proper connection. Test with jumper strap as manufacturer directs.
3. Poor grounding.	Check to ensure that the instrument is properly grounded.
4. Faulty cables, loose connectors or fittings.	Check for a good fit. If any cables, connectors, or fittings are loose or broken, contact manufacturer for service.
5. Faulty pH meter causing a shift in calibration or nonlinear curve.	Contact manufacturer for service.
PCO$_2$ ELECTRODE	
Calibration	
1. Drift or incorrect calibration.	Recalibrate.
2. Improperly certified gas tank.	Use new gas tank with maximum tolerance of 0.05%.
3. Cooling of electrode due to rapid gas flow rate (excessive bubble/sec).	Reduce gas flow rate as manufacturer directs.
4. Idle gas lines not adequately flushed or diffusion of room air into gas tubing lines.	Allow sufficient time for adequate flushing, 5 minutes at a fast flow rate, before reducing to proper flow rate.
5. Large adjustments in current required during calibration.	Clean cathode and change membrane.
Sample Handling	
1. Improper handling of controls.	Introduce a new control sample. a. Be sure sample has been at room temperature for 24 hours before use. b. Shake 10 seconds to equilibrate the gas/liquid phase. c. Break open control sample and use within 1 minute.
2. Insufficient aspiration of sample.	Introduce a new sample. a. If automatic aspiration is used, check for proper suction. b. Replace pump tubing, if necessary. c. Check seals around sample chamber.
3. Entrapped air bubble in measuring chamber.	Remove bubble by suction, flush, and introduce a new sample.
4. Improper or insufficient cleaning of PCO$_2$ system.	Clean as manufacturer directs.
5. Contamination or carry-over from a previous sample.	Flush system thoroughly as manufacturer directs, followed by a rinse.
6. Room air contamination.	a. Check proper syringe techniques or use adaptor. b. Clean aspiration tip; check for pinholes in tubing. c. Check for poor connections or pinholes in internal tubing.

Table 4-2. ELECTRODE TROUBLESHOOTING GUIDES—*cont'd*.

Possible Cause	Corrective Action
Electrodes	
1. Protein buildup on membrane.	Clean as manufacturer directs, or replace membrane.
2. Stretched or folded membrane, or improperly installed membrane.	Replace membrane.
3. Ripped, torn, or hole in PCO_2 membrane.	Clean electrode tip as recommended by manufacturer and replace membrane.
4. Protein contamination of tip of PCO_2 electrode.	Clean electrode tip as recommended by manufacturer and replace membrane.
5. Improperly positioned spacer or spacer not completely wetted.	Remove electrode, remove membrane, reposition and wet spacer, and replace membrane.
6. Improper electrolyte, insufficient amount, or old electrolyte solution.	Remove electrode assembly, replace with fresh electrolyte solution to the proper level.
7. Electrode temperature not at 37° C.	a. Check water level in water bath. b. Check thermometer for break in mercury column; replace if necessary. c. Set instrument temperature to 37° C. d. Allow sufficient time for instrument to *fully* equilibrate to 37° C before use. e. Check circulation of water by pump. f. Reduce gas flow rate as manufacturer directs.
8. Improperly seated electrode causing flush solution or sample to remain in chamber.	a. Remove and reposition electrodes. b. Dry with cotton swab and introduce new sample. c. If leakage continues, call manufacturer.
9. Air bubbles entrapped beneath membrane.	Remove bubbles or replace membrane.
10. Bubbles in newly refilled PCO_2 electrolyte solution.	Remove electrode and gently tilt to dislodge bubbles adhering to membrane or electrode walls.
11. Dehydrated electrode due to aging or improperly hydrated electrode.	See manufacturer's instruction for rehydration of electrode.
12. Defective electrode due to aging or hairline crack or scratches on electrode.	Replace electrode.
13. Room air contamination from leakage around electrode.	Replace O rings and seals. If leakage persists, call manufacturer.
Electrical	
1. Poor grounding on instrument.	Check to ensure that the instrument is properly grounded.
2. Open circuit.	Check all lines to ensure proper connection. Test with jumper strap as manufacturer directs.
3. Faulty cables, loose connectors.	Check for a good fit. If any cables, connectors, or fittings are loose or broken, contact manufacturer for service.
4. Faulty meter causing a shift in calibration or a nonlinear response.	Contact manufacturer for service.
PO_2 ELECTRODE **Calibration**	
1. Drift or incorrect calibration.	Recalibrate.
2. Improperly certified gas tank.	Use new gas tank with maximum tolerance of 0.05%.
3. Cooling of electrode due to rapid gas flow rate (excessive bubble/sec).	Reduce gas flow rate as manufacturer directs.

Continued

Table 4-2.   Electrode Troubleshooting Guides—*cont'd.*

Possible Cause	Corrective Action
4. Idle gas lines not adequately flushed or diffusion of room air into gas tubing lines.	a. Allow sufficient for adequate flushing, 5 minutes at a fast flow rate, before reducing to proper flow rate. b. Keep gas tanks as close to the analyzer as possible, thus reducing the length of tubing needed. c. Tubing specified by manufacturer must be used.
5. Insufficient time allowed for zero setting.	Allow sufficient time for zero setting as manufacturer directs.
Sample Handling	
1. Improper handling of controls.	Introduce a new control sample. a. Be sure sample has been at room temperature 24 hours before use. b. Shake 10 seconds to equilibrate the gas/liquid phase. c. Break open control sample and use within 1 minute.
2. Insufficient aspiration of sample.	Introduce new sample. a. If automatic aspiration is used, check for proper suction. b. Replace pump tubing, if necessary. c. Check seals around sample chamber.
3. Entrapped air bubble in measuring chamber.	Remove bubble by suction, thoroughly flush and introduce a new sample.
4. Contamination or carry-over from a previous sample.	Flush system thoroughly as manufacturer directs, followed by a rinse.
5. Microbial contamination; insufficient cleaning of PO_2 system.	Flush with cleaner as manufacturer directs, followed by a rinse.
6. Room air contamination.	a. Check proper syringe technique or use adapter. b. Clean aspiration tip; check for pinholes in this tubing. c. Check for poor connections or pinholes in internal tubing.
Electrode	
1. Protein buildup on membrane.	Clean as manufacturer directs or replace membrane.
2. Stretched, folded, or improperly positioned membrane on PO_2 electrode.	Replace membrane.
3. Bubbles entrapped under PO_2 membrane.	Remove membrane. Clean or buff top of electrode as manufacturer directs; rinse well, and replace membrane.
4. Improper electrolyte, insufficient amount of old electrolyte solution.	Remove electrode assembly; replace with fresh electrolyte solution to the proper level.
5. Bubbles in newly refilled PO_2 electrolyte solution.	Remove electrode and gently tilt to dislodge bubbles adhering to walls of electrode.
6. Contamination of the platinum tip of the PO_2 electrode.	Clean electrode tip as recommended by manufacturer and replace membrane.

Table 4-2. ELECTRODE TROUBLESHOOTING GUIDES—*cont'd.*

Possible Cause	Corrective Action
7. Electrode temperature not at 37° C.	a. Check water level in water bath.
	b. Check thermometer for break in mercury column; replace if necessary.
	c. Set instrument temperature to 37° C.
	d. Allow sufficient time for instrument to fully equilibrate to 37° C before use.
	e. Check circulation of water by pump.
	f. Reduce gas flow rate as manufacturer directs.
8. Improperly seated electrode causing flush solution or sample to remain in chamber.	Remove and reposition electrode.
	a. Dry with cotton swab and introduce new samples.
	b. If leakage continues, contact manufacturer.
9. Defective electrode due to aging or hairline crack or scratches on electrode.	Replace electrode.
10. Room air contamination from leakage around electrode.	Replace O rings and seals. If leakage persists, call manufacturer.
Electrical	
1. Open circuit.	Check all lines to ensure proper connection. Test with jumper strap as manufacturer directs.
2. Poor grounding on instrument.	Check to ensure that the instrument is properly grounded.
3. Faulty cables, loose connectors.	Check for a good fit. If any cables, connectors, or fittings are loose or broken, contact manufacturer for service.
4. Faulty meter causing a shift in calibration or a nonlinear response.	Contact manufacturer for service.

Gases

Gases have been used as quality control materials for O_2 and CO_2 electrodes in the past in much the same way that they are used as calibration standards. Gases must always be certified regarding their contents if they are to be used for this purpose. Electrodes, however, do not always react to the partial pressure of a gas in a gas mixture and the partial pressure of a gas in a liquid exactly the same way. This phenomenon was alluded to in the discussion of calibration of the PO_2 electrode as the *blood-gas factor*.

Table 4-3. FIVE WESTGARD RULES

No. of Measurements	Variation	Action
1	(±) 2 SD	Closely monitor
1	(±) 3 SD	Correct sensor
2 consecutive	(±) 2 SD	Correct sensor
4 consecutive	(±) 1 SD	Correct sensor
10 consecutive	(all same side mean)	Correct sensor

SD, Standard deviations.
Modified from Hicks, G. H.: Blood gas and acid-base measurement. In Dantzker, D. R., MacIntyre, N. R., Bakow, E. D. (eds): Comprehensive Respiratory Care. Philadelphia, W. B. Saunders, 1995.

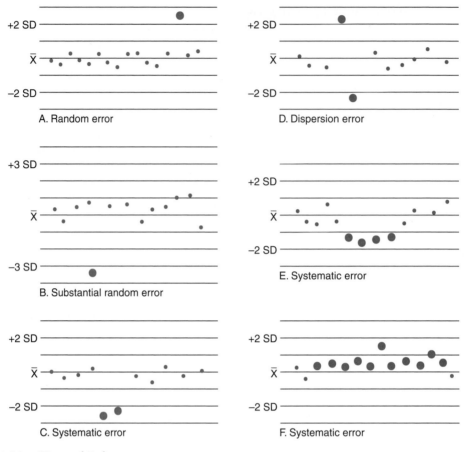

Figure 4-16.   **Westgard Rules.**

Tonometered Liquids

A tonometer is a device that allows for the bubbling of a gas with a known pressure through a liquid until equilibrium is reached. *Tonometry* is the time-tested method for preparing controls and in some institutions may even be the most cost-effective method.[130] The major disadvantage of tonometry is that equilibration with the fluid takes 20 minutes or longer.[130]

Aqueous Buffers

Again, as described under calibration, aqueous (i.e., waterlike) buffers of known pH may be used as controls for evaluation of the pH electrode. However, electrodes have been shown to respond differently to buffers than to blood. Aqueous buffers do not contain protein. They also have different actual buffering capabilities than blood. Finally, they may respond in

a different manner than blood to temperature variations.

Aqueous buffers can be placed in a tonometer and equilibrated with gases to a particular partial pressure. Here again, however, the problems of the aqueous buffers behaving differently compared with blood cannot be avoided.

Whole Blood

Alternatively, whole blood can be placed in the tonometer to eliminate this problem. Nevertheless, the problems associated with handling blood products (e.g., acquired immunodeficiency syndrome, other infections) make this alternative less than optimal.

Emulsions

Emulsions are substances in which two immiscible (non-mixable) liquids are together in solution. One of the liquids is dispersed in the

ON CALL | CASE 4-2 *ABGs and Critical Thinking*

You are the only person available to care for this patient. You must assess the patient/situation and act accordingly.

A 38-year-old woman is admitted to the emergency department with severe pneumonia and a temperature of 41° C.

ARTERIAL BLOOD GASES

SaO$_2$	85%
pH	7.30
PaCO$_2$	41 mm Hg
PaO$_2$	62 mm Hg
[HCO$_3$]	25 mEq/L

(data have been temperature-corrected to 41° C)

ASSESSMENT

Abnormalities: List abnormal data and other noteworthy information.

Explanation: List possible diseases, pathology, or other situations that may have lead to this patient's condition or these laboratory values.

Evaluation: Suggest additional data that would be useful in helping understand the situation or in making a diagnosis.

INTERVENTION

Importance: Prioritize concern(s) of treatment in order of urgency and/or seriousness as you see the overall situation.

Objective: Specifically state the measurable or observable outcomes you would like treatment to accomplish.

Action: Describe your specific plan of action.

other in the form of small droplets. Certain types of emulsions have been shown to behave similarly to blood regarding temperature characteristics and electrode performance. Emulsions could be tonometered and used as controls; however, there is little evidence that this is being done.

Comercially Prepared Controls

The final type of controls and probably the most widely used are commercially prepared controls that are sometimes referred to as *assayed liquids*. Commercial controls are prepared carefully by the manufacturer to ensure concise reproducible results. They are easy to use and eliminate the time-consuming preparation required by tonometry.[137]

Aqueous commercial controls have been widely used in the past. Their precision for pH and PCO$_2$ is good but this is not generally true for PO$_2$.[130] Aqueous controls are temperature-dependent and can be affected simply from the heat of the technician's hand.[138]

Commercially prepared fluorocarbon-based emulsions function more like blood than simply aqueous buffers. Fluorocarbon-based emulsions are probably the best commercially prepared controls.[130]

CONTINUOUS MONITORING OF BLOOD GASES

Introduction

Although the development of blood gas electrodes has greatly enhanced the care of patients, traditional blood gas measurements have distinct limitations. Specifically, they are limited by the fact that they do not provide us with continuous, real-time information. Electrode technology has been restricted historically to a measurement technique. *Measurement* techniques provide the clinician with information about an isolated point in time. Measurement techniques may be compared with *monitoring* techniques such as an electrocardiogram tracing. Monitoring techniques, on the other hand, provide the clinician with continuous information.

Likewise, blood gases are also limited because they do not provide us with *real-time information*. Typically, blood is sampled at one point in time; then, at a later time the blood is analyzed via the blood gas electrodes. Thus, blood gas information is "after the fact" rather than "here and now." Obviously, real-time information is more useful in the evaluation and management of patients. Newer techniques are being explored, however, that allow for continuous, real-time monitoring of blood gases.

Transcutaneous Techniques

The skin PO_2 can be monitored continuously and on a real-time basis via a transcutaneous PO_2 monitor. Skin PO_2, however, is often very different than blood PO_2. Furthermore, these monitors may be associated with complications (e.g., skin burns).

Continuous Intra-Arterial Blood Gases

Research has continued, however, in search of monitoring instruments that can continuously measure blood gases in vivo (i.e., within the body). Several types of in vivo blood gas monitors have been described for this application.[139] In general, these instruments use miniature electrode systems or, more commonly, optodes.

Miniature Electrode Systems

The *electrochemical oxygen probe* consists of a device that could be used to continuously monitor in vivo PO_2.[140] This probe contains a miniature version of the Clark electrode, and the entire probe is small enough that it can be placed within a radial artery catheter.

These miniature electrodes, however, must be temperature-compensated because both PO_2 and electrode current are temperature-sensitive variables. Corrections in temperature may be made manually by entering the patient's temperature into the instrument. Alternatively, corrections in temperature may be accomplished automatically via a special temperature probe attachment.

One concern regarding the electrochemical oxygen probe is that the membrane is susceptible to protein deposits or platelet adhesions. In general, these miniature electrodes are susceptible to a variety of technical problems (e.g., electrode drift, current leakage, corrosion); greater success has been achieved with the use of optode technology.

Optode Technology

Measurement Principles

In contrast to an electrode, an *optode* is a sensor that operates via optical detection of altered light.

The primary blood gas parameters (PO_2, pH, PCO_2) alter photochemical reactions that, in turn, affect light transmission through fiberoptic optical fibers. Fundamentally, the change in light detection is proportional to the blood gas value being measured. Most optodes operate either on the basis of light absorption or fluorescence.[152]

Absorbance optodes, sometimes called transmission optodes, transmit light through an indicator solution and measure the light exiting the solution. The exiting light will be decreased due to the absorption of some of the light by the analyte being measured. The pH or PCO_2 may be measured with this technique. A schematic representation of a CO_2 absorbance or transmission based optode is shown in Figure 4-17.

Fluorescence optodes, on the other hand, measure changes in fluorescence secondary to the analyte being measured. Fluorescence is light emitted from a dye at a lower frequency (i.e., longer wavelength) immediately following cessation of previous light exposure.

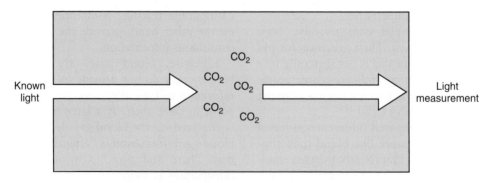

Figure 4-17. **CO_2 Absorption/Transmission Optode.**

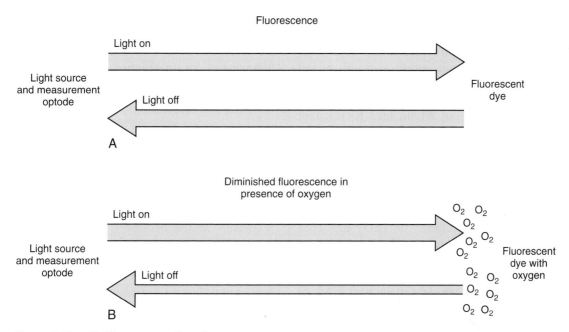

Figure 4-18. O_2 Fluorescence Optode.

PO₂ Measurement

Certain fluorescent dyes decrease their fluorescence in the presence of oxygen.[139] Furthermore, this decrease is in proportion to the amount of oxygen present. Therefore, PO_2 can be determined accurately via fluorescence. A schematic representation of fluorescence (**A**) and diminished fluorescence (**B**) in the presence of increased oxygen is shown in the oxygen optode depicted in Figure 4-18. Fluorescence systems can be made very small and require no direct electrical contact with the patient.

pH Measurement

Measurement of pH may also be accomplished by analyzing the fluorescent properties of certain weak acids at specific light wavelengths. The degree of dissociation of the acid can be determined based on these measurements. Ultimately, the actual pH of the solution can similarly be determined based on the degree of dissociation of the weak acid.

PCO₂ Measurement

A fluorescent CO_2 detector functions much like the fluorescent pH sensor; however, the PCO_2 sensor incorporates a CO_2 permeable membrane between the blood and the actual fluid being measured by fluorescence. Like the Severinghaus electrode system, CO_2 diffuses across the membrane and changes the pH of the fluid being measured. Thus, PCO_2 is determined indirectly based on the measured change in pH.

Monitoring Systems

The *Gas Stat instrument*[141] was the first to use fluorescent methods to monitor arterial and venous blood gases during surgery. Values obtained with the Gas Stat system correlate well with traditional blood gases although the Gas Stat PO_2 is consistently higher.[139] The Gas Stat system may possibly be more accurate than standard electrodes. Standard electrodes tend to underestimate PO_2 at high PaO_2 values, which are often seen during surgery. The Gas Stat system, however, is a large unit that resides away from the patient.

Technical Issues in Continuous Intra-Arterial Blood Gases

The technology of continuous intra-arterial blood gas (CIABG) monitoring devices has now reached a sophisticated level. Devices which are currently available are quite accurate in arterial or venous blood even during periods of severe blood pressure or gas changes.[143,144] In addition, mixed venous gases can be readily monitored with these devices. Continuous monitoring of mixed venous PCO_2 may provide useful information about changes in cardiac output.[144] Because a poor cardiac output would lead to stagnant systemic blood and an increase in PCO_2, an abrupt increase in mixed venous PCO_2 may be the first clue to cardiovascular dysfunction.

Unfortunately, however, CIABG continues to be plagued with a variety of technical problems and a relatively high technical failure rate.[143,145] The accuracy of PaO_2 has been especially in question after large multicenter trials.[142] The accuracy of intravascular PO_2 optodes may be compromised by thrombosis, the "wall effect" (reading tissue wall PO_2), or reduced blood flow in the area of the sensor.[146] Ex vivo, on-demand monitors (described subsequently) that locate optodes outside the body in an arterial line may avoid these problems. There is also a decline in sensor performance over time and they should probably not be used for more than 6 days.[147]

At present, CIABG appears to be of value in carefully selected patient populations. Nevertheless, its invasive nature and high incidence of technical failure are worrisome. In addition, it will ultimately have to withstand a rigorous cost-benefit analysis.

Ex vivo (On-Demand) Systems

Ex vivo (on-demand) blood gas systems are also available that provide reliable, accurate, samples within 90 seconds and avoid some of the pitfalls of CIABG monitors. These systems differ from CIABG in that the measurement devices (e.g., optodes) are located outside of the patient and samples are drawn into the measurement devices on demand typically from the radial artery. Obviously, these are not true continuous monitoring devices but they do facilitate safe, accurate, and expedient sample acquisition on a frequent basis (i.e., as often as every 3 minutes).

Summary

The technology now exists to measure blood gases quickly (e.g., ex vivo) or monitor blood gases continuously (e.g., CIABG) in clinical practice. Care must be taken, however, because important issues remain regarding invasive monitoring techniques, such as the risk of thrombosis or infection and also the cost. Nevertheless, these new techniques may be lifesaving in certain situations and particularly in neonates. The future remains uncertain for continuous in vivo blood gas analysis systems.

POINT-OF-CARE TESTING

A great deal has been written in the last decade regarding point-of-care (POC) laboratory testing. Clearly, there is clinical value in being able to ascertain laboratory values immediately and accurately at the bedside (i.e., the point of care). In most cases, the availability of this instant information will expedite clinical decision-making.[148] At times it can bring about more rapid changes in treatment where timing is "of the essence."[148]

Furthermore, with more and more healthcare being delivered in alternative sites and homes, portable, POC blood gas systems that provide accurate, immediate results would be very beneficial. POC systems are also designed to be very customer-friendly and relatively error-proof for the end user because this person may have a limited understanding of the procedure and potential mistakes. The demand for POC blood gas systems has spawned the development of a variety of accurate and reliable systems.[149] Many of these systems also offer the availability of concurrent electrolyte measurements as well.[149,150] The central blood gas laboratory should carefully monitor the implementation and continued use of POC systems to ensure continued quality control and performance.

The ultimate test for POC systems will be their ability to provide this information accurately and expediently at a reasonable cost. Many clinicians continue to be skeptical of the cost-benefit ratio of these devices because they are often somewhat more expensive to run than traditional blood gas systems. The question will need to be answered: Is the difference in turnaround time clinically significant in measurable outcomes and does it justify the incremental cost?

Many hybrid versions of POC blood gases have also been developed for these very reasons. Certainly, satellite laboratories or the use of pneumatic tubes have also become increasingly popular. In one study, a satellite laboratory in the emergency department was displaced with a computerized pneumatic tube delivery system that proved to be cost-effective.[151] Not surprisingly, it appears that no single solution fits every organization, department, or laboratory. A careful detailed analysis of the procedures and systems that work best in your institution must be carried out. The NCCLS document on POC should be reviewed if POC testing is performed at your institution.

REGULATIONS AND LABORATORY ACCREDITATION

Blood gas laboratories are subject to considerable oversight and regulation. Evaluation of blood gas laboratories is included in site visits and inspections performed by the JCAHO. In addition, there are federal guidelines for blood gas laboratories and personnel that fall under the Clinical Laboratory Improvement Amendments (CLIA) of 1967 and 1988.

Many laboratories are also accredited under the very detailed regulations provided by the CAP. Administration of a blood gas lab requires careful adherence to governmental regulations and the various accreditation bodies and issues. A detailed discussion of these regulations is beyond the scope of this book. The reader is referred to the Internet sites in the Exercises at the end of this chapter.

EXERCISES

Exercise 4-1   Basic Electrical Principles

Fill in the blanks or select the best answer.

1. A type of energy resulting from a flow of electrons is called _____.

2. A negatively charged pole in a battery or generator is called the _____, whereas the positively charged pole is called the _____.

3. The force responsible for pumping electrons is called the _____ force.

4. The unit of measurement of electromotive potential is the (joule/ampere/volt).

5. An instrument that measures an unknown voltage by comparing it with a known reference voltage is a _____.

6. The unit of measurement of electrical current is the (watt/volt/ampere).

7. The unit of electrical resistance is the (watt/ohm/volt).

8. Write the equation for Ohm's law.

9. Electric power consumption is usually measured in (amps/watts/ohms/voltage).

10. A substance through which electrons can flow is called a _____.

Exercise 4-2 Electrodes and Terminology

Fill in the blanks or select the best answer.

1. By using proper chemistry terminology, blood gases are measured by (electrodes/electrochemical cell systems).

2. In this text, the term *electrode* refers to (an entire measuring system for one of the blood gases/an electric conductor or terminal).

3. In this text, a solid site where electrons enter or leave a liquid medium is called an (electrode/electrode terminal).

4. Blood gas electrode terminals may be composed of _____ or _____.

5. A single electrode terminal in contact with an electrolyte solution may also be called a _____.

6. State the two types of half-cells.

7. The half-cell where the actual electrochemical change takes place is called the _____ half-cell.

Exercise 4-3 The PO_2 Electrode

Fill in the blanks or select the best answer.

1. The PO_2 electrode incorporates a/an (ammeter/voltmeter).

2. The electrode terminal in the working half-cell of the PO_2 electrode is usually made of (platinum/silver).

3. The reference electrode terminal in the PO_2 electrode is made of (silver chloride/calomel).

4. When voltage is applied to the cathode of a PO_2 electrode, oxygen reacts with water and (consumes/produces) electrons.

5. PO_2 analysis via the oxygen electrode is often referred to as a _____ technique of gas analysis.

6. The PO_2 electrode that incorporates a semipermeable membrane to prevent contact of the blood with the electrode terminal is called the _____ electrode.

7. Most membranes on modern PO_2 electrodes are made of _____.

8. The chamber that holds the blood sample in the electrode is called the _____.

9. In the electrical system of the Clark electrode, the silver is positively charged and serves as the (cathode/anode).

10. The PO_2 is directly proportional to the electrical current only in a specific (amperage/voltage) range.

Exercise 4-4 The pH Electrode

Fill in the blanks or select the best answer.

1. In the pH electrode, a single unique pH-sensitive, _____ electrode terminal serves as a common electrode terminal for both the reference solution and the solution of unknown pH.

2. The pH-sensitive glass in the pH electrode is the (working/reference) half-cell.

3. There (is/is not) actual flow of electrical current in the pH electrode.

4. The pH electrode works on the (potentiometric/polarographic) principle.

5. The relationship between voltage and pH at a given temperature is described by the modified _____.

6. One of the two major components of the traditional pH electrode has the pH-sensitive glass at the tip and a (silver chloride/calomel) half-cell inside it.

7. The reference half-cell in the pH electrode uses a (silver chloride/calomel) electrode terminal.

8. A calomel electrode terminal is made of _____/_____.

9. A salt or contact bridge may also be referred to as a _____.

10. The (silver chloride/calomel) electrode terminal functions best in KCl solution.

Exercise 4-5 The PCO$_2$ Electrode

Fill in the blanks or select the best answer.

1. In the PCO$_2$ electrode, blood (does/does not) come in direct contact with the pH-sensitive glass.

2. The CO$_2$ permeable membrane of a CO$_2$ electrode is often made of _____.

3. (Bicarbonate/phosphate) solution is in direct contact with the glass electrode and the silver chloride electrode terminal in the PCO$_2$ electrode.

4. The PCO$_2$ electrode has (one/two) AgCl electrode terminals within it.

5. A salt bridge (is/is not) necessary in the PCO$_2$ electrode.

6. The chemical reaction that takes place in the PCO$_2$ electrode is known as the (carbolysis/hydrolysis) reaction.

7. The clinical PCO$_2$ electrode is also known as the _____ electrode.

8. The PCO$_2$ electrode actually measures (voltage/current) change.

9. PCO$_2$ electrodes are accurate to within ±_____ mm Hg.

10. The least accurate of the blood gas electrodes is the (pH/PO$_2$/PCO$_2$) electrode.

Exercise 4-6   Quality Assurance/Preventive Maintenance

Fill in the blanks or select the best answer.

1. Total quality management in the laboratory is currently more focused on (clinical/statistical) decision-making with laboratory results.

2. A systematic procedure used to monitor, document, and regulate the accuracy and reliability of a given procedure or laboratory measurement is called _____.

3. Error that occurs during the actual analysis of the blood gas sample is called _____ error.

4. Failure to mix an iced sample may raise the pH by as much as (0.3/0.1/0.05) units.

5. Most blood gas samples achieve equilibration to 37° C within _____ minutes after introduction into the machine.

Exercise 4-7   Quality Control and Statistics

Fill in the blanks or select the best answer.

1. The periodic checking of an instrument's performance to ensure calibration, stability, and reliability is called _____.

2. External quality control is also known as _____ testing.

3. The _____ is the arithmetic average.

4. A statistical measure of the dispersion of a group of numbers is the _____.

5. In the normal population, _____% of measured values will fall within 1 SD.

6. In the normal population, _____% of measured values will fall within 2 SDs.

7. (PaO_2/$PaCO_2$) has the largest SD.

8. The higher the SD, the (more/less) homogeneous is the group.

9. The most appropriate statistic for comparison of the degree of variation between two measurements with sharply different means is the _____.

10. Coefficient of variation is expressed in units of (%/mm Hg).

Exercise 4-8 **Quality Control Charts-1**

Fill in the blanks or select the best answer.

1. Samples with known blood gas values that are periodically run to ensure that the machine is operating correctly are called _____.

2. It has been recommended that at least _____ levels of controls be run every _____ hour shift.

3. State the two general types of quality control records.

4. Quality control charts are usually referred to as _____ charts or plots.

5. Recurrent measurable deviation away from the mean is called _____ error.

6. Systematic error in which progressive controls steadily increase or decrease is called _____.

7. Systematic error characterized by an *abrupt* change in the measured value followed by clustering or plateauing in the new area is called _____.

8. A single control measurement outside the normal range is called _____.

9. A pattern of frequent random error is referred to as _____.

10. A result falling right on the control line of a Levey-Jennings chart is said to be _____.

Exercise 4-9 **Quality Control Charts-2**

Fill in the blanks or select the best answer.

1. _____ is a measure of how closely measured results reflect the true or actual value.

2. _____ is an index of dispersion of repeated measurements.

3. Dispersion on a Levey-Jennings chart indicates a problem with (accuracy/precision).

4. Shifting on a Levey-Jennings chart indicates a problem with (accuracy/precision).

5. List two potential causes of trending.

6. Drift of the pH electrode, when buffer is left in it, should not exceed _____ units per hour.

7. Buffers remaining in the pH electrode cause (alkaline/acid) drift.

8. Electrode drift should not exceed _____% within 5 minutes.

9. (Results/time) is on the y-axis of a Levey-Jennings chart.

10. (Three/two) levels of controls should be run at least once per shift.

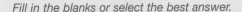

Exercise 4-10   Types of Controls

Fill in the blanks or select the best answer.

1. Gases (do/do not) affect electrodes in the same way that liquids affect them.

2. Aqueous buffers (do/do not) contain protein.

3. A _____ is a device that typically allows for the bubbling of a gas with a known pressure through a liquid until equilibrium is reached.

4. The major disadvantage of tonometry is (time/expense).

5. Whole blood is less than optimal as a control because it is (inaccurate/an infectious risk).

6. _____ are substances in which two immiscible liquids are together in solution, one of the liquids being dispersed in the other in the form of small droplets.

7. (Aqueous fluids/Emulsions) behave similarly to blood.

8. The most widely used types of controls are prepared (commercially/by tonometry).

9. The precision of aqueous commercial controls is not generally good regarding ($pH/PCO_2/PO_2$).

10. Probably the best commercially prepared controls are _____-based emulsions.

Exercise 4-11   Continuous Blood Gas Monitoring

Fill in the blanks or select the best answer.

1. Traditionally, blood gases have been a (monitoring/measurement) technique.

2. Standard blood gases (do/do not) provide us with real-time information about patients.

3. Monitoring that is done within the body is referred to as (in vivo/in vitro).

4. The electrochemical oxygen probe uses the (Clark/fluorescence) principle.

5. In vivo electrodes (must/need not) be temperature corrected.

6. Certain fluorescent dyes decrease their fluorescence in the presence of _____.

7. Continuous monitoring of mixed venous PCO_2 may provide useful information about _____.

8. The first fluorescent blood gas system used in the operating room was the (Gas Stat/CDI 1000) system.

9. Inadvertent reading of tissue wall PO_2 is known as the _____ effect.

10. A blood gas system where the measurement devices are outside the patient but constantly available at the bedside is called a/an (CIABG/ex vivo) system.

Internet Work

1. Please go to the site cms.hhs.gov/clia. Using the FAQ section, write a short description of:
   A) CMS
   B) CLIA

2. Visit the College of American Pathologists site (*cap.org*). Explore the laboratory accreditation site and explain what CAP accreditation means.

3. Visit Westgard.com and describe two current issues of concern regarding quality management systems.

NBRC Challenge 4

Please select the best answer for the following multiple choice questions.

1. When large adjustments in current are required during calibration of the Clark electrode or when the system behaves erratically:
   A) the cathode should be cleaned and the membrane should be changed.
   B) the anode should be de-proteinized.
   C) the water bath temperature should be re-adjusted.
   D) the current should be increased gradually until readings become stable.
   E) the potentiometer should be zeroed and the measurement repeated.
   (RRT EXAM-NBRC Matrix II,B,2,h,4)

2. Running standardized samples from a laboratory outside your institution to see how your lab compares with others is an example of:
   I) internal quality control.
   II) external quality control.
   III) monitoring equipment for precision.
   IV) proficiency testing.
   A) I and III only
   B) II and IV only
   C) I, III, and IV
   D) II,III, and IV
   E) I, II, III, and IV
   (RRT EXAM-NBRC Matrix II,B,3)

3. An aging electrode or protein contamination of the electrode will lead to a Levey-Jennings pattern of:
   A) shifting.
   B) trending.
   C) dispersion.
   D) random error.
   E) stagnatation.
   (RRT EXAM-NBRC MATRIX II,B,1,h,4)

4. When there is an increase in dispersion of values and the standard deviation from the mean increases, there is a problem with measurement _____.
   A) trending
   B) shifting
   C) accuracy
   D) precision
   E) proficiency
   (RRT EXAM-NBRC MATRIX II,B,3,a)

5. A blood gas PaO_2 error due to the "wall effect" could occur with measurements made via:
   A) transcutaneous techniques.
   B) ex vivo methods.
   C) CIABG.
   D) on-demand methods.
   E) POC systems.
   (RRT EXAM-NBRC MATRIX II,B,1,h,4)

Chapter 5

Accuracy Check and Metabolic Acid-Base Indices

Of the three variables in the H-H (Henderson-Hasselbalch) equation, any one obviously can be calculated if the other two are known.

Charles B. Spearman[591]

The problem in acid-base balance has been quantitation of the metabolic, or nonrespiratory, component, as HCO_3^- ion concentration is strongly dependent on the PCO_2.

John W. Severinghaus[588]

Outline

ACCURACY CHECK

The novice in blood gas application must master Chapter 2 before addressing the content in this chapter. Indeed, Chapter 5 deals with the less frequent and more subtle technical nuances of blood gas classification and analysis and may lead to confusion if routine blood gas classification is not fully understood. This chapter is intended for use when the clinician is faced with some real or perceived inconsistency in the reported information.

From an educational perspective, some instructors or clinicians may prefer to skip this chapter until a solid foundation of clinical blood gas interpretation is assured. Again, this chapter addresses primarily the recognition of "exceptions" to normal blood gas classification and interpretation and may be more suitable as supplementary reading, reference, or advanced study.

Fortunately, the types of technical errors discussed herein are less common than in the past.

In most state-of-the-art blood gas laboratories, blood gas results are *directly* printed to a report from the blood gas measurement device. These direct printouts preclude the possibility of human errors in transcription or oral reporting. The data on direct printouts can generally be assumed to be accurate assuming controls and safeguards discussed in previous chapters are adhered to. Notwithstanding, occasional errors still may occur and result in inappropriate diagnosis or treatment if they are not recognized.

The present chapter is included in this text for completeness, comprehensiveness, and critical analysis. Literal life-and-death decisions are made based on blood gas data. Errors in the diagnosis or management of acid-base or oxygenation status may have dire consequences. Therefore, individuals who are responsible for these decisions must have a thorough understanding of each index and the normal interrelationships between them. One must be able

ON CALL | CASE 5-1 *ABGs and Critical Thinking*

You are the only person available to care for this patient. You must assess the patient/situation and act accordingly.

A 55-year-old man in the burn unit suffers a cardiac arrest. Blood gases drawn during the arrest are called to the floor and reported as shown. Due to the negative base excess reported, the patient is given two ampules of sodium bicarbonate.

ARTERIAL BLOOD GASES

SaO$_2$	91%
pH	7.52
PaCO$_2$	47 mm Hg
PaO$_2$	63 mm Hg
[BE]	−11 mEq/L

ASSESSMENT

Abnormalities: List abnormal data and other noteworthy information. Classify ABG.

Explanation: List possible diseases, pathology, or other situations which may have led to this patient's condition.

Evaluation: Suggest additional data which would be useful in helping understand the situation or in making diagnosis.

INTERVENTION

Importance: Prioritize concern(s) of treatment in order of urgency and/or seriousness as you see the overall situation.

---

to detect inaccurate data, or explain and interpret seemingly inconsistent information.

Thus, at some point during the assessment of blood gas data, the clinician should briefly pause and consider the plausibility, consistency, and harmony of the various recorded data. Assessment of the consistency of the reported measurements is recommended in comprehensive and systematic acid-base assessment by most experts.[176] To ensure accuracy, blood gas values should be evaluated for *internal consistency* and *external congruity*.

Internal Consistency

Techniques for Evaluating Internal Consistency

Most often, gross inspection of blood gases facilitates the detection of internal inconsistencies. Conceptually, acidemia (i.e., pH < 7.35) cannot be present in the absence of a causative acidosis (i.e., PaCO$_2$ > 45 mm Hg and/or [HCO$_3$] < 22 mEq/L). Likewise, alkalemia cannot occur without alkalosis. Another type of gross inconsistency might be the presence of a normal pH with concurrent respiratory and metabolic acidosis. Here again, this combination of circumstances is impossible. Once the basic relationship between acidosis and acidemia is understood, most gross errors in blood gas data are easily and readily recognized.

Occasionally, technical error is less obvious. In these cases, the blood gas values generally

make sense but something doesn't seem exactly right. Example 5-1 may serve as an example.

Example 5-1

pH	7.60
PaCO$_2$	30 mm Hg
[HCO$_3$]	23 mEq/L

Example 5-1 is *not* internally consistent. The pH is too high given a PaCO$_2$ of 30 mm Hg and essentially normal metabolic status. Actually, the pH must be approximately 7.50. Failure to detect this inconsistency could have undesirable diagnostic or therapeutic consequences. A pH of 7.60 indicates severe alkalemia and should be cause for serious concern. A pH of 7.50 is common in the intensive care unit and most often requires no intervention.

The following discussion explores four methods that can be used to assess internal consistency when errors may be more subtle. These methods are indirect metabolic assessment, the rule of eights, the modified Henderson equation, and an acid-base map. All of these methods make use of the principle that the three acid-base components (i.e., pH, PaCO$_2$, and [HCO$_3$] or alternatively [BE]) are interrelated such that if two components are known, the third component can be deduced.

Indirect Metabolic Assessment

The metabolic tendency (e.g., presence of metabolic acidosis or metabolic alkalosis) can actually be determined without ever looking at a metabolic index. *Indirect metabolic assessment* is based on the principle that any change in pH must be a result of either the metabolic or the respiratory component because these components are the two sole factors that determine pH. If pH has changed and it is not of respiratory origin, it must be due to a metabolic acid-base change.

Acute PaCO₂–pH Relationship

To simplify these relationships for a moment, assume that all metabolic factors are normal and constant. Under these circumstances, any deviation of pH from normal *must* be a result of a change in respiratory status. If it was known exactly how much a given acute change in $PaCO_2$ would alter pH, then the precise pH that would be present with a given $PaCO_2$ could be predicted.

Assuming normal, constant metabolic status, the amount that pH will change in response to a given $PaCO_2$ change is constant and is termed the *acute PaCO₂–pH relationship*. The acute $PaCO_2$–pH relationship for both increases or decreases in $PaCO_2$ is shown in Table 5-1. A different pH change factor is necessary for a decrease in $PaCO_2$ than for an increase in $PaCO_2$ because of the logarithmic nature of these relationships.

Expected pH

Using a pH of 7.40 and a $PaCO_2$ of 40 mm Hg as our baseline, the expected pH that would result from a specified change in $PaCO_2$ could thus be calculated. For example, if

Table 5-2. Important Landmarks of Acute $PaCO_2$–pH Relationship

PaCO₂	pH
20	7.60
25	7.55
30	7.50
35	7.45
40	7.40
50	7.34
60	7.28
70	7.22
80	7.16
90	7.10

$PaCO_2$ decreases 10 mm Hg (i.e., from 40 to 30 mm Hg), pH increases 0.10 or from 7.40 to 7.50. Conversely, if $PaCO_2$ increased acutely to 50 mm Hg, the expected pH (assuming normal metabolic tendency) would be 7.34.

Important landmarks in the relationship between $PaCO_2$ and pH are shown in Table 5-2. It may be useful for the clinician to memorize these relationships. When a more precise calculation is desired, specific calculation of the *expected pH* for any $PaCO_2$ can also be accomplished by application of the formulas shown in Box 5-1.

Indirect Metabolic Status

After the expected pH has been calculated for a given $PaCO_2$, it can be compared with the actual pH on the blood gas report as a means of "indirect metabolic assessment." Because the acute $PaCO_2$–pH relationship holds true only when metabolic status is normal, if actual pH is equal to the expected pH it can be concluded that metabolic status is, indeed, unchanged and normal.

Table 5-1. Acute $PaCO_2$–pH Relationship

PaCO₂ Change	pH Change
DECREASE	INCREASE
1 mm Hg	0.01
10 mm Hg	0.10
INCREASE	DECREASE
1 mm Hg	0.006
10 mm Hg	0.06

Box 5-1 Calculation of Expected pH

IN HYPOCARBIA

Expected pH = 7.40 + (40 mm Hg – $PaCO_2$) 0.01

IN HYPERCARBIA

Expected pH = 7.40 – ($PaCO_2$ – 40 mm Hg) 0.006

On the other hand, it is likewise true that if the actual pH is not equal to the expected pH, the metabolic status cannot be normal. This is intuitively correct because any alteration in pH that is not of respiratory origin must be metabolic. The clinician should understand that indirect metabolic assessment is only an approximation (albeit a very good one) and that very small differences between actual and expected pH (e.g., ±0.02) can be attributed to slight measurement error. Blood gas electrode error alone may result in discrepancies of at least ±0.01.

For this reason, a ±0.03 comparison factor is recommended. Indirect metabolic assessment using this factor correlates very well with metabolic assessment using the base excess of extracellular fluid [BE]ecf that is described later in this chapter.

The possible outcomes of indirect metabolic assessment based on comparison of actual and expected pH are defined in Table 5-3. When the actual pH is equal to the expected pH ±0.03, the metabolic status must be normal. When the actual pH is significantly more acidic than expected (i.e., more than 0.03 pH units lower), a metabolic acidosis must be present. Conversely, when actual pH is significantly more alkaline (more than 0.03 pH units) than expected, a metabolic alkalosis (nonrespiratory condition tending to cause alkalemia) must be present. These conclusions closely parallel metabolic diagnosis that is made directly with the [BE]ecf to be discussed later in this chapter.

The values in Example 5-1 presented earlier are used to show the application of indirect metabolic assessment to evaluate internal consistency. Based on the acute $PaCO_2$–pH relationship, the expected pH for a $PaCO_2$ of

30 mm Hg is 7.50. Therefore, in a patient with this $PaCO_2$ level and normal metabolic status, one would expect to find an *actual* pH within ±0.03 of 7.50.

The patient's actual pH in Example 5-1 is 7.60, which is much higher than expected. Therefore, the patient *must* also have a concomitant metabolic alkalosis based on the acute $PaCO_2$–pH relationship. The finding of a normal metabolic index (i.e., [HCO_3] 23 mEq/L) is not consistent with the indirect finding. The problem in this case could have been a transcription error. The patient's actual pH should have been 7.50. A pH of 7.50 would make these data internally consistent.

In summary, metabolic status may be accurately assessed indirectly without ever seeing a metabolic index. In fact, using indirect metabolic assessment, a complete blood gas acid-base classification can also be made based on the $PaCO_2$ and pH alone in the event that a metabolic index is, for some reason, unavailable. This technique is likewise a useful tool in attempting to validate or invalidate the internal consistency of a questionable blood gas report.

A lack of internal consistency does not indicate where an error has occurred. Nevertheless, it is clear evidence that an error is present, and the clinician or laboratory diagnostician should be alerted with regard to the need for further investigation and clarification.

Rule of Eights

A similar tool for detecting technical error may be referred to as the *rule of eights*, which provides a mechanism for predicting the plasma bicarbonate when the pH and $PaCO_2$ are known. If the reported bicarbonate differs significantly from the bicarbonate calculated via the rule of eights (e.g., >4 mEq/L difference), a technical error is likely present. To calculate the predicted plasma bicarbonate, the $PaCO_2$ is multiplied by a factor that varies with the pH. The factor to be used with a given pH can be found in Table 5-4.

Modified Henderson Equation

The Henderson equation to be described later in Chapter 8 can be modified to relate [H^+] in nanoequivalents per liter (instead of pH) to

Table 5-3. INDIRECT METABOLIC ASSESSMENT

Actual pH–Expected pH Relationship	Indirect Metabolic Status
Actual pH = expected pH ± 0.03	Normal metabolic status
Actual pH > expected pH + 0.03	Metabolic alkalosis
Actual pH < expected pH − 0.03	Metabolic acidosis

Table 5-4. RULE OF EIGHTS
(Factor × PaCO$_2$) = Predicted bicarbonate

pH	Factor
7.60	8/8
7.50	6/8
7.40	5/8
7.30	4/8
7.20	2.5/8
7.10	2/8

Table 5-5. RELATIONSHIP BETWEEN pH AND [H$^+$]

pH	[H$^+$] nEq/L
7.80	16
7.70	20
7.60	25
7.55	28
7.50	32
7.45	35
7.40	40
7.35	45
7.30	50
7.25	56
7.20	63
7.15	71
7.10	79
7.00	100
6.90	126
6.80	159

PaCO$_2$ and [HCO$_3$] as shown in Equation 5-1. Thus, if any two of these three variables are known the third variable can be calculated.

Equation 5-1

$$[H^+] = 24 \times \frac{PaCO_2}{[HCO_3]}$$

To apply this formula, however, one must be able to convert pH units to hydrogen ion concentration in nanoequivalents per liter (nEq/L). To get an idea of how minute this unit is, a nanoequivalent is one millionth of an equivalent. A milliequivalent is equal to 10^{-3} equivalents. A microequivalent is equal to 10^{-6} equivalents, and a nanoequivalent is equal to 10^{-9} equivalents.

There is a near-linear relationship between [H$^+$] in nEq/L and pH over the pH range (7.20 to 7.50) shown in Table 5-5. It can also be seen that this linear relationship begins to deteriorate quickly beyond this range, especially with acidemia.

A pH of 7.40 is equivalent to a [H$^+$] of 40 nEq/L. As a general rule, for each 0.01 change in pH within the range of 7.20 to 7.50, there is a 1 nEq/L inverse change in [H$^+$]. Thus, a pH of 7.50 is equal to a [H$^+$] of 30 nEq/L, and a pH of 7.30 is equal to a [H$^+$] of 50 nEq/L.

By converting [H$^+$] to pH, Equation 5-1 can be used to check internal consistency of questionable blood gases. This equation is especially useful because it can be used to determine any of the three variables (i.e., pH, PaCO$_2$, or [HCO$_3$]) if the other two variables are known.

With regard to internal consistency, it should also be pointed out that acid-base values can be internally consistent, yet they can still be wrong.

For example, if the pH is measured incorrectly, the [HCO$_3$] is also wrong (although it is internally consistent) because it is calculated in the blood gas machine based on the pH and the PCO$_2$.

Acid-Base Map

The acid-base map is discussed in detail in Chapter 14 (see Fig. 14-1), which addresses the identification of mixed acid-base disturbances. Using an acid-base map, one can easily plot two acid-base variables on the map and determine the third. When readily available, the acid-base map is probably the easiest and most expedient way to assess internal consistency.

External Congruity

In addition to assessing internal consistency, the clinician should also evaluate reported data from other laboratories and the patient's general appearance to ensure external congruity. *External congruity* in this context means ensuring that all laboratory tests and observations are in concert and are harmonious with the blood gas results. A sign of incongruity is when blood gas numbers are not in harmony with the patient's appearance or other laboratory values. Incongruity is often the first clue regarding incorrect and/or misleading laboratory measurements.

Laboratory to Laboratory Congruity

Calculated Bicarbonate

The plasma bicarbonate can be used to evaluate external congruency because it is most often reported by two different, unrelated laboratories. Plasma bicarbonate is reported routinely on the arterial blood gas report. However, the bicarbonate reported on the blood gas report is not directly measured. Rather, it is a calculated value based on the Henderson-Hasselbalch equation.

Total CO_2

The plasma bicarbonate is also usually reported from the chemistry laboratory with standard electrolytes as *total CO_2* ([total CO_2]). Because plasma [HCO_3] comprises approximately 95% of total CO_2, these two measurement may essentially be viewed as being interchangeable.[176,177] One caveat is that total CO_2 is measured in the chemistry laboratory using venous blood, which is typically 2 to 3 mEq/L higher in bicarbonate. Nevertheless, total CO_2 is, for all practical purposes, an index of plasma bicarbonate. Therefore, the electrolyte report may be used as a crosscheck regarding the accuracy of the [HCO_3] reported on the blood gas report.

Historically, total CO_2 was introduced as a clinical metabolic acid-base index before the routine availability of blood gases. Today, total CO_2 is considered to have only minimal value as an isolated index because it must be interpreted in the context of pH and $PaCO_2$. Nevertheless, the [HCO_3] can easily be approximated from the total CO_2, and this value can be compared with the blood gas bicarbonate as a gross index of external congruity. As previously stated, total CO_2 should be expected to be slightly higher than bicarbonate from the blood gas report because it is measured from venous blood.

Total CO_2 Components

As discussed in Chapter 8, CO_2 is transported in the blood as bicarbonate, dissolved CO_2, and carbamino-compounds. Bicarbonate and dissolved CO_2 are responsible for almost all of the CO_2 present in the blood plasma. Therefore, total CO_2, usually reported in mEq/L, is

presumed to be equal to the sum of CO_2 dissolved in the plasma and plasma bicarbonate, which is shown in Equation 5-2. $PaCO_2$ may be multiplied by the conversion factor (0.03 mEq/L/mm Hg) to determine the dissolved CO_2 concentration in mEq/L.

Equation 5-2

$$[\text{Total } CO_2] = [\text{dissolved } CO_2] + [\text{bicarbonate}]$$
$$[\text{Total } CO_2] = (PaCO_2 \times 0.03) + 24$$
$$25.2 = 1.2 + 24 \ (\text{mEq/L})$$

Bicarbonate Calculation from Total CO_2

To calculate the specific [HCO_3], dissolved CO_2 in mEq/L is subtracted from the reported total CO_2 (see Equation 5-3). The difference represents plasma bicarbonate in mEq/L. Because the concentration of dissolved CO_2 in mEq/L is so small (typically 1 to 2 mEq/L) and bicarbonate represents 95% of the total CO_2 value, gross inspection of the total CO_2 provides a reliable estimation of plasma bicarbonate even without this calculation.

Equation 5-3

$$[\text{Total } CO_2] - [\text{dissolved } CO_2] = [\text{bicarbonate}]$$
$$25.2 - (PaCO_2 \times 0.03) = [\text{bicarbonate}]$$
$$25.2 - 1.2 = 24 \ (\text{mEq/L})$$

Keeping in mind the difference between arterial and venous blood bicarbonate, gross differences (e.g., >5 mEq/L) should arouse suspicion of erroneous measurements from one of the laboratories. One should also be aware that the measurement of total CO_2 is fraught with difficulty and the potential for the introduction of error. Blood for total CO_2 measurement should be collected anaerobically and serum promptly separated from whole blood (to avoid effects of metabolism) and stored at 4° C until analyzed. Just as in arterial samples, excessive heparin can dilute the sample and contaminate results. Air contamination is probably one of the most common errors.[176]

Despite the fact that total CO_2 is directly measured and bicarbonate from a blood gas report is a derived calculation, the blood gas is less prone to methodologic errors and is probably more reliable.[176] Notwithstanding, there should normally be a good correlation between these two measurements.

The clinician must also remember that blood gases and electrolytes are very dynamic measurements that may change hourly and even from one minute to another. Therefore, if this crosscheck mechanism is to be used, the blood gases and electrolytes to be compared must have been drawn in relative temporal proximity.

Patient-Laboratory Congruity

The experienced clinician is well aware of the hazards of relying too heavily on laboratory measurements. Any technical measurement is subject to error. The general appearance of the patient is a very important aspect of evaluating external congruence. For example, a pH of 7.10 in an otherwise normal, active, patient should arouse suspicion.

This concept is especially important with regard to oxygenation assessment and hypoxemia. A PaO_2 of 40 mm Hg typically elicits tachycardia, cyanosis, and respiratory distress. When the patient looks remarkably different than the data would suggest, the data must be questioned.

FIO$_2$–PaO$_2$ Incongruity

Most of the information in this chapter deals with acid-base errors rather than oxygenation errors for several reasons. First, more acid-base data are reported with blood gases (e.g., pH, [BE], [HCO_3]) than oxygenation data (e.g., PaO_2, SaO_2). In addition, clinical acid-base relationships are generally more complex and less well understood by many clinicians. Finally, the constant mathematical relationship between pH, [HCO_3], and PCO_2 facilitates the evaluation of internal consistency. No such precise mathematical relationship exists for oxygenation indices.

All this does not mean that the assurance of accurate oxygenation data is any less important. Indeed, a strong argument can be made that these data are in fact more important. Thus, the clinician must also be alert to the potential for errors in oxygenation indices. In particular, the PaO_2 on room air should not exceed 130 mm Hg even with hyperventilation. Also, a PaO_2 that is more than five times higher than the percentage of oxygen being inspired should also arouse suspicion.

For example, if a PaO_2 of 300 mm Hg is reported in a patient who is being mechanically ventilated with an FIO_2 of 0.4, something is wrong. Either the PaO_2 is incorrect or the FIO_2 is really higher than 0.4. In any event, the finding of a PaO_2 more than five times higher than the percentage of inspired oxygen is incongruent, and the source of the error must be sought.

SaO$_2$–SpO$_2$ Incongruity

The SpO_2 represents the oxygen saturation reading displayed by a pulse oximeter. When oxygen saturation of arterial blood (SaO_2) is also measured with an oximeter or a co-oximeter, these two values can be compared for congruency. More commonly, calculated oxygen saturation from a standard blood gas report may be compared with the SpO_2.

A basic understanding of the oxyhemoglobin dissociation curve (discussed in Chapter 7) is also a key to evaluating external congruity. As a rule, *saturation (SpO_2 or SaO_2) should be approximately 90% when PaO_2 is 60 mm Hg.* When one of these values is higher or lower, the other should follow suit in the same direction. For example, a PaO_2 of 50 mm Hg concurrent with an SpO_2 of 95% should arouse suspicion. There are situations (described in Chapter 7) when these relationships will be slightly altered (i.e., shifts of the oxyhemoglobin curve), but as a rule they should remain generally intact.

Sometimes, a discrepancy between two different techniques of saturation measurement is expected (e.g., increased COHb or metHb may lead to falsely elevated SpO_2 as compared to saturation measured via co-oximetry). These situations are described in more detail in other chapters. Notwithstanding, a discrepancy between two measures of oxygen saturation may be the first clue to erroneous values from one of the sources.

METABOLIC ACID-BASE INDICES

Introduction

In Chapter 2, a simple, straightforward method of blood gas classification was presented. Although the step-by-step sequence described in Chapter 2 most often leads to a correct classification, incorrect or misleading results may occur if $PaCO_2$ is significantly abnormal. Example 5-2 may serve as an example.

Example 5-2

pH	7.16
$PaCO_2$	80 mm Hg
[BE]	–4 mEq/L
[HCO_3]	28 mEq/L
Standard [HCO_3]	20 mEq/L
[BE]ecf	0 mEq/L
T_{40} standard [HCO_3]	24 mEq/L

It should be noted that three new metabolic indices have been introduced in this example: standard [HCO_3], T_{40} standard [HCO_3], and [BE]ecf. The value and significance of these indices as well as those presented earlier are explored in the following sections.

Based on the previous discussion of internal consistency, it would appear that the blood gas in Example 5-2 is not internally consistent. The base excess and standard bicarbonate both indicate a laboratory metabolic acidosis, whereas the plasma bicarbonate indicates a laboratory metabolic alkalosis. To further confuse the issue, the [BE]ecf and the T_{40} standard [HCO_3] suggest normal metabolic acid-base status. It turns out, however, that all the values reported on this blood gas are correct.

Shortcomings

The reason that some metabolic indices point in opposite directions is related to flaws or artifacts in the indices themselves. *Many metabolic indices manifest distortions in the presence of notable hypercapnia or hypocapnia.*

In Example 5-2, the [HCO_3] is falsely high as a metabolic acid-base indicator, whereas the standard [HCO_3] and [BE]blood are falsely low. The only metabolic indices that reflect the true normal metabolic status in this example are the [BE]ecf and the standard [HCO_3] T_{40}.

The remainder of this chapter describes the various metabolic indices that may be reported with arterial blood gases and their individual peculiarities. Metabolic acid-base indices are probably the most poorly understood area of clinical acid-base and blood gas application. It is hoped that this discussion may help to unravel some of the mystique and confusion associated with these indices.

Various Indices

All metabolic indices have been introduced into clinical medicine as tools to provide information about the nonrespiratory component of acid-base balance. The $PaCO_2$ is a clear, concise marker of the respiratory acid-base component. An increase in $PaCO_2$ always indicates increased carbonic acid and, conversely, a decrease in $PaCO_2$ always reflects a decrease in carbonic acid levels in the arterial blood. The search for a comparable metabolic index has been fraught with confusion and controversy that persists even presently.

Pre–Blood Gas Indices

Even before the routine availability of arterial blood gases, clinicians were well aware of the usefulness of plasma bicarbonate concentration in assessing the metabolic acid-base component. They understood that the [HCO_3] would tend to increase in metabolic alkalosis and decrease in metabolic acidosis through the buffering mechanism. Furthermore, the more severe the metabolic acidemia, the lower the [HCO_3] would be.

CO_2 Combining Power

The CO_2 *capacity,* often referred to as the CO_2 *combining power,* was described in 1917 by Van Slyke.[178] Venous blood was equilibrated with 5.5% CO_2 after removing the red blood cells. Then, the total CO_2 content of the separated plasma was measured. Because most of the CO_2 in plasma was in the form of bicarbonate, this index was really an indirect measure of plasma bicarbonate. This outmoded index is no longer used today.

Total CO_2

Four years later in 1921, Van Slyke also described the *total CO_2.*[179] With this technique, the CO_2 content of true plasma or serum was determined while taking precautions to prevent the loss of CO_2. As described earlier in this chapter, this index is also a reflection of plasma bicarbonate. Total CO_2 generally replaced the CO_2 combining power as a clinical index because it was much simpler to measure. Total CO_2

remains a standard value reported with most routine serum electrolytes.

Blood Gas Indices

Plasma Bicarbonate

With the development of the PCO_2 and pH electrodes, the plasma bicarbonate could be calculated easily from these measurements by using the Henderson-Hasselbalch equation. Thus, the *plasma bicarbonate* concentration, $[HCO_3]$, became a routine value reported with arterial blood gas results. The plasma bicarbonate is sometimes also called the *actual bicarbonate*.

Underlying Principle. As described in the discussion of buffers in Chapter 8, $NaHCO_3$ is consumed in the buffering of strong fixed acids by the bicarbonate buffer system. Because $NaHCO_3$ is completely ionized, the $[HCO_3]$ decreases in direct proportion to the amount of fixed acid buffered. Conversely, the $[HCO_3]$ increases in the presence of metabolic alkalosis.

Because the weak acid component of the bicarbonate buffer system is carbonic acid, however, this buffer system *cannot* buffer the excess carbonic acid that would build up in a respiratory acidosis. Therefore, from the standpoint of buffering, the $[HCO_3]$ only changes with nonrespiratory acid-base problems. Thus, it would seem to be an ideal indicator of metabolic (nonrespiratory) acid-base changes.

Hydrolysis Effect. It is indeed true that the plasma $[HCO_3]$ does not change as a result of buffering in respiratory acid-base problems. Unfortunately, however, $[HCO_3]$ changes in respiratory acid-base disturbances by another mechanism, the hydrolysis reaction. Because $[HCO_3]$ is one of the constituents of the hydrolysis reaction (see Chapter 8, Equation 4), it tends to increase in respiratory acidosis and decrease in respiratory alkalosis via the law of mass action. Thus, the plasma bicarbonate concentration $[HCO_3]$ is *not* a *pure* metabolic index.

As a rough guide, $[HCO_3]$ increases 1 mEq/L for every 10-mm Hg increase in $PaCO_2$ above 40 mm Hg via the hydrolysis reaction[180] (Box 5-2). The relationship is not linear, however, and when PCO_2 falls 5 mm Hg below normal, $[HCO_3]$ falls approximately 1 mEq/L.[180] For example, let us assume a normal baseline $[HCO_3]$ of 24 mEq/L and $PaCO_2$ of 40 mm Hg in a given individual. If $PaCO_2$ increases to

---

Box 5-2	Effects of PCO_2 Change on $[HCO_3]$

> **HYPERCARBIA**
>
> $[HCO_3]$ increases 1 mEq/L for 10 mm Hg PCO_2 increase
>
> **HYPOCARBIA**
>
> $[HCO_3]$ decreases 1 mEq/L for 5 mm Hg PCO_2 decrease

---

80 mm Hg, $[HCO_3]$ will increase 4 mEq/L (1 mEq/L for every 10-mm Hg $PaCO_2$ increase) to 28 mEq/L. Thus, the increase in $[HCO_3]$ to 28 mEq/L seen in Example 5-2 at the beginning of this section on metabolic indices is simply a result of the hydrolysis reaction. This is, in fact, the $[HCO_3]$ that one would expect to find in any patient with an acute increase in $PaCO_2$ to 80 mm Hg and no compensation. Therefore, the patient in this example has no metabolic (nonrespiratory) acid-base alteration. This is a pure, acute, respiratory acid-base problem.

Standard Bicarbonate

Measurement. The effect of PCO_2 on $[HCO_3]$ has prompted clinicians to seek an alternative to this metabolic index. A logical alternative would be to place the blood sample in a tonometer and to equilibrate the sample to a PCO_2 of 40 mm Hg. This would have the effect of normalizing PCO_2 within the sample and thus eliminating the hydrolysis effect. This procedure has in fact been used, and the resultant measurement is known as the standard bicarbonate.

The *standard bicarbonate* is defined technically as the plasma bicarbonate concentration obtained from blood that has been equilibrated at 37° C with a PCO_2 of 40 mm Hg and a PO_2 sufficient to produce full oxygen saturation.[6]

In Vivo–In Vitro Discrepancy. This procedure of standardizing the bicarbonate is done to the sample in the laboratory under in vitro (laboratory) conditions. Unfortunately, when PCO_2 is returned to 40 mm Hg in the patient, so-called in vivo conditions, a different bicarbonate level results. To understand the reason for this discrepancy, the exchange of bicarbonate that takes place between the plasma and the extravascular (outside the blood vessels) fluid with changes in PCO_2 must be understood.

Figure 5-1,*A* shows approximate normal values for $PaCO_2$, plasma $[HCO_3]$, and $[HCO_3]$ of the extravascular fluid. Actually, the $[HCO_3]$ in the interstitial (extravascular) fluid is slightly higher (approximately 3 mEq/L) than in the plasma (intravascular fluid). Nevertheless, to show the in vivo–in vitro discrepancy, both intravascular and extravascular $[HCO_3]$ are shown as being equal in Figure 5-1.

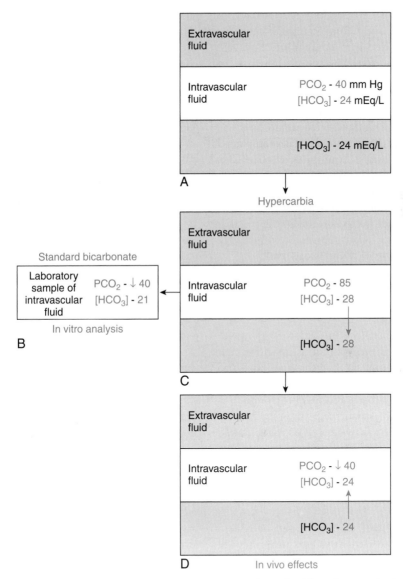

Figure 5-1. **In vivo–in vitro discrepancy in the measurement of standard bicarbonate. A,** Approximate normal values for $PaCO_2$, intravascular plasma $[HCO_3]$, and extravascular-interstitial fluid $[HCO_3]$. **B,** The effects of acute hypercarbia on $[HCO_3]$ in vivo in both intravascular and extravascular fluid spaces. **C,** The results of measuring standard bicarbonate on a blood sample taken at point B. The sample is equilibrated to a PCO_2 of 40 mm Hg in vitro by using a tonometer, and standard bicarbonate reads below normal. The bicarbonate that was lost to the extravascular fluid is unavailable to return to the sample. **D,** When PCO_2 returns to normal in vivo, bicarbonate returns from the interstitial fluid and results in a normal $[HCO_3]$.

As PaCO$_2$ increases acutely, plasma [HCO$_3$] increases via the hydrolysis reaction. A portion of this increased bicarbonate diffuses from within the vascular fluid (i.e., within the blood vessel) to the interstitial fluid. Thus, an increase in both plasma [HCO$_3$] and interstitial fluid [HCO$_3$] accompanies hypercarbia and is shown in Figure 5-1,*B*.

When PaCO$_2$ then quickly returns back to normal in this individual (i.e., 40 mm Hg in vivo), the excess bicarbonate in the extravascular fluid returns to the plasma and the patient manifests a normal [HCO$_3$] (see Fig. 5-1,*D*).

If blood is drawn from the patient at the point shown in Figure 5-1,*B*, plasma [HCO$_3$] is 28 mEq/L. If standard bicarbonate is to be measured on this same sample, it is then placed in a tonometer and is equilibrated to a PCO$_2$ of 40 mm Hg as shown in Figure 5-1,*C*. However, under these laboratory (in vitro) conditions, the bicarbonate that was lost to the interstitial fluid cannot be recaptured in the plasma. Therefore, when PCO$_2$ is returned to 40 mm Hg in vitro, a false low [HCO$_3$] is observed.

Thus, in the presence of hypercarbia, and in direct contrast to the actual bicarbonate, the standard bicarbonate indicates a false low result.

T$_{40}$ Standard Bicarbonate

The T$_{40}$ standard bicarbonate is an index that uses a nomogram to correct the standard bicarbonate for the in vivo–in vitro discrepancy.[181,182] The T$_{40}$ standard bicarbonate is probably the most accurate of the bicarbonate metabolic indices; however, it has not gained widespread popularity, which is probably due at least in part to the technical difficulty in measuring or calculating standard bicarbonate T$_{40}$.

Buffer Base

Description. The bicarbonate buffer system is only one of the buffer systems in the blood. The *whole blood buffer base* [BB], on the other hand, is the sum of *all* the buffer bases in 1 L of blood. Buffer base has the potential to be used as a metabolic index in exactly the same way that [HCO$_3$] is used. In other words, in response to buffering, [BB] decreases in the presence of increased fixed acids (metabolic acidosis) and increases with nonrespiratory (metabolic) alkalosis. Buffer base also has the

purported advantage of showing the effects of all buffering, not just buffering done by the bicarbonate buffer system.

Hemoglobin Dependency. Because hemoglobin is one of the blood buffer bases, its concentration affects the [BB]. At normal [Hb], [BB] is approximately 48 mEq/L.[183] At a [Hb] of 8 g%, the [BB] is approximately 45 mEq/L. In contrast, at a [Hb] of 20 g%, [BB] is 50 mEq/L.[183] Thus, [BB] depends on [Hb], and normal values for [BB] are [Hb]-dependent. Because different individuals have different baselines for [BB], it is not a particularly useful metabolic index.

Base Excess of Blood

Description. A more useful way to look at [BB] is to compare the normal [BB] for a given [Hb] with the observed [BB]. The difference between these two values is called the *base excess of blood* [BE] (Equation 5-4). Actually, if the observed [BB] is less than the normal [BB], the [BE] is a negative value and is technically a base deficit. Nevertheless, it is customary to refer to this index as the base excess, regardless of the actual numeric value.

Equation 5-4
Observed [BB] − normal [BB] = [BE]

In Vivo–In Vitro Discrepancy. Technically, base excess of the blood was determined originally by chemical titration. In other words, the milliequivalents of base or acid that had to be added or extracted from 1 L of whole blood to restore a normal [BB] was measured. In clinical blood gas analysis, however, the base excess of the blood is a value acquired from a Siggard Anderson nomogram based on in vitro chemical titration studies. The nomograms can also correct for different [Hb].

These nomograms, however, were constructed based on in vitro blood conditions. Therefore, the [BE] is subject to the same shortcoming as the standard bicarbonate. Some of the buffer base that diffused into the extravascular fluid compartment is not recaptured in these in vitro titration curves.

Consequently, [BE] of blood manifests false low results in the presence of hypercarbia similar to the standard bicarbonate value. The base excess of blood [BE] is also sometimes called the in vitro base excess ([BE] in vitro); however the term [BE] of blood or [BE]blood is recommended by the National Committee for Clinical Laboratory Standards.[6] In the presence of hypercarbia, the base excess of the blood decreases roughly 1 mEq/L for every 10 mm Hg increase in PCO_2.[177]

Unless otherwise specified, [BE] should be assumed to be [BE]blood. The base excess of the blood was the metabolic index used in the classification examples and exercises in Chapter 2.

Base Excess of Extracellular Fluid

A better index of the change in buffer base in the body would correct for shifts of bases that occur under in vivo conditions between the plasma and the interstitial fluid. In other words, this index would reflect all of the extracellular fluid and not just the blood plasma. There is, in fact, such an index, and it is called the *base excess of the extracellular fluid, [BE]ecf*, compared with the base excess of the blood.

Other symbols and terms that have been used for this index include in vivo base excess ([BE]in vivo), standard base excess ([SBE]), [BE]₃, and [BE]e.[177] The trend in some places is to report the [BE]ecf as simply [BE].[177] Unfortunately, many laboratories do not follow this practice, which leads to additional confusion in that two different values (i.e., base excess of blood and base excess of extracellular fluid) may be reported with the same symbol.

The National Committee for Clinical Laboratory Standards, in their *Standards for Definitions of Quantities and Conventions Related to Blood pH and Gas Analysis*,[6] has suggested that this index should be called the base excess of extracellular fluid, symbolized by [BE]ecf. This practice is followed throughout the remainder of this text.

It has been found that the base excess that would occur under in vivo conditions (e.g., [BE]ecf) is approximately equal to the [BE] value determined by using the base excess of the blood nomogram assuming an [Hb] of 5 g%. Because the buffer line associated with an [Hb] of 5 g% is always used to determine [BE]ecf, there is really no need to know the actual [Hb] of the patient to determine [BE]ecf.

pH–[BE]ecf Relationship. Methods for checking the internal consistency of blood gas data were presented earlier. Henderson's equation and the rule of eights were described as techniques for ensuring accuracy when the plasma bicarbonate was used as the metabolic index. Indirect metabolic assessment was also described and may be useful regardless of the metabolic index being used.

One final relationship that may be useful, especially for those clinicians who prefer the

---

ON CALL | CASE 5-2 *ABGs and Critical Thinking*

You are the only person available to care for this patient. You must assess the patient/situation and act accordingly.

A 25-year-old woman arrives in the emergency department in a coma.

ARTERIAL BLOOD GASES

SaO₂	85%
pH	7.16
PaCO₂	80 mm Hg
PaO₂	52 mm Hg
[BE] blood	−4 mEq/L
[HCO₃]	28 mEq/L

ASSESSMENT

Abnormalities: List abnormal data and other noteworthy information. Classify ABG.

Explanation: List possible disease, pathology, or other situations which may have led to this patient's condition.

Evaluation: Suggest additional data which would be useful in helping understand the situation or in making a diagnosis.

INTERVENTION

Importance: Prioritize concern(s) of treatment in order of urgency and/or seriousness as you see the overall situation.

Table 5-6.   pH–[BE]ECF RELATIONSHIP
(ASSUMING A CONSTANT $PaCO_2$
OF 40 mm Hg)

pH	[BE]ecf (mEq/L)
7.00	−20
7.11	−15
7.22	−10
7.33	−5
7.40	0
7.48	+5
7.55	+10
7.60	+15
7.66	+20

[BE]ecf to the [HCO_3] as a metabolic index, is the [BE]ecf–pH relationship when $PaCO_2$ is held constant at 40 mm Hg. Table 5-6 shows that for every change in [BE]ecf of 5 mEq/L, the pH changes approximately 0.1 units. Knowledge of this relationship may also prove to be useful in an evaluation of internal consistency.

Summary

All of the metabolic acid-base indices that have been used through the years share the characteristic that they are good indicators of metabolic acid-base status when $PaCO_2$ is normal. When $PaCO_2$ is altered significantly, however, many of these indices demonstrate artifacts. In hypercarbia, plasma bicarbonate rises in response to the hydrolysis reaction and the law of mass action. The standard bicarbonate corrects for $PaCO_2$ changes in vitro but suffers from in vivo–in vitro discrepancies. The base excess of the blood has similar drawbacks. Both of these indices are artificially low in the presence of hypercarbia.

Standard bicarbonate T_{40} and base excess of the extracellular fluid correct for both changes in $PaCO_2$ and in vivo–in vitro discrepancies. Therefore, they are the most pure metabolic indices. Overall, these indices are preferred when they are available.

Nevertheless, despite the formidable work done to find the ideal metabolic index, plasma bicarbonate and base excess of the blood are still probably the most common indices reported with arterial blood gases. The clinician should understand the disadvantages of these indices in blood gas classification and interpretation. In the end, however, any of the indices will suffice if the clinician understands their particular nuances and shortcomings.

EXERCISES

Exercise 5-1   Gross Inconsistency

Designate whether the following blood gases are mathematically consistent (C) or inconsistent (I).

	pH	PaCO₂	[BE]
1.	7.42	28	+4
2.	7.30	40	−7
3.	7.40	50	−5
4.	7.25	40	0
5.	7.35	25	0
6.	7.28	60	+1
7.	7.40	50	+5
8.	7.50	30	+1
9.	7.38	30	+5
10.	7.20	25	−18

Exercise 5-2 **Principles of Indirect Metabolic Assessment**

Fill in the blanks or select the best answer.

1. The metabolic tendency (can/cannot) actually be determined without looking at a metabolic index.

2. The pH increases _____ units for every 10 mm Hg decrease in PCO_2 acutely.

3. The pH decreases _____ units for every 10 mm Hg increase in PCO_2 acutely.

4. Acute hyperventilation to a $PaCO_2$ of 20 mm Hg results in a pH of approximately _____.

5. Acute hypoventilation to a $PaCO_2$ of 70 mm Hg results in a pH of approximately _____.

6. If the actual pH is equal to the expected pH, it can be concluded that metabolic status is (normal/alkalosis/acidosis).

7. When actual pH is more than 0.03 pH units *lower* than the expected pH, a metabolic (alkalosis/acidosis) must be present.

8. When actual pH is more than 0.03 pH units *higher* than the expected pH, a metabolic (alkalosis/acidosis) must be present.

9. If actual pH was 7.31 and the expected pH for the given $PaCO_2$ was 7.29, metabolic status would be considered (normal/acidosis).

10. Blood gases (can/cannot) be classified with only the $PaCO_2$ and pH.

Exercise 5-3 **Calculation of Expected pH**

Calculate the expected pH for the following $PaCO_2$ values based on the acute pH–$PaCO_2$ relationship.

	PaCO$_2$	pH
1.	50	
2.	60	
3.	25	
4.	65	
5.	20	
6.	30	
7.	70	
8.	55	
9.	22	
10.	45	

Exercise 5-4 Indirect Metabolic Assessment

Given the pH and PaCO$_2$ shown below, assess the metabolic status indirectly (i.e., the expected pH values that were calculated in the previous exercise should be compared with the actual reported pH values).

	pH	PaCO$_2$
1.	7.34	50
2.	7.30	60
3.	7.52	25
4.	7.15	65
5.	7.62	20
6.	7.56	30
7.	7.38	70
8.	7.20	55
9.	7.48	22
10.	7.34	45

Exercise 5-5 Accuracy Check by Comparing Direct and Indirect Metabolic Status

Determine if the reported data are consistent or inconsistent by comparing the results of indirect metabolic assessment with the value reported directly in the [HCO$_3$] (i.e., direct metabolic assessment). Note that the values for PaCO$_2$ and pH are the same as in the previous two exercises.

	pH	PaCO$_2$	[HCO$_3$]
1.	7.34	50	24
2.	7.30	60	31
3.	7.52	25	18
4.	7.15	65	26
5.	7.62	20	25
6.	7.56	30	30
7.	7.38	70	22
8.	7.20	55	16
9.	7.48	22	24
10.	7.34	45	29

Exercise 5-6   **The Rule of Eights in Accuracy Check**

Apply the Rule of Eights and label the following blood gases as consistent (C) or inconsistent (I).

	pH	PCO_2	$[HCO_3]$
1.	7.28	60	28
2.	7.48	56	40
3.	7.50	30	29
4.	7.20	30	20
5.	7.12	60	25
6.	7.60	40	39
7.	7.30	20	9
8.	7.58	50	30
9.	7.42	30	19
10.	7.08	70	10

Exercise 5-7   **pH–[H$^+$] Conversion**

Calculate the pH given the [H$^+$] in nEq/L.

	[H$^+$] (nEq/L)	pH
1.	45	
2.	56	
3.	32	
4.	30	
5.	48	
6.	80	
7.	60	
8.	39	
9.	28	
10.	51	

Exercise 5-8   Application of Modified Henderson's Equation

Calculate the missing variables given the following:

	pH	[H⁺] (nEq/L)	PaCO₂ (mm Hg)	[HCO₃] (mEq/L)
1.			60	30
2.			55	36
3.			45	33
4.	7.20		50	
5.			40	24
6.	7.30			24
7.			20	16
8.		60		18
9.		40	30	
10.	7.28		40	

Exercise 5-9   Calculation of [HCO₃] from Total CO₂

Given the total CO₂ (i.e., TCO₂), calculate the plasma bicarbonate concentration (i.e., [HCO₃]).

	TCO₂	PCO₂
1.	38	60
2.	26	40
3.	18	50
4.	20	25
5.	21	35

Exercise 5-10 **Metabolic Indices**

Fill in the blanks or select the best answer.

1. List the two metabolic indices most often used before the routine availability of blood gases.

2. The [HCO_3] (does/does not) change in respiratory acid-base disturbances due to buffering.

3. The [HCO_3] (does/does not) change in respiratory acid-base disturbances due to the hydrolysis reaction.

4. As a rough guide, [HCO_3] increases 1 mEq/L for every _____ mm Hg increase in $PaCO_2$.

5. When PCO_2 decreases _____ mm Hg, [HCO_3] decreases approximately 1 mEq/L.

6. The _____ is defined technically as the plasma bicarbonate concentration obtained from blood that has been equilibrated at 37°C with PCO_2 of 40 mm Hg and a PO_2 sufficient to produce full oxygen saturation.

7. In the presence of hypercarbia, the standard bicarbonate indicates a false (high/low) value.

8. The _____ is an index that uses a nomogram to correct the standard bicarbonate for the in vivo–in vitro discrepancy.

9. The _____ is the sum of all the buffer bases in 1 L of blood.

10. The formula: (observed [BB] – normal [BB] =) is used to calculate _____.

11. [BE] of blood manifests false (low/high) values in the presence of hypercarbia.

12. The base excess of the blood is also known as (in vivo/in vitro) base excess.

13. The most accurate form of base excess is ([BE]blood/[BE]ecf).

14. The buffer line associated with an [Hb] of _____ g% is used to determine [BE]ecf.

15. For every change in [BE]ecf of 5 mEq/L, the pH changes approximately _____ units.

Exercise 5-11 **Internet Work**

1. Go to NBRC.org and explain how the multiple-choice questions in this textbook relate to their examinations.

NBRC Challenge 5

Please select the best answer for the following multiple choice questions.

1. The following arterial blood gas is run on an emergency department patient.

   pH   7.52
   PaCO$_2$ 60 mm Hg
   [HCO$_3$]   20 mEq/L
   PaO$_2$ 88 mm Hg

   You should conclude:
   A) the patient needs mechanical ventilation.
   B) the patient needs low flow oxygen therapy.
   C) the blood gas should be checked and/or run again.
   D) the primary alkalosis is respiratory and a sedative is indicated.
   E) the primary alkalosis is metabolic and probably due to diuretic therapy.
   (CRT EXAM-NBRC MATRIX I,B,10,c)

2. A patient who appears to have acute hypoventilation and is on an oxygen mask has a blood gas drawn in the emergency department.

   pH   7.16
   PaCO$_2$ 80 mm Hg
   [HCO$_3$]   28 mEq/L
   PaO$_2$ 88 mm Hg

   The blood gas indicates:
   A) complete acid-base compensation.
   B) significant acid-base compensation by the kidney.
   C) a mixed acid-base disturbance.
   D) technical error.
   E) increased plasma bicarbonate due to hydrolysis.
   (CRT EXAM-NBRC MATRIX I,B,10,c)

3. A patient has a pulse oximeter saturation reading of 86 and a blood gas is ordered. The PaO$_2$ reported is 86 mm Hg. The clinician should conclude:
   A) the blood gas and pulse oximeter readings are perfectly consistent.
   B) the patient is normal.
   C) the patient is hypoventilating.
   D) the blood gas and pulse oximeter readings are incongruent.
   E) the pulse oximeter can be discontinued.
   (CRT EXAM-NBRC MATRIX I,B,10,a)

4. A patient with otherwise normal lungs is inadvertently given a respiratory stimulant. A blood gas is drawn and the PaCO$_2$ is 25 mm Hg. Before looking at the pH, one would expect it to be approximately:
   A) 7.25
   B) 7.35
   C) 7.45
   D) 7.55
   E) 7.65
   (CRT EXAM-NBRC MATRIX I,C,1,e)

5. Which of the following can be concluded from the following arterial blood gas?
   pH   7.16
   PaCO$_2$ 80 mm Hg
   [HCO$_3$]   28 mEq/L
   [BE]   −4 mEq/L
   PaO$_2$ 72 mm Hg
   A) The [HCO$_3$] cannot be correct.
   B) The [BE] cannot be correct.
   C) The change in [BE] and [HCO$_3$] is due to renal compensation.
   D) The change in [BE] and [HCO$_3$] is due to hypercapnia.
   E) The change in [BE] and [HCO$_3$] is due to chronic hyperventilation.
   (RRT EXAM-NBRC MATRIX I,B,10,c)

Basic Physiology

Oxygenation ...
These two systems cooperate (respiratory and cardiovascular) to supply the needs of the tissues. One system supplies air; the other supplies blood. Their ultimate purpose is the transfer of gases between air and all tissue cells.

Julius H. Comroe, Jr.[81]

... and external respiration
The prime function of the lung is to exchange gas ... If its (the lung) thickness were increased to 1 cm and its relative dimensions remained the same, the interface would cover the whole of Connecticut so that its shape is well suited to its gas exchanging function.

John B. West[155]

Outline

INTRODUCTION

The moment-to-moment sustenance of human life depends on a single external substance. This substance is so important that its absence in the environment causes irreversible damage to the human condition in approximately 6 minutes. That substance is, of course, oxygen (O_2), which is essential to each of the billions of cells comprising the human body. O_2 is a colorless, odorless gas that plays a critical role in the efficient production of cellular energy. In its absence, production of cellular energy is grossly inadequate, and the death of the organism ultimately ensues.

Cardiopulmonary System

O_2 cannot directly enter all cells in the body from its atmospheric origin. Simply stated, O_2 cannot penetrate into the body with sufficient

depth and speed to meet all cellular demands; consequently, the human body has evolved a remarkably effective O_2 delivery system that facilitates the transport of atmospheric oxygen to all cells in the body. In addition, this system can vary O_2 delivery to match changing cellular requirements.

It would be only partially correct to state that the respiratory system is the human physiologic system responsible for *cellular oxygenation*. Likewise, it would be false to state that the cardiovascular system assumes full responsibility for cellular oxygenation in the body. Neither of these systems alone can accomplish this life-sustaining function. Rather, it is the combined, cooperative effort of these two systems that is required. Thus, it is valid, both conceptually and clinically, to view these two systems as a single, integrated *cardiopulmonary system*

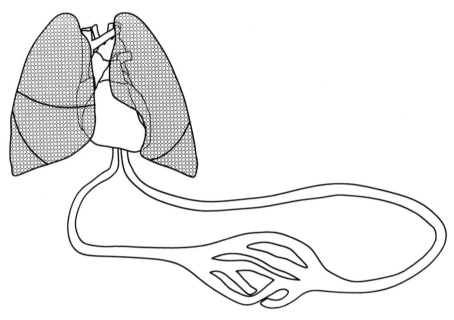

Figure 6-1.   Cardiopulmonary system.

that works to accomplish the ultimate goal of tissue oxygenation and carbon dioxide (CO_2) excretion (Fig. 6-1).

Steps in Tissue Oxygenation

Traditionally, the complete physiologic process of cellular oxygenation and the work of the cardiopulmonary system have been divided into three steps or phases (Fig. 6-2). In step one, ambient O_2 molecules are moved from their atmospheric origin to the blood supply within the lungs. O_2 actually enters the circulatory system via the small blood vessels in the lungs (pulmonary capillaries). O_2 molecules diffuse into the blood from the tiny air sacs in the lung known as *alveoli*. The exchange of O_2 and CO_2 between the alveoli and pulmonary capillaries is called *external respiration* and is the essence of step one (see Fig. 6-2,*A*).

Step two involves the quantitative transport of a sufficient volume of O_2 from the pulmonary capillaries to its cellular destination. This process, which is commonly referred to as O_2 *transport*, requires a normal hemoglobin concentration as well as an adequate cardiac output. *Cardiac output* may be defined as the volume of blood ejected each minute from the heart. The assessment of the adequacy of step two is generally quantitative (i.e., Is a sufficient

volume of O_2 being delivered to the tissues?). This step is depicted in Figure 6-2,*B*.

The final link in the O_2 delivery chain is the diffusion of O_2 from small systemic capillaries in response to cellular metabolic needs. This step, called *internal respiration*, involves both the diffusion of O_2 to the cells and its metabolic utilization by the cells (see Fig. 6-2,*C*). *Internal respiration* is defined technically as the exchange of O_2 and CO_2 between the systemic capillaries and the cells or tissues. In this text, however, the actual metabolism that occurs in the cells is also considered to be part of the process of internal respiration.

The common link throughout this O_2 delivery system is the blood and specifically the hemoglobin within the blood. The blood plays a pivotal role in all three phases. By using the blood or hemoglobin as a focal point, the three steps in the delivery of O_2 can be thought of as simply: O_2 loading (see Fig. 6-2,*A*), O_2 transport (see Fig. 6-2,*B*), and O_2 unloading (see Fig. 6-2,*C*).

Cardiopulmonary Interaction

It is interesting and informative to observe the cooperative effort exerted by the various components in the cardiopulmonary system. In particular, the heart and lungs often complement each other in trying to attain the goal of

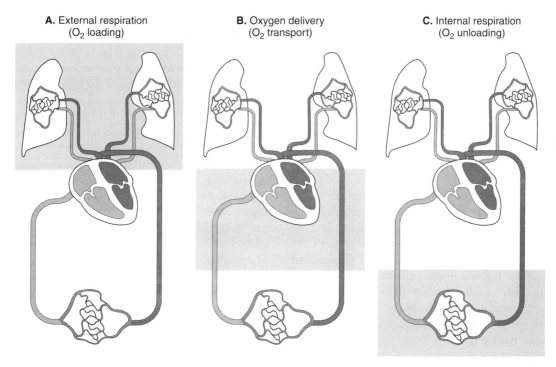

A. External respiration
(O$_2$ loading)

B. Oxygen delivery
(O$_2$ transport)

C. Internal respiration
(O$_2$ unloading)

Figure 6-2. **Steps in oxygen delivery.** The three steps or phases in oxygen delivery to the tissues include: oxygen loading into the blood or external respiration (**A**), oxygen transport or delivery to the tissues (**B**), and oxygen unloading from the blood and utilization by the tissues or internal respiration (**C**).

tissue oxygenation. For example, when breathing is hampered and PaO$_2$ is decreased due to lung disease, hormones are released through the adrenergic system that increase heart rate (tachycardia) and increase blood pressure (hypertension). This response attempts to ensure that sufficient O$_2$ reaches the cells. Thus, the heart may be thought of as compensating for a respiratory deficiency. The novice clinician should be aware that tachycardia and mild hypertension may be secondary to poor oxygenation of the blood via the lungs.

A clinical example of this concept is seen in the monitoring of the discontinuation of a mechanical ventilator from a patient. Here, cardiovascular parameters (e.g., pulse, electrocardiogram, blood pressure) are monitored to assess if spontaneous breathing is adequate. The clinician is alerted to inadequate breathing by *cardiovascular* compensatory changes that accompany it.

Although not really compensatory in nature, rapid or deep ventilation is also common in primary circulatory disturbances. Generally, the heart is effective in compensating for respiratory oxygenation problems. Conversely, the lungs can accomplish little when the initial insult is cardiac in origin. Nevertheless, the circulatory and ventilatory pumps are in intimate collaboration with the common objective of cellular O$_2$ delivery.

Similarly, each of the three steps in cellular oxygenation work in a cooperative manner to ensure tissue oxygenation. For example, when external respiration is impaired due to chronic pulmonary disease or some other condition, mechanisms are triggered in the other two steps to bolster O$_2$ delivery. O$_2$ transport may be improved through the production of more red blood cells and hemoglobin, and the cardiac output may be increased as described above. Increased red blood cells and hemoglobin due to a decreased arterial PO$_2$ is a common clinical finding in chronic pulmonary disease and is called *secondary polycythemia.*

In addition, the body may respond to this problem by increasing chemical 2,3-diphosphoglycerate (DPG) levels. The increased DPG tends to facilitate the release of O_2 from the blood to the cells and thus enhances cellular O_2 delivery. Thus, here again, the concept of cooperative function is evident.

Hypoxemia versus Hypoxia

Hypoxemia has been defined earlier as a below-normal arterial PO_2. Hypoxemia is a *blood* condition. The term *hypoxemia* as used in this text does not consider hemoglobin concentration or saturation; nor does it take into account the red blood cell count. The critical question in oxygenation delivery and assessment pertains not to the blood but rather to the cellular O_2 status. Inadequate O_2 supply to the body tissues is called *tissue hypoxia* or simply *hypoxia.*

Tissue hypoxia may be localized or generalized. *Local tissue hypoxia* may be seen in muscle cells during exercise or in a specific body region that accompanies a local vascular disorder. Examples of local vascular hypoxia and tissue hypoxia include myocardial infarction (i.e., heart attack) and a cerebrovascular accident (i.e., stroke).

Diffuse or generalized tissue hypoxia is an *overall* deficit of O_2 throughout the body tissue (e.g., severe hypoxemia, low cardiac output such as in the patient with congestive heart failure). It is of primary concern in critical care medicine to prevent diffuse hypoxia with its potential for irreversible organ damage. The simple term *hypoxia* that is used in this text refers to diffuse tissue hypoxia, unless otherwise stated. *The foremost goal in the management of oxygenation status is the prevention of tissue hypoxia.*

Severe hypoxemia (i.e., $PaO_2 < 45$ mm Hg) is highly suggestive of concurrent hypoxia. In lesser degrees of hypoxemia, however, hypoxia may not be present. For example, in moderate hypoxemia (i.e., PaO_2 45 to 59 mm Hg), hypoxia often does not occur because the cardiac output is increased and tissue O_2 needs are being met. Thus, *the presence of hypoxemia does not necessarily indicate the presence of hypoxia.*

In other cases, hypoxia may be present in the absence of hypoxemia. In conditions such as severe anemia or shock, the PaO_2 may be quite high; however, the tissue demands for O_2 are not being met. Thus, *hypoxia may be present in the absence of hypoxemia.* Although hypoxemia and hypoxia are closely interrelated, one must be careful to avoid *equating* these distinct entities.

EXTERNAL RESPIRATION

The remainder of this chapter will address the first step in oxygenation, external respiration or oxygen loading (see Fig. 6-2,*A*). The normal function and possible pathologic changes that can occur to disrupt external respiration will be explored.

Three criteria must be met to ensure adequate O_2 loading via external respiration (Fig. 6-3).

Figure 6-3.   **External respiration.** External respiration requires adequate ventilation, ventilation-perfusion matching, and diffusion.

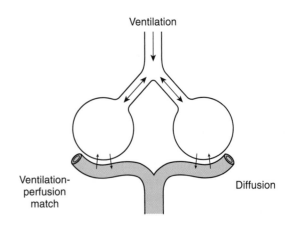

First, an ample supply of O_2 must reach the alveoli, which depends mainly on the adequacy of ventilation. *Ventilation* is the gross movement of air into and out of the lungs.

Second, the fresh O_2 in the alveoli must be exposed to pulmonary capillary blood. This process is often referred to as the *ventilation-perfusion match*. Finally, the ventilation-perfusion interface must exist for a sufficient time to allow for complete *diffusion* and equilibration of O_2.

Ventilation

The total volume of oxygen that enters the alveoli each minute while breathing room air depends on the volume of *alveolar ventilation*. The minute-to-minute regulation of alveolar ventilation, in turn, is controlled by the $PaCO_2$. Under normal circumstances, the body will assume sufficient ventilation to keep the $PaCO_2$ in the normal range of 35 to 45 mm Hg. A problem with ventilation is immediately recognizable because the $PaCO_2$ will be elevated.

Ventilation-Perfusion Matching

Consider for a moment a situation where the volume of lung ventilation is *normal*, but the entire volume enters the left lung. Combine this finding with a normal volume of pulmonary perfusion, but it all goes to the right lung. Obviously, despite a normal volume of ventilation and perfusion, there would be no O_2 loading.

Although this situation is unrealistic clinically, it serves to emphasize the importance of the ventilation-perfusion match. O_2 loading and CO_2 excretion (i.e., external respiration) can occur only in the pulmonary areas where a blood-air interface exists.

To understand the normal ventilation-perfusion match and all the changes that can occur, one must understand the mechanisms that regulate the distribution of ventilation and perfusion in the lungs. The normal distribution of ventilation and perfusion is reviewed first and is followed by a study of the factors that can disrupt the normal pattern of ventilation or perfusion. Finally, the specifics of the ventilation-perfusion match throughout the lungs in health and disease are explored.

Normal Distribution of Pulmonary Perfusion

Gravity Dependence

The volume of blood flow is not uniform throughout all lung segments. Rather, perfusion is preferentially distributed to gravity-dependent lung regions. Thus, in a man or woman placed in an upright position, the lung bases receive the largest proportion of the cardiac output, whereas the lung apices receive the least proportion. When lying supine (on the back), most blood goes to the posterior lung surface while the anterior (front) surface is minimally perfused (Fig. 6-4).

West's Zone Model

West has described a three-zone conceptual model of pulmonary perfusion in which the general regulation and characteristics of perfusion are different in each zone[155] (Fig. 6-5).

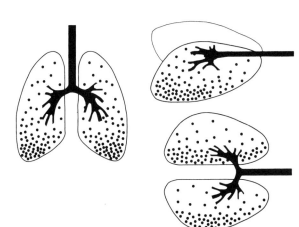

Figure 6-4. **Gravity dependence of perfusion.** Blood flow is greatest to the most gravity-dependent portions of the lungs. Thus, the distribution of pulmonary perfusion depends on the position of the body.

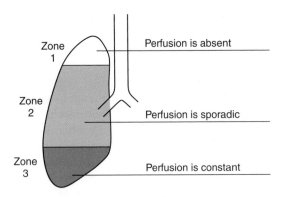

Figure 6-5.   **Pulmonary perfusion zones.**

Zone 1, when it is present, is always in the least gravity-dependent (uppermost) portion of the lung. Conversely, zone 3 is always in the most gravity-dependent (lowest) area of the lung. Of course, zone 2 is between the other two zones. Perfusion is absent in zone 1, sporadic in zone 2, and constant in zone 3.

Zone 1. Zone 1 is a theoretical area of the lung where perfusion is nonexistent because pulmonary arterial pressure is less than alveolar pressure (PA>Pa); consequently, the pulmonary capillary is collapsed (Fig. 6-6). The pulmonary circulation is a low-pressure system (normal pulmonary artery pressure 25/10 mm Hg) and, therefore, there is not a great deal of force available to pump blood to the uppermost areas of the lungs.

In normal humans, however, even the apical areas receive some perfusion, and technically no zone 1 is present. Nevertheless, a decrease in blood volume, cardiac output, or right-sided heart function could lead to the development of pulmonary hypotension and a zone 1 phenomenon in the uppermost lung regions.

Zone 2. Zone 2 is a functional area where the flow of perfusion is moderate. In zone 2, pulmonary arterial pressure is greater than alveolar pressure and, therefore, flow through the capillary is initiated. Zone 2 is also characterized by an alveolar pressure that exceeds pulmonary venous pressure (Pa>PA>Pv). Thus, flow occurs in this area because pulmonary arterial pressure exceeds alveolar pressure. Furthermore, the *amount* of flow depends on the difference between the pulmonary arterial pressure and the alveolar pressure. Because the pulmonary arterial pressure is progressively higher as one moves toward the lower regions of the lung, there is likewise a progressive increase in perfusion as one moves down this zone (see Fig. 6-6).

In certain areas of the lung, perfusion may be limited by the very low pressure at the venous end of the capillary. In these areas, alveolar pressure causes the vessel to constrict

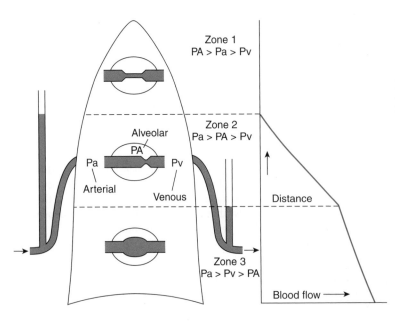

Figure 6-6.   **Three-zone pulmonary perfusion model.** In zone 1, pulmonary perfusion is absent. In zone 2, pulmonary perfusion is intermittent, depends on the cardiac and respiratory cycles, and increases progressively down through the zone. In zone 3, perfusion is heavy and constant.

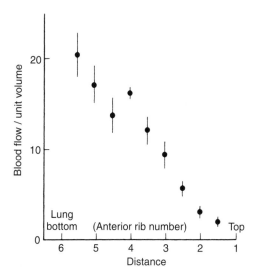

Figure 6-7. **Linear perfusion pattern in the lung.** Distribution of blood flow in the normal upright lung.

and thus to impede the flow of blood. This action is often called the *Starling resistor* or *waterfall effect*. One could surmise that perfusion in zone 2 is vulnerable particularly to the pressure changes that occur during the cardiac and respiratory cycles. The upper lung in a healthy person behaves functionally as a zone 2.

Zone 3. Zone 3 is the most gravity-dependent lung region in which blood flow is heavy and relatively constant. Zone 3 is characterized by a pulmonary venous pressure that exceeds alveolar pressure (Pa > Pv > PA).[155] In zone 3, perfusion is based simply on the difference between arterial and venous pressure, and alveolar pressure is not important. The majority of pulmonary perfusion occurs in zone 3.

Although the zone model may help one to understand the functional characteristics of pulmonary perfusion, it may sometimes be misleading. In the actual lung, there is no clear demarcation of lung perfusion zones. Rather, there is a general, linear increase in perfusion as one moves from the apex to the base of the lung (Fig. 6-7).

Normal Distribution of Ventilation

Basic Principle

The distribution of ventilation throughout the normal lungs, like the distribution of perfusion, is not uniform. The actual distribution of ventilation throughout the lungs can be explained on the basis of regional differences in alveolar compliance and airway resistance throughout the lungs. In other words, air traveling into the lungs always follows the pathway of least resistance and tends to flow to the alveoli with the greatest compliance and lowest airway resistance.

Gas Distribution at Functional Residual Capacity

The volume of gas remaining in the lungs following a normal exhalation is called the *functional residual capacity* (FRC) and is shown in Figure 6-8. At normal FRC, more gas resides in the upper lung zones (apices) and less in the lung bases. As shown in Figure 6-9, alveoli are larger in the apices and smaller in the bases.

This regional variation in FRC volume can be explained by regional differences in transpulmonary pressure. *Transpulmonary pressure* (PL) is the difference in pressure across the lung. It is defined as the pressure inside the lung minus the pressure immediately outside the lung in the pleural space. At the alveolar level, transpulmonary pressure is equal to the pressure within the alveolus (PAlv) minus the intrapleural pressure (Ppl). Intrapleural pressure is the pressure within the pleural cavity that surrounds the lungs. Thus, the formula for calculating transpulmonary pressure is shown in Equation 6-1.

$$\text{Equation 6-1}$$
$$PL = PAlv - Ppl$$

It is common in the literature to refer to the normal intrapleural pressure at rest as a single negative number such as (-4 cm H_2O).[81] This is slightly misleading, however, because this single number is the *average* intrapleural pressure throughout the intrapleural space. Actually, the intrapleural pressure at the base of the lung is almost 8 cm H_2O higher than that in the apex (Fig. 6-10).[155] This increase is probably related to the increased blood present in the bases. Intrapleural pressure increases linearly at a rate of approximately 0.25 cm H_2O for every centimeter of distance down the lung.[155]

Alveolar size is directly related to transpulmonary pressure. This is because the higher the numeric transpulmonary pressure, the greater

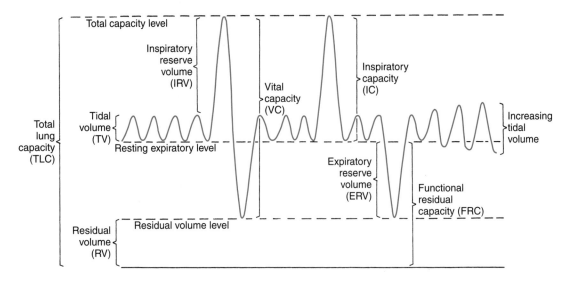

Figure 6-8.   Lung volumes and capacities. The maximum volume of gas the lung can hold is called the total lung capacity (TLC). The gas normally resident in the lungs between breaths is called the functional residual capacity (FRC). The FRC consists of the residual volume (RV) and the expiratory reserve volume (ERV). The RV cannot be exhaled even with maximal exhalation. The inspiratory capacity (IC) consists of the inspiratory reserve volume (IRV) and the tidal volume (TV). The vital capacity (VC) is the maximum volume that can be exhaled after a maximal inhalation.

the *distending* force. Conversely, a negative transpulmonary pressure is a net *compressive* force and may lead to alveolar or small airway collapse. The net effect of any transpulmonary force depends on the actual numeric value and the forces opposing it (e.g., elastic recoil, airway structural support).

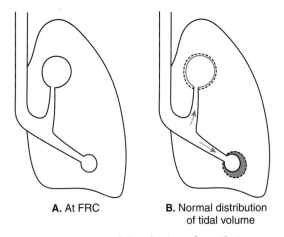

A. At FRC   **B.** Normal distribution of tidal volume

Figure 6-9.   Normal distribution of ventilation. A, The volume of gas resident in the lungs at FRC is greatest in the apices. **B,** Most of the tidal volume at FRC is distributed to the bases in healthy people.

Figure 6-10 shows the transpulmonary pressure across the alveoli in the lung apex compared with the transpulmonary pressure across the alveoli in the lung base at normal resting lung volume.

Normal Distribution of Tidal Volume

As additional air is added to the lung beyond FRC (i.e., tidal volume [VT]), it will preferentially ventilate the lung bases. At normal FRC, compliance of basilar alveoli is greater than compliance of apical alveoli, which are more distended. Thus, *most of the gas inhaled during normal breathing actually ventilates the bases* (see Fig. 6-9,B). In addition, the lower intercostal muscles and the diaphragm are displaced more than the upper part of the chest during normal inspiration, which may further facilitate basilar expansion.[156]

The actual distribution of tidal ventilation in the upright lung is shown in Figure 6-11. Clearly, ventilation is greatest in the lung bases. On the other hand, if one inhales more deeply than usual (large VT), and particularly when inspiratory hold is used, VT is distributed more evenly throughout the entire lungs.[156]

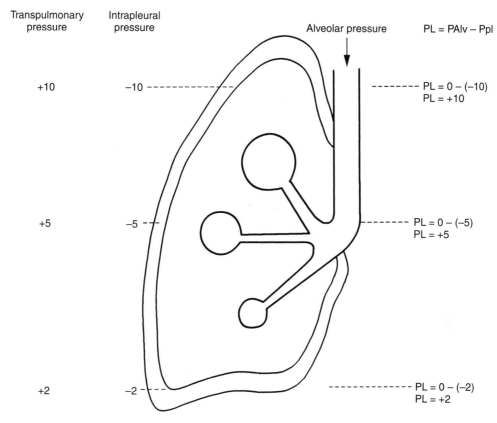

Figure 6-10. Variable transpulmonary pressure in the lung. Transpulmonary pressure is higher in the least gravity-dependent portions of the lung because intrapleural pressure is lower. Thus, at resting lung volume, alveoli are progressively larger as one moves up the lung.

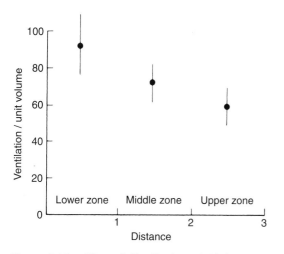

Figure 6-11. Normal distribution of tidal ventilation. Distribution of ventilation in the upright human lung.

Summary

Most normal VT ventilation is distributed to the gravity-dependent areas of the lungs, and the distribution decreases linearly as one moves up the lung. When VT is very large or when breath hold is applied, the distribution of ventilation throughout the lung is more uniform. Also, when FRC is below normal, the distribution of ventilation may be preferentially to the upper lung zones or the reverse of normal tidal distribution.

Abnormal Distribution of Pulmonary Perfusion

The normal distribution of perfusion is shown in Figure 6-12,*A*. A number of factors are known to alter this normal pattern of pulmonary perfusion. For convenience, these mechanisms are classified as primary or compensatory mechanisms. *Primary disturbances* are simply pathologic

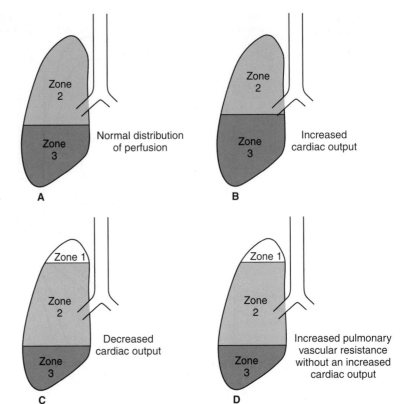

Figure 6-12. Generalized disturbances of pulmonary perfusion.

changes in pulmonary perfusion. *Compensatory disturbances* are changes in the pattern of pulmonary perfusion in response to a change in pulmonary ventilation. Compensatory changes attempt to improve or to restore ventilation-perfusion matching.

Primary Disturbances

Primary disturbances of perfusion may be localized or generalized. Serious local primary disturbances may be caused by pulmonary emboli or vascular tumors that affect the pattern of perfusion. Drugs such as isoproterenol, nitroglycerin, or propranolol may also alter the pattern of perfusion and may affect the PaO_2.[157,158] Most commonly, however, primary disturbances are the result of a generalized increase or decrease in pulmonary perfusion.

Generalized Increase in Pulmonary Perfusion

A generalized increase in pulmonary perfusion tends to move the borders of the perfusion zones upward and has an overall tendency to distribute perfusion more equally throughout the entire lung (see Fig. 6-12,*B*). The volume of blood present in the lungs may be increased because a greater amount is pumped to the lungs from the right side of the heart (e.g., increased cardiac output). Alternatively, pulmonary blood volume may be increased due to backpressure from poor left-sided heart function (e.g., mitral stenosis, left-sided heart failure) and pooling of blood in the lungs.

Generalized Decrease in Pulmonary Perfusion

Conversely, a generalized decrease in pulmonary perfusion results if the cardiac output decreases due to inadequate blood volume or heart (pump) failure. A decrease in the quantity of pulmonary perfusion causes the upper margins of the lung zones to move downward (see Fig. 6-12,*C*), which, in turn, may precipitate the development of a zone 1 area where ventilation is present without perfusion. It is noteworthy that the application of positive pressure ventilation may be associated with a similar shifting of the pulmonary perfusion zones downward.

Overall, pulmonary perfusion could likewise decrease if the pulmonary blood vessels constrict (increased pulmonary vascular resistance) and the heart is unable to pump blood throughout the entire lung (see Fig. 6-12,*D*). Normally, increased pulmonary vascular resistance (PVR) is countered with an increased right-sided heart pumping force. Thus, the normal distribution of pulmonary perfusion is usually maintained despite an increase in PVR. However, when the heart is unable to increase its pumping force because it is weak or damaged, increased PVR may result in a generalized decrease in perfusion.

PVR may increase acutely due to hypoxemia or acidemia. Remarkably, the pulmonary vessels are the only blood vessels in the body that react to low O_2 levels by constriction rather than dilation, although the reason for this is still unclear.[159,160]

PVR may similarly increase in certain chronic conditions, such as pulmonary fibrosis. Nevertheless, regardless of the cause or the duration of onset, a generalized decrease in pulmonary perfusion may lead to a pulmonary perfusion zone 1.

Compensatory Disturbances

To a certain extent, perfusion seems to distribute to areas of maximal ventilation in the lung. It has been described earlier how both ventilation and perfusion are preferentially distributed to the lung bases in a normal upright human at normal FRC.

Macroscopic Changes

It can also be shown on a macroscopic level that as lung volume decreases, relatively more perfusion is distributed to nondependent lung regions. If FRC is allowed to fall completely to residual volume (RV), blood flow is actually greater at the second rib level than at the lung bases in an upright person.[155] Again, this appears to maximize the ventilation-perfusion interface because at low lung volume the distribution of ventilation is similar. Furthermore, because dependent lung zones are particularly prone to pathologic alveolar collapse or consolidation, an upward shift of perfusion in these situations seems to be especially beneficial.

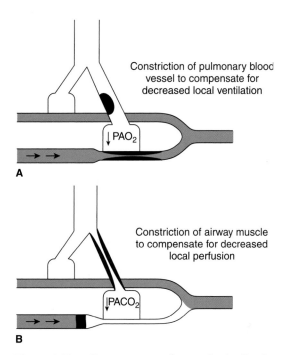

Figure 6-13. Compensatory changes in the distribution of ventilation and perfusion.

Local Changes

On a local level, the partial pressure of O_2 in the alveoli (PAO_2) serves as the primary regulatory mechanism.[158] Decreases in PAO_2 that result from poor ventilation to a specific lung area result in profound arteriolar and venule constriction and thus minimize perfusion to a poorly ventilated space (Fig. 6-13,*A*). The release of histamine from hypoxic mast cells has been suggested as a potential mediator of this response,[156] but regardless of the mechanism, the net effect is to improve the ventilation-perfusion match.

Abnormal Distribution of Ventilation

As described previously, ventilation is distributed throughout the lung based on regional differences in compliance and resistance. Any pulmonary disorder that leads to a change in compliance or resistance likewise leads to a change in the distribution of ventilation. Alterations in the distribution of ventilation may be primary or compensatory.

Primary Disturbances

Increased Airway Resistance. The single most common cause of abnormal distribution of

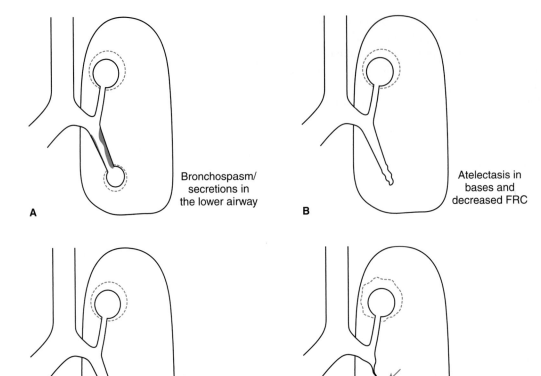

A   Bronchospasm/
      secretions in
      the lower airway

B   Atelectasis in
      bases and
      decreased FRC

C   Mechanical
      ventilation

D   Airway
      closure

Figure 6-14.   **Abnormal distribution of ventilation.**

ventilation is increased pulmonary secretions. The accumulation of secretions leads to decreased airway diameter and turbulent gas flow, both of which increase airway resistance. Other causes of increased airway resistance include bronchospasm, mucosal edema, artificial airways, and external compression of the airways by an abnormal tumor or fluid space. The effects of increased secretions or bronchospasm in the lower airway on the distribution of ventilation are shown in Figure 6-14,*A*.

Abnormal Functional Residual Capacity. An abnormal FRC also leads to the abnormal distribution of ventilation, which is true regardless of whether the FRC is increased or decreased. Both situations lead to changes in alveolar compliances throughout the lung and changes in the distribution of inspired gas. The effect of atelectasis and a decreased FRC on the distribution of ventilation is shown in Figure 6-14,*B*.

Positive-Pressure Ventilation. The application of positive-pressure ventilation disturbs the normal distribution of ventilation (see Fig. 6-14,*C*). Positive-pressure ventilation increases the distribution of ventilation to upper lung zones while simultaneously decreasing perfusion to these areas. Thus, the application of mechanical ventilation interferes with ventilation-perfusion matching and normal external respiration.

Airway Closure. Finally, a less recognized clinical problem in ventilation distribution is the phenomenon of *airway closure*. When the lung is compressed, such as during forced expiration, a point in the expiratory phase can be shown at which gravity-dependent lung zones cease to ventilate (see Figure 6-14,*D*). *Dependent lung regions* are the lung zones that are most affected by gravity. The actual anatomic location of these regions varies with body position.

As exhalation continues beyond the point of airway closure, gas is expired only from non-dependent lung regions. Presumably, this is because small airways in dependent lung regions are collapsed. Furthermore, the distribution of ventilation of the following breath is abnormal because gas is unable to enter collapsed regions or regions that are unable to empty normally.

The mechanism for this airway closure is related to the positive intrapleural pressure generated during forced expiration. Positive intrapleural pressure tends to decrease transpulmonary pressure and creates a compressive effect on the airway. Airways that are not well supported with cartilage, and diseased small airways in particular, eventually collapse. Collapse occurs first in dependent lung zones because this region is subjected to the lowest transpulmonary pressure.

Regional airway collapse during forced expiration was the basis for the *closing volume study*, a pulmonary diagnostic test that gained popularity in the 1970s for its purported ability to detect lung disease at a very early stage.[161] It was speculated that individual knowledge of the presence of early lung disease (i.e., premature airway closure) would serve as a deterrent to smoking. However, no data are available to substantiate this claim.

In healthy young individuals, airway closure does not occur until very near residual volume (RV) and in some is not seen at all. RV is, of course, the volume of gas remaining in the lungs after maximal expiration. In certain individuals (e.g., the elderly, children, obese, and smokers) and particularly in the presence of certain predisposing factors (e.g., reduced bronchial muscle tone, small airway disease, pulmonary edema, decreased elastic recoil in lungs, forced expiration), airway closure occurs at much higher lung volume.[161-163] In fact, basal airway closure above FRC is common in patients with pulmonary emphysema.[155]

Of clinical concern, airway closure may occur in susceptible individuals during normal tidal ventilation, particularly when the FRC is reduced. The FRC, in turn, has been reported as decreased in the following: supine position,

under anesthesia,[164] pain, obesity, smoking, and prolonged bedrest.[165] Simple assumption of the supine position may in itself decrease FRC (300 to 800 mL).[165] Thus, in individuals prone to airway closure or in those with diminished FRC, the clinician should strongly suspect this gas exchange problem. In healthy individuals older than 65 years of age, airway closure during tidal ventilation is likely to occur.[165] Furthermore, the decrease in FRC associated with the supine position would allow this to happen at 44 years of age in healthy people.[165]

Compensatory Disturbances. Compensatory disturbances in the distribution of ventilation are in response to some primary change in the distribution of perfusion. In general, the body attempts to match ventilation to perfusion in given lung segments.

The compensatory change in the distribution of ventilation is mediated primarily through local changes in airway resistance. In the absence of perfusion to a particular lung segment, local airway resistance increases and ventilation to that region is reduced. The decrease in the alveolar CO_2 partial pressure ($PACO_2$) that accompanies a decrease in perfusion appears to be the chemical mechanism responsible for constriction of muscle in the airways (see Fig. 6-13,*B*).[155] In addition, decreased surfactant production secondary to poor pulmonary perfusion may also contribute to decreased regional ventilation.

Ventilation-Perfusion Match

The volume of blood ejected by the heart each minute is called the *cardiac minute output* ($\dot{Q}$). With very minor exceptions, all of this blood passes through the pulmonary capillaries and has the opportunity to participate in gas exchange via external respiration. On the ventilation side, the volume of fresh gas reaching the alveoli each minute is called the *alveolar minute ventilation* ($\dot{V}A$).

The volume of blood perfusing the lungs each minute (4 to 5 L) is approximately equivalent to the amount of fresh gas reaching the alveoli each minute (4 to 5 L). In a gas exchange system that perfectly matched ventilation with perfusion, one would expect the volume of blood perfusing a given alveolar-capillary (AC)

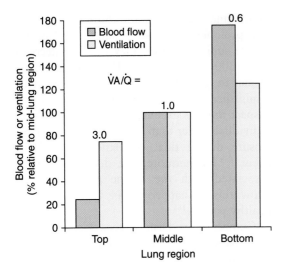

Figure 6-15. **Regional ventilation-perfusion relationships.** Relative ventilation, blood flow, and V̇/Q̇ relationships in three areas of the vertical lung. Alveoli at the bottom of the lung receive more blood flow than ventilation and therefore have a V̇/Q̇ less than 1.0. Alveoli near the top of the lung receive somewhat less ventilation than the bases, however they receive **much** less blood flow.

ideal unit, because the matching of blood and gas is perfect.

Although the general patterns of ventilation and perfusion are similar in the normal lung, the ventilation-perfusion ratios in specific AC units are rarely equal to 1. The reason is that perfusion is almost 20 times greater in the lung bases than the apices of an upright man or woman, whereas ventilation is only four times greater in the bases than the apices.[156] Thus, although the general distribution of both perfusion *and* ventilation is greatest in the lung bases, there is *relatively* more perfusion than ventilation in the lung bases and *relatively* more ventilation than perfusion in the lung apices.

As shown in Figures 6-15 and 6-16, ventilation volumes may be three times higher than perfusion volumes near the top of the normal lung (i.e., ventilation-perfusion ratio = 3). Conversely, perfusion volumes normally exceed ventilation volumes in the lung bases, and ventilation-perfusion ratios may be as low as 0.6. Thus, the range of ventilation-perfusion values seen throughout the lungs of a normal upright human is approximately 0.6 to 3.3, and the average ventilation-perfusion is approximately 0.85.[155] This range represents the normal ventilation-perfusion mismatch in humans.[166] In chronic obstructive lung disease, which is characterized by an abnormal distribution of ventilation, the range of ventilation-perfusion ratios throughout the lung is greater (e.g., 0.1 to 10).

unit to be exactly equal to the volume of ventilation to that unit. For example, if an AC unit received 1 mL of ventilation, it should likewise receive 1 mL of perfusion. If this were indeed the case, the *ventilation-perfusion ratio* (V̇/Q̇) of that AC unit would be equal to *one.* An AC unit with a V̇/Q̇ of 1 is called an

Figure 6-16. **Ventilation and perfusion in the normal lung.** Regional blood flow and ventilation. Both ventilation and blood flow decrease from bottom to top but the ratio between them changes so that the upper regions are overventilated in relation to their perfusion and the lower regions are relatively underventilated.

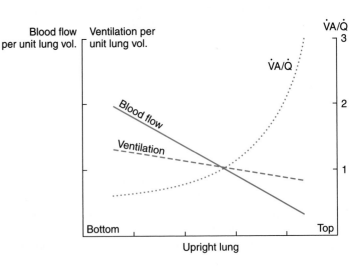

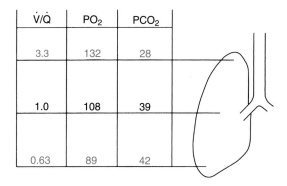

V̇/Q̇	PO₂	PCO₂
3.3	132	28
1.0	108	39
0.63	89	42

Figure 6-17. **Regional gas exchange in the normal lung.**

The exchange of gases in different regions of the lung likewise varies according to the local ventilation-perfusion ratio (Fig. 6-17). The PO₂ of blood leaving the lung apices may be greater than 130 mm Hg, whereas the PO₂ of blood leaving the lung bases may be less than 90 mm Hg.[156]

As stated previously, the ideal AC unit would have a ventilation-perfusion ratio of 1. Indeed, the ideal lung would have ventilation-perfusion ratios of 1 throughout. The further ventilation-perfusion ratios deviate from 1, the more inefficient gas exchange becomes. Even in the normal lung, there is a certain degree of inefficiency or ventilation-perfusion mismatch. The range of ventilation-perfusion ratios that may be present in cardiopulmonary disease, however, is virtually infinite. Table 6-1 shows some examples of these ratios that could exist in various AC units. Also, terminology that is used frequently to describe a particular

ventilation-perfusion relationship is likewise given.

An ideal ventilation-perfusion unit and the two utmost extremes are shown in Figure 6-18. Alveolar ventilation in the absence of perfusion (ventilation-perfusion ratio = infinity) is *true alveolar deadspace.* Conversely, perfusion in the absence of ventilation (ventilation-perfusion ratio = 0) is called *true capillary shunting.* The concepts of pulmonary deadspace and shunting are explored in the following section. All the various components that comprise total deadspace and total shunting are shown in Figure 6-19.

Deadspace and Shunting

Deadspace

In external respiration, the term *deadspace* is used to refer to ventilation that does not participate in gas exchange. Energy is consumed in moving this gas in and out of the lungs; however, there is virtually no benefit in terms of gas exchange. It is useful to think of deadspace as simply *wasted ventilation.* Basically, ventilation may be wasted if it fails to reach an alveolus (anatomic deadspace) or if it reaches an alveolus that is not adequately perfused (alveolar deadspace). Alveolar deadspace may be further subdivided into *true* alveolar deadspace and *relative* alveolar deadspace.

True Alveolar Deadspace

An alveolus that is ventilated but not perfused is called a *true alveolar deadspace unit* (see Fig. 6-19,*F*). The V̇/Q̇ of a true alveolar deadspace unit is infinity, which is true regardless of the actual quantity of ventilation because any number divided by zero is equal to infinity.

Table 6-1. SPECTRUM OF VENTILATION-PERFUSION UNITS (V̇/Q̇)

Ventilation (mL)	Perfusion (mL)	V̇/Q̇	Unit
10	0	∞	Absolute deadspace
10	1	10	Relative deadspace
3	1	3	Relative deadspace
1	1	1	Ideal unit
0.5	1	0.5	Relative shunt
0.1	1	0.1	Relative shunt
0	10	0	Absolute shunt
0	0	0	Silent unit

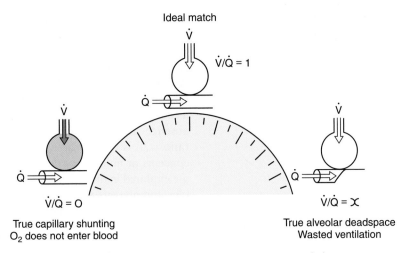

Figure 6-18.   **The extremes of V̇/Q̇ mismatch.** In true capillary shunting (V̇/Q̇ = 0), blood does not pick up O_2 as it passes through the lungs and therefore remains at the mixed venous PO_2 level. In true alveolar deadspace (V̇/Q̇ = infinity), ventilation is wasted.

This type of deadspace may be described as true or absolute because not a single molecule entering the alveolus partakes in gas exchange. In healthy people, there is no significant true alveolar deadspace because even the apical lung receives some perfusion.[155]

Relative Alveolar Deadspace

It should likewise be apparent that any (V̇/Q̇ > 1) represents some surplus of ventilation even in AC units where gas exchange is taking place. This pseudo-deadspace may be referred to as *relative alveolar deadspace* and is shown in Figure 6-19,*E.*

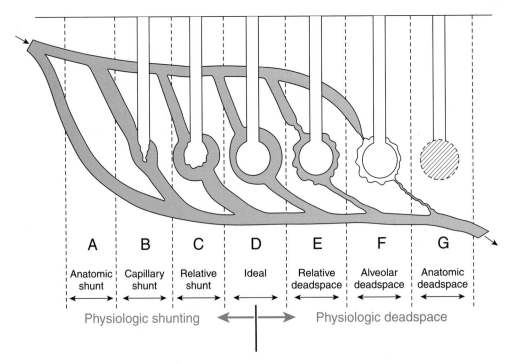

Figure 6-19.   **Components of physiologic shunting and deadspace.**

Anatomic Deadspace

Our discussion of deadspace has been confined to only ventilation that reaches the alveoli but does not partake in gas exchange. Another form of wasted ventilation is the portion of the inspired gas that never reaches the alveoli. The gas remaining in the *airway* at the end of each breath (see Fig. 6-19,*G*) is sometimes referred to as the *anatomic deadspace*. The quantity of anatomic deadspace in an individual can be approximated as 1 mL/lb of ideal body weight, or approximately one third of the tidal volume. Thus, anatomic deadspace in an average 150-lb individual would be approximately 150 mL.

In a given individual, the volume of anatomic deadspace is a constant that is present with each breath, regardless of VT. If the VT were to fall below the volume of anatomic deadspace, *all* ventilation would appear to be wasted. In reality, jet ventilation has shown that some portion of this ventilation may still reach the alveoli.

Normally, however, for external respiration to take place, VT must exceed anatomic deadspace volume. The volume of ventilation in excess of deadspace is called *effective alveolar ventilation*. Gas exchange is proportional to the volume of alveolar ventilation.

Breathing Pattern

Low tidal volumes are inefficient regarding alveolar ventilation because a large percentage of each breath is wasted as anatomic deadspace. On the other hand, large tidal volumes are more efficient because all ventilation in excess of anatomic deadspace represents alveolar ventilation. Obviously then, a rapid, shallow breathing pattern does not facilitate gas exchange in external respiration. With this pattern, a greater percentage of the total ventilation must be wasted as anatomic deadspace ventilation. A more detailed discussion of the effects of deadspace on alveolar ventilation and PaCO₂ is included in Chapter 8.

When a patient is breathing through an artificial airway (e.g., via tracheostomy tube or endotube), the volume of anatomic deadspace depends on the dimensions of the artificial airway. Generally, the use of artificial airways reduces the total anatomic deadspace volume.

Mechanical Deadspace

Additionally, when an individual is connected to some type of breathing appliance (e.g., mechanical ventilator, oxygen mask), another form of deadspace may also be present. The volume of any breathing apparatus in which exhaled gas remains and is inspired on the next breath is called *mechanical deadspace*. Functionally, mechanical deadspace represents an extension of the anatomic deadspace.

Physiologic Deadspace

The sum of all alveolar and anatomic deadspace is called *physiologic deadspace* (VD). In Figure 6-19, this would represent the sum of E + F + G. Physiologic deadspace is expressed normally as a percentage of tidal volume (VD/VT).

Measurement. At the bedside, the VD/VT may be calculated by using the Enghoff modification of the Bohr equation shown in Equation 6-2. Data necessary to use Equation 6-2 can be obtained via arterial blood gases (PaCO₂) and collection of mean expired gas samples (P̄ECO₂). Mean expired gas samples may be collected by using a large reservoir bag (e.g., a Douglas bag) connected to the exhalation port of a breathing circuit.

$$\text{Equation 6-2}$$

$$\frac{\text{VD}}{\text{VT}} = \text{PaCO}_2 - \frac{\text{P}\overline{\text{E}}\text{CO}_2}{\text{PaCO}_2}$$

Normal Values. The normal VD/VT in the spontaneously breathing individual is less than 0.4. During mechanical ventilation, however, an increase in VD/VT is expected owing to changes in the distribution of ventilation and perfusion. The normal VD/VT in the patient on a mechanical ventilator is less than 0.6.[10]

Clinical Significance. The major clinical significance of increased physiologic deadspace is that ventilation of that deadspace is wasted. If gas exchange in external respiration is to remain adequate in the face of increased deadspace, the total volume of ventilation must increase beyond normal. An increase in total ventilation can be accomplished only with a concomitant increase in the work of breathing and consumption of O₂ which, in turn, places further demands on the supply of O₂ via external respiration.

Clinical Assessment. In many clinical situations, measurement of the VD/VT is not practical. The fact that an increase in total ventilation is required to maintain adequate alveolar ventilation in the presence of increased physiologic deadspace, however, may provide useful diagnostic information. When ventilation is excessive while the $PaCO_2$ remains remarkably high or normal, increased physiologic deadspace should be suspected.

In normal humans, a total expired ventilation ($\dot{V}E$) of approximately 5 L/min results in a $PaCO_2$ of approximately 40 mm Hg. Doubling the minute ventilation to approximately 10 L/minute lowers $PaCO_2$ to approximately 30 mm Hg. Quadrupling ventilation (i.e., 20 L/minute) lowers $PaCO_2$ to almost 20 mm Hg.

If a patient's measured $\dot{V}E$ was 10 L/minute and measured $PaCO_2$ was 45 mm Hg, increased deadspace may be present. With this volume of ventilation, $PaCO_2$ should be approximately 30 mm Hg. The high $PaCO_2$ may be evidence of greater than normal wasted ventilation (i.e., increased deadspace component). Alternatively, this situation could reflect an increased CO_2 production.

When available, another good index of physiologic deadspace is the difference between the $PaCO_2$ and the end-tidal partial pressure of CO_2. The end-tidal partial pressure of CO_2 ($PetCO_2$) may be measured via capnometry, which is described later. The arterial end-tidal PCO_2 difference $[P(a-et)CO_2]$ is normally only 2 to 3 mm Hg. A high $P(a-et)CO_2$ is evidence of increased physiologic deadspace.

Deadspace Disorders

An increase in deadspace (wasted ventilation) results in an increased work of breathing and the clinical cause should be identified. As described previously, anatomic deadspace becomes a significant factor in rapid, shallow breathing.

True alveolar deadspace is typically the result of a pulmonary embolus or decreased pulmonary perfusion (e.g., decreased cardiac output). Finally, relative alveolar deadspace is increased when the distribution of ventilation is abnormal such as in chronic obstructive pulmonary disease or positive-pressure ventilation.

Table 6-2.   COMMON CAUSES OF INCREASED DEADSPACE

Anatomic: Rapid, shallow breathing
Alveolar
True: Pulmonary emboli
Decreased cardiac output
Relative: Chronic obstructive pulmonary disease
Positive-pressure ventilation

Table 6-2 lists the common causes of increased deadspace.

Shunting

In the cardiopulmonary system, *pulmonary shunting* is the phrase used to describe blood that passes through the lungs without participating in external respiration. Shunted blood enters and leaves the lungs with identical blood gases because it does not have the opportunity for gas exchange. This blood behaves as though it was diverted (shunted) around the lungs rather than passed through the lungs.

There are two general mechanisms by which shunting may occur. First, it occurs if blood on its way to the lungs bypasses the pulmonary capillaries and returns to the heart through some other vessel (anatomic shunting). Alternatively, shunting occurs when blood passes through an AC lung unit that does not contain fresh alveolar ventilation (capillary shunting). Perhaps the alveolus in this unit is collapsed or filled with fluid and is, therefore, not functional. Capillary shunting may be further subdivided into true and relative capillary shunting.

True Capillary Shunting

As described previously, a *true* or *absolute capillary shunt* is an AC unit in which there is no alveolar ventilation (see Fig. 6-19,*B*). The $\dot{V}/\dot{Q}$ of a true capillary shunt unit is 0. True capillary shunting is virtually absent in the normal human.

Pulmonary edema (e.g., left heart failure [Fig. 6-20] or acute respiratory distress syndrome) may result in true capillary shunting by causing alveoli to fill with fluid. Pneumonia may cause a similar phenomenon with infectious liquid filling alveoli. The collapse of alveoli

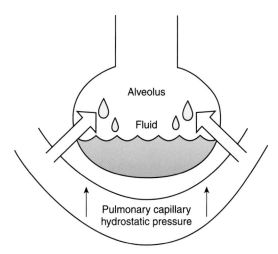

Figure 6-20. **Pulmonary edema and capillary shunting in left heart failure.**

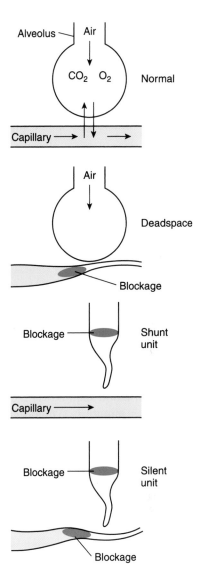

Figure 6-21. **Blockage of ventilation or perfusion.**

(atelectasis) may likewise result in a true capillary shunt. The primary pathologic mechanism in true capillary shunting is the *loss of functional alveoli.*

An AC unit with no ventilation or perfusion is called a *silent unit.* Silent units normally have no direct effects on external respiration; however, they do represent a loss of functional surface area available for gas exchange. The ventilation-perfusion effects of blockage of ventilation or perfusion in a given AC unit are shown in Figure 6-21.

Relative Capillary Shunting

An AC unit in which the volume of perfusion exceeds the volume of ventilation may be referred to as a *relative capillary shunt.* A relative shunt differs from a true shunt in that *some*, albeit not enough, ventilation is present in this type of unit. A relative capillary shunt unit has a V̇/Q̇ of less than 1, but it is greater than 0 (see Fig. 6-19,C).

Blood traversing a relative capillary shunt unit cannot be oxygenated completely because the supply of fresh alveolar gas is insufficient in proportion to the supply of perfusion. The lung bases in a normal human may be characterized as relative shunt units.

Conceptually, one could surmise that the alveolus would be depleted of O_2 before all the blood perfusing that unit were fully oxygenated. This can be visualized as though the

initial blood perfusing the capillary is normally oxygenated, whereas the final blood to perfuse the capillary would receive no O_2. Thus, this final blood behaves as though it had never passed an AC unit or *as if it were shunted past the lungs.* This theoretical explanation is of course an oversimplification, because gas exchange does not actually stop. Nonetheless, it may help to show the major clinical consequence of relative shunting (i.e., low ventilation-perfusion units); that is, an insufficient alveolar O_2 supply.

Anatomic Shunting

Some blood that leaves the heart on its way to the lungs never even passes through a pulmonary capillary. It is not that this blood passes a nonfunctional alveolus, this blood never passes an alveolus at all (see Fig. 6-19,A). This form of true/absolute shunting is called *anatomic shunting*.

In normal humans, approximately 2% of the cardiac output follows this anatomic course. Vessels involved in the normal anatomic shunt include the pleural, thebesian, and bronchial veins. Congenital anomalies and other disorders of the cardiovascular system may cause substantial increases in the anatomic shunt.

Physiologic Shunting

The *physiologic shunt* is the combined shunt that results from the additive effects of the anatomic and capillary shunts in a given individual. The physiologic shunt includes both the true and relative shunt components. In Figure 6-19, the physiologic shunt is the sum of A, B, and C.

The volume of blood shunted via the physiologic shunt each minute is symbolized $\dot{Q}sp$. The physiologic shunt is usually expressed as a percentage of the total cardiac output ($\dot{Q}T$). Thus, the symbol for the physiologic shunt is $\dot{Q}sp/\dot{Q}T$. When relative shunting is ignored and only the percentage of true shunt is measured, the symbol is $\dot{Q}s/\dot{Q}T$.

Measurement. The $\dot{Q}sp/\dot{Q}T$ can be calculated at the patient's bedside by using the classic shunt formula shown in Equation 6-3. Formulas for determining O_2 content in various blood vessels are described in Chapter 7. It is noteworthy, however, that several variables must be measured to calculate O_2 contents accurately. These variables include: PaO_2, SaO_2, PvO_2, mixed venous O_2 saturation (SvO_2), and hemoglobin concentration [Hb].

Also, capillary O_2 content cannot be measured directly; therefore, it is estimated based on certain theoretical assumptions. The ideal end capillary PO_2 ($P\dot{c}O_2$) is assumed to be equal to the PAO_2, and capillary blood is assumed to be completely saturated (i.e., SO_2 100%). Furthermore, calculation of mixed venous O_2 content requires the acquisition of a mixed venous blood sample through a special catheter placed in the heart (i.e., Swan-Ganz catheter).

Equation 6-3

$$\frac{\dot{Q}sp}{\dot{Q}T} = \frac{[C\dot{c}O_2 - CaO_2]}{[C\dot{c}O_2 - C\bar{v}O_2]}$$

$C\dot{c}O_2$ = oxygen content of ideal capillary blood
CaO_2 = oxygen content of arterial blood
$C\bar{v}O_2$ = oxygen content of mixed venous blood

Normal Values. In normal humans, there is no true capillary shunting, and relative capillary shunting is equivalent to approximately 1% of the cardiac output.[155] The normal anatomic shunt accounts for another (1% to 2%) of the cardiac output. Thus, the normal physiologic shunt is approximately 3% of the cardiac output.

Clinical Significance. In the clinical arena, even a $\dot{Q}sp/\dot{Q}T$ as high as 15% is not usually of major clinical consequence. Notwithstanding, the most important clinical result of increased physiologic shunting is failure of the shunted blood to pick up O_2 as it passes through the lungs. Thus, *shunting tends to cause primarily hypoxemia* (Fig. 6-22).

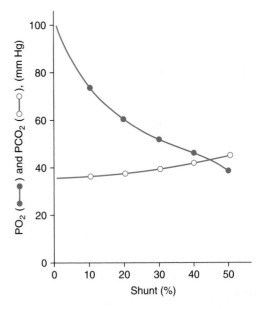

Figure 6-22.   **Effect of increasing shunt on PaO_2 and $PaCO_2$.** The PaO_2 (*closed circles*) falls precipitously, whereas $PaCO_2$ (*open circles*) is hardly affected.

Mild-to-moderate increases in physiologic shunting do not affect the ability of the lungs to excrete CO_2 (see Fig. 6-22). Only when the increase in physiologic shunting is huge are abnormal amounts of CO_2 retained in the arterial blood. The reason why moderate physiologic shunting affects arterial O_2 levels but not CO_2 levels is related to the different mechanisms by which these two gases are transported in the blood (see Chapter 7).

It is also noteworthy that the body responds to hypoxemia caused by increased physiologic shunting by augmenting the cardiac output, which has the effect of minimizing the fall in arterial PaO_2.

Clinical Assessment. As shown earlier, calculation of the physiologic shunt requires measurement of several blood gas variables. Furthermore, acquisition of mixed venous blood is necessary for its determination. For these reasons, various other indices that are easier to measure or calculate have been used by clinicians to estimate physiologic shunting. These indices include $P(A-a)O_2$, PaO_2/PAO_2, and PaO_2/FIO_2. The application of these various indices is explored in Chapter 9 in the assessment and management of hypoxemia. Presently, it is sufficient to say that various other indices are

Table 6-3. COMMON CAUSES OF INCREASED SHUNTING

Anatomic: Congenital heart defects
Capillary
      True: Congestive heart failure
            Acute respiratory distress syndrome
            Pneumonia
            Atelectasis
      Relative: Pulmonary secretions
                Positive-pressure ventilation

sometimes used as gross estimates of pulmonary shunting.

Shunting Disorders

An increase in pulmonary shunting leads to hypoxemia breathing room air. As described previously, an increased abnormal anatomic shunt is most often the result of a congenital heart defect.

True capillary shunting is typically the result of fluid filling alveoli (e.g., acute respiratory distress syndrome, congestive heart failure, pneumonia) or alveolar collapse (atelectasis). Finally, relative capillary shunting is seen with abnormal distribution of ventilation such as may accompany accumulation of pulmonary secretions or bronchospasm. Table 6-3 lists some of the common causes of shunt disorders.

ON CALL | CASE 6-1 *ABGs and Critical Thinking*

You are the only person available to care for this patient. You must assess the patient/situation and act accordingly.

A 72-year-old woman undergoes surgery for a leg fracture following a fall. Three days later, she has an acute onset of severe shortness of breath, hemoptysis, and chest pain.

Temp	37° C
Minute ventilation	18 L/min

ASSESSMENT

Abnormalities: List abnormal data and other noteworthy information. Classify ABG.

Explanation: List possible diseases, pathology, or other situations that may have led to this patient's condition.

Evaluation: Suggest additional data that would be useful in helping understand the situation or in making a diagnosis.

ARTERIAL BLOOD GASES

SaO_2	88%
pH	7.41
$PaCO_2$	38 mm Hg
PaO_2	50 mm Hg
$[HCO_3]$	24 mEq/L

INTERVENTION

Importance: Prioritize concern(s) of treatment in order of urgency and/or seriousness as you see the overall situation.

VITAL SIGNS

B/P	135/90 mm Hg
RR	30/min
HR	112/min

ON CALL | CASE 6-2 *ABGs and Critical Thinking*

You are the only person available to care for this patient. You must assess the patient/situation and act accordingly.

A previously healthy 47-year-old man returns from the operating room following abdominal surgery and presents with the following ABGs and vital signs 48 hours after returning to the unit. He also has diminished breath sounds in the lung bases.

ARTERIAL BLOOD GASES

SaO_2	86%
pH	7.51
$PaCO_2$	29 mm Hg
PaO_2	52 mm Hg
$[HCO_3]$	22 mEq/L

VITAL SIGNS

B/P	140/90 mm Hg
RR	24/min
HR	106/min
Temp	39° C

ASSESSMENT

Abnormalities: List abnormal data and other noteworthy information. Classify ABG.

Explanation: List possible diseases, pathology, or other situations which may have led to this patient's condition.

Evaluation: Suggest additional data which would be useful in helping understand the situation or in making a diagnosis.

INTERVENTION

Importance: Prioritize concern(s) of treatment in order of urgency and/or seriousness as you see the overall situation.

Objective: Specifically state the measurable or observable outcomes you would like treatment to accomplish.

Action: Describe your specific plan of action.

Diffusion

Appropriate external respiration requires both an adequate volume of ventilation and the matching of this ventilation with perfusion. The final prerequisite for effective external respiration is normal *diffusion*. There are two major requirements for successful pulmonary diffusion. First, there must be sufficient time available to allow for the *complete equilibration* of gases between the alveolus and the pulmonary capillary blood. Second, there must be a sufficient number of functional AC units (surface area) to allow for an adequate volume of gas exchange.

Equilibration

Available Time

The time available for gas equilibration in the AC unit is sometimes referred to as the *pulmonary capillary transit time*; this is the time that it takes for blood in the pulmonary capillaries to pass the alveolus or the time during which the AC interface is maintained. Pulmonary capillary transit time in normal resting humans is approximately 0.75 seconds.[155,166] Thus, diffusion must be completed (complete equilibration) during this period.

Speed of Diffusion

The speed of gas diffusion through the AC membrane depends on a variety of factors including: molecular size, solubility coefficients, Graham's Law, and driving pressures.

Molecular Size. One factor that determines the speed of diffusion of a particular gas is its molecular weight. Lighter molecules move and therefore diffuse more quickly. Because O_2 molecules are lighter than CO_2 molecules, O_2 molecules diffuse more quickly *in a gaseous phase*.

Solubility Coefficient. In a *liquid* medium, however, an additional property comes into play; that is, the solubility of the gas in the liquid. Gases that are more soluble in a given liquid diffuse faster throughout that liquid. This is precisely why CO_2 (a larger molecule) diffuses about 20 times faster than O_2 across the AC membrane, which is essentially a liquid membrane.

Graham's Law. This law summarizes these relationships by stating that diffusion of a gas through a liquid is directly proportional to its solubility coefficient and inversely proportional to the square root of its density.

Driving Pressure. The speed of diffusion also varies directly with the driving pressure of a gas across the AC membrane. The driving pressure across the AC membrane for a given gas is equal to the difference between its partial pressure in the alveolus and its partial pressure in the mixed venous blood entering the capillary. As shown in Figure 6-23, the driving pressure for O_2 is approximately 63 mm Hg ($PAO_2 - P\bar{v}O_2$) whereas the driving pressure for CO_2 is only 6 mm Hg ($P\bar{v}CO_2 - PACO_2$).

The calculation of driving pressure in this example represents the *ideal* driving pressure as blood *enters* the AC unit. Actually, the driving pressure must decrease progressively as blood travels through the capillary until theoretically it is equal to zero. Nevertheless, calculation of the initial driving pressure is a reasonable method to evaluate the speed

of equilibration because the speed of equilibration varies directly with this value. Administration of supplemental O_2 increases the driving pressure and the speed of diffusion.

Complete Equilibration

From a clinical standpoint, the complete equilibration of CO_2 between the alveoli and blood is never a problem because of the high solubility coefficient of CO_2. Similarly, complete equilibration of O_2 should not be a problem under ordinary circumstances. In healthy people, O_2 equilibration across the AC unit takes approximately 0.25 seconds.[155,166] Thus, O_2 equilibration occurs during the first one third of pulmonary capillary transit time (0.75 seconds), as shown in Figure 6-23. This provides for a large amount of reserve time for equilibration in normal resting humans.

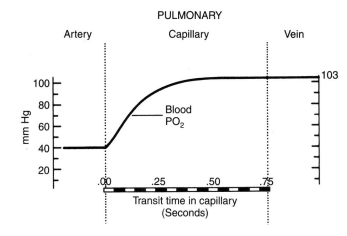

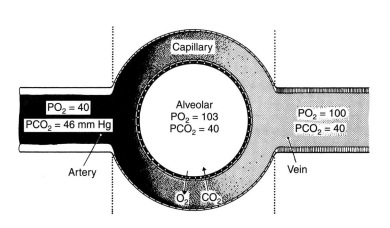

Figure 6-23. **O_2 diffusion across the AC membrane.** The PO_2 in the capillary normally equilibrates with the alveolar PO_2 within one third of pulmonary capillary transit time at rest.

Diffusion Barriers

As is discussed in Chapter 7, most of the O_2 in the blood is carried within the red blood cells. Thus, the functional barriers to diffusion of O_2 include all the microscopic anatomic layers between the alveolus and the red blood cells, as shown in Figure 6-24. These layers include the alveolar membrane, the interstitial fluid, the capillary membrane, plasma, and the red blood cell.

Thickening of the AC Membrane

Excluding the red blood cell and plasma, the normal thickness of the AC membrane is approximately 1 μm (1/1000 mm).[81,155] Significant thickening of this membrane may occur in pulmonary fibrosis or pulmonary edema, which is associated with an increased volume of interstitial fluid. Thickening of the membrane, of course, would increase the diffusion distance and prolong equilibration time.

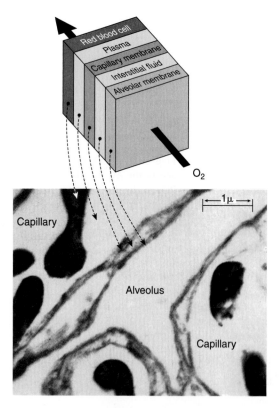

Figure 6-24.   **O_2 diffusion barriers in external respiration.** The barriers to AC diffusion as seen via electron microscopy in the rat lung.

Doubling the thickness of the AC membrane would double equilibration time (e.g., 0.25 to 0.5 seconds). Nevertheless, the long time available for O_2 equilibration (0.75 seconds), as shown in Figure 6-23, ensures that complete equilibration would still take place with normal pulmonary capillary transit time.

Decreased Driving Pressure

Ascent to high altitude with the resultant decrease in PAO_2 and drop in the driving pressure for O_2 across the AC membrane may likewise prolong equilibration. Nevertheless, here again, the large reserve of extra time available for diffusion allows for complete equilibration.

Incomplete Equilibration

Incomplete equilibration may occur, however, if a reduced driving pressure or thickening of the alveolar capillary membrane is *combined* with a reduced pulmonary capillary transit time. A reduced pulmonary capillary transit time accompanies an increased cardiac output because the speed of perfusion is increased. Specifically, pulmonary capillary transit time may be as low as 0.34 seconds during exercise.[81] Thus, the net effects of exercise at high altitude may lead to severe hypoxemia even in healthy subjects because of the low driving pressure combined with the decreased pulmonary capillary transit time.[155]

Similarly, incomplete O_2 equilibration may be observed during exercise in the patient with thickening of the AC membrane. Specifically, if complete equilibration requires 0.5 seconds due to AC thickening, and pulmonary capillary transit time falls to 0.4 seconds, equilibration will not occur.

Clinical Considerations

Diminished pulmonary capillary transit time leading to incomplete equilibration is largely responsible for the hypoxemia and shortness of breath seen on exertion in patients with pulmonary fibrosis. When hypoxemia is present in these patients at rest, the mechanism is most likely increased physiologic shunting rather than incomplete equilibration.[155]

The presence of a thickened AC membrane is sometimes referred to as an AC *block* or a *diffusion defect*; however, use of these terms is discouraged because a thickened AC membrane alone does not lead to incomplete equilibration of O_2.[155] One should remember that alveolar capillary thickening may lead to incomplete equilibration and hypoxemia only when combined with a decreased pulmonary capillary transit time. This may occur during exercise or in the critically ill patient with an increased cardiac output.

Less obvious factors may also present barriers to diffusion. These factors include situations where O_2 would not normally diffuse through red blood cell membranes or combine with hemoglobin. The clinical significance of these considerations, however, appears to be minimal.

Surface Area

Also important in the quantitative exchange of gases in external respiration is an adequate number of functional AC units. The normal alveolar surface area that is exposed to pulmonary capillary blood is approximately 70 m^2 or approximately the size of a tennis court. Because the volume of blood undergoing gas exchange in the lungs is only approximately 70 mL,[155] there is about 1 m^2 of surface area for every milliliter of blood. If one could imagine 1 mL of blood spread out over a square meter, the vast gas exchanging capability of the lungs could be appreciated.

Pulmonary diseases that affect the architecture of the lung (e.g., emphysema, pneumonectomy, tumors) may result in the loss of functional AC units. Thus, the quantitative ability of the cardiopulmonary system to load O_2 into the pulmonary capillary blood is reduced. This phenomenon can be detected through pulmonary function diffusion studies.

EXERCISES

Exercise 6-1   Introduction to Oxygenation

Fill in the blanks or select the best answer.

1. The system responsible for cellular oxygenation in the human is the (respiratory/cardiovascular/cardiopulmonary) system.

2. Define external respiration.

3. Define O_2 transport.

4. Define internal respiration.

5. The assessment of O_2 transport is (qualitative/quantitative) in nature.

6. List the three phases in oxygenation using blood as the reference point.

7. The heart is (less/more) effective in compensating for respiratory oxygenation problems than the lungs in compensating for cardiovascular oxygenation problems.

8. The body increases the amount of red blood cells and hemoglobin in the blood in response to diminished O_2 loading. The result of this response is called _____.

9. Hypoxemia is a (blood/tissue) condition.

10. The utmost goal in the management of oxygenation status is the prevention of (hypoxemia/hypoxia).

11. Hypoxemia (may be/is never) present in the absence of hypoxia.

12. Hypoxia (may be/is never) present in the absence of hypoxemia.

Exercise 6-2 External Respiration and Normal Pulmonary Perfusion

Fill in the blanks or select the best answer.

1. State the three criteria that must be met to ensure adequate O_2 loading.

2. The minute-to-minute control of ventilation in normal humans is mediated via the (PaO_2/$PaCO_2$).

3. Normal ventilation ensures an adequate supply of O_2 to the alveoli unless the FIO_2 or the _____ of the inspired gas is low.

4. A significant direct stimulation of ventilation in response to hypoxemia occurs only when PaO_2 is less than approximately _____ mm Hg.

5. Most pulmonary perfusion is normally distributed to the (most/least) gravity-dependent lung regions.

6. Pulmonary perfusion in zone 1 of West's model is (vast/minimal/absent).

7. A pulmonary perfusion zone 1 (is/is not) present in normal healthy humans.

8. The upper lung zones in healthy upright people function as a pulmonary perfusion zone (1/2/3).

9. Most pulmonary perfusion occurs in zone _____.

10. Hypotension may lead to the development of a pulmonary perfusion zone _____.

Exercise 6-3 Normal Distribution of Ventilation

Fill in the blanks or select the best answer.

1. The distribution of ventilation in the lung depends on regional differences in _____ and _____.

2. At residual volume, most gas entering the lung would go to the (apices/bases).

3. The intrapleural pressure in the apices is (more/less) negative than it is in the bases of an upright individual.

4. Calculate the transpulmonary pressure given an intrapulmonary pressure of 2 cm H_2O and an intrapleural pressure of −8 cm H_2O.

5. At resting FRC, the apical alveoli are (larger/smaller) than the basal alveoli.

6. A negative PL is a net (compressive/distending) force on the lungs.

7. Transpulmonary pressure is (higher/lower) in the lung apices of an upright individual than in the bases.

8. Most gas inhaled during normal breathing from normal FRC enters the (apices/bases).

9. The amount of air moved in and out of the lungs during normal breathing is called the _____.

10. Large tidal volumes tend to make the distribution of ventilation (more/less) even throughout the lungs.

Exercise 6-4 **Abnormal Pulmonary Perfusion**

Fill in the blanks or select the best answer.

1. Changes in the pattern of pulmonary perfusion in response to a change in pulmonary ventilation are called (primary/compensatory) disturbances.

2. Most primary disturbances of pulmonary perfusion are (localized/generalized) in nature.

3. The upper borders of the pulmonary perfusion zones tend to move (higher/lower) due to an increased cardiac output.

4. List two situations that may shift the upper borders of the pulmonary perfusion zones downward.

5. Cite a situation when an increased pulmonary vascular resistance could result in a generalized decrease in pulmonary perfusion.

6. List two blood gas conditions that can increase pulmonary vascular resistance acutely.

7. Suggest a clinical disease entity that could increase generalized pulmonary vascular resistance chronically.

8. The most potent regulator of the distribution of pulmonary perfusion on the local level is the _____.

Exercise 6-5 **Abnormal Distribution of Ventilation**

Fill in the blanks or select the best answer.

1. A change in FRC (will/will not) affect the distribution of ventilation.

2. State the single most common cause of abnormal distribution of ventilation.

3. Accumulated pulmonary secretions affect the distribution of ventilation primarily through their effects on pulmonary (compliance/airway resistance).

4. Bronchospasm and mucosal edema primarily affect pulmonary (compliance/airway resistance).

5. Airway closure occurs first in (gravity/nongravity) dependent lung regions.

6. Forced expiration tends to (increase/decrease) PL.

7. Airway closure occurs prematurely in (obese/thin) patients.

8. Airway closure occurs prematurely in (smokers/nonsmokers).

9. The FRC may be reduced in the (supine/sitting) position.

10. Airway closure has been reported to occur in normal individuals in the supine position at age _____.

11. Compensatory changes in the distribution of ventilation are mediated by changes in (PAO_2/$PACO_2$).

Exercise 6-6   Ventilation-Perfusion Matching

Fill in the blanks or select the best answer.

1. The volume of blood ejected by the heart each minute is called the _____.

2. The volume of fresh gas reaching the alveoli each minute is called the _____.

3. The ventilation-perfusion ratio of an ideal AC unit is approximately _____.

4. Although perfusion and ventilation are both greatest in the lung bases, perfusion is relatively (less/more) than ventilation in this region.

5. The average ventilation-perfusion ratio in the lung is approximately (0.8/0.4).

6. The ventilation-perfusion ratios in the apex of the normal erect lung are about (10/3).

7. The $\dot{V}/\dot{Q}$ in the base of the normal erect lung are approximately (0.6/0.2).

8. The PaO_2 of blood leaving the lung apices is approximately (100/130) mm Hg.

9. A $\dot{V}/\dot{Q}$ of zero is associated with a unit called a _____.

10. A $\dot{V}/\dot{Q}$ of infinity is associated with a unit called a _____ unit.

Exercise 6-7   Physiologic Deadspace

Fill in the blanks or select the best answer.

1. In healthy people, there is (some/no) absolute alveolar deadspace.

2. The (higher/lower) the numeric value of a $\dot{V}/\dot{Q}$, the more wasted ventilation is present.

3. Normal anatomic deadspace ventilation per breath in a 200-lb adult is approximately _____ mL.

4. Anatomic deadspace ventilation increases in significance when VT is (high/low).

5. The sum of all types of deadspace expressed as a percentage of VT is called _____ deadspace.

6. Calculate VD/VT given:
   $PaCO_2$ = 60 mm Hg
   $P\bar{E}CO_2$ = 30 mm Hg

7. The physiologic deadspace equation uses (mean/end tidal) expired PCO_2.

8. The normal VD/VT in the spontaneously breathing individual is _____.

9. The normal VD/VT in the patient receiving mechanical ventilation is _____.

10. The volume of any breathing apparatus in which exhaled gas remains and is inspired on the next breath is called _____.

11. The major clinical consequence of increased physiologic deadspace is that ventilation of that deadspace is _____.

12. Increased deadspace ventilation will (increase/decrease) the work of breathing.

13. Increased deadspace ventilation (will/will not) directly cause hypoxemia.

14. A minute ventilation of 10 L/min in healthy people should result in a $PaCO_2$ of approximately (20/30) mm Hg.

15. A minute ventilation of 15 L/min and a $PaCO_2$ of 40 mm Hg suggests (normal deadspace/increased physiologic deadspace).

16. A $PaCO_2$ of 25 mm Hg and a minute ventilation of 15 L/minute suggests (normal deadspace/increased physiologic deadspace).

17. The difference in partial pressures between end-tidal and arterial (O_2/CO_2) is a good index of physiologic deadspace.

Exercise 6-8 **Physiologic Shunting**

Fill in the blanks or select the best answer.

1. The (lower/higher) the $\dot{V}/\dot{Q}$, the lower is the PO_2 that leaves the unit.

2. A ventilation-perfusion unit with no perfusion or ventilation is called a _____ unit.

3. The two forms of absolute shunting are _____ shunts and _____ shunts.

4. The normal anatomic shunt is approximately _____% of the cardiac output.

5. List three veins that contribute to the normal anatomic shunt.

6. Capillary shunting may be subdivided further into _____ and _____ capillary shunting.

7. Another term for true capillary shunting is _____ capillary shunting.

8. State two clinical causes of increased true capillary shunting.

9. The normal percentage of the physiologic shunt that passes relative capillary shunt units is _____%.

10. The major clinical consequence of increased physiologic shunting is _____.

Exercise 6-9 **Diffusion**

Fill in the blanks or select the best answer.

1. State the two major concerns regarding the adequacy of diffusion in the lung.

2. The time that it takes blood to pass the alveolus during which the AC interface is maintained is called the _____ time.

3. Pulmonary capillary transit time in a normal resting human is _____ seconds.

4. Normal O_2 equilibration time with a normal AC membrane is _____ seconds.

5. In a gaseous phase, (larger/smaller) molecules diffuse faster.

6. CO_2 diffuses 20 times (faster/slower) than O_2 across the liquid AC membrane.

7. What law states that diffusion of a gas through a liquid is directly proportional to its solubility coefficient and inversely proportional to the square root of its density?

8. Normal AC membrane thickness is approximately _____ μm.

9. A decreased O_2 driving pressure or a thickened AC membrane may result in hypoxemia if pulmonary capillary transit time were (increased/decreased) as occurs during exercise.

10. The normal alveolar surface area is approximately _____ m^2.

1. Go to google.com and do an image search on the following: (a) $\dot{V}/\dot{Q}$, (b) lungs, and (c) alveolar-capillary gas exchange. Print out the one picture on each topic that best illustrates each topic.

NBRC Challenge 6

Please select the best answer for the following multiple-choice questions.

1. A VD/VT study is performed on a patient in the critical care unit. The VD/VT is determined to be 0.6. Which of the following may explain the patient's status?
   I. Decreased cardiac output
   II. Atelectasis
   III. Mechanical ventilation
   A) I only
   B) II only
   C) I, II only
   D) I, III only
   E) I, II, and III
   (RRT EXAMINATION — NBRC
   MATRIX I,C,2,c)

2. To calculate VD/VT, one would need to simultaneously measure $PaCO_2$ and:
   A) cardiac output.
   B) end-tidal CO_2.
   C) PAO_2.
   D) alveolar ventilation.
   E) mean exhaled CO_2.
   (RRT EXAMINATION — NBRC
   MATRIX I,B,9,c)

3. Which of the following disorders would typically lead to a $\dot{Q}s/\dot{Q}T$ calculation of 24%?
   I. Pulmonary embolus
   II. Acute respiratory distress syndrome
   III. Congenital heart defect
   A) I only
   B) II only
   C) I and II only
   D) II and III only
   E) I, II, and III
   (RRT EXAMINATION — NBRC
   MATRIX I,C,1,c)

4. A suspected tuberculosis patient has increased crackles in both lung apices. Tuberculosis is more likely to be seen in the _____ lung zones because of the _____.
   A) upper, higher PaO_2
   B) upper, lower $PaCO_2$
   C) upper, higher $PaCO_2$
   D) lower, lower PaO_2
   E) lower, lower $PaCO_2$
   (RRT EXAMINATION — NBRC
   MATRIX I,B,4,a)

5. A normal PaO_2 at rest that decreases during exercise may suggest the presence of:
   A) pulmonary embolus.
   B) pneumonia.
   C) pulmonary fibrosis.
   D) adult respiratory distress syndrome.
   E) atelectasis.
   (RRT EXAMINATION — NBRC
   MATRIX I,C,1,a)

Chapter 7

Oxygen Transport and Internal Respiration

Oxygen transport ...
... a proper type and quality of hemoglobin are also necessary for optimal loading and unloading of O$_2$, and the heart and vessels are necessary to deliver the proper amount of oxygenated blood to all tissues in proportion to their need.

Julius H. Comroe[81]

... and internal respiration
The pulmonary gas exchange system is not an end in itself. It exists to meet the needs of organs, tissues, and cells.

Julius H. Comroe[81]

Outline

INTRODUCTION

The first step in delivering oxygen to the tissues, external respiration and oxygen loading into the blood, has been discussed in detail in Chapter 6. The second step in tissue oxygenation is oxygen transport as shown in Figure 7-1,*B*. In this chapter, we will explore basic physiology and pathology as it relates to oxygen transport. Finally, in the last section of this chapter, we will explore internal respiration, the final link in the oxygenation system. Internal respiration and oxygen unloading to the tissues will include the release and use of oxygen by the cells (see Fig. 7-1,*C*).

BLOOD OXYGEN COMPARTMENTS

Life-sustaining oxygen molecules may be present in the blood in one of two forms or compartments. Oxygen may be carried in the dissolved state or it may be carried in the *combined* state.

Dissolved Oxygen
Solubility Coefficients

As described in Chapter 3, gases may diffuse freely between liquid and gaseous phases depending on the difference in partial pressure between the two phases. This principle is important in external respiration because the alveolar-capillary unit is essentially a liquid-gas interface.

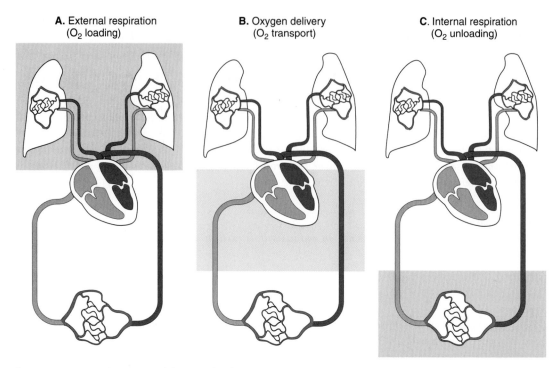

A. External respiration
(O₂ loading)

B. Oxygen delivery
(O₂ transport)

C. Internal respiration
(O₂ unloading)

Figure 7-1.   **Steps in oxygen delivery.** The three steps or phases in oxygen delivery to the tissues include: oxygen loading into the blood or external respiration (**A**), oxygen transport or delivery to the tissues (**B**), and oxygen unloading from the blood and utilization by the tissues or internal respiration (**C**).

The partial pressure of oxygen in a freshly ventilated alveolus is greater than the partial pressure of oxygen in the blood. Thus, when blood is exposed to alveolar gas, the partial pressure of oxygen increases in the blood until it equilibrates with the alveolus. Oxygen present in the blood in this uncombined or free state is referred to as *dissolved oxygen* or oxygen in physical solution.

The **volume** of gas that dissolves in a given liquid, however, depends on the *solubility coefficient* of the gas in that particular liquid. A gas with a high solubility coefficient has a greater *volume* of gas dissolved in a particular fluid than a gas with a low solubility coefficient, despite the fact that both gases may have the same partial pressure.

The solubility coefficient of oxygen in blood at 37° C is

0.003 mL of O₂/100 mL of blood/mm Hg

As shown in Figure 7-2, this means that in a 100-mL blood sample, 0.003 mL of oxygen are dissolved for every 1 mm Hg of oxygen

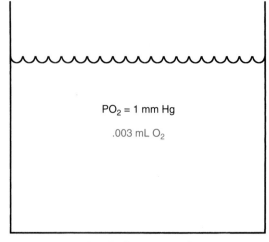

$PO_2 = 1$ mm Hg

.003 mL O₂

100 mL of blood at 37° C

Figure 7-2.   **Solubility coefficient of oxygen in blood at 37° C.** The solubility coefficient of oxygen in blood at 37° C is 0.003 mL O₂/100 mL of blood/mm Hg or 0.003 vol%/mm Hg.

partial pressure. The unit vol% is usually used instead of the more cumbersome milliliters of gas per 100 mL of blood. Thus, 2 vol% of oxygen in the blood is equivalent to 2 mL of oxygen in 100 mL of blood.

The solubility coefficient of a gas in a particular fluid also depends on temperature. As a rule, gases become less soluble as temperature increases, which is the reason why small bubbles can be observed escaping water as it is being heated but before it comes to a boil. Solubility coefficients expressed for clinical practice are generally expressed at body temperature, ambient pressure, saturated (BTPS).

Linear PO₂–Dissolved Oxygen Relationship

There is a linear relationship between arterial PO_2 and the volume of oxygen dissolved in arterial blood. If 0.003 vol% is present when the PO_2 is 1 mm Hg, 0.006 vol% is present when the PO_2 is 2 mm Hg (0.003 vol% × 2). It follows then that 0.3 vol% of oxygen is present when PO_2 is 100 mm Hg. The direct, linear relationship between PO_2 and the volume of oxygen dissolved in the blood persists as PO_2 increases still further to very high levels (Fig. 7-3).

Significance of the PaO₂

The previous discussion described the relationship between the *volume* of gas dissolved in a liquid and the *partial pressure* of a gas dissolved in a liquid. The volume is the critical component regarding quantitative oxygen delivery to the cells. Nevertheless, partial pressure is not without important physiologic significance in its own right. The partial pressure of oxygen controls the driving pressure for diffusion of oxygen throughout the body and to the cells and for the combination of oxygen with hemoglobin.

Combined Oxygen

Hemoglobin

The volume of *dissolved oxygen* is clearly inadequate to meet the body's metabolic needs. We are fortunate, however, because we have a substance present in our blood that loosely binds with oxygen in sufficient quantities to meet the body's needs while at the same time it easily releases this oxygen to the tissues. This unique substance is called *hemoglobin* (Hb). Even more remarkable, this same miracle molecule can also carry carbon dioxide and protect the pH through buffering. Oxygen present in the blood in combination with hemoglobin is called *combined oxygen* or *oxyhemoglobin.*

Chemically, normal adult hemoglobin (HbA) is made up of a heme group and a protein group (globin). The Hb molecule is very large and has a molecular weight of 64,500.

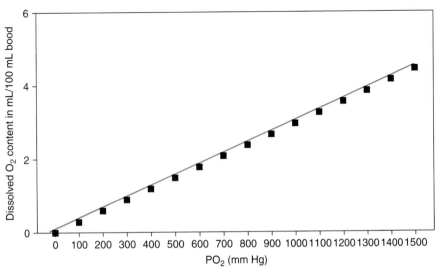

Figure 7-3. **PO₂–dissolved oxygen content.** There is a direct, linear relationship between PO_2 and the *volume* of oxygen dissolved in the blood.

Globin alone consists of four chains of amino acids: two alpha chains, each made up of 141 amino acids; and two beta chains, each comprised of 146 amino acids. These long rows of amino acids are called polypeptide chains. The four independent polypeptide chains are shown schematically in Figure 7-4,*B,* and also their integration into globin (see Fig. 7-4,*A*).

A heme group is combined with each one of these amino acid chains. Each heme group, in turn, is made up of a porphyrin and iron (Fe). Oxygen actually combines with hemoglobin at the site of this iron. Oxygen and iron form a loose bond in this reversible reaction because iron remains in the ferrous (Fe^{2+}) state. Because there are four iron sites, each Hb molecule can carry four oxygen molecules (see Fig. 7-4,*C* and *D*). A further simplified schematic of normal HbA is shown in Figure 7-5.

Hb resides in red blood cells (*erythrocytes*) where it accounts for approximately one third of the intracellular space. This pigment (i.e., Hb) is also responsible for giving blood its characteristic red color. It is in tremendous supply in

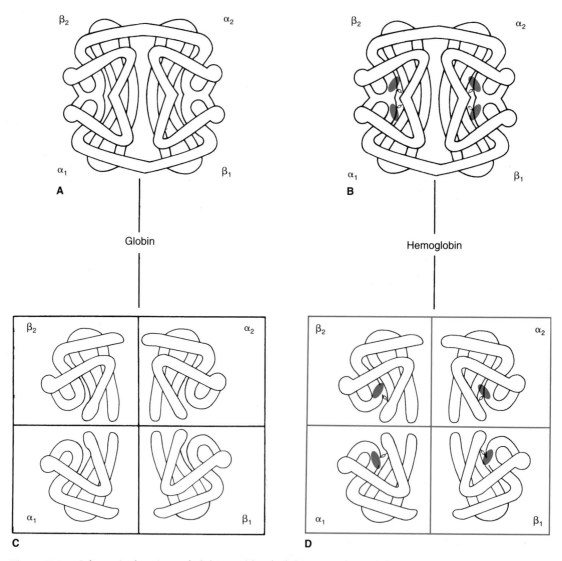

Figure 7-4. **Schematic drawings of globin and hemoglobin.** A and B, Globin is made up of four polypeptide chains (two alpha chains and two beta chains). C and D, Each of the four polypeptide chains is combined with a heme group. Oxygen combines with hemoglobin at the Fe site of each heme group.

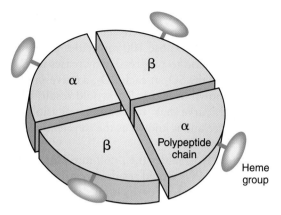

Figure 7-5. **Schematic of normal human hemoglobin A.**

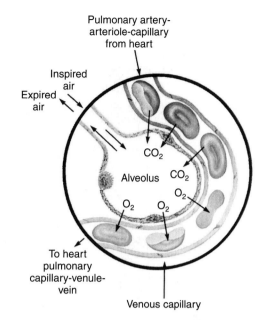

Figure 7-6. **Erythrocytes passing through capillaries single-file.**

the body, and one erythrocyte contains as many as 280 million molecules.[10] The normal concentration of hemoglobin [Hb] is 15 g/100 mL blood in men and 13 to 14 g/100 mL blood in women.

The erythrocytes are biconcave discs approximately 7 μm in diameter. Technically, they are corpuscles rather than cells because they extrude their nuclei just before they mature. Remarkably, the size and flexibility of erythrocytes allow them to pass through the pulmonary capillaries in single file. Figure 7-6 shows erythrocytes passing through a capillary single file. Due to their flexibility, as they pass through, they actually assume a parachute-like shape (Fig. 7-7).

Approximately 2 to 10 million erythrocytes are produced each second, and the life span of an erythrocyte is nearly 120 days. The normal count is approximately 5.4 million cells/mm³ in men and 4.7 million cells/mm³ of blood in women. A decrease in either the erythrocyte count or the [Hb] is called *anemia.*

In the adult, erythrocytes are produced primarily in the bone marrow under the control of the hormone *erythropoietin.* Erythropoietin is secreted primarily in the kidney; however, small quantities are also produced in the liver.[222] The secretion of erythropoietin may increase 100-fold or more in the presence of anemia.[223]

Molecular biologists have been able to synthesize erythropoietin; recombinant human erythropoietin (Epoetin) became available in 1985.[223] Recombinant human erythropoietin has been shown to be effective in the treatment of anemia secondary to renal (kidney) failure.[222] Moreover, synthetic erythropoietin has also shown promise in the treatment of sickle cell

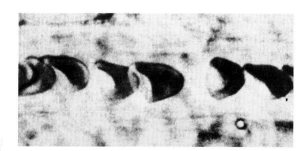

Figure 7-7. **Single-file movement of erythrocytes through pulmonary capillaries.**

disease, anemia of prematurity, and even as a substitute for transfusion.[224–226] Its effectiveness has even caused concern related to its potential abuse to enhance athletic performance.[227]

Saturation

As stated earlier, each hemoglobin molecule is capable of combining with four oxygen molecules. The affinity of hemoglobin for additional oxygen molecules is increased after combination with each single oxygen molecule.[81] Thus, hemoglobin tends to combine with either four oxygen molecules or none (i.e., it is either carrying oxygen or it is not). Thus, we can think of hemoglobin as being either *saturated* (oxygenated) or *desaturated* (unoxygenated). Oxygenated hemoglobin is called *oxyhemoglobin*. Unoxygenated hemoglobin is called *deoxyhemoglobin* or *reduced hemoglobin*, although the latter term is chemically incorrect.[10,81]

The percentage of hemoglobin that is carrying oxygen in arterial blood is called *oxygen saturation of arterial blood* (SaO_2) or simply *saturation* (Fig. 7-8). Saturation is a measure of oxygen in the combined state. One must remember, however, that this is only a percentage of *available* hemoglobin and is in no way a measure of the actual quantity of hemoglobin present.

Oxyhemoglobin Dissociation Curve

The percentage of hemoglobin that actually carries oxygen depends on several factors, but most importantly on the partial pressure of oxygen (PO_2) in the blood. There is a direct, but not linear, relationship between PaO_2 and SaO_2. If one were to expose 100 molecules of hemoglobin in blood to progressive increases in PO_2 and to plot the SO_2 at each PO_2, a curve similar to that shown in Figure 7-9 would result. This S-shaped curve has tremendous physiologic significance and is known as the *oxyhemoglobin dissociation curve*.

At low PO_2 values (i.e., <60 mm Hg), small increases in PO_2 would result in relatively large increases in SO_2. For example, 50% of the hemoglobin molecules would be oxygenated at a PO_2 of only 26 mm Hg (Fig. 7-10). As PO_2 is elevated to 40 mm Hg, saturation increases substantially to approximately 75%. Furthermore, this general trend continues as PO_2 increases to 60 mm Hg where the corresponding saturation is 90%. Beyond a PO_2 of 60 mm Hg, however, saturation increases very slowly and does not reach 100% until approximately 250 mm Hg.[81]

The oxyhemoglobin dissociation curve closely approximates two straight lines (Fig. 7-11); a rather steep line from PO_2, 0 to 60 mm Hg, and a straight flat line above 60 mm Hg. The critical difference between the two portions is that on the steep lower portion of the curve, a small change in PO_2 is associated with a large change in oxygen saturation. Conversely, on the flat upper portion, a large change in PO_2 is associated with only a small change in SO_2. The effect of PO_2 on saturation may be more

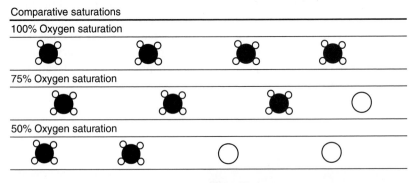

Figure 7-8.   **Comparative saturations.** Saturation is equal to the percentage of hemoglobin that is carrying oxygen. Hemoglobin can be carrying either four molecules of oxygen (oxygenated) or none (deoxygenated).

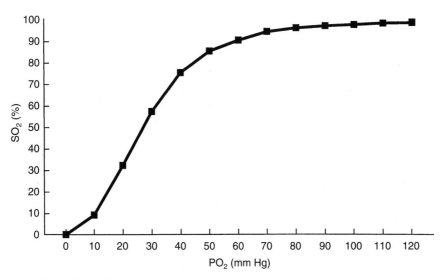

Figure 7-9.   Oxyhemoglobin dissociation curve.

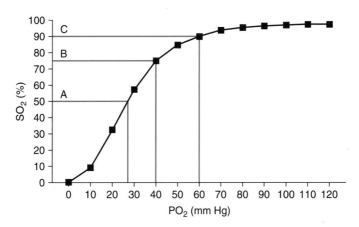

Figure 7-10.   **Key landmarks on the oxyhemoglobin dissociation curve. A,** In the normal oxyhemoglobin curve, the hemoglobin is 50% saturated at a PO_2 of approximately 26 mm Hg. The PO_2 necessary to obtain 50% saturation is called the P_{50}. **B,** The normal PO_2 of mixed venous blood is 40 mm Hg. Therefore, the normal saturation of mixed venous blood is 75%. **C,** A critical point to remember in clinical practice is that at a PO_2 of 60 mm Hg, saturation is still 90%. Saturation falls quickly when PO_2 falls below 60 mm Hg.

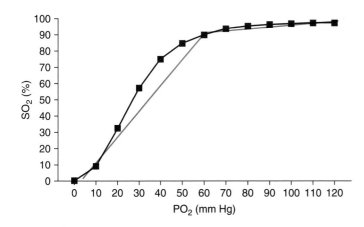

Figure 7-11.   **The oxyhemoglobin curve as two straight lines.** The oxy-hemoglobin curve has two distinct portions: a steep lower portion and a flat upper portion. Because the end of oxygen loading into the blood occurs on the upper portion, it may be called the association portion. The end of oxygen unloading to the tissues occurs on the steep portion, thus it may be called the dissociation portion.

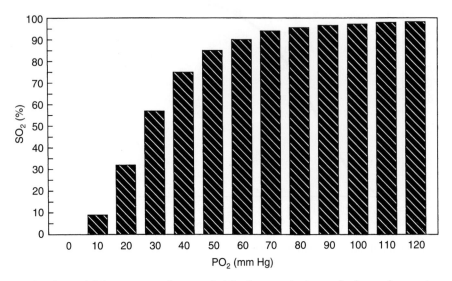

Figure 7-12.   **Oxyhemoglobin curve as a bar graph.** The bar graph shows the large changes in saturation that accompany PO_2 changes on the steep lower portion of the curve. On the upper flat portion of the curve, large changes in PO_2 only slightly change saturation because it is almost 100%.

readily visualized when saturation is plotted as a bar graph, as shown in Figure 7-12.

This concept can be further illustrated if we compare the effect on saturation of an identical PO_2 change on the two portions of the curve (Fig. 7-13). When PO_2 increases 40 mm Hg from 20 to 60 mm Hg, saturation increases from approximately 35% to 90% (total of 55%). Thus, on the steep lower portion of the curve there is a large change (55%) in saturation for a relatively small change (40 mm Hg) in PO_2. Conversely, when PO_2 increases 40 mm Hg from 60 to 100 mm Hg, saturation increases from 90% to 97% (total 7%). Thus, on the flat

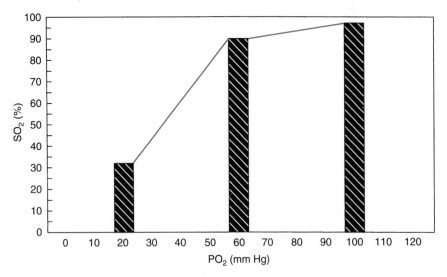

Figure 7-13.   **Significance of PO_2 changes on different portions of the curve.** Saturation increases 55% as PO_2 increases by 40 mm Hg on the steep portion of the curve, whereas saturation increases by only 7% when PO_2 increases by 40 mm Hg on the flat portion of the curve.

upper portion of the curve there is a small change (7%) in saturation for a relatively large change (40 mm Hg) in PO_2. Obviously, this same principle holds true when PO_2 decreases on the respective portions of the curve. Comprehending this critical difference is the essence of understanding the physiologic implications of this curve.

Association/Dissociation Portions

The association (i.e., combination) of oxygen with hemoglobin occurs in the lungs as the PO_2 increases from 40 mm Hg in mixed venous blood to approximately 100 mm Hg. Because the *end* of oxygen loading into the blood occurs on the flat, upper portion of the curve, it is sometimes referred to as the *association portion* of the curve. Conversely, the steep lower portion of the curve is sometimes referred to as the *dissociation portion* of the curve because the *end* of oxygen unloading occurs on this portion as PaO_2 decreases from 100 to 40 mm Hg in the systemic capillaries (see Fig. 7-11). The association part of the curve is important in the lungs, whereas the dissociation part of the curve is important in the tissues.

Association Portion. Normal adult PaO_2 is approximately 100 mm Hg. Normal SaO_2 is approximately 97% to 98%. At normal PaO_2 while breathing room air, hemoglobin is almost 100% saturated. This is generally considered to be a physiologic advantage because the ability of the hemoglobin to carry oxygen is maximized under ordinary conditions. Conversely, however, the association portion of the curve could be viewed as a physiologic disadvantage if the body was trying to add additional amounts of oxygen to the blood. Increasing the PO_2 above normal does relatively little to add more oxygen to the blood because the hemoglobin is already maximally saturated.

It is likewise interesting that PO_2 can decrease by 40 mm Hg below normal down to a PaO_2 of 60 mm Hg while SaO_2 remains at 90%. This serves as an excellent defense mechanism in that the PaO_2 may decrease substantially while the combination of oxygen with hemoglobin will be only slightly decreased. Thus, the decrease in PaO_2 observed at high altitude, or during the aging process, does not significantly decrease the SaO_2 when one remains on the flat

portion of the curve. The amount of oxygen in the combined state remains relatively constant. A diagnostic advantage of the association portion of the curve is that early pulmonary disease can be detected by a decrease in PaO_2, and this can be accomplished before SaO_2 decreases appreciably.

Dissociation Portion. The end of oxygen unloading from the blood to the tissues occurs on the dissociation (steep) portion of the curve. Because, on this portion, a small change in PO_2 greatly affects saturation, a large amount of additional oxygen can be supplied to the tissues by allowing venous PO_2 to fall to levels just slightly below normal. For example, a large amount of oxygen would move from the blood to the tissues as venous PO_2 decreased from 40 to 30 mm Hg. Thus, a mechanism exists to easily deliver additional oxygen to the cells if metabolism increases or if supply of oxygen is compromised, such as during a decline in cardiac output.

Comprehension of this portion of the oxyhemoglobin dissociation curve is also essential for understanding the value and goal of low percentages of oxygen therapy in chronic obstructive pulmonary disease (COPD). Because most patients with COPD and acute pulmonary problems have PaO_2 values on the steep portion of the curve, any small increase in PaO_2 greatly increases SaO_2 values. Thus, the volume of oxygen combined with hemoglobin can be increased substantially with only a small increase in PaO_2. This is important in COPD patients to avoid the adverse effects of PaO_2 greater than 60 mm Hg on ventilation that may occur.

Oxyhemoglobin Affinity/P₅₀

P_{50}. The oxyhemoglobin dissociation curve is a graphic representation of how PO_2 normally affects the combination of oxygen with hemoglobin. The specific affinity of oxygen for hemoglobin can be quantitated by evaluating what partial pressure of oxygen is necessary to achieve 50% saturation. This standardized index of Hb-O_2 affinity that is measured at 37° C, PCO_2 of 40 mm Hg, and a pH of 7.40 is called the P_{50}.[184] Normal P_{50} is about 26 mm Hg, approximately 27 mm Hg in women and 25 mm Hg in men.[185] In other words, 26 mm Hg of oxygen pressure is normally

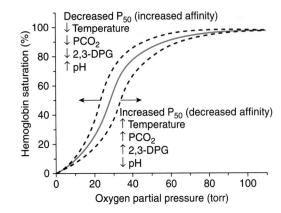

Figure 7-14. **Oxyhemoglobin affinity**. The affinity of hemoglobin for oxygen is expressed as the P_{50}. Increases in PCO_2, temperature, or DPG; and decreases in pH shift the curve to the right (increased P_{50} = decreased affinity). Opposite changes shift the curve to the left (decreased P_{50} = increased affinity).

required to oxygenate 50% of the hemoglobin (see Fig. 7-10).

Shifts of the Curve

At least four factors are known to alter Hb-O_2 affinity. As shown in Figure 7-14, temperature, pH, or PCO_2 may shift the oxyhemoglobin curve. In addition, the concentration of the substance 2,3-diphosphoglycerate (DPG) within the erythrocyte is similarly known to affect Hb-O_2 affinity.

Affinity of oxygen for hemoglobin increases when there is a *decrease* in temperature, hydrogen ion concentration, PCO_2, or DPG (Box 7-1). A decrease in hydrogen ion concentration is associated with an increased pH. Conversely (see Fig. 7-14), Hb-O_2 affinity is decreased when there is an *increase* in temperature, hydrogen ion (decreased pH), PCO_2, or DPG (Box 7-2).

Box 7-1 Increased Hb-O_2 Affinity/ Left Shift of Hb-O_2 Curve

A *decrease* in any of the following will *increase* Hb-O_2 affinity and will shift the oxyhemoglobin dissociation curve to the *left*.
1. Temperature
2. Hydrogen ion concentration ($\uparrow$ pH)
3. PCO_2
4. DPG

Box 7-2 Decreased Hb-O_2 Affinity/ Right Shift of Hb-O_2 Curve

A *increase* in any of the following will *decrease* Hb-O_2 affinity and will shift the oxyhemoglobin dissociation curve to the *right*.
1. Temperature
2. Hydrogen ion concentration ($\downarrow$ pH)
3. PCO_2
4. DPG

The fact that high PCO_2 and low pH decreases Hb-O_2 affinity is known as the *Bohr effect*. An increase in oxygen similarly decreases hemoglobin affinity for CO_2, and this is known as the *Haldane effect*.

Clinical Effects of Hb-O_2 Curve Shifts

A shift of the curve to the left and increased Hb-O_2 affinity would appear to benefit the patient because hemoglobin could more easily pick up oxygen. However, hemoglobin is 97% saturated with normal Hb-O_2 affinity; therefore, oxygen loading is not enhanced appreciably with a shift of the curve to the left. Furthermore, this increased Hb-O_2 affinity impedes the release of oxygen to the tissues and generally has a net detrimental effect.

Decreased Hb-O_2 affinity and a shift of the curve to the right, on the other hand, generally enhances oxygen delivery to the tissues and is often a valuable compensatory mechanism. Figure 7-15 shows the amount of oxygen that is released to the tissues with various positions of the curve and assuming a normal PaO_2 and mixed venous PO_2 ($P\bar{v}O_2$). The amount of oxygen released to the tissues is least when the curve is shifted to the left (see Fig. 7-15,*B*). Conversely, the amount of oxygen released to the tissues is greatest when the curve is shifted to the right (see Fig. 7-15,*C*). A shift of the curve to the right in an individual with a PaO_2 of 90 mm Hg and a normal $P\bar{v}O_2$ of 40 mm Hg could enhance oxygen release to the tissues by as much as 60%.[186]

In conclusion, although a shift of the curve to the left tends to enhance the combination of hemoglobin with oxygen, it may be detrimental to the patient because the release of oxygen to the tissues will be impeded. On the other hand, a shift to the right is usually beneficial because

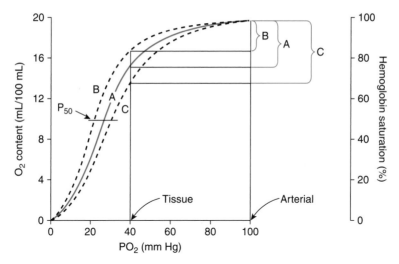

Figure 7-15.   Effects of shifts of curve on tissue oxygen delivery. *A*, The normal Hb-O_2 curve and the amount of oxygen released to the tissues from hemoglobin. *B*, A left shift tends to decrease tissue oxygen release. *C*, A shift to the right tends to increase oxygen release to the tissues.

the release of oxygen to the tissues is enhanced. This benefit may be negated, however, when PaO_2 is less than 60 mm Hg. When hypoxemia is present, shifts of the curve to the right may substantially decrease oxygen loading into the blood, and this factor may outweigh any benefits in terms of oxygen unloading.[186]

2,3-Diphosphoglycerate

Organic phosphates represent a chemical group normally present in erythrocytes. These organic phosphates tend to bind with hemoglobin and thus reduce affinity of hemoglobin for oxygen.[187,188] A decrease in Hb-O_2 affinity will, of course, shift the oxyhemoglobin dissociation curve to the right. Therefore, the large amounts of organic phosphates present within the erythrocytes are generally considered to be beneficial. The most important inorganic phosphate is DPG, primarily because it is the most abundant.[185,189]

Furthermore, changes in DPG tend to have a sustained effect on Hb-O_2 affinity whereas the shift of the curve to the right that accompanies an increased hydrogen ion concentration, for example, lasts for only a few hours.[185]

Increased 2,3-Diphosphoglycerate. A twofold increase in DPG, which could occur clinically, would greatly enhance oxygen unloading to the tissues. A twofold increase in DPG

would increase P_{50} by 10 mm Hg (e.g., $P_{50} = 36$ mm Hg). DPG increases in various situations and appears generally to be an adaptive mechanism in hypoxic insults. Several conditions that have been associated with *high* DPG levels are shown in Box 7-3.

DPG increases relatively quickly as a compensatory mechanism. Measurable increases in DPG may be seen within 60 minutes after strenuous exercise.[189] The increase in DPG enhances oxygen unloading and helps to offset deficiencies in the transport or loading of oxygen.

Decreased 2,3-Diphosphoglycerate. Conversely, DPG concentrations may be *less* than normal in several conditions such as those shown in Box 7-4. Septic shock is a cardiovascular problem associated with bacterial infection of the blood. Acidemia is a below-normal pH

Box 7-3	Conditions Associated with Increased DPG

Anemia
Hyperthyroidism
Hypoxemia associated with COPD
Congenital heart disease
Ascent to high altitude
Low output heart failure
Healthy subjects after strenuous exercise

Box 7-4   Conditions Associated with Decreased DPG

Septic shock
Certain enzyme deficiencies
Acidemia
Blood stored in ACD

---

of the blood. The fact that acidemia decreases DPG levels probably explains why high DPG levels are not seen consistently in acute crisis of patients with COPD.[190] The increased DPG associated with hypoxemia in these patients may be offset by the decreased DPG associated with acidemia.

Probably the most common clinical cause of DPG deficiency, however, is the intravenous infusion of stored blood into a patient. DPG decreases rapidly in blood stored in acid-citrate dextrose preservative and falls to approximately one-third of normal after approximately 1 week of storage.[191] Within 2 weeks of storage at 4° C, DPG is almost completely absent.[192] Nevertheless, low DPG levels would not preclude a transfusion in a patient who is anemic.

It is possible to restore DPG in stored blood to normal levels within 30 minutes, which can be accomplished by incubating the blood with inosine, pyruvate, and phosphate.[192] This procedure is not clinically useful, however, because inosine has been associated with adverse effects when administered intravenously.[189] Furthermore, DPG levels increase to approximately 50% of normal in approximately 24 hours after the administration of the blood.[193]

Oxygen Content

Arterial Oxygen Content

The total *volume* of oxygen present in arterial blood is called *arterial oxygen content* (CaO_2). The oxygen content can be calculated by adding the volume of oxygen present in the two blood compartments, as shown in Box 7-5. The volume of dissolved oxygen in arterial blood is calculated by multiplying the PaO_2 by the solubility coefficient of oxygen in blood ($CsO_2 = 0.003$ mL O_2/100 mL blood/mm Hg). The normal volume of oxygen dissolved in arterial blood is approximately 0.3 vol% (0.3 mL O_2/100 mL of blood), which is calculated in Box 7-6.

Box 7-5   Arterial Oxygen Content

$$\frac{\text{Volume of dissolved oxygen} + \text{Volume of combined oxygen}}{\text{TOTAL OXYGEN CONTENT}}$$

To calculate the volume of combined oxygen in arterial blood, one must know the hemoglobin concentration [Hb], arterial oxygen saturation (SaO_2), and the oxygen-carrying capacity of hemoglobin. The oxygen-carrying capacity of hemoglobin is a constant value of 1.34 mL O_2/g HbO_2.[81] Theoretical calculations suggest that this value should be 1.39 mL O_2/g HbO_2; however, this amount is never achieved in humans because of the presence of hemoglobin variants.[185] Thus, in calculations here, it is assumed that for every gram of oxygenated hemoglobin, 1.34 mL O_2 is present.

The formula for calculating the volume of combined oxygen is shown in Box 7-7. SaO_2 is multiplied by the [Hb] to determine the amount of oxygenated hemoglobin present. Then, the HbO_2 in grams is multiplied by the oxygen-carrying capacity of hemoglobin to determine the volume of oxygen in the combined state. Assuming a normal [Hb] of 15 g% and an SaO_2 of 98%, the volume of combined oxygen in arterial blood is approximately 19.7 vol%.

Finally, the CaO_2 is equal to the sum of dissolved and combined oxygen (Box 7-8). Normal CaO_2 is approximately 20 vol%. Approximately 98% of the oxygen in the blood is in the combined state (Fig. 7-16). For this reason, CaO_2 correlates very closely with SaO_2 and the oxyhemoglobin dissociation curve as shown in Figure 7-17. PaO_2, on the other hand, only reflects blood oxygen volume indirectly.

Mixed Venous Oxygen Content

Obviously, venous blood returning to the heart will contain less oxygen than arterial blood.

Box 7-6   Normal Volume of Oxygen Dissolved in Arterial Blood

$PaO_2 \times CsO_2$ = volume of dissolved O_2
(100 mm Hg) × (0.003 vol%/mm Hg)
    = 0.3 vol% O_2

Box 7-7	Normal Volume of Oxygen Combined in Arterial Blood

$[Hb] \times SaO_2 \times 1.34 \text{ mL } O_2/g \text{ HbO}_2 = \text{volume of combined } O_2$
$(15 \text{ g}/100 \text{ mL blood}) \times (0.98) \times 1.34 \text{ mL } O_2/g \text{ HbO}_2 = 19.7 \text{ vol}\%$

Box 7-8	Normal CaO$_2$

$\text{Dissolved } O_2 + \text{Combined } O_2 = CaO_2$
$0.3 \text{ vol}\% + 19.7 \text{ vol}\% = 20 \text{ vol}\%$

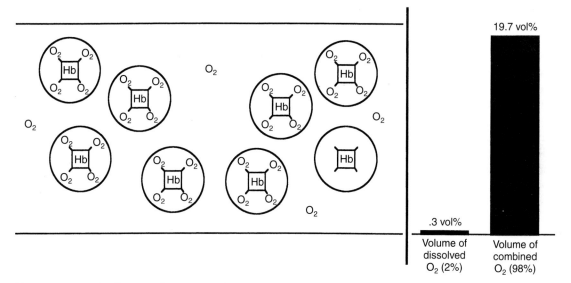

Figure 7-16.   **Distribution of oxygen in the blood.**

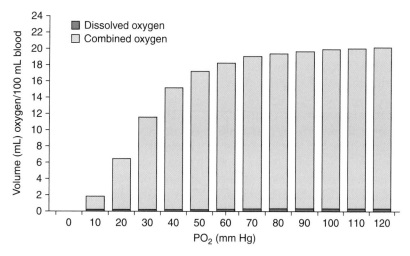

Figure 7-17.   **Oxygen content by compartment.** The total oxygen content of the blood is primarily a result of the degree of saturation of hemoglobin. Thus, this bar graph of oxygen content closely resembles the oxyhemoglobin curve. There is, however, a small linear increase in dissolved oxygen content with increased PO$_2$. At normal PO$_2$ of 100 mm Hg, 98% of oxygen is in the combined form.

Box 7-9 | Mixed Venous Oxygen Content

$$\text{Dissolved } O_2 = P\bar{v}O_2 \times CsO_2$$
$$\text{Dissolved } O_2 = (40 \text{ mm Hg}) \times (0.003 \text{ vol\%/mm Hg}) = 0.12 \text{ vol\%}$$
$$\text{Combined } O_2 = [\text{Hb}] \times S\bar{v}O_2 \times O_2 \text{ carrying capacity}$$
$$\text{Combined } O_2 = (15 \text{ g\%}) (0.75) (1.34 \text{ mL } O_2/\text{g}) = 15.08 \text{ vol\%}$$
$$\text{Oxygen content} = \text{dissolved } O_2 + \text{combined } O_2$$
$$\text{Oxygen content} = (0.12 \text{ vol\%}) + (15.08 \text{ vol\%}) = \underline{15.2 \text{ vol\%}}$$

As discussed in Chapter 3, peripheral venous blood varies in its oxygen volume depending on the specific tissue it is returning from. *Mixed* venous blood, however (available only from a pulmonary artery catheter), is an average of all venous blood and normally has a $P\bar{v}O_2$ of approximately 40 mm Hg and an $S\bar{v}O_2$ of 75% (see Fig. 7-10). The oxygen content of mixed venous blood can thus be calculated by adding dissolved oxygen and combined oxygen, which is shown in Box 7-9.

Arteriovenous Oxygen Content Difference

The difference in oxygen content between arterial and mixed venous blood $C(a-\bar{v})O_2$ is approximately 5 vol% and is shown in Box 7-10. Thus, for every 100 mL of blood that perfuses the tissues, approximately 5 mL of oxygen is normally released to the cells. The *Fick equation* (Box 7-11) shows the relationship between cardiac minute output ($\dot{Q}$), arteriovenous oxygen content difference $C(a-\bar{v})O_2$, and oxygen consumption ($\dot{V}O_2$). Given a normal cardiac output of approximately 5 L/min and an arteriovenous oxygen content difference of 5 vol%, the total amount of oxygen delivered and consumed by the tissues is approximately 250 mL/min.

In some clinical situations, oxygen consumption is constant over short periods; thus making cardiac output and the $C(a-\bar{v})O_2$ inversely proportional. Indeed, $C(a-\bar{v})O_2$ was often used in the past as an indicator of cardiac output; high gradients indicated a decrease in cardiac output, whereas low gradients supposedly reflected an increased cardiac output. For example, a $C(a-\bar{v})O_2$ of 10 vol% suggests a low cardiac output, whereas a $C(a-\bar{v})O_2$ of 2.5 vol% suggests an increased cardiac output.

More recently, however, it has been shown that oxygen consumption is not constant in critically ill patients, even over short periods. Therefore, the $C(a-\bar{v})O_2$ should not be considered to be a reliable indicator of cardiac output.

The $C(a-\bar{v})O_2$ divided by CaO_2 is called the *oxygen extraction ratio* or the *oxygen utilization coefficient*. The normal oxygen extraction ratio is 25% (5 vol% divided by 20 vol%). This index may be useful for monitoring and predicting outcome in critically ill patients.[228]

Cyanosis

Cyanosis is a clinical condition in which a patient's skin, mucous membranes, or nailbeds appear blue or gray. Blue discoloration of the skin is sometimes referred to as *peripheral cyanosis*, whereas discoloration of the mucous membranes may be called *central cyanosis*. Peripheral cyanosis is difficult to detect in dark-skinned individuals. Cyanosis has long been a clinical sign known to be frequently associated with inadequate oxygenation status and hypoxia.

The color observed is a result of the increased quantity of *desaturated* hemoglobin present in many types of oxygenation disturbances. The percentage of desaturated hemoglobin is the difference between total hemoglobin (100%) and oxygenated hemoglobin (SO_2). For example, if SO_2 is 90%, then the percentage of desaturated hemoglobin (Hb %desat) is the remainder or 10%.

Cyanosis can usually be observed when the average quantity of desaturated hemoglobin in the capillaries is approximately 5 g/100 mL of blood. The unit usually used in place of

---

Box 7-10 | Normal $C(a-\bar{v})O_2$

$$CaO_2 - C\bar{v}O_2 = C(a-\bar{v})O_2$$
$$20 \text{ vol\%} - 15.2 \text{ vol\%} = 4.8 \text{ vol\%}$$

Box 7-11 Fick Equation

Cardiac output × arteriovenous oxygen content difference = O_2 consumption

$$\dot{Q} \times C(a - \bar{v}) \, O_2 = \dot{V}O_2$$

$$(5000 \text{ mL blood/min}) \times (5 \text{ mL } O_2/100 \text{ mL blood}) = 250 \text{ mL } O_2/\text{min}$$

---

g/100 mL of blood is g%. Thus, cyanosis is observed in the presence of an average of 5 g% of desaturated hemoglobin in the capillaries.

The *average* quantity of desaturated hemoglobin in the capillary can be calculated by averaging the amount of desaturated hemoglobin entering the capillary (i.e., arterial blood) with the amount of desaturated hemoglobin leaving the capillary (i.e., venous blood), which is shown in Box 7-12. Normally, [Hb] is 15 g%, SaO_2 is approximately 98%, and $S\bar{v}O_2$ is 75%. Thus, (Hb %desat) of arterial blood is about 2% (i.e., 100% − 98% = 2%), and (Hb %desat) of venous blood is approximately 25% (i.e., 100% − 75% = 25%). Thus, the normal average amount of desaturated Hb (Hb desat) is approximately 2 g% (Box 7-13).

Obviously, if arterial or venous blood is poorly oxygenated (highly desaturated), at some point, there will be an average of 5 g% of desaturated hemoglobin and cyanosis will be evident. It has also been observed that cyanosis is typically seen when SaO_2 decreases to approximately 85%.[194]

It is important to realize, however, that cyanosis is only present when a certain *quantity* of desaturated hemoglobin is present. Thus, in the presence of anemia, an individual may be very poorly oxygenated yet cyanosis will not be seen. Conversely, in the presence of polycythemia, cyanosis may be present even though the individual is adequately oxygenated.

In summary, although cyanosis may suggest hypoxia, its presence or absence must always be interpreted in light of the patient's actual [Hb].

QUANTITATIVE OXYGEN TRANSPORT

Dissolved Oxygen Transport

Oxygen transport, sometimes referred to as *oxygen delivery*, is defined as the volume of oxygen leaving the left ventricle of the heart each minute. Assuming that a patient had no hemoglobin and could carry oxygen only in the dissolved state, oxygen transport would be calculated (Box 7-14). Under basal metabolic conditions, the average young man consumes approximately 250 mL O_2/minute, whereas women consume slightly less. Basal metabolic conditions exist when an individual is resting and fasting but is not asleep.[185] Dissolved oxygen transport (15 mL O_2/minute) is clearly inadequate to meet the tissue oxygen requirements of humans even at rest.

The quantity of oxygen transported in the dissolved state could be increased only by increasing one of the factors in the formula shown in Box 7-14. To meet tissue requirements, cardiac output would have to increase to 83 L/minute at rest and 166 L/minute during exercise, assuming the volume of dissolved oxygen remained constant.[81] This, of course, is impossible because the maximum cardiac output even during exercise in a well-conditioned athlete may be only 30 to 40 L/minute.[229]

Alternatively, dissolved oxygen transport could be increased by increasing dissolved

---

Box 7-12 Calculation of Average Desaturated Hemoglobin in Capillaries

$$\frac{[\text{Hb}] \times \text{arterial (Hb %desat)} + [\text{Hb}] \times \text{venous (Hb %desat)}}{2}$$

Box 7-13 Calculation of the Normal Average Desaturated Hemoglobin in Capillaries

$$\frac{[\text{Hb}] \times \text{arterial (Hb %desat)} + [\text{Hb}] \times \text{venous (Hb %desat)}}{2}$$

$$= \frac{(15 \text{ g%}) \times (0.02) + (15 \text{ g%}) \times (0.25)}{2}$$

$$= \frac{(0.3 \text{ g%}) + (3.7 \text{ g%})}{2} = 2 \text{ g% (Hb desat)}$$

Box 7-14   Dissolved Oxygen Transport

(Cardiac output) × (volume of dissolved O_2) = dissolved O_2 transport
(5000 mL blood/min) × (0.3 mL O_2/100 mL blood) = 15 mL O_2/min

---

Box 7-15   Combined Oxygen Transport

(Cardiac output) × (volume of combined O_2) = combined O_2 transport
(5000 mL of blood/min) × (19.7 mL O_2/100 mL blood) = 985 mL O_2/min

---

Box 7-16   Total Oxygen Transport

(Cardiac output) × (CaO_2) = O_2 transport
(5000 mL of blood/min) × (20 mL O_2/100 mL blood) = 1000 mL O_2/min

---

oxygen content, which depends on the PaO_2 and the solubility coefficient for oxygen in blood. An increase in either of these factors would directly enhance oxygen transport. Because PO_2 and oxygen content are directly related, tissue oxygen demands could be met if PO_2 was sufficiently high. Unfortunately, PO_2 would need to be approximately 2000 mm Hg to meet basal metabolic needs. Although a PaO_2 in this range could be achieved through the administration of FIO_2 1.0 at 3 atm in a hyperbaric chamber, these devices are often not available and high FIO_2 values may lead to oxygen toxicity.

Finally, certain blood substitutes with very high solubility coefficients may be administered, although their use has been limited.

Combined Oxygen Transport

The volume of *combined oxygen transport* can be calculated as shown in Box 7-15. Using the normal volume of combined oxygen in the arterial blood, which was calculated in Box 7-7, combined oxygen transport is approximately 985 mL O_2/minute. This amount is almost four times that of oxygen required under basal conditions (i.e., 250 mL O_2/minute). Furthermore, during heavy exercise, oxygen consumption may increase 10-fold.[239] Thus, the tremendous value of hemoglobin in oxygen transport can be appreciated.

Total Oxygen Transport

Total oxygen transport, or simply oxygen transport, is a quantitative measure of *all* the oxygen that is transported out to the tissues each minute regardless of the method in which it is carried. The formula for oxygen transport is shown in Box 7-16. The phrase *oxygen delivery* is synonymous with oxygen transport.

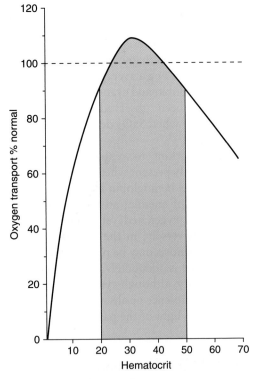

Figure 7-18.   **Oxygen transport vs. hematocrit level.** Slight elevations in hematocrit increase oxygen transport above normal due to increased oxygen carrying capacity. Large increases in hematocrit diminish oxygen transport secondary to increased blood viscosity and decreased cardiac output.

One can see through these calculations that as [Hb] increases there will be a corresponding increase in oxygen transport as long as cardiac output remains constant. Notwithstanding, however, as [Hb] increases, there will be a corresponding increase in blood viscosity, which, in turn, may decrease cardiac output. Figure 7-18 illustrates how oxygen transport tends to increase up to a hematocrit of approximately 33% but beyond this level, oxygen transport actually tends to decline because of a decreased cardiac output secondary to increased blood viscosity.

HEMOGLOBIN ABNORMALITIES

Carboxyhemoglobin

Carbon monoxide (CO) is a colorless, odorless, tasteless *toxic* gas that competes with oxygen for the same molecular site on the hemoglobin molecule. CO has almost 245 times more affinity for hemoglobin than does oxygen.[230] Given 100 available molecules of hemoglobin in 21% oxygen and 0.01% CO, half of the molecules would combine with oxygen and half would combine with CO despite the much lower concentration of CO. Hemoglobin combined with CO forms the substance *carboxyhemoglobin* (HbCO).

HbCO levels are expressed usually as a percentage of total hemoglobin. Levels as high as 10% may be observed in heavy cigarette smokers. Crack smoking has also been associated with increased HbCO levels, which could further aggravate cocaine-induced cardiac problems.[195]

Carbon monoxide is produced by the incomplete combustion of carbonaceous substances. Thus, critically high HbCO levels generally only occur after inhalation of gasoline engine exhaust, or in conjunction with injuries caused by smoke inhalation (e.g., fires, etc.). Indeed, 60% to 80% of early smoke inhalation deaths are due to HbCO rather than cutaneous burns.[196] Typically HbCO toxicity occurs when exposed to high levels of CO in a closed or poorly ventilated environment. Occasionally, however, high levels and even fatalities have been reported *outdoors* following prolonged use of gasoline- or oil-burning equipment.[203]

Traditionally, HbCO has been considered to be harmful to cellular oxygenation in two ways. First, hemoglobin combined with CO is incapable of carrying oxygen at that molecular site. Second, HbCO shifts the oxyhemoglobin curve to the left and makes oxygen unloading to the tissues more difficult. The leftward shift

---

ON CALL | CASE 7-1 *ABGs and Critical Thinking*

You are the only person available to care for this patient. You must assess the patient/situation and act accordingly.

A postoperative 55-year-old woman arrives in the recovery room following cardiac surgery. She appears pale and uncomfortable.

HR	90/min
RR	25/min
Temp	37° C

ARTERIAL BLOOD GASES

FIO$_2$	0.60
SaO$_2$	95%
pH	7.30
PaCO$_2$	37 mm Hg
PaO$_2$	94 mm Hg
[HCO$_3$]	20 mEq/L

LABORATORY WORK

[Hb]	5 g%
[WBC]	8000 mm^3

VITAL SIGNS

BP	130/85

ASSESSMENT

Abnormalities: List abnormal data and other noteworthy information. Classify ABG

Explanation: List possible diseases, pathology, or other situations that may have led to this patient's condition.

Evaluation: Suggest additional data that would be useful in helping understand the situation or in making a diagnosis.

INTERVENTION

Importance: Prioritize concern(s) of treatment in order of urgency and/or seriousness as you see the overall situation.

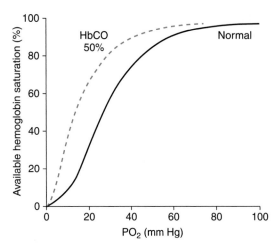

Figure 7-19. **Effect of HbCO on oxyhemoglobin affinity.** In addition to occupying heme sites in place of oxygen, carboxyhemoglobin also increases the affinity of Hb for oxygen and shifts the oxyhemoglobin curve to the left.

of the curve is often depicted as shown in Figure 7-19; however, Figure 7-20 is probably a better way to illustrate the decrease in oxygenation because the available [Hb] is likewise decreased with the formation of HbCO.[197]

Although toxicity is typically measured as HbCO%, substantial evidence suggests that the toxicity of CO may be due primarily to the direct metabolic effects of dissolved CO in the plasma rather than to the HbCO concentration per se.[198] The highly variable toxicity in patients with comparable HbCO levels is consistent with this theory.[199] Some patients are severely toxic at HbCO levels of only 20%, whereas other patients are nearly asymptomatic (e.g., headaches) at levels as high as 50%.[200]

Regardless of the exact mechanism and in the absence of a simple alternative, HbCO levels, which are easily attained with CO-oximetry, still probably provide the best markers of the degree of CO toxicity.[201] Notwithstanding, one should always focus treatment on the total patient picture versus simply the laboratory value.[199]

Administration of FIO_2 1.0 is very effective in the treatment of high HbCO levels. FIO_2 1.0 is effective because it reduces the half-life of HbCO from 5 hours and 20 minutes to approximately 1 hour and 20 minutes.[202] In addition, a secondary benefit is a slight increase in dissolved oxygen content because of the increased PaO_2. Hyperbaric oxygen, when available, is even more effective in the treatment of CO poisoning because it reduces the half-life of HbCO to 23 minutes.[202]

Hemoglobin Variants

The hemoglobin described earlier is normal adult hemoglobin (HbA). More than 120 variations of hemoglobin, however, have been identified. Any small change in the sequence of amino

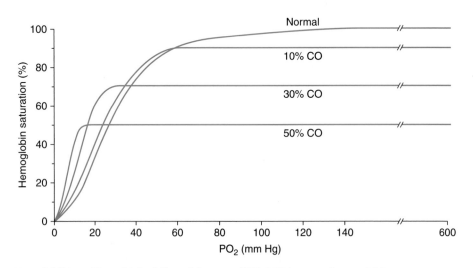

Figure 7-20. **Additive effect of left shift and increased HbCO% on oxyhemoglobin curve.**

acids in the hemoglobin molecule results in a different form of hemoglobin that may have very different chemical properties. Originally, as new forms of Hb were recognized, they were named according to the letters of the alphabet (e.g., HbS, HbM, etc.). It soon became apparent, however, that there would be more than 26 types of hemoglobin; therefore, new forms of hemoglobin were named according to the geographic region where they were first discovered (e.g., Hb Kansas, Hb Beth Israel).

Several hemoglobin variants have an altered affinity for oxygen. For example, Hb Kansas has a P_{50} of 70 mm Hg, whereas Hb Rainier has a P_{50} of 12 mm Hg (Fig. 7-21). HbH has 12 times more affinity for oxygen than HbA and cannot release oxygen to the tissues. The three hemoglobin variants of common clinical significance are HbF, HbM, and HbS. These species of hemoglobin are discussed in the following sections.

Fetal Hemoglobin

Fetal hemoglobin (HbF) is found in the fetus and has a greater affinity for oxygen than HbA, presumably because it is less affected by DPG.[81] The P_{50} of normal HbF is about 20 mm Hg.[231] In premature infants, P_{50} is approximately 18 mm Hg and in infant respiratory distress

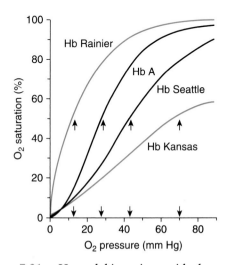

Figure 7-21. Hemoglobin variants with abnormal affinity. Hb Kansas has decreased oxygen affinity and a P_{50} of 70 mm Hg. Hb Rainier has increased affinity for oxygen and a P_{50} of 12 mm Hg.

syndrome, it is lower still at nearly 16 mm Hg.[232] Thus, through HbF, the fetus can attract oxygen from maternal HbA because of its greater affinity. Furthermore, oxygen transport is further enhanced in the infant because of a higher hemoglobin concentration ([Hb] 18 g% in a term infant).

Ninety-five percent of hemoglobin present in the fetus at 10 weeks' gestation is HbF.[231] At approximately 30 weeks' gestation, the concentration of HbF begins to decline; and at term the concentration of HbF is roughly 80%. HbF should continue to decline after birth, falling to 50% at 1 to 2 months and 5% at 6 months. Often, HbF may even fall to normal adult levels (<2%) after the first 6 months of life.[233]

Failure of HbF to decline has been observed in certain pathologic conditions, such as beta thalassemia.[231] More recently, elevated levels of HbF have been shown in sudden infant death syndrome and may help to shed some light on this disorder, although the significance of this finding remains unclear.[234]

Methemoglobin

A small portion of hemoglobin in the red blood cell normally undergoes a slight chemical change and forms methemoglobin (metHb). This change occurs when the ferrous ion loses an electron and is thus transformed to the ferric state. In this event, hemoglobin is *oxidized* (i.e., loss of an electron) rather than *oxygenated*. Methemoglobin is useless in the transport of oxygen. Normal metHb concentration is approximately 1%.

Methemoglobinemia is defined usually as a metHb concentration exceeding 1% to 2%. High levels of metHb may be acquired or congenital. Methemoglobinemia may be caused by ingestion of amyl nitrate or nitroglycerin. Amyl nitrite, "snappers," and other volatile nitrites are sometimes used as a recreational drugs for stimulant, aphrodisiac, or psychedelic effects.[204] These drugs may lead to rapid onset of severe methemoglobinemia (30% to 70% metHb) and an individual who presents to the emergency department incoherent and with severe cyanosis.[204,205]

Topical anesthetics have frequently been implicated in the abrupt onset of methemoglobinemia. Twenty-percent benzocaine (e.g., Hurricaine spray) and prilocaine have been implicated in several cases of acute onset severe methemoglobinemia especially when the normal dose is exceeded.[209,210]

Infants younger than 6 months of age are particularly vulnerable to dietary methemoglobinemia, especially when exposed to well water that contains nitrates.[235] Nitrates may be converted to nitrites by bacteria in the intestines, thus leading to methemoglobinemia.[204] Likewise, infants exposed to topical anesthetics used as teething gels for the relief of pain have also developed severe methemoglobinemia.[207,208] Hemoglobin M is a congenital hemoglobin variant that is functionally the same as metHb in that it too is oxidized when exposed to oxygen.

Abrupt onset of severe cyanosis, especially following administration of topical anesthetics, should alert one to the possibility of methemoglobinemia. Cyanosis typically appears with metHb levels of approximately 15%.[211] Other researchers have described the clinical presentation as cyanosis with a normal or high PaO_2[206,211] or, in the case of inherited methemoglobinemias, as being more blue than sick.[236]

Another clue to the onset of methemoglobinemia may be a modest decrease in SpO_2 via pulse oximetry (e.g., 98% falling to 94%).[212] Interestingly, however, with increasing levels of methemoglobin, the pulse oximeter tends to migrate towards an SpO_2 reading of 85% (Fig. 7-22).[213] Blood with elevated metHb will typically appear brown, rusty, or even black and this too may be a useful clue to diagnosis. Ultimately, laboratory analysis via spectrophotometry confirms the diagnosis.

Methylene blue accelerates the reduction of metHb and may be useful in the treatment of some forms of this disorder. Methylene blue is usually administered intravenously at a rate of 1 to 2 mg/kg in adults and 2 mg/kg in infants; it should be administered slowly over 5 minutes and repeated if cyanosis persists for 1 hour.[204] Often, relatively high levels of metHb (i.e., >35%) are fairly well tolerated, and treatment may not be necessary.

Although less common, another type of abnormal hemoglobin, sulfhemoglobinemia, may be mistaken for methemoglobinemia.

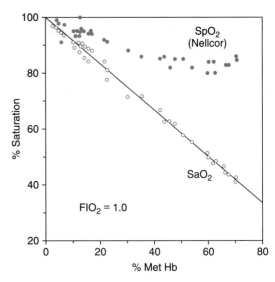

Figure 7-22. **Comparison of pulse oximetry readings at various levels of metHb%.** With increasing concentrations of metHb, the pulse oximeter readings tend to plateau around 85%.

Sulfhemoglobin is present if oxyhemoglobin combines with hydrogen sulfide. The blood may also appear chocolate and measurements via co-oximetry may indicate high levels of methemoglobin because the absorption characteristics are similar. Even low doses of sulfhemoglobin may cause severe cyanosis. Sulfhemoglobin appears to be less toxic than methemoglobin probably because it shifts the oxyhemoglobin curve to the right. Sulfhemoglobin should be suspected when the patient with presumed methemoglobinemia does not respond to methylene blue.[214]

Hemoglobin S

Hemoglobin S is identical to HbA with the exception that one of the 146 amino acids in the beta chains of globin is different. HbS results when glutamate is substituted for valine on position 6 of the beta chain.[215] This seemingly minute difference, however, is responsible for the pathophysiology of sickle cell disease.

Sickle cell anemia is an inherited disorder observed in patients who are homozygous (i.e., inherited from both parents) for HbS. Sickle cell anemia is present in nearly 1% of African Americans.[215] The frequent painful episodes

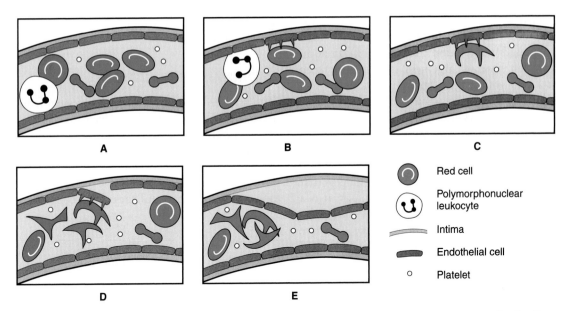

Figure 7-23.   **Pathophysiologic progression in sickle cell disease.** A, Normal circulation. B, Red cell adherence to vessel wall. C, Sickling of bound cell. D, Sickled red cells obstruct flow. E, Narrowing of vessel.

with sickle cell anemia is referred to in some African countries as the "state of suffering,"[216] and the typical life span for these individuals is often less than 50 years.[217] An individual experiencing one of the recurrent painful episodes that affect almost every part of the body is said to be in *"sickle cell crisis."*

A purported sequence of vascular pathophysiology associated with sickle cell anemia is shown in Figure 7-23.[216] Figure 7-23,*A* shows a normal vessel with circulating red blood cells. Figure 7-23,*B* illustrates initial attachment and lingering of a red blood cell to the vascular internal (endothelial) wall.

This is followed by sickling of the red blood cell as shown in Figure 7-23,*C*. Sickling occurs because HbS has unique chemical properties and is less soluble than HbA in the absence of oxygen and tends to crystallize in the cells. Figure 7-24 illustrates the characteristic sickle shape of red blood cells observed under microscope. Specifically, HbS is 50 times less soluble than HbA in the deoxygenated form.[216] Low oxygen pressure, acidosis, and hypothermia all tend to increase the sickling phenomenon.[216] Interestingly, the presence of increased HbF tends to diminish sickling and enhance prognosis.[218,219]

Once the sickling phenomenon begins, additional cells begin to sickle and obstruct blood flow (see Fig. 7-23,*D*). Vaso-occlusion leads to severe pain, destruction of endothelium, and ultimately narrowing of the vessel (see Fig. 7-23,*E*).

Vaso-occlusion often leads to cerebrovascular accident, which is one of the most devastating consequences of the disease.[220] Another very frequent occurrence in those with sickle cell disease is "acute chest syndrome." *Acute chest*

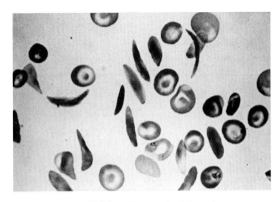

Figure 7-24.   **Sickle cell anemia.** Note the presence of abnormal sickle-shaped erythrocytes. These sickle cells are less pliable and are easily subject to rupture (hemolysis).

syndrome is a term coined in 1979 to describe episodes of chest pain, fever, and leukocytosis (increased white blood cell counts).[221] In addition, left heart enlargement is frequently seen at a very young age in many individuals.[216]

The drug hydroxyurea is often used in the treatment of sickle cell disease. Hydroxyurea increases the production of HbF which, in turn, appears to decrease sickling and vaso-occlusion. Because the life span of these blood cells is only approximately 10% as long as that for normal red blood cells, anemia is also a common finding and transfusions may be a mainstay of treatment. Although there is no cure for sickle cell anemia, most individuals can lead relatively normal lives.

When an individual is heterozygous (i.e., inherited from only one parent), he or she possesses *sickle cell trait*. Nearly 10% of African Americans possess sickle cell trait. Sickle cell trait is not associated with anemia and is generally considered to be a benign condition. Notwithstanding, the sickling phenomenon may occur in these individuals in the presence of prolonged hypoxia. In addition, it has been suggested that the presence of sickle cell trait may be associated with an increased incidence of sudden unexplained death.[223]

INTERNAL RESPIRATION

The final link in the transport of oxygen from the atmosphere to the cells is referred to as *internal respiration* (Fig. 7-25). Although internal respiration has been defined specifically as the exchange of gases between the systemic capillaries and the cells, both cellular oxygen supply and cellular oxygen utilization are considered in this section.

Cellular Oxygen Supply

Although all arteries in the body carry virtually identical concentrations of oxygen, not all cells in the body are supplied with equal amounts of oxygen, which is because not all cells in the body are exposed to the same amount of *blood*. Several factors determine the availability of oxygen to a given cell (Fig. 7-26). Obviously, some cells are simply closer to capillaries than others. Because movement of oxygen depends on pressure gradients, the cells furthest away are most vulnerable to hypoxia.

On Call | CASE 7-2 *ABGs and Critical Thinking*

You are the only person available to care for this patient. You must assess the patient/situation and act accordingly.

A 62-year-old man appears in acute distress with shortness of breath and is cold and clammy.

HR	132/min
RR	22/min
Temp	37° C

ARTERIAL BLOOD GASES

FIO$_2$	0.40
SaO$_2$	93%
pH	7.32
PaCO$_2$	28 mm Hg
PaO$_2$	74 mm Hg
[HCO$_3$]	18 mEq/L

LABORATORY WORK

[Hb]	13 g%
[WBC]	9000 mm^3

VITAL SIGNS

BP	85/P

ASSESSMENT

Abnormalities: List abnormal data and other noteworthy information. Classify ABG.

Explanation: List possible diseases, pathology, or other situations that may have led to this patient's condition.

Evaluation: Suggest additional data that would be useful in helping understand the situation or in making a diagnosis.

INTERVENTION

Importance: Prioritize concern(s) of treatment in order of urgency and/or seriousness as you see the overall situation.

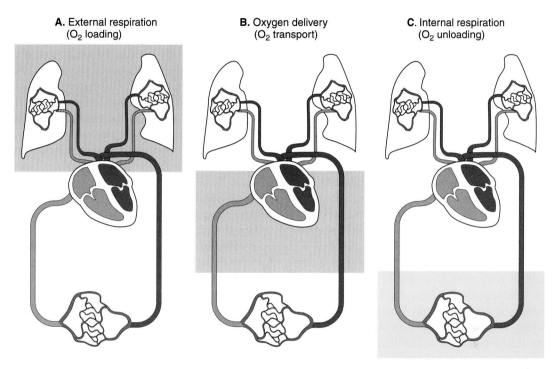

A. External respiration
(O$_2$ loading)

B. Oxygen delivery
(O$_2$ transport)

C. Internal respiration
(O$_2$ unloading)

Figure 7-25.   **Three steps in oxygen delivery to the tissues.**

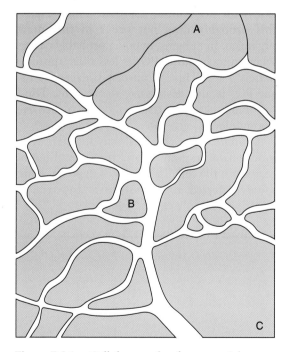

Figure 7-26.   **Cellular supply of oxygen.** Schema showing intercapillary distances. Oxygen from blood flowing through tissue capillaries must diffuse over a longer path to reach cells *A* and *C*. Oxygen has a short path to cell A when its capillary is open and a much longer one when it is closed.

Distance From Capillary

As previously described, the distance of a given cell from a capillary is not constant. Many capillaries are normally closed and open only when gross perfusion to that particular region increases. For example, actively contracting muscle may have as many as 10 times more open capillaries than resting muscle.[81] The gatekeeper of blood supply to a capillary network is the local arteriole.

Arteriolar Constriction/Dilation

Arterioles may dilate or constrict in response to the various factors that regulate them. Arterioles are subject to both local and central influences. Locally, arterioles dilate in response to decreased oxygen supply, increased CO_2, increased temperature, and decreased pH. All these changes are typically the result of increased metabolism that necessitates increased oxygen supply.

The release of epinephrine is a central mechanism that attempts to preferentially distribute blood to the vital organs when oxygen is in short supply in the body. When the body is confronted with an overall deficit in oxygen, both central and local mechanisms are stimulated. In the short term, central effects tend to predominate. If the oxygen shortage persists, however, local effects ultimately override and generalized vascular dilation is seen.

Cellular Oxygen Utilization

Variable Oxygen Extraction

Earlier in this chapter the normal $C(a-\bar{v})O_2$ was calculated at about 5 vol%, which means that, on the average, about 5 mL O_2 is taken up and used by the tissues for every 100 mL of perfusion. It should be noted, however, that the arteriovenous difference observed in specific organs and tissues may vary considerably (Table 7-1). For example, the arteriovenous oxygen difference in the heart is about 11 vol% whereas the arteriovenous difference in the skin and kidneys is approximately 1 vol%. Apparently, tissues with high blood flow and low oxygen requirements use the additional blood flow for nonoxygenation processes, such as glomerular filtration or temperature regulation.

To further complicate matters, some tissues are capable of increasing oxygen extraction when additional oxygen is needed. Skeletal muscle can extract almost all of the blood oxygen during maximal exercise; however, heart muscle is unable to increase oxygen extraction despite its normally high extraction ratio.[81]

Biochemical Respiration

In biochemistry, *respiration* refers to the oxidation of pyruvic acid in the Krebs cycle (Fig. 7-27). This series of reactions takes place in the mitochondria of the cells and results in the production of 36 adenosine triphosphate (ATP) molecules. ATP molecules, in turn, contain the high energy bonds that are so essential for life itself. The availability of oxygen is crucial in the production of ATP from adenosine diphosphate (ADP) in the Krebs cycle. The actual process of ATP formation is called *oxidative phosphorylation*, because phosphate is added to ADP by using the energy from oxidation.

Anaerobic Glycolysis

In the absence of oxygen, metabolism is less efficient and only two molecules of ATP are generated in the metabolism of glucose without oxygen (anaerobic glycolysis). Furthermore, anaerobic metabolism results in the production of lactic acid, which may in turn lead to metabolic acidemia.

Hypoxia

Tissue hypoxia exists when the cellular needs for oxygen are not met. Although isolated mitochondria maintain oxidative phosphorylation with PO_2 values less than 1 mm Hg,[237] this probably does not occur in the intact organism. In humans, hypoxia probably occurs when mitochondrial PO_2 is less than approximately 7 mm Hg.[238] Conversely, excessive tissue PO_2 is also destructive to the cells. Thus, one must carefully titrate oxygen to achieve optimal levels.

Cyanide or amobarbital may interfere with biochemical respiration and the normal use of oxygen in the cell. This form of hypoxia, commonly referred to as *histotoxic hypoxia*, is

Table 7-1. LOCAL VARIATIONS IN THE DISTRIBUTION OF BLOOD FLOW AND O_2 UTILIZATION

Site	Blood Flow (%)	O_2 Used (%)	$C(a-\bar{v})\,O_2$ (vol%)	$P\bar{v}O_2$ (mm Hg)
Heart	4	11	11	23
Skeletal muscle	21	30	8	34
Brain	13	20	6	33
Liver	24	25	4	43
Kidneys	19	7	1	56
Skin	9	2	1	60
Other	10	5	5	40
Total	*100*	*100*	*5*	*40*

Modified 2005 with permission from Finch, C.A., and Lenfant, C.: O_2 transport in man. N. Engl. J. Med., *286*:407, 1972. Copyright © Massachusetts Medical Society. All rights reserved.

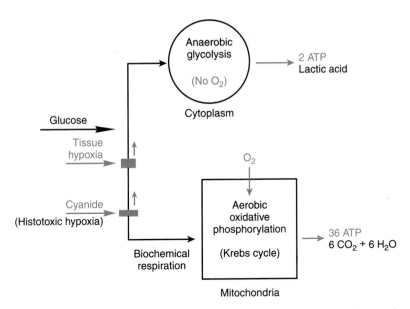

Figure 7-27. **Aerobic metabolism via oxidative phosphorylation in the mitochondria produces 19 times more energy (ATP) than anaerobic glycolysis.** Normal aerobic metabolism decreases in the presence of tissue hypoxia or cyanide poison. When aerobic metabolism cannot proceed, anaerobic metabolism increases with the subsequent buildup of lactic acid.

unique because the primary defect occurs at the site of internal respiration.

Another factor that may alter oxygen requirements is the patient's temperature. Oxygen consumption increases approximately 10% for each degree increase celsius.[10]

Respiratory Quotient

The respiratory quotient (RQ) quantitates the relationship between production of CO_2 and the consumption of oxygen. Specifically, it is the ratio of CO_2 produced each minute to oxygen consumed ($\dot{V}CO_2/\dot{V}O_2$). In pure carbohydrate metabolism, the RQ is 1.0 because six molecules of CO_2 are produced for every six molecules of oxygen consumed (Equation 7-1).

Equation 7-1

$$C_6H_{12}O_6 + 6\ O_2 \rightarrow 6\ H_2O + 6\ CO_2 + energy$$

Fat metabolism, on the other hand, produces less CO_2 and the RQ is approximately 0.7. The RQ of protein metabolism is near 0.8. The RQ of alcohol is approximately 0.7 and the RQ during lipogenesis may be as high as 1.0 to 1.3.

Indeed, an RQ greater than 1.0 suggests lipogenesis secondary to excessive carbohydrate intake and conversion of carbohydrates into fat.[240] Finally, the combined RQ of the body that reflects a composite of all types of metabolism is normally approximately 0.8.

CO_2 excretion via the lungs and oxygen uptake through the lungs may be measured as a reflection of the RQ. The ratio of CO_2 excretion to oxygen uptake is sometimes referred to as the *respiratory exchange ratio*. During steady-state conditions, the respiratory exchange ratio is equal to the respiratory quotient.

In critically ill patients in whom the work of breathing is a matter of concern, the RQ is sometimes monitored by a device called an *indirect calorimeter* or *metabolic cart*. The goal is to try to keep the RQ low via a low carbohydrate diet, which, in turn, minimizes CO_2 production and diminishes the work required for CO_2 excretion via ventilation. This technique may be useful when an attempt is made to decrease the work of breathing in patients who are being gradually weaned off mechanical ventilators.

EXERCISES

Exercise 7-1   Oxygen Transport

Fill in the blanks or select the best answer.

1. State the two forms in which oxygen is carried in the blood.

2. State the solubility coefficient for oxygen in blood at 37° C.

3. Milliliters of a substance in 100 mL of blood is usually referred to as _____.

4. Solubility of gases will (increase/decrease) as temperature increases.

5. The relationship between PO_2 and the volume of dissolved oxygen is direct and (logarithmic/linear).

6. Combined oxygen is carried in combination with _____.

7. A heme group is made up of _____ and _____.

8. Each molecule of hemoglobin is capable of combining with _____ molecules of oxygen.

9. The percentage of available hemoglobin molecules that are carrying oxygen in arterial blood is symbolized as _____.

10. For all practical purposes, SaO_2 refers to (combined/dissolved) oxygen.

Exercise 7-2   Oxyhemoglobin Dissociation Curve

Fill in the blanks or select the best answer.

1. The most important physiologic variable that determines SaO_2 is the _____.

2. The relationship between PaO_2 and SaO_2 is direct and (linear/nonlinear).

3. What PaO_2 values are normally associated with the following SaO_2 values:
   SaO_2 (%) PaO_2 (mm Hg)
   50
   90
   100

4. At low PaO_2 values, small changes in PaO_2 are associated with (small/large) changes in SaO_2.

5. On the flat upper portion of the curve, large changes in PaO_2 values are associated with (large/small) changes in SaO_2 values.

6. The flat upper portion of the curve is known as the (association/dissociation) portion of the curve.

7. The dissociation portion of the curve is so-named because the (beginning/end) of oxygen unloading occurs on this portion of the curve.

8. Normal SaO_2 is approximately _____%.

9. If PaO_2 were to decrease from 100 to 60 mm Hg, SaO_2 would decrease from 97% to _____%.

10. The end of oxygen loading occurs on the (upper/lower) portion of the curve and the end of oxygen unloading occurs on the (upper/lower) portion of the curve.

Exercise 7-3 Oxyhemoglobin Affinity

Fill in the blanks or select the best answer.

1. The standardized index of oxyhemoglobin affinity is _____.

2. Normal P_{50} is approximately _____ mm Hg.

3. List four factors known to alter the affinity of hemoglobin for oxygen (excluding PO_2).

4. Increased PCO_2 and temperature shift the oxyhemoglobin curve to the (right/left) because $Hb-O_2$ affinity is (increased/decreased).

5. The fact that increasing PCO_2 decreases the affinity of oxygen for hemoglobin is known as the _____ effect.

6. In humans with a normal PaO_2, increased $Hb-O_2$ affinity usually has a net (beneficial/detrimental) effect.

7. A shift of the oxyhemoglobin curve to the right is usually beneficial because it enhances oxygen (loading/unloading).

8. The oxyhemoglobin curve will shift to the left owing to a/an (increase/decrease) in hydrogen ions; or stated another way, a/an (increase/decrease) in pH.

9. The P_{50} is measured at a pH of _____ and a PCO_2 of _____ mm Hg.

10. The P_{50} is slightly lower in (men/women).

Exercise 7-4 2,3-Diphosphoglycerate

Fill in the blanks or select the best answer.

1. The presence of DPG (increases/decreases) the affinity of hemoglobin for oxygen.

2. The most important organic phosphate in the erythrocyte is DPG because it is the most (diffusible/abundant).

3. DPG enhances oxygen (loading/unloading).

4. Anemia is associated with a/an (increase/decrease) in DPG.

5. Probably the most common cause of decreased DPG is (hypoxemia/infusion of stored blood).

6. It is (possible/not possible) to restore DPG levels in stored blood.

7. DPG levels return to 50% of normal within _____ hours after the administration of stored blood.

8. (Increased/decreased) pH tends to decrease DPG levels.

9. Changes in DPG levels tend to have a (short-term/sustained) effect on $Hb-O_2$ affinity.

10. Blood DPG levels tend to decrease to approximately one-third that of normal after blood storage for 1 week in the preservative _____.

Exercise 7-5   Oxygen Content

Fill in the blanks or select the best answer.

1. The symbol for the total volume of oxygen present in arterial blood is _____.

2. Calculate the volume of oxygen in the dissolved state (vol%) in the blood given the following PaO_2 values:
   100 mm Hg
   60 mm Hg
   400 mm Hg

3. Calculate the volume of oxygen in the combined state (vol%) given the following:

[Hb] (g%)	SaO_2 (%)
15	95
12	90
10	80

4. Calculate CaO_2 given:

[Hb] (g%)	SaO_2 (%)	PaO_2 (mm Hg)
10	94	70
14	98	65
7	97	80

5. The normal CaO_2 is approximately _____ vol%.

6. Normal mixed venous PO_2 is approximately _____ mm Hg, and normal mixed venous oxygen saturation is approximately _____%.

7. Normal $C(a-\bar{v})O_2$ is approximately _____ vol%.

8. The relationship between the cardiac output, the oxygen consumption, and the difference in arteriovenous oxygen content is expressed in the _____ equation.

9. When cardiac output decreases, $C(a-\bar{v})O_2$ (increases/decreases).

10. Normal oxygen consumption under basal metabolic conditions in a 70 Kg young man is _____ mL/min.

Exercise 7-6   Cyanosis

Fill in the blanks or select the best answer.

1. The bluish color seen in certain oxygenation disturbances is called _____.

2. A bluish hue of the skin is called _____ cyanosis.

3. Central cyanosis may be observed on the _____.

4. When SO_2 is 80%, the percentage of desaturated hemoglobin is _____%.

5. Cyanosis is usually evident when there is _____ g% average desaturated hemoglobin in the (artery/capillary).

6. Normally, the average quantity of desaturated hemoglobin in the capillaries is approximately _____ g%.

7. Cyanosis is unlikely in (anemia/polycythemia).

8. Cyanosis may be of less immediate concern in (anemia/polycythemia).

9. Calculate the average amount of desaturated hemoglobin given the following data, and state whether this individual (would/would not) be cyanotic.
   Given: [Hb] = 20 g%
               SaO_2 = 80%
               $S\bar{v}O_2$ = 60%

10. Calculate the average amount of desaturated hemoglobin given the following data, and state whether this individual (would/would not) be cyanotic.
    Given: [Hb] = 10 g%
                SaO_2 = 80%
                $S\bar{v}O_2$ = 60%

Exercise 7-7   Oxygen Transport/HbCO/HbF

Fill in the blanks or select the best answer.

1. Dissolved oxygen transport is normally approximately _____ mL/min.

2. Normal total oxygen transport is approximately _____ mL/min.

3. Calculate total oxygen transport given:

PaO_2 (mm Hg)	[Hb] (g%)	SaO_2 (%)	$\dot{Q}$(L/min)
70	12	92	5
100	15	98	2.5
80	6	97	5.2

4. CO has _____ times the affinity for hemoglobin compared with oxygen.

5. CO in chemical combination with hemoglobin is known as _____.

6. Classically, HbCO has been considered to be harmful to oxygenation by what two mechanisms?

7. The P_{50} of HbF is approximately _____ mm Hg.

8. HbF has a (greater/lesser) affinity for oxygen than HbA within the body.

9. HbCO can be accurately measured with a (pulse oximeter/CO-oximeter).

10. The concentration of HbF in the term infant is approximately _____%.

Exercise 7-8   Methemoglobinemia and Sickle Cell Disease

Fill in the blanks or select the best answer.

1. When hemoglobin is oxidized rather than oxygenated, it is called _____.

2. Chocolate-colored blood is often seen with (hemoglobin S/methemoglobinemia).

3. Sulfhemoglobinemia may be mistaken for (methemoglobinemia/sickle cell disease)

4. Treatment for methemoglobinemia is intravenous (hydroxyurea/methylene blue).

5. Benzocaine spray for local anesthesia has been implicated in abrupt (cyanosis/flushing of mucous membranes).

6. Sickling appears to decrease in the presence of (HbF/HbM).

7. State the three components of "acute chest syndrome."

8. The SpO_2 reading with severe methemoglobinemia tends to migrate toward ____%.

9. Amyl nitrate tends to cause increased (HbS/metHb).

10. Sickle cell trait is present in ___% of African Americans.

Exercise 7-9   Internal Respiration

Fill in the blanks or select the best answer.

1. State the four factors known to cause local vasodilation.

2. The normal arteriovenous oxygen content difference is _____ vol% in the heart and _____ vol% in the skin.

3. Actual utilization of oxygen takes place in the (Golgi bodies/mitochondria) within the cells.

4. Oxygen consumption increases approximately _____% for every degree centigrade increase in temperature.

5. The normal respiratory quotient for the entire body is _____.

6. The RQ of carbohydrate metabolism is _____.

7. Actively contracting muscle may have as many as _____ times the ordinary number of open capillaries.

8. Most energy is produced in the cell during (glycolysis/the Krebs cycle).

9. Anaerobic metabolism results in the accumulation of _____ _____.

10. Concerning control of peripheral arterioles, (central/peripheral) effects predominate in the short term.

11. Lipogenesis will result in an RQ as high as ___.

Internet Work

1. Visit www.austin.cc.tx.us/~emeyerth/hemoglob.htm. How many Hb molecules are in 100 mL of blood?

NBRC Challenge 7

Please select the best answer for the following multiple choice questions.

1. A patient is treated with 20% benzocaine spray as a topical anesthetic prior to bronchoscopy. The patient becomes suddenly very cyanotic. What laboratory test should be performed?
   A) P_{50}
   B) Arterial blood gases
   C) Serum electrolytes
   D) CO-oximetry
   E) H&H
   (RRT CSE EXAM—NBRC MATRIX III,B,1,h)

2. The treatment of choice for methemoglobinemia is:
   A) Mechanical ventilation
   B) Methylene blue I.V.
   C) Potassium I.V.
   D) Hyperbaric oxygenation
   E) Biphasic Positive Airway Pressure
   (RRT CSE EXAM—NBRC MATRIX I,C,1,b)

3. A patient with a pulse oximetry reading of 82% and a PaO_2 of 60 mm Hg may have:
   I. hypothermia.
   II. hypercapnia.
   III. acidemia.
   IV. abnormal Hb.
   A) I and II only
   B) I and IV only
   C) II and III only
   D) II and IV only
   E) II, III, and IV only
   (RRT EXAM—NBRC MATRIX I,C,2,b)

4. A $(Ca - \bar{v})O_2$ of 10 vol% suggests:
   A) a high cardiac stroke volume.
   B) a low cardiac output.
   C) polycythemia.
   D) methemoglobinemia.
   E) sickle cell crisis.
   (RRT EXAM—NBRC MATRIX I,C,2,c)

5. An RQ measurement of 1.2 suggests:
   A) technical error using indirect calorimetry.
   B) alcohol intoxication.
   C) excessive fat metabolism.
   D) diabetes mellitus.
   E) lipogenesis.
   (RRT EXAM—NBRC MATRIX I,C,2,g)

The body's defenses against blood pH changes operate at different time rates. Chemical buffering is almost instantaneous; pulmonary responses occur in minutes; renal responses in hours to days.

Giles F. Filley[2]

Acid-base physiology is inherently a slightly confusing subject, but clinical acid-base terminology makes it very confusing.

Giles F. Filley[2]

Outline

HYDROGEN IONS AND pH

Free Hydrogen Ions

Clinical Significance

The free hydrogen ion concentration [H⁺] in the blood must be maintained within very narrow limits to maintain life. Seemingly slight alterations in the free [H⁺] may have profound, life-threatening effects on the chemistry of the body. This unusual degree of reactivity is probably related to the small size of the H⁺ that affords it reaction sites unapproachable by larger ions.

Description

Only hydrogen in *free ionic form*, however, possesses this chemical potential and is part of the measurement of free hydrogen ion concentration. Hydrogen in chemical combination with other elements (e.g., H_2O, HCO_3) is not part of the *free* [H⁺].

Technically, however, in an aqueous solution, even "free" hydrogen ions are combined chemically with water to form *hydronium ions* (e.g., H_3O^+, H_5O^+). Nevertheless, the distinction between free hydrogen ions and hydronium ions is not important for clinical purposes.

Sometimes, a comparison is also made between H^+ activity and H^+ concentration. Most hydrogen ion analyzers measure activity rather than actual concentration. Here again, however, there is little clinical significance to this differentiation. Thus, the term *hydrogen ion concentration* is used to refer to hydrogen ion measurements throughout this text.

pH

Definition

The actual $[H^+]$ in the blood is very low, approximately 0.00000004 equivalents per liter (Eq/L). Obviously, monitoring clinical changes using these units would be a very difficult and cumbersome process. Therefore, it has become customary to express $[H^+]$ as pH. The definition of pH is the *negative log of the free $[H^+]$*. Although this definition appears to be complex, pH is a less cumbersome method of assessing the amount of H^+ present in a given fluid. The normal range for pH in arterial blood is 7.35 to 7.45.

Relationship Between pH and $[H^+]$

It is important to understand the relationship between $[H^+]$ and pH, however, because it is not a simple direct one. Because the pH is the *negative* log of the free hydrogen ion concentration, the relationship between pH and $[H^+]$ is *inverse*. An increase in pH reflects a decrease in $[H^+]$, whereas a decrease in pH is associated with a increase of hydrogen ions.

Also, because the relationship is logarithmic, a relatively large change in hydrogen ion concentration only slightly alters the numeric value of pH. For example, *doubling* of the normal $[H^+]$ only results in a 0.3 unit decrease in pH.[2]

Acid-Base Balance

Acids

Free hydrogen ions enter the blood on their release from other chemical substances. Any chemical substance capable of releasing a H^+ into solution is defined as an *acid*. Therefore, the greater the number and quantity of acids present in solution, the higher the $[H^+]$ (and lower the pH) will be. A variety of acids are normally present in the blood, and these acids serve as the source of free hydrogen ions.

Bases

All hydrogen ions released in solution, however, do not remain free. Many hydrogen ions are attracted to and combine with other chemical substances that are present in the blood. Any substance capable of combining with or accepting a hydrogen ion in solution is called a *base*.

Thus, from a chemical standpoint, *the blood pH is a result of the balance of acids and bases (i.e., acid-base balance) at any given moment.*

pH Homeostasis

Human cells and organs function best under constant internal conditions including normal pH. Maintenance of a constant internal environment is called *homeostasis*. Both acids and bases must be regulated closely to ensure stable levels and a normal pH. Maintenance of a constant pH may be called *pH homeostasis*.

The dynamic regulation of blood pH is accomplished through the interaction of the lungs, the kidneys, and the blood buffers. The lungs and kidneys precisely maintain levels of acids and bases present in the blood. The blood buffers serve primarily a protective role, preventing large changes in pH when abnormal conditions expose the blood to acid-base abnormalities.

Acid Homeostasis

Normal body metabolism tends to result in an accumulation of excess acid. Thus, it is important that the body excrete acid at a rate equivalent to its production to maintain pH homeostasis.

Acid Excretion

Two major organ systems are responsible for the excretion of acids: the kidneys and the lungs. Although the kidneys are often the first organs thought of when considering acid excretion, *the lungs are actually the major organs of acid excretion.*

In normal humans, the lungs excrete approximately 13,000 mEq/day of carbonic acid.[363] However, the kidneys of an average American adult excrete only 40 to 80 mEq/day of acid.[363] Thus, the lungs are the single most important organs involved in the moment-to-moment regulation of acid-base status and pH.

Acid Groups

The kidneys and the lungs each excrete a different general chemical group of acids. The lungs excrete volatile acid. *Volatile acids* are those that can be converted from a liquid form to a gaseous form to facilitate excretion. For all practical purposes, carbonic acid (H_2CO_3) is the only volatile acid excreted by the lungs under ordinary conditions.

The kidneys, on the other hand, excrete fixed acids such as sulfuric acid and phosphoric acid. *Fixed acids* cannot be converted into a gas and therefore must be excreted in a fixed (liquid) state in the urine.

Base Homeostasis

Like acids, the bases in the bloodstream must also be maintained in a constant balance. The organ responsible for the regulation of blood bases is the kidney. The plasma bicarbonate concentration [HCO_3] is the major blood base of clinical significance. The [HCO_3] is carefully controlled in the nephron, which is the functional unit of the kidney.

THE LUNGS AND REGULATION OF VOLATILE ACID

Underlying Chemistry

The role of the lungs in human acid-base balance and pH homeostasis is to maintain the concentration of carbonic acid [H_2CO_3] at constant levels in the arterial blood. As described earlier, the lungs are the major organs of volatile acid (i.e., H_2CO_3) excretion. Therefore, it is the exclusive responsibility of the respiratory system to excrete carbonic acid in quantities that are exactly in proportion to its production.

Some fundamental principles and chemical relationships must be grasped to fully understand the mechanisms involved in H_2CO_3 homeostasis. These basic chemical relationships and principles include chemical equilibrium, the law of mass action, the hydrolysis reaction, and the direct, linear relationship between dissolved CO_2 and H_2CO_3.

Chemical Equilibrium

A reversible chemical reaction can proceed in either direction. In reversible chemical reactions, chemical equilibrium exists when the rate of the reaction in one direction is equal to the rate of the reaction in the opposing direction. Chemical equilibrium does *not* mean that the concentrations of constituents on both sides of an equation are equal.

A *closed chemical system* is one in which all the reactants and products in a chemical reaction must remain within that system. Once chemical equilibrium for a particular reaction is reached in a closed system, the concentrations of the various constituents do not change. The reaction continues to proceed in both directions but a state of *dynamic* equilibrium is maintained.

When the *concentration* of the substances on the left side of a chemical reaction at equilibrium is greater than the concentration of the constituents on the right side, the reaction is said to be shifted to the left. For example, the equation shown in Equation 8-1 is said to be shifted to the left because the concentration of reactants on the left is greater than the concentration of H_2CO_3. Nevertheless, the reaction is still at equilibrium. Also note that the arrow pointing to the left is longer than the arrow pointing to the right. This designation shows that the reaction is shifted to the left at equilibrium.

$$\textbf{Equation 8-1}$$
$$H_2O + CO_2 \xrightleftharpoons{} H_2CO_3$$
$$(340) + (340) \xrightleftharpoons{} (1)$$

Law of Mass Action

Once achieved, a reaction remains at equilibrium in a closed system. If an additional amount of one of the constituents is added to the closed system from an external source, however, a new equilibrium is established. This new equilibrium partially counteracts the initial imbalance in the equilibrium caused by the constituent that has been added. The change in equilibrium in response to a change in the amount of one of the reaction constituents is referred to as the *law of mass action*.

Thus, if there is an increase in one of the reactants on the right side of the equation, the law of mass action causes the equilibrium point to shift to the left to partially counteract the disturbance. For example, in Equation 8-1, if 5 units of external H_2CO_3 were *added* to this equilibrium in a closed system, the equilibrium would shift to the left to partially counteract the alteration. The change in units shown in Equation 8-2 shows the direction of changes that would occur in response to the additional H_2CO_3 in the system. Conceptually, the increase in mass on the right side of the equation pushes the reaction to the left side of the equation.

Equation 8-2

$$H_2O + CO_2 \underset{\rightarrow}{\longleftarrow} H_2CO_3$$

$$(343) + (343) \underset{\rightarrow}{\longleftarrow} (3)$$

A similar phenomenon occurs if one of the constituents is *removed* from the closed system. In this case, however, the change in equilibrium is an attempt to restore the lost constituent. If CO_2 is removed from Equation 8-2, the equilibrium would shift slightly to the left to attempt to restore the lost CO_2. The change in units in Equation 8-3 shows the general direction of changes that would accompany the loss of CO_2. Note that the removal of CO_2 from the system leads to a fall in H_2CO_3 concentration due to the law of mass action.

Equation 8-3

$$H_2O + CO_2 \underset{\rightarrow}{\longleftarrow} H_2CO_3$$

$$(344) + (340) \underset{\rightarrow}{\longleftarrow} (2)$$

Hydrolysis Reaction

CO_2 is produced continuously in the cells of the body as an end product of aerobic metabolism. This CO_2 then diffuses to the systemic circulation where some of it reacts with water to form carbonic acid. This reaction, shown in Equation 8-4, is called the *hydrolysis reaction* because water (hydro) is broken down (lysed) as it reacts with dissolved CO_2 to form carbonic acid. Because all acids are capable of releasing hydrogen ions, the release of free H^+ from carbonic acid is also shown in Equation 8-4.

Equation 8-4

$$H_2O + CO_2 \underset{\rightarrow}{\longleftarrow} H_2CO_3 \underset{\rightarrow}{\longleftarrow} HCO_3^- + H^+$$

Direct Relationship between [CO₂] and [H₂CO₃]

Because of their common involvement in the hydrolysis reaction, there is a direct, linear relationship between the concentration of dissolved

CO_2 and the concentration of carbonic acid $[H_2CO_3]$ in the blood. At 37° C, each H_2CO_3 molecule in solution is in equilibrium with approximately 340 CO_2 molecules, as shown in Equation 8-1.[364] Earlier estimates reported that the ratio was greater than 700 to 1; however, improved methods suggest the ratio given here. When blood PCO_2 levels increase, blood levels of H_2CO_3 likewise increase. Thus, PCO_2 can be used as a marker of blood volatile acid (i.e., H_2CO_3) levels.

Carbonic Acid Production

Based on the law of mass action, the CO_2 that builds up at the tissues leads to a parallel increase in carbonic acid and ultimately hydrogen ions (Fig. 8-1). Thus, there is an increase in the amount of carbonic acid present in the blood as it passes the tissues and CO_2 enters. Venous blood has more CO_2 and carbonic acid than arterial blood. In fact, that is why venous blood is slightly more acidic (pH = 7.38) compared with arterial blood (pH = 7.40). Actually, the difference in pH would be more substantial were it not for the many effective buffer systems in the blood.

Carbonic Acid Excretion

When the venous blood reaches the lungs, the increased CO_2 and carbonic acid that entered the blood at the tissues must be excreted. This is precisely the role of the lungs in acid-base balance: to excrete CO_2 and carbonic acid at the

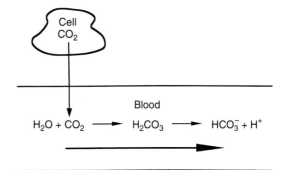

Figure 8-1. **Carbonic acid production at the tissues.** Hydrogen ions are produced in the blood at the cells as CO_2 reacts with water in the hydrolysis reaction.

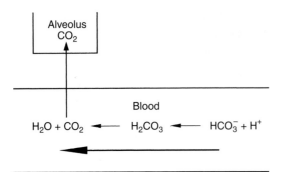

Figure 8-2.   **Carbonic acid excretion in the lungs.** Hydrogen ions are removed from the blood in the lungs as CO_2 is excreted into the alveoli.

same rate that it is being produced. Figure 8-2 shows that as CO_2 diffuses into the alveoli, the law of mass action forces the hydrolysis reaction to the left. The net effect of this action is a reduction in carbonic acid and a decrease in the number of hydrogen ions in the blood. Thus, as CO_2 is excreted via the lungs, the body is functionally excreting H_2CO_3.

CO_2 Homeostasis

It has been shown that carbonic acid levels in the blood closely parallel dissolved CO_2 levels. Dissolved CO_2 is maintained at constant internal levels both because of its direct effect on pH and for other physiologic reasons. The maintenance of constant arterial blood PCO_2 levels can also be called CO_2 *homeostasis*. The physiologic and metabolic processes that ultimately determine blood CO_2 levels are explored.

The arterial PCO_2 at any given moment depends on the quantity of CO_2 entering the blood from the tissues and the quantity of CO_2 leaving the blood via the lungs. The amount of CO_2 entering the blood, in turn, depends on the metabolic rate and the substrate being metabolized. The volume of CO_2 produced per minute (i.e., CO_2 production) is designated as the $\dot{V}CO_2$.

Excretion of CO_2, on the other hand, depends on alveolar ventilation. *Alveolar minute ventilation* is the amount of fresh gas that reaches functional (i.e., perfused) alveoli each minute. The symbol for alveolar ventilation per minute is $\dot{V}A$. The balance of $\dot{V}CO_2$

and $\dot{V}A$ determines the arterial $PaCO_2$ at any given instant, which is shown in Proportion 8-1.

Proportion 8-1. CO_2 HOMEOSTASIS

$$\frac{\dot{V}CO_2}{\dot{V}A} \approx PaCO_2$$

CO_2 Production

CO_2 production depends on both the quantity and the nature of metabolism. The quantity of metabolism varies directly with body temperature. Metabolism increases as an individual's body temperature increases. The nature of metabolism depends on the type of foodstuff (e.g., fat, protein, carbohydrate) being metabolized. For example, carbohydrate metabolism produces more CO_2 than does fat metabolism.

In normal humans, increases in CO_2 production, such as during exercise, are balanced physiologically by increasing alveolar ventilation proportionately. Sometimes, however, increases in CO_2 production cannot be offset by increased ventilation. This finding may occur when CO_2 production is high (e.g., patients with burns, total parenteral nutrition, sepsis) or when the ventilatory system is compromised.

Large increases in metabolism and CO_2 production sufficient to result in $PaCO_2$ elevation may occur occasionally in patients with sepsis (blood infection) or massive burns. Also, an increase in blood $PaCO_2$ can occur after intravenous administration of the drug sodium bicarbonate ($NaHCO_3$) to a patient who is unable to increase alveolar ventilation.[365] Because bicarbonate is one of the factors in the hydrolysis reaction, its presence in increased quantities pushes the reaction to the left, which, in turn, has the effect of increasing dissolved CO_2 and H_2CO_3 levels in the blood.

The individual with a normal respiratory system responds to the increased CO_2 with a parallel rise in alveolar ventilation and CO_2 excretion. The inability to increase alveolar ventilation may be seen, however, when central nervous system ventilatory control mechanisms are not intact or when the respiratory muscles are paralyzed. Paralysis of the ventilatory muscles may occur after trauma or pharmacologic intervention for control of mechanical ventilation. Thus, in these situations the clinician should try to minimize CO_2 loading in the blood or to provide the patient with some type of ventilatory support to aid in excretion of the additional CO_2 load.

CO_2 Excretion

In the clinical setting, increased CO_2 production is usually balanced by increasing alveolar ventilation. Furthermore, most clinical changes in $PaCO_2$ are a result of changes in alveolar ventilation. Nevertheless, it is becoming increasingly clear that changes in CO_2 production can also lead to $PaCO_2$ alterations.

To show the inverse relationship between alveolar ventilation and $PaCO_2$, Proportion 8-1 is sometimes simplified to the form shown in Proportion 8-2. In this proportion, $\dot{V}CO_2$ is considered to be a constant and the number one is substituted in the numerator. The proportion becomes simply an inverse relationship between $PaCO_2$ and alveolar ventilation. *An increase in alveolar ventilation results in a decreased PaCO₂.* Conversely, a decrease in alveolar ventilation causes an increased $PaCO_2$.

Proportion 8-2. SIMPLIFIED CO_2 HOMEOSTASIS

$$\frac{1}{\dot{V}A} \approx PaCO_2$$

Minute Ventilation

The amount of gas moving in and out of the lungs with each breath is called the tidal volume (VT). The number of breaths taken each minute is often referred to as the frequency or respiratory rate (RR). Exhaled minute ventilation ($\dot{V}E$) can be calculated as shown in Equation 8-5.

Equation 8-5
$$VT \times RR = \dot{V}E$$

Minute ventilation, however, is *not* a very reliable index of the adequacy of ventilation. The drawback of minute ventilation is that it does not tell us if the lungs are excreting CO_2

in correct proportion to its production. To assess the adequacy of ventilation one must get an arterial blood gas and evaluate the $PaCO_2$. The $PaCO_2$ is the best index available to assess the adequacy of ventilation relative to CO_2 production. If the lungs are maintaining CO_2 homeostasis, the $PaCO_2$ is maintained within the normal range (i.e., $PaCO_2$ 35 to 45 mm Hg).

Alveolar Ventilation

As shown in Proportion 8-2, $PaCO_2$ is inversely proportional to alveolar ventilation. Alveolar ventilation differs from minute ventilation in that only the gas that reaches functional (i.e., perfused) alveoli is considered alveolar ventilation; in other words, deadspace volume (VD) (see Chapter 6) is subtracted from the tidal volume (VT) to determine alveolar ventilation ($\dot{V}A$). The formula for calculation of alveolar minute ventilation is shown in Equation 8-6.

Equation 8-6
$$\dot{V}A = (VT - VD) \times RR$$

One can readily see that any increase in tidal volume or RR (or a decrease in deadspace) increases alveolar ventilation, assuming of course that all other variables remain constant. An increase in alveolar ventilation, in turn, lowers $PaCO_2$. Conversely, a fall in RR or tidal volume (or an increase in deadspace) decreases alveolar ventilation and increases $PaCO_2$. When a change in $PaCO_2$ is seen clinically, Equation 8-6 should be analyzed to determine what variable has resulted in the change in the patient's ability to excrete CO_2.

Minute Ventilation versus Alveolar Ventilation

Table 8-1 shows three sets of parameters where the minute ventilation is the same (6000 mL/min); however, alveolar ventilation and CO_2 excretion are grossly different. Figure 8-3 similarly illustrates how alveolar ventilation and

Table 8-1. MINUTE VENTILATION VERSUS ALVEOLAR VENTILATION

VT (mL)	RR (bpm)	VD (mL)	$\dot{V}$ (mL/min)	VA (mL/min)	PaCO₂ (mm Hg)
500	12	150	6000	4200	40
250	24	150	6000	2400	80
1000	6	150	6000	5100	30

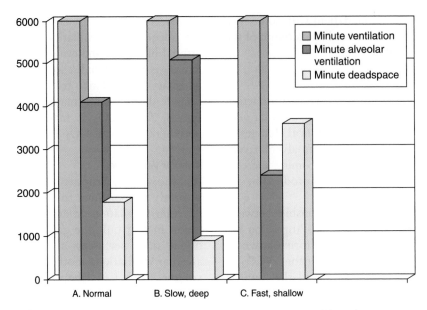

Figure 8-3.   **Effect of breathing pattern on alveolar ventilation. A,** Normal breathing pattern. **B,** Slow deep breathing. **C,** Rapid shallow breathing.

deadspace ventilation would be impacted by the breathing patterns in Table 8-1. During normal breathing (see Fig. 8-3,*A*), most ventilation is effective alveolar ventilation. If minute volume remains constant, alveolar ventilation will increase with larger tidal volumes and a slower respiratory rate (see Fig. 8-3,*B*). Finally, if breathing is very rapid and shallow, deadspace ventilation can actually exceed alveolar ventilation (see Fig. 8-3,*C*) despite a constant minute ventilation.

Note likewise that the $PaCO_2$ varies inversely with the alveolar ventilation. The inadequacy of minute ventilation as an index of the adequacy

---

ON CALL | CASE **8-1**   *ABGs and Critical Thinking*

You are the only person available to care for this patient. You must assess the patient/situation and act accordingly.

A 52-year-old patient with acute respiratory distress syndrome is being mechanically ventilated in the control mode in the critical care unit. The patient is being pharmacologically paralyzed to facilitate mechanical ventilation. Previous blood gases had shown a normal $PaCO_2$ and PaO_2 with a severe metabolic acidosis (pH 7.12) secondary to renal failure. Two ampules of sodium bicarbonate are administered IV to correct the metabolic acidosis and the following blood gas is obtained.

ARTERIAL BLOOD GASES

SaO_2	70%
pH	7.10
$PaCO_2$	56 mm Hg

PaO_2	52 mm Hg
$[HCO_3]$	16 mEq/L
FIO_2	0.50

ASSESSMENT

Abnormalities: List abnormal data and other noteworthy information. Classify ABG.

Explanation: List possible diseases, pathology, or other situations that may have led to this patient's condition.

INTERVENTION

Importance: Prioritize concern(s) of treatment in order of urgency and/or seriousness as you see the overall situation.

of ventilation is clearly shown in Table 8-1 and Figure 8-3. *The $PaCO_2$ is the only reliable index of the adequacy of ventilation.*

It should also be noted that in Table 8-1 and Figure 8-3, deadspace is considered a constant 150 mL/breath. In these sets, changes in alveolar ventilation are due to alterations in VT and RR. In many disease states, deadspace varies considerably from this value. Thus, even when tidal volume and RR are known, the blood gas and specifically the $PaCO_2$ are necessary to assess the adequacy of V̇A and the ability of the body to maintain CO_2 homeostasis.

CO_2 Transport

CO_2 is transported in the blood in both the plasma and within the red blood cells (erythrocytes). The mechanisms by which CO_2 is actually carried in these two compartments are reviewed. The transport of CO_2 in the blood is related intimately to acid-base status and homeostasis. CO_2 is carried in the blood in four basic forms: dissolved CO_2, carbonic acid (H_2CO_3), bicarbonate (HCO_3^-), and carbamino compounds.

Dissolved CO_2

As described in Chapter 3, gases dissolve in liquids in direct proportion to their partial pressures. Furthermore, the volume of gas dissolved in a given liquid depends on the solubility coefficient of that gas in that particular fluid. The solubility coefficient of CO_2 in blood is approximately 0.072 vol%/mm Hg, which, of course, is much higher than the solubility coefficient of O_2 (0.003 vol%/mm Hg). Given a normal $PaCO_2$ of 40 mm Hg, the normal volume of dissolved CO_2 in the arterial blood is approximately 2.9 vol%.

In comparison with O_2, however, CO_2 is sometimes reported in units of mEq/L. The solubility coefficient of CO_2 in units of mEq/L is 0.03 mEq/L/mm Hg. Thus, given a normal arterial PCO_2 of 40 mm Hg, the normal volume of dissolved CO_2 in the plasma is (40 mm Hg × 0.03 mEq/L/mm Hg) 1.2 mEq/L. Dissolved CO_2 transport accounts for only approximately 8% of the total volume of CO_2 transported from the tissues to the lungs. The factor for converting CO_2 in vol% to mEq/L is (vol%/2.23 = mEq/L).

Carbonic Acid

As shown previously in Equation 8-1, the concentration of carbonic acid [H_2CO_3] in the blood varies directly with the quantity of dissolved CO_2, because these two substances are related directly via the hydrolysis reaction. The amount of actual H_2CO_3 in the blood, however, is minute (0.006%) in comparison with total CO_2 transport.

The reason for this unbalanced relationship is that the chemical equilibrium point of the reaction is such that the ratio of dissolved [CO_2] to [H_2CO_3] is approximately 340 to 1 (see Equation 8-1).[364] In other words, the reaction is shifted far to the left. Thus, although the quantitative relationship between dissolved CO_2 and H_2CO_3 is very important from an acid-base perspective, the volume of CO_2 being transported in the form of H_2CO_3 is negligible.

In some texts, H_2CO_3 is excluded as a mechanism of CO_2 transport because of its nominal role. Nevertheless, it is included here for completeness and to reinforce understanding of the direct relationship between the quantities of dissolved CO_2 and H_2CO_3.

Bicarbonate

Plasma Bicarbonate Formation

Equation 8-4 showed that not only is carbonic acid in equilibrium with dissolved CO_2, but it is also in equilibrium with bicarbonate (HCO_3^-). Thus, some of the CO_2 that enters the blood ultimately forms HCO_3^-. The amount of HCO_3 formed in the plasma, however, tends to be very small for two reasons. First, the accumulation of the products of the hydrolysis reaction tends to halt the reaction. Second, the hydrolysis reaction itself occurs at a very slow rate in the plasma, which is because there is no enzyme available to catalyze (speed up) the reaction.

Thus, based on these limitations, one would expect the amount of CO_2 to be transported as HCO_3 to be very small. Surprisingly, HCO_3 is actually the major mechanism of CO_2 transport and accounts for approximately 80% of the CO_2 transport from tissues to the lungs. This is because of an interesting phenomenon known as the chloride shift.

Chloride Shift

As CO_2 enters the blood from the tissues, it accumulates in the blood plasma. Because CO_2 readily diffuses through cell membranes, CO_2 levels also increase within the erythrocytes. Therefore, the hydrolysis reaction also takes place within the erythrocyte.

Inside the erythrocyte, however, the hydrolysis reaction can occur at a much faster pace (13,000 times faster)[81] than in the plasma for two reasons. First, the presence of the enzyme *carbonic anhydrase* speeds up the hydrolysis reaction. Second, the products of the hydrolysis reaction (i.e., HCO_3^- and H^+) are not permitted to accumulate within the erythrocytes. Hydrogen ions promptly combine with (are buffered by) desaturated hemoglobin to prevent their accumulation and a substantial change in intracellular pH. Simultaneously, bicarbonate ions are transported through the erythrocyte membrane into the plasma.

The large quantity of bicarbonate (negative anion) migrating from the erythrocyte to the plasma sets up an electrostatic gradient between the intracellular fluid and the plasma. This electrical gradient in turn results in the movement of chloride anions into the erythrocyte from the plasma. This exchange of bicarbonate ions for chloride anions across the erythrocyte membrane is known as the *chloride shift* or the *Hamburger phenomenon* (Fig. 8-4).

Chloride Shift at the Tissues

At the tissues, chloride enters the erythrocytes as bicarbonate enters the plasma. Thus, the vast majority of CO_2 transport is in the form of HCO_3. This HCO_3^- is produced in the erythrocytes but is transported from the tissues to the lungs in the plasma.

Chloride Shift in the Lungs

As CO_2 diffuses from the blood to the alveoli in the lungs, the chloride shift occurs in the opposite direction (Fig. 8-5). In other words, Cl^- returns to the plasma in exchange for the return of bicarbonate ions to the erythrocyte. Inside the cells, HCO_3 is converted back to dissolved CO_2. In this gaseous form, it can be excreted from the plasma into the alveoli.

Carbamino Compounds

Plasma Carbamino Compounds

A small amount of CO_2 is also transported in the plasma in combination with protein. In this case, CO_2 reacts with the amino acid groups present on the protein molecule. Protein in combination with CO_2 is called a *carbamino compound*. Carbamino compounds in the plasma account for only approximately 2% of CO_2 transport.

Carbamino-Hemoglobin

Because the hemoglobin molecule contains the protein globin, CO_2 can combine with hemoglobin. The combined form of hemoglobin and CO_2 is called carbamino-hemoglobin. It should be understood that the hemoglobin combination with CO_2 does not occur at the same site

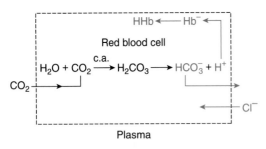

Figure 8-4.   Chloride shift at the tissues. Chloride enters the erythrocytes at the tissues in exchange for the bicarbonate produced via the hydrolysis reaction. The hydrolysis reaction is accelerated in the erythrocyte due to the presence of carbonic anhydrase. The hydrogen ion produced via the hydrolysis reaction is buffered by hemoglobin.

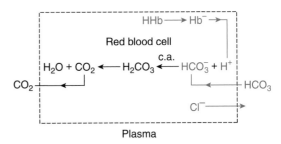

Figure 8-5.   Chloride shift in the lungs. Chloride returns to the plasma in exchange for bicarbonate. Bicarbonate is needed inside the cells to replenish stores that are used up via the hydrolysis reaction as CO_2 is excreted.

as the hemoglobin combination with O_2. Whereas O_2 combines with hemoglobin at the heme site, CO_2 combines with the amino groups of proteins.[81] It is indeed possible for the hemoglobin molecule to carry O_2 and CO_2 at the same time. Notwithstanding, however, the affinity of hemoglobin for CO_2 is greater when it is not combined with O_2. This result is the well-known *Haldane effect*. Conversely, when hemoglobin is already carrying CO_2, its affinity for O_2 decreases (i.e., Bohr effect).

The percentage of CO_2 transport in the form of carbamino-hemoglobin is approximately 10%. Thus, the total amount of CO_2 transported as carbamino compounds is 12%.

Summary

A summary of quantitative CO_2 transport is shown in Table 8-2.[96] These percentages are based solely on CO_2 added to the blood at the tissue and transported to the lungs to be excreted. The normal stores of CO_2 continuously present in the blood are not reflected in these numbers. Also, the percentage of CO_2 transport in the chemical form of H_2CO_3 is so small that it is not included in Table 8-2.

THE KIDNEYS AND ACID-BASE BALANCE

The kidneys (renal system) are second only to the lungs in their role of controlling blood pH. The kidneys serve two major functions in acid-base homeostasis: fixed acid excretion and normal regulation of the bicarbonate concentration $[HCO_3^-]$ in the blood. Bicarbonate is an important blood base.

Regulation of Fixed Acids in the Blood

Nonvolatile or fixed acids are produced through normal body metabolism. These fixed acids cannot be converted into gases and excreted via the lungs. Therefore, the kidneys are responsible for maintaining normal fixed acid homeostasis.

Furthermore, several conditions (e.g., diabetes, hypoxia) can result in an abnormal increase in fixed acid production. In these situations, the kidneys accelerate acid excretion and attempt to maintain homeostasis.

Origin of Fixed Acids

Metabolism

Fixed acids are a common product of metabolism. The specific fixed acid accumulating in the blood plasma at the tissues depends on the type of substance being metabolized. The conditions surrounding metabolism (e.g., presence of O_2) may also affect the products that result. The most common fixed acids that may accumulate in the blood are shown in Table 8-3. The type of substance that metabolizes into each specific acid is also shown.

Protein metabolism results in the production of inorganic (not containing carbon) phosphoric and sulfuric acid. The incomplete metabolism of lipids or carbohydrates results in the accumulation of organic (containing carbon) acids. Specifically, lipid metabolism in the absence of insulin produces a buildup of acetoacetic and beta-hydroxybutyric acid. These two acids are often referred to collectively as the ketoacids. On the other hand, in the absence of O_2, carbohydrate metabolism produces an accumulation of lactic acid.

Normally, the amount of fixed acid produced each day is small, approximately 50 to 60 mEq.

Table 8-2. PERCENTAGES OF CO_2 TRANSPORT FROM TISSUES TO LUNGS

Mechanism	%
Bicarbonate	80
Carbamino compounds	12
Dissolved	8
Total	**100**

Table 8-3. VARIOUS TYPES OF METABOLISM WITH ASSOCIATED FIXED ACIDS

Substance	Fixed Acids
Protein catabolism	Sulfuric acid (H_2SO_4) Phosphoric acid (H_3PO_4)
Incomplete lipid metabolism	(*Ketoacids*) Acetoacetic acid Beta-hydroxybutyric acid
Carbohydrate metabolism (in the absence of O_2)	Lactic acid

In the presence of disease (e.g., diabetic ketoacidosis), however, fixed acid production may increase tremendously (e.g., 2000 mEq/day).[366]

Nonmetabolic Origin

Occasionally, an increase in fixed acids in the blood may originate from a cause other than metabolism. This finding occurs typically when a salt such as ammonium chloride (NH_4Cl) is administered intravenously to a patient, such as in the treatment of severe metabolic alkalosis. Ammonium chloride is metabolized by the liver and results in the production of hydrochloric acid (HCl).

Excretion of Fixed Acids

Because the amount of fixed acid the kidneys must normally excrete is small, there is usually no problem in maintaining homeostasis. Nevertheless, in the presence of renal disease, retention of fixed acids may occur.

When the fixed acid load is unusually high, even the normal kidney is unable to excrete them over the short term. This finding may occur when large quantities of organic acids are being produced due to incomplete metabolism or when a chloride salt is administered.

In any event, a large abnormal fixed acid load leads to an excess of hydrogen ions in the blood. This nonrespiratory (metabolic) acid-base disturbance results in a decrease in blood pH.

Regulation of Bicarbonate Concentration in the Blood

As is shown in the section on buffering, strong bases can be converted into the base (HCO_3^-) in the blood. The bicarbonate concentration, in turn, is precisely regulated by the kidneys. The kidneys can both excrete excess bicarbonate and produce bicarbonate when needed. Clear comprehension of the renal regulation of [HCO_3^-] is crucial to understanding the role of the kidneys in acid-base balance.

The specific mechanisms through which the kidneys control bicarbonate are complex. These mechanisms are affected by certain blood electrolytes, hormones, and drugs. Due to the complex nature of this regulation, this subject is discussed in more detail in Chapter 12.

BUFFER SYSTEMS

Central features of the lungs and the kidneys regarding acid-base homeostasis have been

---

ON CALL | CASE 8-2 *ABGs and Critical Thinking*

You are the only person available to care for this patient. You must assess the patient/situation and act accordingly.

A patient who has had cardiac surgery is being mechanically ventilated in the assist/control mode following surgery. Earlier blood gases had shown a significant respiratory alkalosis ($PaCO_2$ was 26 mm Hg / pH 7.54). The physician overseeing the patient was concerned about the respiratory alkalemia because the electrocardiograph was very unstable. Therefore, the physician added increased mechanical deadspace to try to increase the $PaCO_2$. You go up to see the patient just as blood gases are reported after the mechanical deadspace had been applied.

ARTERIAL BLOOD GASES

SaO_2	98%
pH	7.61
$PaCO_2$	20 mm Hg
PaO_2	94 mm Hg

[HCO_3]	22 mEq/L
FIO_2	0.4

ASSESSMENT

Abnormalities: List abnormal data and other noteworthy information. Classify ABG.

Explanation: List possible diseases, pathology, or other situations that may have led to this patient's condition.

Evaluation: Suggest additional data that would be useful in helping understand the situation or in making a diagnosis.

INTERVENTION

Importance: Prioritize concern(s) of treatment in order of urgency and/or seriousness as you see the overall situation.

Objective: Specifically state the measurable or observable outcomes you would like treatment to accomplish.

Action: Describe your specific plan of action.

discussed. Another important aspect of acid-base homeostasis is the blood buffer system. This remarkable system tends to stabilize the body's pH despite substantial alterations in the concentrations of acids or bases.

Basic Chemistry

A brief review of some additional chemical fundamentals helps to ensure a solid theoretical base for understanding the body buffers.

Conjugate Acid-Base Pairs

Acids, by definition, release hydrogen ions in solution. The hydrogen ions are said to *dissociate* from the acid. The generic formula for dissociation of an acid is shown in Equation 8-7. Note that on dissociation, a hydrogen ion (H^+) is released and a base (A^-) is present. Because all dissociation reactions are reversible equations, bases can combine (associate) with a hydrogen ion to form the acid.

Equation 8-7

$$HA \rightleftarrows H^+ + A^-$$

Thus, every acid must have a related base that will be present on dissociation of the hydrogen ion. An acid in conjunction with its associated base is sometimes referred to as a *conjugate acid-base pair*. Equation 8-8 shows the dissociation reaction for hydrochloric acid. In this reaction, the conjugate acid-base pair is HCl and Cl^-. In other words, the conjugate base of HCl is chloride (Cl^-). Similarly, the conjugate base of carbonic acid (H_2CO_3) is bicarbonate (HCO_3^-).

Equation 8-8

$$HCl \xrightleftharpoons{} H^+ + Cl^-$$

Degree of Dissociation

Given an identical quantity of two different acids in solution, however, the number of hydrogen ions that dissociate into a free state at equilibrium is not identical. Different acids have different degrees of dissociation. The greater the degree of dissociation of a given acid, the stronger that acid is said to be. *Strong acids have a high degree of dissociation, whereas weak acids have a low degree of dissociation.*

For example, Figure 8-6 compares the degree of dissociation between a strong acid (e.g., HCl) and a weak acid (e.g., H_2CO_3). The actual numbers used in this example are not accurate but they are used only to show this concept. Ten molecules of hydrochloric acid are added to one solution, and 10 molecules of carbonic acid are added to the other. Most of the HCl dissociates (eight of 10 molecules), and many free hydrogen ions are seen. However, only two molecules of carbonic acid dissociate. Thus, although both HCl and H_2CO_3 are acids, HCl is a stronger acid because it has a higher degree of dissociation.

Symbolically, the degree of dissociation is shown in the dissociation reaction by the size or length of the arrows in the reversible reaction. A longer arrow in one direction indicates that the concentrations of substances on that side of the equation are greater at equilibrium. Note the length of the arrow to the right in

Figure 8-6. **Comparison of strong and weak acids.** Although both containers are filled with 10 acid molecules, the HCl solution has many more free hydrogen ions due to its degree of dissociation. Therefore, HCl is a much stronger acid.

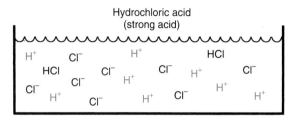

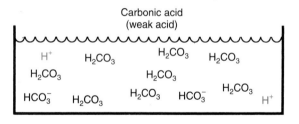

Table 8-4.   ACIDS IN DECREASING STRENGTH

Strength	Acid
Strongest	$HCl \rightarrow H^+ + Cl^-$
	$HHbO_2 \rightarrow H^+ + HbO_2^-$
	$HHb \rightarrow H^+ + Hb^-$
	$NH_4 \leftarrow H^+ + NH_3^-$
Weakest	$H_2O \leftarrow H^+ + OH^-$

Equation 8-8, denoting a high degree of dissociation and a strong acid.

Table 8-4 contains a list of some common acids arranged in order of decreasing strength. The conjugate bases are shown in ascending order of strength. In other words, the conjugate base OH^- has the strongest affinity for the H^+, and the conjugate base Cl^- has the least affinity for the hydrogen ion. Weak acids are associated with strong bases, whereas strong acids are associated with weak bases.

It may also be noted that hemoglobin may function as an acid or a base in the blood. A substance that can act as either an acid or as a base is sometimes referred to as an *amphoteric* substance or an ampholyte.[81] Also, both oxygenated and deoxygenated hemoglobin are included on the list. It can be seen, however, that the conjugate base of deoxygenated hemoglobin (Hb^-) is a stronger base than the conjugate base of oxygenated hemoglobin (HbO_2^-). Thus, deoxygenated hemoglobin more readily picks up hydrogen ions than oxygenated hemoglobin.

This characteristic of hemoglobin serves as an advantage at the body tissues. After releasing O_2, hemoglobin more readily accepts the excess of hydrogen ions generated by the increased CO_2 levels and the hydrolysis reaction.

Buffer Solutions

A buffer solution is a solution in which the pH tends to be stable. The pH of a buffer solution is less affected by the addition of acid or base than a nonbuffer solution. If large quantities of acid are added to a nonbuffer solution, the pH decreases sharply. If the same amount of acid is added to the same solution containing buffers, the pH does not fall to the same extent. Nevertheless, it would still decrease.

Therefore, buffer solutions do not prevent pH change. Rather, buffer solutions minimize pH change. Buffer solutions accomplish this by converting strong acids into weaker acids or by converting strong bases into weaker bases.

Chemical Components

Chemically, a buffer solution consists of two substances in a common solution: a weak acid, and a salt of its conjugate base. For example, carbonic acid is a weak acid. The conjugate base of carbonic acid is bicarbonate (HCO_3). A salt of bicarbonate is sodium bicarbonate ($NaHCO_3$). Salts are completely dissociated into two charged ions (e.g., Na^+ and HCO_3^-). Thus, a buffer solution could be prepared by placing carbonic acid in solution with $NaHCO_3$, which is shown in Proportion 8-3.

Proportion 8-3. BICARBONATE BUFFER
SYSTEM
$$\frac{H_2CO_3}{NaHCO_3}$$

Buffering Reactions

When a strong acid is introduced into the buffer solution, it reacts with the conjugate base (salt) portion of the buffer pair. Equation 8-9 shows how the strong acid HCl would react with the $NaHCO_3$ in this buffer system. The result of this reaction is that one molecule of the strong, highly dissociated acid HCl is converted to one molecule of the weak, poorly dissociated acid H_2CO_3. In addition, one molecule of the salt NaCl is produced.

Equation 8-9
$$\frac{H_2CO_3}{HCl + NaHCO_3} \rightarrow NaCl + H_2CO_3$$

When a strong base such as sodium hydroxide (NaOH) is added to a buffer solution, it reacts with the weak acid portion of the buffer pair as shown in Equation 8-10. In this reaction, the strong OH^- base is converted to the weaker base bicarbonate (HCO_3). Another product of this reaction is water (H_2O).

Equation 8-10
$$\frac{H_2CO_3}{NaOH + NaHCO_3} \rightarrow NaHCO_3 + H_2O$$

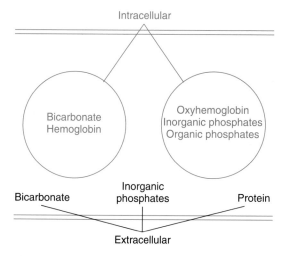

Figure 8-7. **Blood buffer compartments.** The various intracellular and extracellular buffers are shown in their respective fluid compartments.

Blood Buffers

The blood consists of many buffer systems including the bicarbonate buffer system. These buffer systems constitute the first line of defense against abrupt changes in blood pH. The blood buffers work quickly and effectively to minimize alterations in pH.

The various blood buffers may be divided based on their physical location. Blood buffer systems exist both within cells (intracellular fluid) and within the plasma (extracellular fluid). Figure 8-7 and Box 8-1 show the various buffers located in these two fluid compartments. Each buffer contains a weak acid and a salt of its conjugate base.

Box 8-1	Buffers in the Blood

EXTRACELLULAR FLUID BUFFERS

Plasma bicarbonate
Plasma proteins (e.g., albumin, globulin)
Inorganic phosphates

INTRACELLULAR FLUID BUFFERS

Bicarbonate
Hemoglobin
Oxyhemoglobin
Inorganic phoshates
Organic phosphates

Buffer Effectiveness

The effectiveness of a given buffer system depends on three factors: the quantity of buffer available, the pK of the buffer system, and whether the buffer functions in an open or closed system.

Quantity

Obviously, the larger the quantity of a given buffer that is available, the more acid or base it can buffer. Hemoglobin is the most important intracellular fluid buffer because of its tremendous concentration.

pK of the Buffer System

A buffer functions best when the pH of the solution is equal to the pK of the weak acid of the buffer system. The pK of a weak acid is the pH at which 50% of the acid is dissociated and 50% is undissociated. Figure 8-8 shows the pK of carbonic acid, which is approximately 6.1 in the blood. Because strong acids are buffered by the dissociated portion of the buffer pair (e.g., $NaHCO_3$) and strong bases are buffered by the undissociated portion (e.g., H_2CO_3), it follows that *both* bases and acids could be buffered equally well when the buffer system is at its pK.

Buffers are generally considered to function well within 1 pH unit of their pK. Because the pK of the bicarbonate buffer system in blood is 6.1, this buffer functions best in the pH range of 5.1 to 7.1. The blood, however, has a pH of 7.4. Thus, considering only the pK, the bicarbonate buffer is not particularly effective in the blood. For reasons described in the following section, however, the bicarbonate buffer is still a very important blood buffer.

Open versus Closed Buffer Systems

In a closed chemical system, a buffer becomes less and less effective as the products of buffering accumulate, which is indeed the case for most of the blood buffers. Buffering effectiveness is compared in an open versus a closed system in Figure 8-9. The hemoglobin buffer functions in a closed system. As hydrogen ions are buffered by hemoglobin, acid hemoglobin (HHb) accumulates. The buildup of HHb in turn slows the buffering reaction due to the law of mass action.

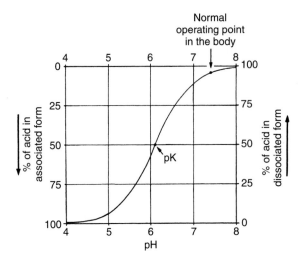

Figure 8-8.   **The pK of carbonic acid.** The pK is the pH at which an acid is 50% dissociated. The pK of carbonic acid in blood is 6.1.

This is not the case, however, for the bicarbonate buffer system. Due to the hydrolysis reaction and the law of mass action, the bicarbonate buffer system has the unique ability to excrete carbonic acid via the lungs as it accumulates through buffering. CO_2 does not accumulate in the blood; rather, any excess of CO_2 is excreted to maintain CO_2 homeostasis. Thus, the bicarbonate buffer is the only blood buffer that functions in an *open system*. For this reason, the bicarbonate buffer system is the most important extracellular fluid buffer.

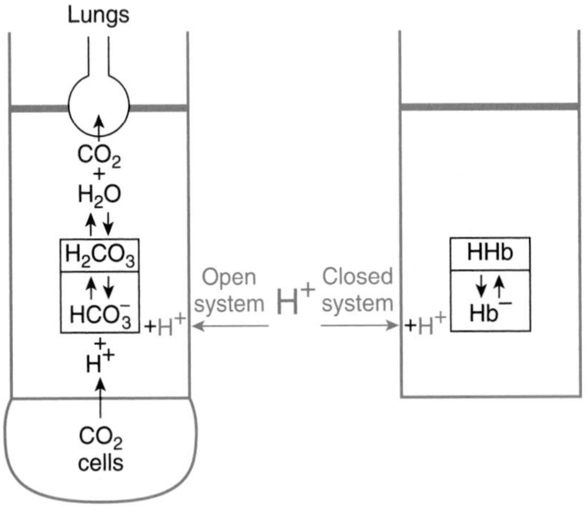

Buffer Interactions

Quantitatively, the extracellular and intracellular fluids share the buffering of an acute acid load almost equally, although the extracellular buffering occurs more quickly. The bicarbonate buffer system alone is responsible for more than 50% of total buffering.[367]

The various blood buffers do not really function independently in the blood. They are, in fact, all chemically interdependent because the hydrogen ion is common to all buffer reactions. This principle of inter-relationship is sometimes referred to as the *isohydric principle.* Guyton stated that "the buffer systems actually buffer each other."[173]

HENDERSON-HASSELBALCH EQUATION

A discussion of acid-base homeostasis would be incomplete without some mention of the famous Henderson-Hasselbalch equation. This chemical equation provides the basis for determining many common blood gas measurements (e.g., PCO_2, $[HCO_3]$). This equation describes the fixed inter-relationships between PCO_2, pH, and $[HCO_3]$. A brief historical perspective of the development of this equation is presented, followed by a mathematical calculation of

Figure 8-9.   **Open versus closed system buffering.** The bicarbonate buffer system is the most effective extracellular buffer because it functions as an open system. CO_2, the product of acid buffering, does not accumulate in the blood and slow the buffering process. Also, CO_2 that is used up when carbonic acid is consumed in buffering bases is replenished easily through metabolism.

pH, and finally the clinical application of this equation.

Henderson's Equation

Chemists have known for a long time that there was a constant mathematical relationship between the various substances present in the dissociation reaction of an acid. If the concentration of the products of dissociation (right side of the dissociation reaction) is divided by the concentration of the undissociated acid (left side of the equation), a constant number would always result for a given acid. This constant number is called the dissociation constant of that particular acid, and each acid has its own distinctive constant. Calculation of the dissociation constant for carbonic acid is shown in Equation 8-11.

Equation 8-11

$$Kc = \frac{[H^+][HCO_3]}{[H_2CO_3]}$$

Kc = dissociation constant for carbonic acid

Henderson simply took this equation (see Equation 8-11) and solved it for the $[H^+]$ (Equation 8-12). The dissociation constant for H_2CO_3 is a known value that can be substituted into the equation. If the $[HCO_3]$ and the $[H_2CO_3^-]$ could then be measured, the equation could be solved for the $[H^+]$. Unfortunately, the normal hydrogen ion concentration in the blood is a very small and awkward number (0.00000004 Eq/L). Therefore, a different method of reporting this measurement was sought.

Equation 8-12

$$[H^+] = \frac{Kc[H_2CO_3]}{[HCO_3]}$$

Hasselbalch's Modification

Hasselbalch addressed this problem by taking the negative log of both sides of the Henderson equation. The symbol for the negative log of a substance is *p*. Thus, the negative log of the free hydrogen ion concentration becomes simply pH. The equation that results after this manipulation is called the Henderson-Hasselbalch equation and is shown

in Equation 8-13. By using the negative log, the normal value for the free hydrogen ion concentration (pH) in the arterial blood becomes simply 7.35 to 7.45.

Equation 8-13

$$pH = pKc + \log \frac{[HCO_3]}{[H_2CO_3]}$$

pKc = negative log of the dissociation constant of carbonic acid

In practice, it is very difficult to measure the $[H_2CO_3]$ because it is so minute. An alternative, however, is to substitute the dissolved CO_2 concentration in place of $[H_2CO_3]$ because the two are related directly and linearly. The modified form of the Henderson-Hasselbalch equation that results is shown in Equation 8-14.

Equation 8-14

$$pH = pKc + \log \frac{[HCO_3]}{[\text{diss } CO_2]}$$

[diss CO_2] = dissolved CO_2 concentration in mEq/L

Numeric Calculation

The normal blood pH can be calculated by substituting the normal values for the factors given in the modified Henderson-Hasselbalch equation. Normal pKc within the blood is a constant value of 6.1. The normal $[HCO_3^-]$ in the plasma is approximately 24 mEq/L.

The dissolved CO_2 concentration in mEq/L can be calculated by multiplying $PaCO_2$ (mm Hg) by the conversion factor (0.03 mEq/L/mm Hg). Because the normal $PaCO_2$ is approximately 40 mm Hg, this value becomes (40 mm Hg × 0.03 mEq/L/mm Hg) 1.2 mEq/L of dissolved CO_2. The result of substitution of these values into Equation 8-14 is shown in Equation 8-15.

One can see that the normal ratio of bicarbonate to dissolved CO_2 in units of mEq/L is approximately 20:1. Preservation of this ratio is essential to maintain a normal pH. Figure 8-10 shows the effect that alterations in this ratio have on the pH. Extreme alterations have a substantial effect on pH and can ultimately result in death.

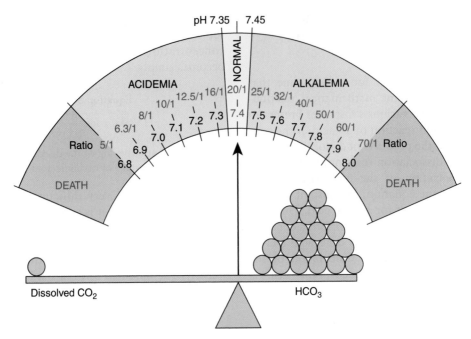

Figure 8-10. **Normal 20:1 ratio of bicarbonate to dissolved CO$_2$ in milliequivalents per liter.** The normal ratio of [HCO$_3$] to dissolved CO$_2$ in mEq/L is 20:1. Alteration of this ratio changes the pH and may lead to death in severe cases.

Finally, Equation 8-15 shows that the log of 20 is 1.3. Therefore, adding 1.3 to the normal pKc of 6.1 results in the normal arterial pH of 7.4.

Equation 8-15

$$pH = (6.1) + \log \frac{24 \text{ mEq/L}}{1.2 \text{ mEq/L}}$$

$$pH = (6.1) + \log 20$$

$$pH = (6.1) + 1.3$$

$$pH = 7.4$$

Clinical Application

[HCO$_3$]/PaCO$_2$ Ratio

If all of the constants are eliminated from the Henderson-Hasselbalch equation, it is reduced to the simple relationship shown in Proportion 8-4. The unit that [HCO$_3$] is usually reported in is mEq/L. The unit that PaCO$_2$ is typically reported in is mm Hg. Technically, from a mathematical standpoint, different units in the numerator and denominator should not be used. Rather, both should be converted to mEq/L, which was described earlier. Nevertheless, the gross effect of a change in PaCO$_2$ or [HCO$_3$] on pH can still be appreciated if these quantities are left in their normally recorded units. Using the normally reported units, the ratio is simply 24/40 ([HCO$_3$] in mEq/L and PaCO$_2$ in mm Hg).

Proportion 8-4. [HCO$_3$]/PaCO$_2$ RATIO

$$pH \approx \frac{[HCO_3]}{PaCO_2} \approx \frac{\text{kidneys}}{\text{lungs}}$$

The denominator in Proportion 8-4 (i.e., PaCO$_2$) is, of course, primarily a product of respiratory lung function. The numerator, on the other hand, [HCO$_3$], is affected by buffering and other nonrespiratory acid-base changes. The organs with primary responsibility for [HCO$_3$] regulation are the kidneys.

Metabolic Disturbances

Based on Proportion 8-4, an increase in the numerator, [HCO$_3$], tends to increase blood pH. When analyzing blood gas data, a specific, measured acid-base condition that tends to increase blood pH may be called a *laboratory alkalosis*. When the term *alkalosis* is used to infer a patient's diagnosis, however, it should be used only to indicate an abnormal, *primary* acid-base condition and not compensatory responses.

Thus, a distinction should be made between a laboratory alkalosis (e.g., increased [HCO$_3$]), and an actual patient's diagnosis of alkalosis (e.g., vomiting that resulted in an increased [HCO$_3$]).

On the other hand, a decrease in the numerator tends to decrease blood pH. A specific, measured acid-base condition that tends to lower blood pH may be called a *laboratory acidosis*. Here again, the distinction should be made between a laboratory acidosis (e.g., decreased [HCO$_3$]) and an actual patient's diagnosis of acidosis (e.g., renal failure leading to a decreased [HCO$_3$]). A more detailed discussion of this acid-base terminology appears at the end of this chapter.

The terms *acidosis* or *alkalosis* can be further clarified based on their origin. A condition originating from the respiratory system is called a *respiratory acid-base condition* (acidosis/alkalosis). A nonrespiratory condition is called a *metabolic acid-base condition*.

Respiratory Disturbances

A change in the denominator of the [HCO$_3$]/PaCO$_2$ also tends to change blood pH. An increase in the denominator (i.e., PaCO$_2$) tends to decrease blood pH. In comparison, a decrease in PaCO$_2$ tends to increase pH.

The proportion points out that it is the ***ratio*** of bicarbonate to PaCO$_2$ that determines blood pH, not the absolute value of either of the factors. For example, if both [HCO$_3$] and PaCO$_2$ increase proportionately, the ratio and therefore blood pH will be normal.

Acid-Base Compensation

When acid-base disturbances occur, the human organism takes advantage of this ratio (i.e., [HCO$_3$]/PaCO$_2$) in an attempt to normalize pH. In other words, when the denominator increases, the body responds by increasing the numerator, which has the effect of normalizing the [HCO$_3$]/PaCO$_2$ ratio and pH. This process of altering the unaffected component in the ratio in an attempt to normalize the overall ratio is called *acid-base compensation*.

The organs involved in acid-base compensation are the lungs and the kidneys. The lungs regulate PaCO$_2$, the denominator of the ratio. The kidneys regulate [HCO$_3$], the numerator of the ratio. The lungs can modify PaCO$_2$ in

response to a change in the numerator within minutes. Nevertheless, the maximal respiratory response may take up to 24 hours.[368,369] In comparison, the compensatory response of the kidneys is slow. The kidneys require 48 to 72 hours to achieve maximal compensation.

The initial, abnormal acid-base disturbance that occurs in a particular patient is sometimes referred to as the *primary* disturbance or problem. The acid-base change that occurs during compensation for the primary problem is sometimes referred to as a *secondary* or *compensatory* acid-base condition.

Respiratory Disturbances

Figure 8-11,*A* shows the normal [HCO$_3$]/PaCO$_2$ ratio of 24/40. In ordinary circumstances this reflects a normal balance of acids and bases within the body and a normal pH. Figure 8-11,*B* shows a *primary respiratory acidosis*. This condition is associated with a rise in PaCO$_2$ and carbonic acid. A narcotic drug overdose could lead to poor ventilation and to this condition. Acute (abrupt onset) respiratory acidosis increases the denominator of the ratio and decreases pH.

The kidneys, however, respond to this situation by increasing blood [HCO$_3$] and thus increasing the numerator of the ratio. This result represents the secondary acid-base change. Figures 8-11,*C* and *D* show progressive compensation. Ultimately, in Figure 8-11,*D*, compensation is complete and the ratio is restored.

In patients, complete compensation to a pH of 7.40 is probably never achieved. Complete compensation is shown here, however, to show the concept of progressive compensation. Also remember that renal (kidney) compensation is not complete for 2 to 3 days. Figures 8-12,*A* to *D* show the same chain of events that occur in the development and compensation for a primary *respiratory alkalosis*.

Metabolic Disturbances

Figures 8-13,*A* to *D* show the onset and progressive compensation of nonrespiratory (metabolic) acidosis. In this particular case, *metabolic acidosis* is shown to have resulted from a loss of blood base (i.e., HCO$_3$). Metabolic acidosis may also develop due to an accumulation of fixed acid in the blood. In either event, however, bicarbonate (the numerator)

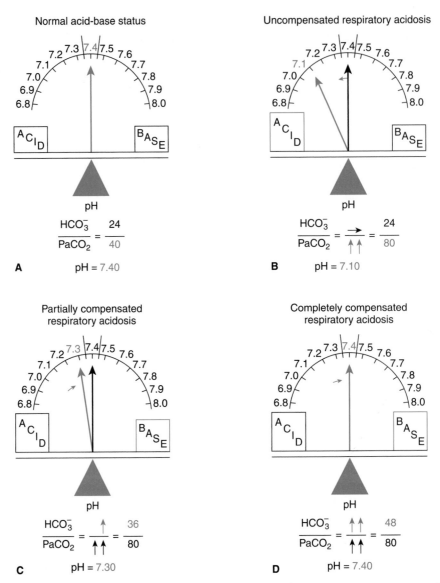

Figure 8-11. **Compensation for respiratory acidosis. A,** The normal [HCO₃]/PaCO₂ is associated with a normal pH and acid-base balance. **B,** Increased PaCO₂ is associated with an increase in volatile acid [H₂CO₃] and a decreased pH. **C,** Renal compensation increases the blood [HCO₃] and tends to normalize the ratio. **D,** A normal pH would result if the ratio were restored to normal.

concentration decreases. In the case of increased fixed acids, bicarbonate is used up in the buffering reaction of the bicarbonate buffer system.

Finally, Figures 8-14,*A* to *D* show the onset and compensation for *metabolic alkalosis*. Metabolic alkalosis is shown to result from the accumulation of blood base, although theoretically it could also result from the excessive loss of fixed acids. Compensation for metabolic

acid-base problems is accomplished quickly via the lungs. Nevertheless, like the kidneys, the lungs rarely achieve complete compensation back to a pH of 7.40.

In clinical situations, what appears to be acid-base compensation may actually represent two distinct acid-base problems. These mixed acid-base disturbances are discussed in greater detail in Chapter 14.

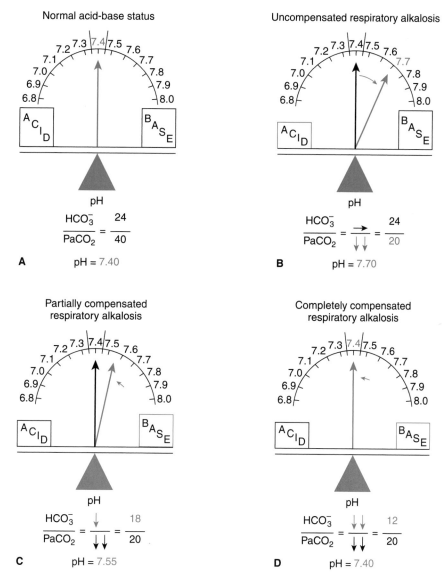

Figure 8-12.   **Compensation for respiratory alkalosis. A,** The normal $[HCO_3]/PaCO_2$ is associated with a normal pH and acid-base balance. **B,** Decreased $PaCO_2$ is associated with a decrease in volatile acid $[H_2CO_3]$ and an increased pH. **C,** Renal compensation decreases the blood $[HCO_3]$ and tends to normalize the ratio. **D,** A normal pH would result if the ratio were restored to normal.

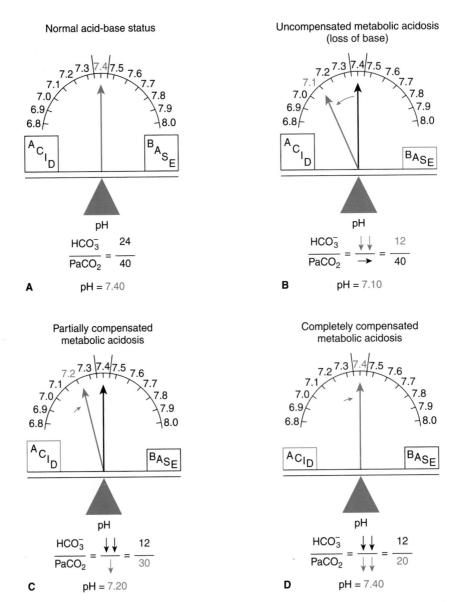

Figure 8-13.   Compensation for metabolic acidosis. A, The normal [HCO3]/PaCO2 is associated with a normal pH and acid-base balance. **B,** Decreased [HCO3] is associated with a decrease in blood base and a decreased pH. **C,** Respiratory compensation decreases the blood volatile acid through hyperventilation and tends to normalize the ratio. **D,** A normal pH would result if the ratio were restored to normal.

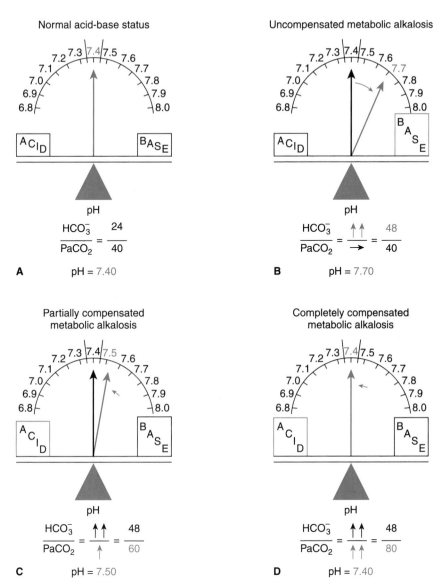

Figure 8-14. Compensation for metabolic alkalosis. A, The normal [HCO$_3$]/PaCO$_2$ is associated with a normal pH and acid-base balance. **B,** Increased [HCO$_3$] is associated with an increase in blood base and an increased pH. **C,** Respiratory compensation increases the blood volatile acid through hypoventilation and tends to normalize the ratio. **D,** A normal pH would result if the ratio were restored to normal.

Acid-Base Terminology

In 1964, the International Conference on Acid-Base Terminology was sponsored by the New York Academy of Sciences in an attempt to standardize acid-base terminology.[370] Most of the controversy at that time (and I might add presently) surrounded the appropriate use of the terms *acidosis* and *alkalosis*. One school thought that the term *acidosis* should be used

for abnormal laboratory acid-base measurements (e.g., [HCO$_3$], [BE], etc.). Conversely, the other school thought that the term *acidosis* should not represent a specific laboratory measurement but rather a *primary* abnormal acid-base process or condition.

Despite considerable disagreement,[371] the conferees recommended in their report that the terms *acidosis* and *alkalosis* be used *only* for primary, abnormal acid-base processes, which is consistent with the usual use of the suffix *osis* which means "pathologic condition."[372] Thus, according to their recommendations, a *compensatory* increase in [HCO_3] in a particular patient should not technically be called a metabolic alkalosis because it is not a primary acid-base disturbance. In the past (and in many circles in the present), it was common to refer to a secondary increase in bicarbonate as a *compensatory metabolic alkalosis*, which, of course, is inconsistent with recommendations of the International Conference on Acid-Base Terminology.

Unfortunately, however, the committee did not recommend an alternative terminology for what is sometimes referred to as a compensatory or secondary acidosis/alkalosis, which, I might add, are often very useful terms in blood

gas classification.[371] The terms *hyperbasemia* and *hypobasemia* have been used by several authors,[373–375] but this terminology is cumbersome and is not standard in the literature or in my clinic.

Therefore, in this text, I have chosen to use the terms *acidosis* and *alkalosis* to indicate *measured* laboratory changes in [HCO_3] and $PaCO_2$. I believe that naming abnormal laboratory values in this manner greatly aids the novice in blood gas classification.

When referring to the patient (compared with the blood gas), however, the terms *acidosis* and *alkalosis* should be used only to indicate primary, abnormal acid-base processes. In comparison, a laboratory metabolic acidosis (e.g., decreased [HCO_3]), may represent either a *primary* or a *secondary* acid-base condition.

EXERCISES

Exercise 8-1 Hydrogen Ions and pH

Fill in the blanks or select the best answer.

1. Hydrogen in chemical combination with other elements (is/is not) part of the pH measurement.
2. The definition of pH is the _____.
3. The normal range for pH in arterial blood is _____.
4. The relationship between pH and [H^+] is (direct/inverse) and (linear/logarithmic).
5. Doubling of the normal [H^+] results in a (0.03/0.3) unit decrease in pH.
6. Any chemical substance capable of releasing a H^+ into solution is defined as a/an _____.
7. Any substance capable of combining with or accepting a hydrogen ion in solution is called a _____.
8. Maintenance of a constant internal environment is called _____.
9. State the two organs primarily responsible for acid-base balance.
10. Normal body metabolism tends to result in an accumulation of excess (acid/base).
11. The (kidneys/lungs) are the major organs of acid excretion.
12. The lungs excrete (volatile/fixed) acid.
13. Normally, _____ is the only volatile acid excreted by the lungs under ordinary conditions.
14. The organs responsible for the regulation of blood bases is the (lungs/kidneys).
15. The major blood base of clinical significance in blood gas interpretation is _____.

Exercise 8-2 Underlying Chemistry of H_2CO_3 Regulation

Fill in the blanks or select the best answer.

1. Chemical equilibrium (does/does not) mean that the concentrations of constituents on both sides of an equation are equal.

2. A/an (open/closed) chemical system is one in which all the reactants and products in a chemical reaction must remain within that system.

3. The chemical reaction below is said to be shifted to the (left/right).

   $H_2O + CO_2 \underset{\longleftarrow}{\overset{\rightarrow}{\quad}} H_2CO_3$

   $(800) + (800) \underset{\longleftarrow}{\overset{\rightarrow}{\quad}} (1)$

4. The change in equilibrium in response to a change in the amount of one of the reaction constituents is referred to as the law of _____.

5. If there is an increase in one of the reactants on the right side of a reversible chemical equation, the law of mass action causes the equilibrium to shift to the (right/left).

6. Write the hydrolysis reaction.

7. There is a (direct/inverse) and (linear/logarithmic) relationship between the concentration of dissolved CO_2 and the concentration of carbonic acid [H_2CO_3] in the blood.

8. _____ can be used as a marker of blood volatile acid (i.e., [H_2CO_3]) levels in the arterial blood.

9. There is a/an (increase/decrease/no change) in the amount of carbonic acid present in the blood as it passes the tissues.

10. Venous blood is slightly more (acidic/alkaline) compared with arterial blood.

Exercise 8-3 CO_2 Homeostasis

Fill in the blanks or select the best answer.

1. The amount of CO_2 entering the blood depends primarily on the _____.

2. The volume of CO_2 produced per minute is designated as the _____.

3. _____ is the amount of fresh gas that reaches functional alveoli.

4. The symbol for alveolar ventilation per minute is _____.

5. State two conditions in which a large increase in metabolism and CO_2 production may result in increased $PaCO_2$.

6. An increase in blood $PaCO_2$ can occur after intravenous administration of the drug _____ to a patient unable to increase his or her alveolar ventilation.

7. An increase in alveolar ventilation results in a/an (increased/decreased) $PaCO_2$.

8. The amount of gas moving in and out of the lungs with each breath is called the _____.

9. Write the formula for minute ventilation.

10. Minute ventilation (is/is not) a reliable index of the adequacy of ventilation.

11. The _____ is the best index available to assess the adequacy of ventilation.

12. Write the formula for alveolar minute ventilation.

13. Alveolar ventilation is (directly/inversely) proportional to $PaCO_2$.

14. An increase in physiologic deadspace may (increase/decrease) $PaCO_2$.

15. A decrease in respiratory rate or tidal volume (increases/decreases) alveolar ventilation.

Exercise 8-4 CO_2 Transport

Fill in the blanks or select the best answer.

1. State the four mechanisms through which CO_2 is carried in the blood.

2. In blood, the solubility coefficient of CO_2 is (higher/lower) than the solubility coefficient of O_2.

3. The solubility coefficient of CO_2 in blood is _____ mEq/L/mm Hg.

4. A $PaCO_2$ of 80 mm Hg is equal to _____ mEq/L of CO_2.

5. The volume of CO_2 being transported in the form of H_2CO_3 (is/is not) negligible.

6. The hydrolysis reaction occurs at a very (slow/fast) rate in the plasma.

7. Of the CO_2 transport from tissues to the lungs, 80% is in the form of (dissolved CO_2/ carbonic acid/bicarbonate).

8. Inside the erythrocyte, the hydrolysis reaction occurs at a much (faster/slower) rate than in the plasma.

9. The enzyme that speeds up the hydrolysis reaction is called _____.

10. Hydrogen ions generated by the hydrolysis reaction within erythrocytes are buffered by (bicarbonate/hemoglobin).

11. Bicarbonate ions are transported through the cell membrane in exchange for (Cl^-/PO_4^-/K^+).

12. The chloride shift is sometimes referred to as the _____ phenomenon.

13. Most of the HCO_3 transporting CO_2 from the tissues to the lungs originates in the (erythrocytes/plasma).

14. Protein in combination with CO_2 is called a/an _____.

15. The combined form of hemoglobin and CO_2 is called _____.

16. Hemoglobin combination with CO_2 (does/does not) occur at the same chemical site as hemoglobin combination with O_2.

17. The affinity of hemoglobin for CO_2 is (greater/less) when it is combined with O_2.

18. The decreased affinity of hemoglobin for CO_2 when it is already carrying O_2 is known as the _____ effect.

19. The percentage of CO_2 transport in the form of carbamino-hemoglobin is approximately _____%.

20. Carbamino compounds in the plasma account for only approximately _____% of CO_2 transport.

Exercise 8-5 The Kidney and Acid-Base Balance

Fill in the blanks or select the best answer.

1. State the two major acid-base functions of the kidney.

2. Fixed acids (can/cannot) be converted into gases and excreted via the lungs.

3. (Protein/carbohydrate/lipid) metabolism results in the production of inorganic phosphoric and sulfuric acid.

4. (Protein/carbohydrate/lipid) metabolism in the absence of insulin produces a buildup of acetoacetic and beta-hydroxybutyric acid.

5. Acetoacetic and beta-hydroxybutyric acid are often referred to collectively as the _____.

6. In the absence of O_2, carbohydrate metabolism produces an accumulation of _____ acid.

7. Normally, the amount of fixed acid produced each day is small, approximately _____ mEq.

8. Ammonium chloride is metabolized by the liver, resulting in the production of _____.

9. The kidneys can (excrete/produce/excrete and produce) bicarbonate ions.

10. The regulation of ([HCO_3]/CO_2) is the single most important role of the kidneys in acid-base balance.

Exercise 8-6 Basic Chemistry Related to Buffers

Fill in the blanks or select the best answer.

1. Every acid must have a related _____ that is present on dissociation of the hydrogen ion.

2. An acid in conjunction with its associated base is sometimes referred to as a _____.

3. The conjugate base of H_2CO_3 is _____, and the conjugate base of HHb is _____.

4. All acids have (different/similar) degrees of dissociation.

5. Strong acids have a (high/low) degree of dissociation.

6. A longer arrow in one direction of a dissociation reaction indicates that the concentrations of substances on that side of the equation are (greater/lower) at equilibrium.

7. In general, the stronger the acid, the (stronger/weaker) is its conjugate base.

8. (Deoxygenated/oxygenated) hemoglobin most readily picks up hydrogen ions.

9. The reaction: $HCl \rightleftharpoons H^+ + Cl^-$ shows a (strong/weak) acid.

10. Hemoglobin may function as an (acid/base/acid or a base) in the blood and is sometimes referred to as a/an _____ substance.

Exercise 8-7   Blood Buffer Systems

Fill in the blanks or select the best answer.

1. Buffer solutions (do/do not) prevent pH change.

2. Buffer solutions minimize pH change by converting strong acids into (bases/weaker acids).

3. State the two chemical substances that must be present in a buffer solution.

4. When a strong acid is introduced into the buffer solution, it reacts with the (salt/weak acid) portion of the buffer pair.

5. State the two chemical components of the plasma bicarbonate buffer system in the blood.

6. If HCl is added to a bicarbonate buffer system, the results of the buffering are the chemical substances _____ and _____.

7. Fill in the products of the following buffer reaction:
   $NaOH + H_2CO_3/NaHCO_3 \rightarrow$ _____.

8. State the three plasma buffers in the blood.

9. List the three factors that determine buffer effectiveness.

10. The pK of a weak acid is the pH at which _____% of the acid is dissociated.

11. (Open/closed) system buffers are most effective.

12. Buffers are generally considered to function well within (1/2/3) pH unit(s) of their pK.

13. The most important buffer system in the plasma is the (protein/bicarbonate) system.

14. The most important intracellular buffer is _____.

15. The principle of inter-relationship of the different buffer systems is sometimes referred to as the _____ principle.

Exercise 8-8   Henderson-Hasselbalch Equation

Fill in the blanks or select the best answer.

1. State the name of the following equation:

   $[H^+] = Kc\ [H_2CO_3]/[HCO_3]$

2. The symbol for the negative log of a substance is _____.

3. Write the formula for the Henderson-Hasselbalch equation.

4. Normal pKc is a constant value of _____.

5. The normal $[HCO_3]$ in the arterial plasma is _____ mEq/L.

6. The normal volume of dissolved CO_2 in the arterial blood in mEq/L is _____.

7. The normal ratio of $[HCO_3]$/dissolved CO_2 in mEq/L is _____.

8. The log of 20 is _____.

9. Write the proportion that results if all constants are removed from the Henderson-Hasselbalch equation.

10. Respiratory conditions alter the (numerator/denominator) of the Henderson-Hasselbalch proportion.

11. The most important aspect of the Henderson-Hasselbalch proportion is the (numerator/denominator/ratio between the numerator and denominator).

12. The process of altering the unaffected acid-base component in the Henderson-Hasselbalch ratio in an attempt to normalize the overall ratio is called acid-base _____.

13. The normal $[HCO_3]/PaCO_2$ is _____.

Exercise 8-9   Acid-Base Physiology and Terminology

Fill in the blanks or select the best answer.

1. The primary organ system responsible for the $[HCO_3]$ is the (renal/respiratory) system.

2. A measured acid-base condition that tends to increase blood pH is termed a/an _____.

3. A measured acid-base condition that tends to lower blood pH is termed a/an _____.

4. A nonrespiratory acid-base condition is called a/an _____ acid-base disturbance.

5. The kidneys require approximately _____ hours to achieve maximal compensation.

6. In actual patients, complete compensation to a pH of 7.4 is (usually/rarely) achieved.

7. Classify the laboratory acid-base status associated with the following $[HCO_3]/PaCO_2$ ratios as (metabolic acidosis/metabolic alkalosis/respiratory acidosis/respiratory alkalosis):

   a. 14/40
   b. 24/80
   c. 24/20
   d. 36/40

8. According to the International Conference on Acid-Base Terminology, the term *acidosis* should be reserved for (primary/compensatory) disturbances.

9. In this text, a compensatory increase in bicarbonate is called a/an _____ metabolic alkalosis.

10. A term used by some authors to indicate decreased blood bicarbonate is _____.

Exercise 8-10   Internet Work

1. Perform a web search using Clinical Acid-Base Balance. Visit sites listed under:
   Acid Base Balance: Interactive teaching tools
   Acid Base Balance: Introduction
   Acid Base Balance: Clinical Considerations
   pH of the Blood – M.J. Bookallil

2. Write a summary of two new points regarding acid-base balance learned at each site.

NBRC Challenge 8

Please select the best answer for the following multiple-choice questions.

1. A 63-year-old man presents to the emergency department with the following arterial blood gases:

   pH   7.35
   $PaCO_2$ 59 mm Hg
   $[HCO_3]$ 30 mEq/L
   PaO_2 61 mm Hg

   The patient appears to have:
   I.   chronic renal acid-base compensation.
   II. COPD.
   III. acute respiratory acidosis.
   A) I only
   B) II only
   C) I and II only
   D) II and III only
   E) I, II, and III
   (CRT EXAMINATION — NBRC
       MATRIX I,C,2,c)

2. In reviewing the patient's chart you note that measured venous bicarbonate on the electrolyte report is 28 mEq/L whereas the bicarbonate on the blood gas report is 25 mEq/L. You should conclude:
   A) there is a technical error on the electrolyte report.
   B) there is a technical error on the blood gas report.
   C) the lab tests must have been done at different points in time.
   D) the patient must have COPD.
   E) these results are consistent and expected.
   (RRT EXAMINATION — NBRC
       MATRIX I,C,2,f)

3. A 40-year-old man presents to the emergency department with the following arterial blood gases:

   pH   7.56
   $PaCO_2$ 52 mm Hg
   $[HCO_3]$ 48 mEq/L
   PaO_2 71 mm Hg

   You can conclude:
   A) the patient has COPD.
   B) the patient has mild hypoxemia secondary to pneumonia.
   C) the patient needs mechanical ventilation.
   D) the hypoxemia indicates a pulmonary problem.
   E) the pulmonary changes suggest compensation for a metabolic alkalosis.
   (RRT EXAMINATION — NBRC
       MATRIX I,B,10,c)

4. A burn patient is being mechanically ventilated with a minute ventilation of 15 LPM and his $PaCO_2$ is 52 mm Hg. A probable explanation is:
   A) increased CO_2 production.
   B) decreased CO_2 production.
   C) the Haldane Effect.
   D) the Bohr Effect.
   E) excessive fat metabolism.
   (RRT EXAMINATION — NBRC
       MATRIX I,C,2,b)

5. A patient is inadvertently given a small amount of a strong acid intravenously. Blood gases are immediately drawn and pH is 7.31. A large swing in pH was most likely prevented because of:
   A) renal compensation.
   B) hypoventilation.
   C) blood buffers.
   D) the hydrolysis reaction.
   E) carbamino compounds.
   (RRT EXAMINATION — NBRC
       MATRIX I,B,10,c)

Clinical Oxygenation

Chapter 9

Assessment and Treatment of Hypoxemia and Shunting

Hypoxemia...

...cardiac output, oxygen consumption, hemoglobin content, alveolar ventilation or lung disease can each change, sometimes simultaneously and in opposite directions, so as to complexly alter the PaO₂.

Peter D. Wagner[243]

Outline

OVERVIEW

The ability of the lungs to transfer oxygen from the atmosphere to the pulmonary capillary blood (i.e., external respiration) is the first critical step in the overall process of oxygenation. The clinical assessment of oxygen transfer in the lungs is a two-part evaluation.

First, the *adequacy* of oxygen transfer must be evaluated. Assessment of the adequacy of oxygen transfer in the lungs is essentially *hypoxemic* (i.e., PaO₂) evaluation. An adequate PaO₂ is one that is sufficiently high so as not to suggest the likelihood of tissue hypoxia.

Second, the *efficiency* of oxygen transfer through the lungs should be considered. In other words, "Is the PaO₂ appropriate for the given FIO₂?" Thus, the second part of oxygen transfer evaluation is essentially an assessment of pulmonary shunting.

The first section of this chapter briefly describes the classification and assessment of hypoxemia. Special reference is also made to the effects of cardiac output and mixed venous blood on PaO₂. The next portion of this chapter addresses the evaluation and quantification of pulmonary shunting. The various clinical indices that have been used to estimate and quantify pulmonary shunting are surveyed. The use of some of these indices in the differential diagnosis of clinical hypoxemia is also discussed.

This is followed by a description of the clinical signs and symptoms associated with hypoxemia, hypercapnia, and hyperoxemia. Finally, methods for treating hypoxemia are discussed. The value and clinical indications for oxygen therapy, body positioning, mechanical ventilation, and the use of positive end-expiratory pressure (PEEP) are explored.

ASSESSMENT OF HYPOXEMIA

Hypoxemia is defined in this text as a below-normal PaO_2 in the blood. The severity of hypoxemia is an important indicator of the likelihood of hypoxia concomitant with the hypoxemia. Table 2-7 is provided in Chapter 2 for classification of the severity of hypoxemia.

Five mechanisms by which hypoxemia may occur are shown in Figure 9-1. Hypoxemia may be due to a low partial pressure of inhaled oxygen (PIO_2) (which is present at high altitude), when exhaled gas is rebreathed continuously in a confined area, or when a gas with less than 21% oxygen is inspired (see Fig. 9-1,B). This mechanism, however, is rarely responsible for hypoxemia in the acute care setting.

| Box 9-1 | Mechanisms of Hypoxemia |

1. Hypoventilation
2. Absolute shunting
3. Relative shunting
4. Diffusion defects

In the hospital, there are really only four potential causes of hypoxemia (Box 9-1). These causes include hypoventilation (see Fig. 9-1,C); absolute shunting (see Fig. 9-1,D); relative shunting, commonly referred to as ventilation/perfusion mismatch (see Fig. 9-1,E); and diffusion defects (see Fig. 9-1,F). Almost all hypoxemia (excluding changes in cardiac output) in the hospital setting may be presumed to be due to one or more of these four mechanisms. The differential diagnosis of hypoxemia is discussed in a subsequent section of this chapter.

EFFECTS OF CARDIAC OUTPUT ON PaO_2

A decrease in cardiac output is not generally considered to be a primary cause of hypoxemia,

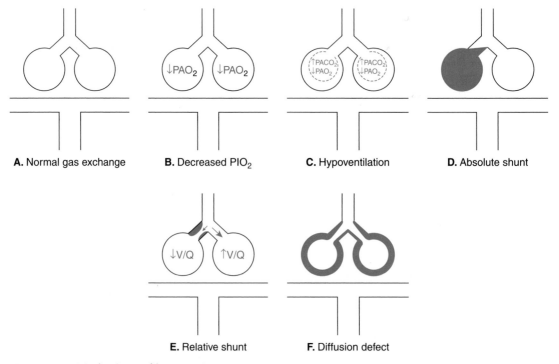

Figure 9-1. **Mechanisms of hypoxemia.**

and no mention of cardiac output is made in Box 9-1 regarding the causes of hypoxemia. Notwithstanding, it is not correct to presume that the cardiac output has *no* effect on PaO_2. The relative influence of cardiac output on PaO_2 in various clinical situations is explored.

Arterial Blood as a Mixture

The clinician must always keep in mind that arterial blood is a *mixture* of blood from two sources. *Oxygenated blood* is leaving functional alveolar-capillary units and entering the arteries. Also, some *mixed venous blood* is always entering the arterial circulation via the normal anatomic shunt (Fig. 9-2).

Note that, in a healthy individual breathing room air, the PaO_2 (100 mm Hg) is slightly *lower* than the average partial pressure of oxygen in the average alveolus (i.e., $PAO_2 \cong$ 105 mm Hg) and significantly higher than the mixed venous partial pressure of oxygen (i.e., $P\bar{v}O_2$, which is approximately 40 mm Hg). Arterial PaO_2 nearly approximates alveolar PAO_2 because roughly 95% of arterial blood originates from normally functioning alveolar-capillary units where the blood end-capillary PO_2 ($P\acute{c}O_2$ equilibrates with the PAO_2). In contrast, less than 5% of the arterial mixture is comprised of $P\bar{v}O_2$ contributed from the shunted blood.

Throughout the discussion regarding the effects of cardiac output on PaO_2, the amount of oxygen in the shunted blood is shown as a *pressure* measurement (e.g., $P\bar{v}O_2$). Actually, the oxygen content of mixed venous blood ($C\bar{v}O_2$) more accurately reflects the amount of oxygen present in this blood and, therefore, how much it affects the arterial PO_2. Nevertheless, $P\bar{v}O_2$ is used here to illustrate this concept in the most straightforward manner.

Changes in Cardiac Output or Shunting

Decreased Cardiac Output with a Normal Shunt

A decrease in $P\bar{v}O_2$ typically accompanies a decrease in cardiac output if oxygen consumption remains constant. Because tissues are exposed to less blood, they must extract more oxygen from available blood, which results in a lower $P\bar{v}O_2$. Thus, when cardiac output falls, shunted blood entering the arterial circulation will have a lower $P\bar{v}O_2$ than shunted blood when cardiac output is normal (Fig. 9-3). Nevertheless, it is important to note that in otherwise normal lungs, a decrease in cardiac output lowers PaO_2 only slightly *because shunted blood accounts for only 5% of the total arterial blood mixture.* Thus, although PaO_2 decreases slightly with a decrease in cardiac output, the effect of a decreased cardiac output on PaO_2 in the normal lung is minute.

Increased Shunting with Normal Cardiac Output

In the individual with an abnormally high pulmonary shunt, the $P\bar{v}O_2$ of the shunted blood has a more substantial impact on PaO_2 as shown in Figure 9-4. The low PaO_2 that accompanies increased physiologic shunting is a result of the ***large percentage*** of venous

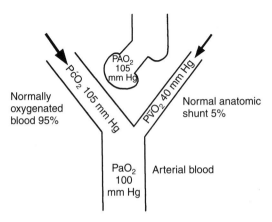

Figure 9-2. **Arterial blood is a mixture of oxygenated and shunted blood.**

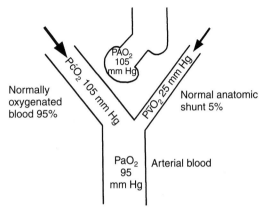

Figure 9-3. **Effects of decreased cardiac output on PaO_2 in humans with normal physiologic shunting.**

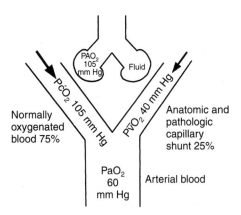

Figure 9-4.   Effect of substantial physiologic shunting on PaO₂.

blood entering the arterial circulation. Note that, in this case, the cardiac output and P̄vO₂ are still normal. Increased shunting is the most common mechanism responsible for the development of hypoxemia.

Decreased Cardiac Output with an Increased Shunt

When substantial shunting is present, any change in cardiac output has a *more profound* effect on PaO₂. This is because changes in cardiac output affect the PO₂ of the shunted blood, and the larger the physiologic shunt, the greater is the percentage of shunted blood entering the arterial circulation.

Figure 9-5 shows how a decline in cardiac output affects PaO₂ in the patient compromised with preexisting pathologic shunting. Note the lower PaO₂ shown in Figure 9-5 compared with Figure 9-4, despite identical shunt fractions of 25%. Note also that a decrease in cardiac output has a greater impact on PaO₂ in the individual with increased physiologic shunting (see Fig. 9-5), compared with the individual who has only a normal anatomic shunt (see Fig. 9-3). It has in fact been shown that a decrease in P̄vO₂ from 40 to 30 mm Hg with a constant 30% shunt decreases PaO₂ from 55 mm Hg to approximately 45 mm Hg.[244]

Increased Cardiac Output with an Increased Shunt

In the presence of a large physiologic shunt and hypoxemia, cardiac output is more likely to increase rather than decrease in the individual with an intact cardiovascular system.[245] The increase in cardiac output is due at least partly to stimulation of the peripheral chemoreceptors secondary to the hypoxemia. Cardiac output tends to increase quickly, due primarily to an increased heart rate, and in a dose-response fashion.[245] In other words, the more severe the hypoxemia, the greater the increase in cardiac output.

Increasing cardiac output tends to enhance tissue oxygenation both by an increase in the blood reaching the tissues and, to a lesser extent, by increasing PaO₂. The increase in cardiac output improves PaO₂ by increasing P̄vO₂,

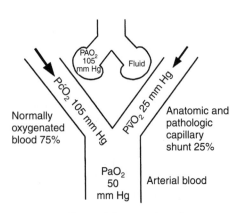

Figure 9-5.   Effects of decreased cardiac output on PaO₂ in the patient with increased physiologic shunting.

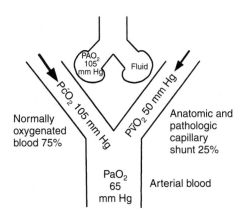

Figure 9-6.   Effects of increased cardiac output on PaO₂ in the patient with increased physiologic shunting.

which is shown in Figure 9-6. This result is the opposite effect to that shown in Figure 9-5 where cardiac output is decreased.

Clinical Implications

In clinical practice, the PaO_2 is often used as a crude index of pulmonary shunting. When the fractional concentration of inspired oxygen (FIO_2) is held constant, an increase in PaO_2 is usually attributed to an improvement in lung function and the pulmonary shunt. Conversely, a decline in PaO_2 suggests further deterioration in pulmonary gas exchange and worsening of the pulmonary shunt.

The logic of these assumptions is sound, and most often these assumptions prove to be correct. Sometimes, however—particularly in the critically ill patient with substantial pulmonary dysfunction—a change in PaO_2 may be primarily due to a nonpulmonary change.[246] As has been shown, cardiac output has a notable effect on PaO_2 in patients with increased physiologic shunts. Furthermore, the influence of cardiac output on PaO_2 is related directly to the size of the shunt.

It is wise to suspect a change in cardiac output when **abrupt, unexplained hypoxemia is observed in the critically ill patient with *apparently stable pulmonary status*.** Cardiac output can be measured directly in the patient with a pulmonary artery catheter in place. In the absence of a pulmonary catheter, the patient should be monitored for signs of low cardiac output, such as those described in Chapter 10.

Other Mechanisms of Decreased $P\bar{v}O_2$

The clinician should understand that the preceding discussion about how cardiac output affects PaO_2 is really an oversimplification. First, as stated previously, the actual PaO_2 that results from the mixture of oxygenated and shunted blood depends more on the oxygen content of the two components than on their respective oxygen tensions.

Second, it should be understood that the mixed venous oxygen content or tension does not depend solely on cardiac output. Anemia, increased metabolism, and abnormal distribution of systemic perfusion are only some of the other factors that can significantly affect mixed venous oxygen levels and, consequently, the PaO_2. It has been shown, however, that cardiac output is probably a primary factor in many clinical situations.

ON CALL | CASE 9-1 *ABGs and Critical Thinking*

You are the only person available to care for this patient. You must assess the patient/situation and act accordingly.

Shortly before 11:00 AM, acute chest pain, shortness of breath, frequent arrhythmias, and hypotension develop in a 52-year-old woman with severe pneumonia. Interpret the blood gases and patient condition at 11:00 AM.

ARTERIAL BLOOD GASES 10:00 AM

SaO_2	93%
pH	7.37
$PaCO_2$	37 mm Hg
PaO_2	72 mm Hg
$[HCO_3]$	25 mEq/L
FIO_2	0.50

ARTERIAL BLOOD GASES 11:00 AM

SaO_2	84%
pH	7.28
$PaCO_2$	29 mm Hg
PaO_2	49 mm Hg
$[HCO_3]$	13 mEq/L
FIO_2	0.50

ASSESSMENT

Abnormalities: List abnormal data and other noteworthy information. Classify ABG.

Explanation: List possible diseases, pathology, or other situations that may have led to this patient's condition.

Evaluation: Suggest additional data that would be useful in helping understand the situation or in making a diagnosis.

INTERVENTION

Importance: Prioritize concern(s) of treatment in order of urgency and/or seriousness as you see the overall situation.

ASSESSMENT OF PHYSIOLOGIC SHUNTING

Introduction

It is often useful in the clinic to quantitate the efficiency of oxygen transfer in external respiration. Analysis of oxygen-loading efficiency can aid the clinician in the differential diagnosis of lung disease and can provide valuable information about severity or progression of pulmonary disease. In addition, some indices of oxygen loading can be useful in guiding oxygen therapy and related treatment of lung disorders.

The PaO_2 alone provides little information regarding the efficiency of oxygen loading into the pulmonary capillary blood. The *physiologic shunt*, on the other hand, is the percentage of the venous blood that remains unoxygenated after traveling from the right side of the heart to the left side of the heart. It includes blood that is absolutely shunted (i.e., anatomic shunts and true capillary shunts) and alveolar-capillary units in which perfusion exceeds ventilation (i.e., relative shunts). Thus, monitoring physiologic shunting is an excellent way to quantitate the efficiency of oxygen uptake via the lungs. The indices that can be used to measure or to estimate physiologic shunting are shown in Box 9-2.

Indices of Physiologic Shunting

Classic Shunt Equation

The classic shunt equation for calculation of physiologic shunting ($\dot{Q}sp/\dot{Q}T$) was described in Chapter 6 (Equation 6-3). It is noteworthy that the classic shunt equation corrects for any nonpulmonary (e.g., $P\bar{v}O_2$) mediated effects on arterial oxygenation, which have been described earlier in this chapter. This is accomplished by directly measuring mixed venous oxygen content and by using this value in the denominator of the equation. In fact, the classic shunt calculation is the only index of oxygen-loading efficiency of those shown in Box 9-2 that takes into account these *nonpulmonary factors*.

Calculation of ($\dot{Q}sp/\dot{Q}T$) via the classic shunt equation is thus the only accurate way to measure physiologic shunting when cardiac output is unstable. Also, by using this index, the clinician can distinguish between PaO_2 disturbances of pulmonary versus cardiovascular origin.

Box 9-2	Indices to Evaluate the Physiologic Shunt

1. Classic shunt calculation
2. Modified shunt equations
3. $P(A-a)O_2$
4. PaO_2/PAO_2
5. PaO_2/FIO_2

The physiologic shunt as calculated via the classic shunt equation is therefore the most sophisticated and accurate measure of the efficiency of the lungs to transfer oxygen. **The classic shunt equation and measurement is therefore the *gold standard* in the measurement of the efficiency of oxygen uptake by the lungs.**

Probably the most notable deterrent to routine measurement of the physiologic shunt is the requirement for mixed venous blood samples. Mixed venous blood samples are available only when a pulmonary artery (Swan-Ganz) catheter is in place.

It should also be noted that $\dot{Q}sp/\dot{Q}T$ changes somewhat depending on the FIO_2 at which it is measured. The pulmonary shunt tends to decrease as FIO_2 is increased from 0.21 to 0.40, remains constant from FIO_2 0.40 to 0.70, then increases as FIO_2 moves above 0.70.[253]

Nevertheless, $\dot{Q}sp/\dot{Q}T$, which is calculated through the classic shunt equation, is the measurement of choice whenever a pulmonary artery catheter is in place. Similarly, when precise monitoring of pulmonary shunting is indicated, such as in the patient with severe pulmonary shunting (e.g., PaO_2 of 60 mm Hg on FIO_2 of 0.60), some clinicians recommend pulmonary catheterization to facilitate accurate monitoring of the physiologic shunt.[247]

Estimated Shunt Equations

When mixed venous blood is unavailable, a modified version of the classic shunt equation is sometimes used to estimate physiologic shunting. Estimated shunt equations assume a given arteriovenous oxygen content difference ($C[a-\bar{v}]O_2$) in their calculations. In some versions of the equation, the difference is assumed to be the normal 5 vol%.[248,249] Because it is common for critically ill patients to have a higher cardiac output or lower oxygen extraction than normal (and therefore a lower arteriovenous difference), in some versions, a difference of 3.5 vol% is deemed more accurate.[250] A lower $C(a-\bar{v})O_2$ has also been demonstrated in patients with hepatopulmonary syndrome and should be used when calculating estimated shunt in this group.[282]

An example of an estimated shunt equation using a $C(a-\bar{v})O_2$ difference of 3.5 vol% is shown in Equation 9-1. Also note that the equation has been rearranged to accommodate inclusion of the arteriovenous difference.

Equation 9-1

$$\dot{Q}sp/\dot{Q}T = (C\acute{c}O_2 - CaO_2)/(C\acute{c}O_2 - C\bar{a}O_2) + 3.5$$

When mixed venous blood gases are unavailable, the estimated shunt equation is probably the best alternative to the classic shunt formula.[248,251] Notwithstanding, however, there are really no true substitutes for actually measuring mixed venous oxygen contents in critically ill patients.[252]

The $P(A-a)O_2$

Normal Values
The alveolar-arterial oxygen tension gradient, or $P(A-a)O_2$, is a well-known noninvasive bedside index that is used to quantitate the efficiency of oxygen loading. If the blood and alveolar gas were perfectly matched, the efficiency of oxygen loading would be high and little or no difference would exist between the mean alveolar PO_2 and the arterial PO_2. On the other hand, an increase in $P(A-a)O_2$ suggests an increase in the physiologic shunt.

The mean normal $P(A-a)O_2$ is approximately 10 mm Hg in adults younger than 60 years of age breathing room air.[254] Individual variations, however, may be great. The upper limit of normal for adults younger than 60 years of age is approximately 20 mm Hg.[254,255]

Unfortunately, $P(A-a)O_2$ increases with advancing age and may be as high as 35 mm Hg in the healthy individual older than 60 years of age.[254] Furthermore, in some individuals, $P(A-a)O_2$ may also change with body position. In individuals older than 44 years of age, $P(A-a)O_2$ increases with the assumption of the supine position.[256,257]

Calculation
Obviously, only two measurements (PaO_2 and PAO_2) are needed to calculate the gradient. PaO_2 is reported with the arterial blood gas data. The PAO_2 represents the *ideal or mean alveolar oxygen tension*. Equation 9-2 is referred to as the *clinical alveolar air equation* and represents the best formula to calculate clinical PAO_2 when FIO_2 is 0.6 or less.[258] Other forms of this equation have been shown to be less accurate and should be avoided.[258] Equation 9-2 roughly assumes a respiratory quotient (RQ) of 0.8, which has been shown to be a reasonable clinical assumption.[259,260]

Equation 9-2

$$PAO_2 = PIO_2 - 1.2(PaCO_2)$$

When an individual is breathing an FIO_2 greater than 0.6, the form of the clinical alveolar air equation shown in Equation 9-3 should be used for this calculation.[258]

Equation 9-3

$$PAO_2 = PIO_2 - PaCO_2$$

The PIO_2 can be determined by multiplying the FIO_2 by the barometric pressure minus water vapor pressure (Equation 9-4). Equation 9-5 shows that when breathing room air at sea level, PIO_2 is approximately 150 mm Hg.

Equation 9-4

$$PIO_2 = (PB - PH_2O) \times FIO_2$$

where:
PB = barometric pressure, and
PH_2O = water vapor pressure at 37° C.

Equation 9-5

$$\begin{aligned}PIO_2 &= (PB - PH_2O) \times FIO_2 \\ &= (760 \text{ mm Hg} - 47 \text{ mm Hg}) \times 0.21 \\ &= 150 \text{ mm Hg}\end{aligned}$$

A shortcut that can be used to calculate $P(A-a)O_2$ is to subtract the sum of PaO_2 and $PaCO_2$ from the normal sum of PAO_2 and $PACO_2$ for the pertinent altitude.[258] At sea level, the normal sum of alveolar PO_2 and PCO_2 is approximately 140 mm Hg. Thus, at sea level, Equation 9-6 can be used to calculate $P(A-a)O_2$.

Equation 9-6

$$P(A-a)O_2 = 140 \text{ mm Hg} - (PaCO_2 + PaO_2)$$

Limitations

The $P(A-a)O_2$ is not particularly useful for monitoring the progress of pulmonary dysfunction at various values of FIO_2.[253] $P(A-a)O_2$ varies with both age and FIO_2. In one study, the $P(A-a)O_2$ escalated with increasing FIO_2 up to 0.6. Above FIO_2 of 0.6, no further increase in $P(A-a)O_2$ was observed.[254] In the same study, mean $P(A-a)O_2$ was 38 mm Hg for individuals 40 to 50 years old with FIO_2 at 0.4.[254] At FIO_2 of 0.6, the mean $P(A-a)O_2$ for all age groups was 50 mm Hg. Most importantly, $P(A-a)O_2$ correlates poorly with changes in pulmonary shunting.[253]

Furthermore, the $P(A-a)O_2$ does not provide the clinician with information regarding the selection of the most appropriate FIO_2 level when treating the patient. Some indices discussed later in this chapter are purported to be valuable in this regard. Overall, the $P(A-a)O_2$ has limited use when supplemental oxygen is being administered. The normal $P(A-a)O_2$ does not remain constant at different FIO_2 levels, nor is the normal range well established for many given FIO_2 levels.

The $P(A-a)O_2$ may be somewhat useful in evaluating pulmonary shunting in the patient breathing room air who is also hypoventilating. This application will be described later in this chapter.

The PaO_2/PAO_2

Description

Limitations of the $P(A-a)O_2$ have led to the introduction of other indices to evaluate oxygen transfer across the lungs. An alternative way to look at the efficiency of pulmonary oxygenation is to determine what percentage of the PAO_2 that is delivered to the alveoli actually reaches the arterial blood. Thus, instead of looking at the absolute numeric alveolar-arterial oxygen tension difference, one is evaluating the *percentage of successful oxygen transfer*. A clinical index that may be used for this purpose is the PaO_2/PAO_2.

Theoretically, assuming constant lung function, the percentage of the PAO_2 that is successfully transferred across the lung should remain constant regardless of FIO_2. Thus, as one might expect, the arterial/alveolar PO_2 ratio has been shown to be more stable than the $P(A-a)O_2$

with changing values of FIO_2.[261] Due to its increased stability, the PaO_2/PAO_2 appears to have several advantages in clinical and research application, compared with the $P(A-a)O_2$.[253,262]

Evaluation of Lung Function

Because, unlike $P(A-a)O_2$, the PaO_2/PAO_2 is relatively constant with changes in FIO_2, the progressive evaluation of lung function is more readily accomplished. The PaO_2/PAO_2 has also been shown to parallel disease severity and shunt fraction in neonatal respiratory distress syndrome patients.[263] Similarly, PaO_2/PAO_2 can be used to compare oxygen-loading efficiency in patients on different FIO_2 levels. The findings may have potential research application.

Guide to Oxygen Therapy

Under certain clinical conditions (see the following section on *stability*), the PaO_2/PAO_2 may also be useful to the clinician as a guide for selecting appropriate oxygen therapy. However, this method of selecting oxygen therapy is only accurate in the patient with unchanging cardiopulmonary status.

When PaO_2/PAO_2 is calculated for a given patient at a given FIO_2, the PaO_2 that will result from a change in FIO_2 can be reasonably approximated. Similarly, the FIO_2 required to achieve a specific target PaO_2 can also be calculated if the initial PaO_2/PAO_2 is known. In one study, a nomogram based on the PaO_2/PAO_2 was shown to be quite accurate in predicting the required FIO_2 level to achieve a desired PaO_2.[264]

Normal Values

The *lower limit of normal* for PaO_2/PAO_2 appears to be 0.75.[261,265] In other words, 75% of the oxygen partial pressure that is delivered to the alveoli normally reaches the arterial blood. Obviously, a low percentage (e.g., 0.30) indicates poor oxygen transfer and increased physiologic shunting. Generally, the lower the percentage, the greater the shunt. It must always be remembered, however, that these simplified indices of shunting do *not* take into account changes in cardiac output and may be misleading in the patient with cardiovascular instability.

Stability

As the FIO_2 is changed, the PaO_2/PAO_2 shows the most stability when the FIO_2 is greater than 0.3 and when the PaO_2 is less than 100 mm Hg.[262] Therefore, the ratio is most accurate for predicting PaO_2 for a given FIO_2 when values before and after the change fall within this range. The ratio also seems to be particularly constant in patients with fairly substantial shunts (i.e., those patients with ratios <0.55).[261,265] Interestingly, a large relative shunt component (many low but finite $\dot{V}/\dot{Q}$) seems to diminish stability and is associated with an abrupt increase in the ratio at some point as the FIO_2 increases.[262] The precise FIO_2 level at which this spike occurs is unpredictable; however, the more severe the ventilation/perfusion mismatch, the closer this FIO_2 level is to 1.0.[262]

The PaO_2/FIO_2

The PaO_2/FIO_2, which is a simplified version of the PaO_2/PAO_2, has been used by many clinicians as an index of pulmonary oxygen exchange efficiency.[266-268] This index is easier to calculate because changes in arterial $PaCO_2$ are disregarded and the clinical alveolar air equation is not needed. Because normal PaO_2 on room air (≈ 0.2 FIO_2) in adults is 80 to 100 mm Hg, it follows that the normal PaO_2/FIO_2 is approximately 400 to 500 mm Hg.

Oxygenation Ratio

In 1972, Lecky and Ominsky reported the denominator of the PaO_2/FIO_2 ratio as a percentage (i.e., $PaO_2/\%FIO_2$) and called this *the oxygenation ratio*.[269] Using percentage in the denominator, the normal range for the oxygenation ratio is simply 4.0 to 5.0. These workers concluded that this index was the most simple, understandable, and useful method for training a novice to relate arterial to inspired oxygen levels and to interpret this relationship.[269]

Index of Shunting

The PaO_2/FIO_2 and oxygenation ratio have been criticized because they do not always reflect changes in shunting.[270,271] However, in critically ill patients with compromised cardiovascular status, none of the shunt indices except the actual shunt measurement should be expected to parallel closely the actual shunting. Any index

of shunting that fails to account for cardiac output and venous blood gas values is inherently inaccurate.[253,272] When a precise measure of shunting is indicated, the physiologic shunt should be measured.

Surprisingly, several studies have suggested that the PaO_2/FIO_2 is actually more accurate than the PaO_2/PAO_2 as an index of pulmonary shunting.[247,248,273] A PaO_2/FIO_2 less than 200 most often indicates a shunt greater than 20%.[247,270,272] Furthermore, a low PaO_2/FIO_2 ratio on a relatively high FIO_2 (e.g., PaO_2/FIO_2 of 60 at FIO_2 of 0.6) is clear evidence of a poor response to oxygen therapy and the presence of absolute shunting.

$PaCO_2$ Changes

A notable limitation of the PaO_2/FIO_2 is that it does not take into account changes in $PaCO_2$. For example, if a patient's PaO_2 fell to 60 mm Hg due to hypoventilation (e.g., $PaCO_2 = 80$ mm Hg) while breathing room air, the oxygenation ratio would decrease from a normal value of 5.0 to approximately 3.0. This oxygenation ratio implies that the intrinsic ability of the lungs to transfer oxygen is impaired. In fact, physiologic shunting is normal; the hypoxemia is solely the result of hypoventilation.

Therefore, the oxygenation ratio should not be used as an index of physiologic shunting with low FIO_2 levels (e.g., <0.3). At low FIO_2 levels, changes in $PaCO_2$ tend to have a considerable effect on the ratio. On the other hand, in many clinical situations, and particularly in patients receiving mechanical ventilation, the $PaCO_2$ does not usually change substantially between blood gases,[274,275] and the oxygenation ratio is a useful gross indicator of pulmonary oxygenation efficiency.

The entire issue regarding the effects of changes in $PaCO_2$ is further clouded because changes in $PaCO_2$ directly influence cardiac output and PaO_2.[276] Decreases in $PaCO_2$ levels have been shown to significantly decrease cardiac output.[277,278] Thus, changes in $PaCO_2$ should be expected to alter oxygen-loading efficiency. Because of the complex nature of these interactions, high levels of precision in these clinical indices are difficult, if not impossible, to obtain.

Summary

The search continues for a noninvasive index of true venous admixture. However, one may not exist.
                                W. M. Granger[253]

The ideal method to assess the physiologic shunt is to measure the necessary values and calculate it. Mixed venous blood is essential to make these calculations; therefore, blood must be sampled via a pulmonary artery catheter. The second best method to assess pulmonary shunting is calculation of an estimated shunt, based on an assumed arteriovenous oxygen content difference.

All shunt calculations are rather cumbersome; however, a pocket computer can be programmed for easy calculation. When shunt calculations are unavailable, other indices of pulmonary oxygenation efficiency, based on arterial PO_2 and alveolar PO_2, are often used. All of these indices may be somewhat inaccurate because PaO_2, PAO_2, and FIO_2 values have similarly questionable precision.

The PaO_2 is the least accurate of blood gas measurements, and the oxygen electrode may be especially inaccurate at high PaO_2.[279] Similarly, the level of FIO_2 that a given patient is presumed to be receiving is often very different from the level that actual measurements have indicated.[280,281] Finally, it has been shown that precise calculation of PAO_2 is virtually impossible, given the assumptions and inaccuracies implicit in the clinical alveolar air equation.

Despite these limitations, these indices are often useful as gross indicators of the efficiency of pulmonary oxygen uptake. Using these indices, impairment of pulmonary gas exchange can be tracked, and may provide crude guidelines to appropriate oxygen therapy.

DIFFERENTIAL DIAGNOSIS OF HYPOXEMIA

In the presence of clinical hypoxemia or increased physiologic shunting, the pathologic mechanism in gas exchange should be sought. Ultimately, the primary disease process or mechanism should be identified, and a comprehensive care plan should be formulated. Until this comprehensive treatment plan can completely correct the problem, *supportive therapy* must be provided to ensure adequate oxygen delivery to the tissues at minimum energy expense.

Although it is desirable to try to isolate a single mechanism responsible for hypoxemia in a given patient, this is often not possible. Frequently, hypoxemia is due to a combination of the four mechanisms shown in Box 9-1. For example, the patient with pneumonia typically has both true and relative shunting. In fact, it is unlikely that absolute capillary shunting is ever present without some degree of relative shunting. Nonetheless, it is beneficial to determine the *major* mechanism causing hypoxemia because treatment that is focused on the primary problem is more likely to be effective.

In approaching the differential diagnosis of hypoxemia, each of the potential hypoxemic mechanisms shown in Box 9-1 should be respectively considered. Clinical evidence should then be sought to support or rule out the presence of that mechanism.

Hypoventilation

Evaluation

Alveolar hypoventilation while breathing room air leads to hypoxemia as carbon dioxide replaces oxygen in the alveoli. This mechanism should be evaluated first because its presence or absence can be determined quickly and accurately via $PaCO_2$ assessment. Alveolar hypoventilation is easily recognized as an arterial PCO_2 higher than normal (i.e., $PaCO_2 > 45$ mm Hg). When hypoventilation is observed in an individual with hypoxemia, the hypoventilation is responsible, at least in part, for the hypoxemia.

Hypoventilation with Increased Shunting

In disease states, other hypoxemic mechanisms commonly accompany hypoventilation. Calculation of the alveolar-arterial oxygen tension gradient ($P[A-a]O_2$) while the patient is breathing room air is a useful tool for determining if the hypoxemia is due to hypoventilation alone or to hypoventilation in combination with increased physiologic shunting.[283-285]

In individuals younger than 60 years of age, a $P(A-a)O_2$ less than 20 mm Hg while breathing room air is indicative of relatively normal oxygen uptake by the lungs. Conversely, a $P(A-a)O_2$ in excess of 20 mm Hg is abnormal and suggests increased physiologic shunting. Some authors consider 10 to 15 mm Hg to be a normal range for $P(A-a)O_2$ while breathing room air.[286] A normal gradient of up to 20 mm Hg is used here because this includes approximately 2 standard deviations from the mean of the adult population.[287]

Hypoventilation Secondary to Hemodialysis

Somewhat surprisingly, hemodialysis has been associated with the development of hypoventilation and hypoxemia. Apparently, the dialysis acts like a second set of lungs in that carbon dioxide is excreted. The pseudo-hypoventilation that ensues reduces ventilation to the actual lungs with resultant hypoxemia although actual $PaCO_2$ remains normal.[290]

Absolute Shunting

Blood passing from the right side to the left side of the heart without being exposed to alveolar oxygen constitutes an absolute shunt. Absolute, or true, shunts may be anatomic or capillary in nature (see Chapter 6). *Absolute shunting responds poorly to administration of supplemental oxygen, because the oxygen does not come in contact with the shunted blood.*

Capillary Shunting

Absolute capillary shunting results from *alveolar consolidation* (filling with fluid) or *collapse*. Alveolar consolidation appears as a "white-out" on the chest radiograph. Conditions known to be associated with absolute capillary shunting should alert the clinician to its likelihood. These include acute respiratory distress syndrome, left-sided heart failure, pneumonia, and atelectasis. Pulmonary edema, whether cardiogenic (left-sided heart failure) or noncardiogenic, is probably the single greatest cause of severe, absolute capillary shunting in critical care units.

Anatomic Shunting

Congenital cardiovascular anomalies are often accompanied by increased anatomic shunting. Similarly, newborn infants with persistent fetal circulation also have anatomic shunts. Generally, pulmonary intervention is ineffective in the treatment of these problems. In the case of persistent fetal circulation, however, decreasing the pulmonary vascular resistance

may result in profound improvement in arterial oxygenation. Substantial anatomic shunting often requires surgical intervention.

The 100% O₂ Test

The 100% O_2 test, which compares the $P(A-a)O_2$ of an individual breathing room air with the $P(A-a)O_2$ on FIO_2 of 1.0, is useful in differentiating true capillary shunting from relative capillary shunting.[262] Both absolute and relative capillary shunting will show an increased $P(A-a)O_2$ on room air; however, when FIO_2 1.0 is administered for approximately 20 minutes, the $P(A-a)O_2$ remains abnormal only if absolute shunting is present.

Hypoxemia due to relative capillary shunting is caused by an inadequate oxygen supply in the poorly ventilated alveoli (i.e., low $\dot{V}/\dot{Q}$). Administration of FIO_2 of 1.0 provides sufficient oxygen to all alveoli regardless of the actual volume of ventilation. Thus, FIO_2 of 1.0 totally corrects hypoxemia due to relative capillary shunting.

The normal $P(A-a)O_2$ at FIO_2 of 1.0 is less than 50 mm Hg. Therefore, at FIO_2 of 1.0, a $P(A-a)O_2$ greater than 50 mm Hg indicates the presence of absolute shunting; conversely, when it is less than 50 mm Hg, there is no abnormal *absolute* shunt component. In this case, shunting observed on room air must be due to the *relative* shunt effect.

Actual performance of the 100% O_2 test is presently rarely done because it has been shown that breathing FIO_2 of 1.0 leads in itself to absorption atelectasis and to increased true capillary shunting.[288] The absolute shunt measured in normal individuals may even exceed 10% after breathing FIO_2 of 1.0. This shunt inducing effect is undesirable, particularly in patients already compromised by increased physiologic shunting.

Nevertheless, the basic theory underlying the 100% O_2 test may be clinically useful. That is, the general degree of PaO_2 responsiveness to oxygen therapy may help to differentiate true from relative shunting.[286] A substantial increase in PaO_2 after elevation of FIO_2 suggests relative shunting, whereas a poor response to oxygen therapy is typical of absolute shunting.

Relative Shunting

Relative shunting is often referred to as *ventilation-perfusion mismatch* or simply perfusion in excess of ventilation. Hypoxemia is observed on room air when a substantial quantity of pulmonary perfusion is to areas with below-normal V̇/Q̇. In contrast to absolute shunting, relative shunting is characterized by a good PaO_2 response to small increments of oxygen therapy.

Relative shunting in the clinic is most often the result of uneven distribution of ventilation secondary to increased pulmonary secretions. It represents the major hypoxemic mechanism in uncomplicated chronic obstructive pulmonary disease. A relatively abrupt onset of relative shunting and increased hypoxemia often accompanies hemodialysis (see discussion under hypoventilation) or the administration of bronchodilators (e.g., albuterol, levalbuterol, salmeterol, isoproterenol) or nitrates (e.g., nitroprusside, nitroglycerin).[289]

Increased relative shunting and hypoxemia may also be seen in patients with chronic liver disease or cirrhosis.[291] The hypoxemia of liver disease appears to be due to ascites, which may alter the distribution of ventilation, and abnormalities in pulmonary perfusion.[291,292] Overall, relative shunting is, in all likelihood, the most common clinical hypoxemic mechanism and is probably evident to some degree in all patients who manifest hypoxemia.

Diffusion Defects

A *diffusion defect* is a structural impedance to oxygen transfer in the lungs, due to a thickened alveolar-capillary membrane. However, it is unlikely that diffusion defects alone result in hypoxemia at sea level in humans with normal cardiac output. Most of the hypoxemia at rest observed in patients with diffusion defects is believed to be mainly a result of concurrent relative shunting.[288] These patients may, however, manifest hypoxemia during exercise, which may facilitate the diagnosis.

In any event, hypoxemia associated with diffusion defects responds to oxygen therapy. Thus, regarding supportive treatment, it is reasonable to include these patients under the category of relative shunting.

Effects of Altitude and Air Travel in Hypoxemia

As previously described, the partial pressure of inspired oxygen will decrease as altitude increases. Likewise, the partial pressure of arterial oxygen will decrease in a corresponding manner with increasing altitude.

Not surprisingly, the converse is also true; that is, PaO_2 will tend to increase as one descends below sea level (760 mm Hg). Indeed, individuals

---

ON CALL | CASE 9-2 *ABGs and Critical Thinking*

You are the only person available to care for this patient. You must assess the patient/situation and act accordingly.

A 28-year-old woman is admitted semi-comatose due to a drug overdose and possible aspiration.

ARTERIAL BLOOD GASES

SaO_2	86%
pH	7.22
$PaCO_2$	50 mm Hg
PaO_2	62 mm Hg
$[HCO_3]$	20 mEq/L
FIO_2	room air

ASSESSMENT

Abnormalities: List abnormal data and other noteworthy information. Classify ABG.

Explanation: List possible diseases, pathology, or other situations that may have led to this patient's condition.

Evaluation: Suggest additional data that would be useful in helping understand the situation or in making a diagnosis.

INTERVENTION

Importance: Prioritize concern(s) of treatment in order of urgency and/or seriousness as you see the overall situation.

with end-stage lung disease manifested an increase in PaO_2, increased exercise capability, and felt better subjectively after descent to a barometric pressure of 798 mm Hg at the Dead Sea, the lowest altitude on earth.[293]

Because air travel occurs at a high altitude, airplane cabins are pressurized to equate to an altitude of approximately 5000 ft. In some cases, cabin pressures may equate to even higher altitudes but the Federal Aviation Administration requires equilibration to no higher than 8000-ft altitude.[695] At 8000 ft, even healthy people will likely have PaO_2s less than 60 mm Hg and SaO_2s less than 90%. Roughly, one can expect a PaO_2 decrease of approximately 4 mm Hg per 1000-ft increase in elevation.[695]

The decrease in PaO_2 associated with air travel is of particular concern to the individual with chronic lung disease, decreased ventilatory reserve, and chronic hypoxemia. Therefore, oxygen supplementation should be administered in these individuals especially if the PaO_2 is expected to fall below 50 mm Hg.[295,296]

Summary

Methods for differentiation of the four mechanisms of hypoxemia have been discussed. Application of $P(A-a)O_2$ in making the differential diagnosis has also been presented. The role of $P(A-a)O_2$ in the differential diagnosis of hypoxemia is summarized in Table 9-1. Limitations of the $P(A-a)O_2$ have also been discussed. The purpose of the differential diagnosis

is to enhance our understanding of the pathologic mechanisms that predominate in a given patient, which, in turn, should assist us in the development of a sound therapeutic plan.

CLINICAL APPEARANCE OF THE PATIENT WITH HYPOXEMIA/HYPERCAPNIA

The clinical appearance of the patient may be the first clue with regard to the onset or worsening of hypoxemia or hypercapnia. Some of the most important signs and symptoms commonly associated with hypoxemia or hypercapnia are shown in Box 9-3. The body will typically respond to hypoxemia with increased cardiac output in a dose-response manner,[301] but cardiac output may sometimes decrease with severe hypoxemia.

Sometimes the hypoxemic patient is relatively asymptomatic, and hypoxemia can only be determined by blood gas analysis or pulse oximetry. In the acute emergency, the patient's airway, respiratory, and circulatory status must be quickly evaluated and, if necessary, corrective action should be undertaken.

HYPEROXEMIA

Not only hypoxemia but also *hyperoxemia* (an excessive amount of oxygen in the blood) is undesirable. When the PaO_2 exceeds 100 mm Hg, very little benefit is accrued in terms

Table 9-1. DIFFERENTIAL DIAGNOSIS OF HYPOXEMIA

Abnormality	Arterial PO₂	Arterial PCO₂	Alveolar-Arterial PO₂ Difference	
			Room Air	*100% O₂*
Hypoventilation	Decreased	Increased	Normal	Normal
Absolute shunt	Decreased	Normal or decreased*	Increased	Increased
Relative shunt	Decreased	Normal, increased, or decreased*	Increased	Normal
Diffusion defect	Normal at rest Decreased during exercise	Normal or decreased*	Normal at rest Increased during exercise	Normal

*Attributable to hyperventilation from secondary causes.
From Hinshaw, H.C., Murray, J. F.: Diseases of the Chest, 4th ed. Philadelphia, W. B. Saunders, 1980, p. 960.

| **Box** 9-3 | Signs and Symptoms of Hypoxemia and Hypercapnia |

Hypoxemia
    Muscular incoordination
    Confusion
    Loss of judgment
    Extreme restlessness, combative behavior
    Tachycardia
    Mild hypertension
    Peripheral vasoconstriction
    Cyanosis
    Bradycardia*
    Bradyarrhythmias*
    Hypotension*
Hypercapnia
    Progressive somnolence
    Disorientation
    Mucosal, scleral, conjunctival hyperemia
    Diaphoresis
    Tachycardia
    Hypertension

*Associated with severe hypoxemia.
From Glauser F. L., Polatty R.C., and Sessler C.N.: Worsening oxygenation in the mechanically ventilated patient. Am. Rev. Resp. Dis., 138:458–465, 1988.

of additional blood oxygen content, whereas the risk of complications increases.

Excluding mild elevations of PaO_2 (up to a maximum of about 130 mm Hg),[81] hyperoxemia is always the result of excessive FIO_2. Occasionally unexpectedly high PaO_2 levels may provide the first clue of erroneous laboratory data or technical error.

In certain cases in which the patient is believed to be hypoxic from nonpulmonary factors, hyperoxemia may be used therapeutically. For example, tissue oxygenation may improve slightly when there is severe anemia or cardiovascular failure. Hyperoxemia is particularly valuable in the treatment of carboxyhemoglobinemia (carbon monoxide poisoning) because it accelerates the destruction of the pathologic carboxyhemoglobin.

In general, the clinician should realize that the gain in blood oxygen content with hyperoxemia is only modest and that this measure is only a stopgap to mitigate the impact of severe hypoxia in the short term. Ultimately, therapy must address the actual cause of the hypoxia.

EXERCISES

Exercise 9-1   Hypoxemia and the Role of Cardiac Output

Fill in the blanks or select the best answer.

1. The PaO_2 is a measure of oxygen-loading (adequacy/efficiency) in the lungs, whereas the $P(A-a)O_2$ is a measure of oxygen-loading (adequacy/efficiency).

2. State the four mechanisms of hypoxemia usually observed in the hospital setting.

3. (Relative shunting/absolute shunting) is commonly referred to as $\dot{V}/\dot{Q}$ mismatch.

4. Venous blood (sometimes/always) mixes with oxygenated blood to form arterial blood.

5. In the patient with a normal shunt, changes in cardiac output will have (no/minimal/substantial) effects on PaO_2.

6. The PaO_2 is always slightly (higher/lower) than the average $P\acute{c}O_2$ from well-oxygenated alveolar-capillary units.

7. A decrease in cardiac output is associated typically with a (rise/fall) in $P\bar{v}O_2$.

8. In a patient with normal cardiac output and a substantial shunt, PaO_2 decreases because of (low $P\bar{v}O_2$/a large percentage of venous blood entering the arteries).

9. When PaO_2 decreases from 55 to 45 mm Hg in a patient with a previously measured $\dot{Q}sp/\dot{Q}T$ of 30%, it (can/cannot) be presumed that shunting has increased.

10. Cardiac output affects PaO_2 levels most in the individual with (normal/increased) physiologic shunting.

Exercise 9-2 Alveolar-Arterial O₂ Gradients

Fill in the blanks or select the best answer.

1. The symbol for the alveolar-arterial oxygen tension gradient is _____.

2. The mean normal $P(A-a)O_2$ in adults breathing room air is approximately _____ mm Hg, and the upper limit of normal is _____ mm Hg.

3. The $P(A-a)O_2$ reflects primarily (ventilation-perfusion mismatch/cardiac output).

4. The PAO_2 calculated in the alveolar air equation represents the (actual/mean) PAO_2 in all alveoli.

5. Write the clinical form of the alveolar air equation that should be used when FIO_2 is less than or equal to 0.60.

6. Write the formula for calculation of PIO_2.

7. Normal maximum $P(A-a)O_2$ while breathing FIO_2 of 1.0 in adults is _____ mm Hg.

8. Administration of 100% O_2 may lead to increased true shunting through the development of _____.

9. The $P(A-a)O_2$ (increases/decreases/does not change) with advancing age.

10. Write the clinical form of the alveolar air equation that should be used to calculate PAO_2 when FIO_2 is greater than 0.6.

Exercise 9-3 Oxygenation Ratios

Fill in the blanks or select the best answer.

1. The PaO_2/PAO_2 is (more/less) stable than the $P(A-a)O_2$ at varying FIO_2 levels.

2. The lower limit of normal for PaO_2/PAO_2 in adults is a value of _____.

3. The PaO_2/PAO_2 is most stable in critically ill patients when FIO_2 is in the range of _____ to _____.

4. The PaO_2/PAO_2 is most stable in critically ill patients when the PaO_2 is less than _____ mm Hg.

5. The normal PaO_2/FIO_2 is a value greater than _____.

6. The $PaO_2/\%FIO_2$ is called the _____ ratio.

7. A PaO_2/FIO_2 of 200 is equivalent to an oxygenation ratio of _____.

8. The PaO_2/FIO_2 (does/does not) account for changes in $PaCO_2$.

9. The (PaO_2/PAO_2 or $P[A-a]O_2$) may be useful to the clinician as a guide for selecting appropriate oxygen therapy.

10. Changes in $PaCO_2$ (do/do not) influence cardiac output and PaO_2.

Exercise 9-4   Indices of Physiologic Shunting

Fill in the blanks or select the best answer.

1. The classic shunt equation (corrects/does not correct) for any nonpulmonary (e.g., $P\bar{v}O_2$) mediated effects on arterial oxygenation.

2. Calculation of $\dot{Q}sp/\dot{Q}T$ via the (classic/estimated) shunt equation is the only accurate measurement of physiologic shunting when cardiac output is unstable.

3. The most notable deterrent to routine measurement of the physiologic shunt is the requirement for (arterial oxygen content/mixed venous blood).

4. The $\dot{Q}sp/\dot{Q}T$, as calculated through the classic shunt equation, is the measurement of choice whenever a/an (arterial catheter/pulmonary artery catheter) is in place.

5. Estimated shunt equations assume a given _____ in their calculations.

6. The gold standard in evaluation of shunting is the measurement of the ($\dot{Q}sp/\dot{Q}T$ or $P[A-a]O_2$).

7. The best index to use to differentiate simple hypoventilation from hypoventilation with increased physiologic shunting is the _____ with the patient breathing room air.

8. The oxygenation index used in the 100% O_2 test is the _____ with FIO_2 of 1.0.

9. The simplest oxygenation index to use that does not require calculation of the alveolar PO_2 is the _____.

10. A PaO_2/FIO_2 of less than 200 almost always indicates a shunt greater than _____%.

Differential Diagnosis of Hypoxemia and Effects of Altitude on Hypoxemia

Fill in the blanks or select the best answer.

1. In most clinical situations, (a single mechanism is/multiple mechanisms are) responsible for a given decrease in PaO_2.

2. The first mechanism to rule out in the presence of hypoxemia is (absolute shunting/hypoventilation).

3. Absolute shunting is characterized by a (poor/good) response to oxygen therapy.

4. Absolute shunting is characterized by a (white-out/darkening) of the chest radiograph.

5. Pulmonary (embolus/edema) is probably the single most common cause of severe absolute shunting in critical care units.

6. It is wise to suspect (diffusion defect/decreased cardiac output) when there is abrupt onset of hypoxemia in a critically ill patient with apparently stable lungs.

7. State the two potential causes of hyperoxemia.

8. The (relative/absolute) shunt phenomenon is commonly referred to as V̇/Q̇ mismatch.

9. The maximum PaO_2 attainable on room air is approximately (130/150) mm Hg.

10. Name two general groups of drugs that have been associated with the onset of relative shunting after their administration.

11. A form of pseudo-hypoventilation may occur in the patient with (hemodialysis/nitrate therapy).

12. Hypoxemia is often seen in conjunction with chronic (renal/liver) failure.

13. PaO_2 will tend to (increase/decrease) at the Dead Sea.

14. Airplane cabins tend to be pressurized equivalent to approximately (5000/12,000) feet.

15. PaO_2 will typically decrease approximately _____ mm Hg per 1000-ft. elevation.

Exercise 9-6 The P(A−a)O₂ in Differential Diagnosis

Determine whether the hypoxemia in the following cases (1 to 5) is due to simple hypoventilation or hypoventilation with increased physiologic shunting. All blood gases were drawn at FIO₂ of 0.21.

Case	PaO_2 (mm Hg)	$PaCO_2$ (mm Hg)
1.	40	60
2.	62	50
3.	68	60
4.	40	80
5.	59	55

Assuming an abnormal P(A−a)O₂ on room air and given the P(A−a)O₂ at FIO₂ of 1.0, determine whether the primary hypoxemic mechanism is true or relative shunting.

Case	$P(A-a)O_2$ (mm Hg)
6.	360
7.	47
8.	240
9.	30
10.	90

Exercise 9-7 Internet Work

1. Search the web by entering arterial-alveolar oxygen gradient. List two sources that provide useful information or examples and critique them.

NBRC Challenge 9

Please select the best answer for the following multiple-choice questions.

1. A 45-year-old patient has a $P(A-a)O_2$ of 35 on room air. This value is consistent with a diagnosis of:
   A) deadspace disease.
   B) pneumonia.
   C) low cardiac output.
   D) high cardiac output.
   E) acute renal failure.
   (CRT EXAMINATION — NBRC
   MATRIX I,B,10,c)

2. A patient has an increased $PaCO_2$, a normal $P(A-a)O_2$, and hypoxemia. The hypoxemia is due to:
   A) hypoventilation.
   B) V/Q mismatch.
   C) absolute shunting.
   D) diffusion defect.
   E) high altitude exposure.
   (CRT EXAMINATION — NBRC
   MATRIX I,C,2,c)

3. A patient with a pulmonary shunt fraction of 30% has a sudden decrease in $P\bar{v}O_2$. This will result in a decrease in:
   A) physiologic deadspace.
   B) physiologic shunting.
   C) potassium.

   D) PaO_2.
   E) tidal volume.
   (RRT EXAMINATION — NBRC
   MATRIX I,C,2,c)

4. A patient with a normal physiologic shunt has a sudden decrease in cardiac output. One would expect PaO_2 to:
   A) increase sharply.
   B) increase slightly.
   C) increase substantially over the next few hours.
   D) decrease sharply.
   E) decrease very slightly or not at all.
   (RRT EXAMINATION — NBRC
   MATRIX I,B,9,c)

5. If the PaO_2/PAO_2 decreased, $P(A-a)O_2$ would _____ and $\dot{Q}sp/\dot{Q}T$ would _____.
   A) increase, increase
   B) increase, decrease
   C) decrease, increase
   D) decrease, decrease
   E) decrease, not change
   (RRT EXAMINATION — NBRC
   MATRIX III,A,1,m,1)

10

Treatment of Hypoxemia and Shunting

I believe the frequent forceful encouragement to cough and raise sputum supplemented by a degree of bullying and buffeting is often more relevant than all the paraphernalia of O_2 masks, intubation, ventilators, and blood gas measurements put together.

E. J. Campbell[297]

Outline

TREATMENT

There are two primary objectives in the treatment of hypoxemia (i.e., decreased PaO_2) and increased pulmonary shunting. Foremost is the maintenance of an *adequate* PaO_2 to prevent hypoxia (decreased cellular oxygenation). When the presence of hypoxia is likely, such as in severe hypoxemia, this objective requires immediate attention. The maintenance of adequate oxygenation is considered to be supportive,

or *palliative*, treatment. Supportive treatment does not aim to correct the underlying problem; rather, its aim is to support the patient until correction of the underlying problem can take place.

Equally important, albeit less urgent, is the reversal or correction of the underlying defect. Thus, the initial priority is to ensure an adequate PaO_2 and to prevent tissue hypoxia. The long-term focus is correction or control of the basic pathologic insults.

Acute Hypoxemia

The management and control of acute hypoxemia and chronic hypoxemia are different. Obviously, the goals and objectives of oxygen therapy in the chronic patient are less urgent and focused more on the long term. The management of acute hypoxemia certainly has a more emergent focus and will be discussed first.

As stated previously, the prevention of tissue hypoxia is foremost. A precise PaO_2 that will result in hypoxia in all individuals cannot be identified, because various factors (e.g., hemoglobin concentration, oxyhemoglobin affinity, cardiac output) interrelate in a complex manner to deliver oxygen to the tissues. Nevertheless, it is prudent to make a few clinical assumptions based solely on the PaO_2.

Tissue hypoxia is likely in the presence of *severe hypoxemia* (i.e., PaO_2 <45 mm Hg). Therefore, severe hypoxemia must be corrected immediately. *Moderate hypoxemia* (PaO_2 45 to 59 mm Hg) may be associated with hypoxia if the cardiovascular system is unable to compensate. Thus, the likelihood of hypoxia in conjunction with moderate hypoxemia depends primarily on the integrity of the cardiovascular system.

In clinical practice, moderate hypoxemia is usually corrected, which minimizes the compensatory stress placed on the cardiovascular system and ensures that hypoxia does not occur. Although *mild hypoxemia* (PaO_2 60 to 79 mm Hg) is generally not associated with hypoxia, oxygen therapy may be used to minimize the strain on the cardiopulmonary system and to make the patient more comfortable. Notwithstanding, liberal use of oxygen therapy has recently been challenged.[696] It has been purported that oxygen administration may delay application of appropriate respiratory care.[696]

The types of palliative therapy commonly used for acute PaO_2 support are shown in Box 10-1. The most appropriate measures for a particular patient depend on the specific nature of the oxygen-loading problem. For example, when hypoxemia results from severe hypoventilation, mechanical ventilation will likely be necessary. On the other hand, when the hypoxemic mechanism is predominantly relative shunting, oxygen therapy may be all that is needed.

Box 10-1   Options for Treatment of Hypoxemia
Oxygen therapy
Mechanical ventilation
PEEP/CPAP
Alveolar recruitment maneuvers
Body positioning
Nitric oxide

Finally, with substantial absolute capillary shunting, therapy with positive end-expiratory pressure or continuous positive airway pressure (PEEP/CPAP) and/or alveolar recruitment maneuvers will probably be necessary.

Frequently, a combination of these therapies is administered to a given patient. This is simply because most cases of hypoxemia will have more than one mechanism. The optimal supportive plan for each patient must be individualized, based on the pulmonary pathology present and a thorough understanding of the value and role of each supportive modality.

OXYGEN THERAPY

Mechanism of Effectiveness

Relative Shunting

The effectiveness of oxygen therapy in relieving hypoxemia depends primarily on the nature of the mechanism responsible for the hypoxemia in the first place. For example, oxygen therapy is very effective in reversing the hypoxemia caused by relative shunting. As illustrated in Figure 10-1, relative shunts are alveolar-capillary units that have low but finite ventilation-perfusion ratios. The gas exchange problem in these units is that the quantity of oxygen available is insufficient (i.e., decreased partial pressure of alveolar oxygen [PAO_2]) to oxygenate completely the volume of blood perfusing them.

The effectiveness of oxygen therapy is related to its effects on alveolar-capillary units with low V/Q ratios. Administration of oxygen increases the alveolar oxygen supply and partial pressure in these units (see Fig. 10-1). It should be understood that the administration of oxygen does not change the ventilation-perfusion ratio or improve lung function. Nevertheless, despite low ventilation with respect to perfusion, alveolar oxygen delivery and PaO_2 are increased.

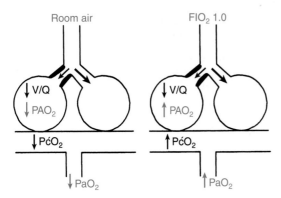

Figure 10-1.   **Response of relative shunting to O_2 therapy.** O_2 therapy increases the PAO_2 of the alveolar-capillary units with low $\dot{V}/\dot{Q}$ and thus corrects this form of hypoxemia.

Diffusion Defects

Oxygen therapy is also effective in the presence of diffusion defects. The increased PAO_2 associated with oxygen therapy increases the driving pressure of oxygen across the alveolar-capillary membrane and thereby speeds up equilibration. Pulmonary diffusion is discussed in detail in Chapter 6.

Hypoventilation

Oxygen therapy corrects the hypoxemia associated with hypoventilation by replenishing the alveolar oxygen supply. Oxygen therapy alone in the treatment of hypoventilation, however, is inadequate, because it does not correct the hypercarbia and acidemia that are also present.

Absolute Shunting

Oxygen therapy is generally ineffective in relieving hypoxemia resulting from true capillary shunting. This finding should not be surprising, because the increased partial pressure of inhaled oxygen (PIO_2) associated with oxygen therapy never reaches blood that is perfusing consolidated or collapsed alveoli. Despite its relative ineffectiveness, however, oxygen therapy is administered to all patients with hypoxemia, because there is probably some relative shunt component in *all* hypoxemia and oxygen therapy is likely too add some additional volume of oxygen to the blood.

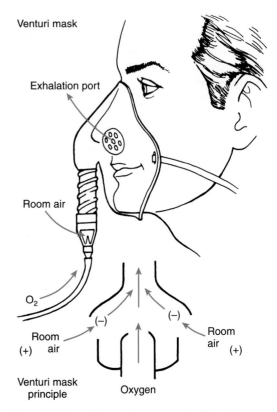

Figure 10-2.   **Air-entrainment mask.** The air-entrainment mask is a high-flow oxygen administration system that makes use of the Venturi principle.

Oxygen Administration Devices

There are two general types of oxygen administration devices: low-flow systems and high-flow systems.

High-Flow Systems

High-flow systems, sometimes referred to as fixed performance systems, are defined as oxygen administration devices that provide gas flow rates that are high enough to *completely* satisfy the patient's inspiratory demand.[298] Ventilators and low fraction of inspired oxygen (FIO_2) air-entrainment masks (Fig. 10-2) are examples of high-flow systems. High-flow systems offer the advantage of delivering accurate, controlled levels of FIO_2. Furthermore, they often provide control of temperature and humidity of the inspired gas. A disadvantage of high-flow systems is that they are often noisy, bulky, and uncomfortable.

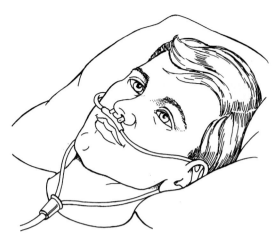

Figure 10-3. Nasal cannula. The nasal cannula is a low-flow system for delivering oxygen.

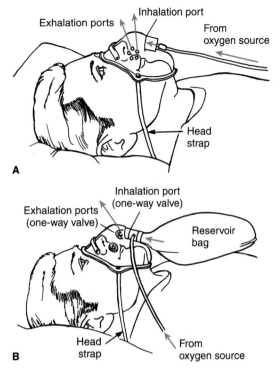

Figure 10-4. Types of oxygen masks.
A, A simple oxygen mask delivers an FIO$_2$ of approximately 0.5. **B,** Partial and rebreathing masks tend to provide an FIO$_2$ of approximately 0.40 to 0.70.

Low-Flow Systems

Low-flow systems, sometimes referred to as variable performance systems, supply oxygen at flow rates that are less than the patient's inspiratory flow demand. The specific level of FIO$_2$ delivered may be high or low. Examples include the nasal cannula (Fig. 10-3), the simple mask (Fig. 10-4,*A*), and partial and non-rebreathing masks. A non-rebreathing mask is shown in Figure 10-4,*B*. Advantages of low-flow systems include simplicity and patient tolerance. A disadvantage is that control of FIO$_2$ levels with low-flow systems is less precise, because levels may vary with changes in ventilatory pattern.

Low-flow systems that use reservoir bags (e.g., partial rebreathing masks and non-rebreathing masks) allow for some rebreathing of the first portion of exhaled gas and delivery of higher rates of FIO$_2$. With the partial rebreathing mask, the first one-third of exhaled gas is captured in the reservoir bag during expiration and is re-inhaled on the following breath. Because this gas is rich in oxygen, FIO$_2$ levels increase.

The approximate levels of FIO$_2$ that are delivered with a specific apparatus set on a given flow rate are shown in Table 10-1. One must remember, however, that these approximations apply only to individuals with a *normal* breathing pattern (e.g., tidal volume $\cong$ 500 mL, respiratory rate $\cong$ 12 breaths per minute). When a patient breathes more rapidly or deeper than

normal, the actual FIO$_2$ level delivered is less than that shown in Table 10-1. Conversely, with slow, shallow ventilation, FIO$_2$ levels may be much higher than those shown in Table 10-1.

Non-rebreathing masks that incorporate one-way valves to prevent inspiration of room air have been traditionally thought to provide a higher FIO$_2$ (i.e., 0.6 to 0.8) than partial rebreathing masks (i.e., 0.4 to 0.7).[302] There is some evidence to suggest only very minimal FIO$_2$ differences between these two types of masks under normal clinical circumstances.[303,698,699]

It is interesting to note that, as a variable system, FIO$_2$ delivered via a nasal cannula could theoretically increase from 0.44 at a tidal volume of 500 mL, to 0.68 if tidal volume fell to 250 mL.[10] Therefore, it must not be assumed that low flow rates of oxygen from devices such as nasal cannulas always deliver low FIO$_2$ levels. One must always keep in mind the effects of breathing pattern on FIO$_2$ when using

Table 10-1. APPROXIMATE FIO_2 LEVELS WITH LOW-FLOW DEVICES

Device	Flow (L/min)	FIO_2
Nasal Cannula	1	0.24
	2	0.28
	3	0.32
	4	0.36
	5	0.40
	6	0.44
Simple mask	6	0.40
	7	0.50
	8	0.60
Partial rebreathing mask	6–10	0.60

Adapted from Ziment, I.: Respiratory Pharmacology and Therapeutics. Philadelphia, W.B. Saunders, 1978.

low-flow oxygen administration systems. To further complicate matters, there is evidence to suggest that oxygen concentration may be higher during nasal breathing versus mouth breathing when using nasal cannulas,[315] although this finding is controversial.[302]

Despite the fact that high-flow systems are more accurate and that their use is advocated by some clinicians,[300] low-flow systems have more widespread use because of their simplicity and comfort.

Oxygen Therapy in the Spontaneously Breathing Patient

Since the early nineteenth century, when Thomas Beddoes opened the Pneumatic Institute of Bristol, oxygen therapy has played a vital role in healthcare. Without exception, oxygen therapy is the first-line clinical treatment for acute hypoxemia regardless of the mechanism or underlying cause. Immediate application of oxygen therapy is essential in the treatment of *severe hypoxemia* or when there is a high probability of *tissue hypoxia*.

Recommendations by the American Association for Respiratory Care[302] as well as the American College of Chest Physicians and the National Heart and Blood Institute state that oxygen therapy should be used when PaO_2 is less than 60 mm Hg or SaO_2 is less than 90%.[298] A summary of key recommendations for oxygen therapy in the acute care hospital are shown in Box 10-2. Box 10-3 outlines key

factors to consider when applying oxygen therapy in preterms and neonates.[302,304]

Goals in Oxygen Therapy

The traditional goals of oxygen therapy are to maintain an adequate PaO_2, to minimize cardiopulmonary work, and to prevent or alleviate hypoxia. Although PaO_2 has historically been the single most important parameter used to gauge the appropriateness of oxygen therapy, it should not be the sole criterion. Vital organ function, general clinical appearance of the patient, and indices of cardiovascular stress such as heart rate and arterial blood pressure must also be incorporated into decision making.

For example, oxygen therapy may be deemed beneficial if it is accompanied by an improving blood pressure or heart rate even if the PaO_2 failed to increase significantly. As stated by Campbell, "Oxygen therapy is too serious to be left to electrodes alone."[297] Evaluation of the need for oxygen must include an assessment of the entire cardiopulmonary system as well as complete hypoxic assessment as discussed in Chapter 11.

It is noteworthy that analysis of arterial blood gases is not always indicated simply because oxygen is being briefly administered. The cost of arterial blood analysis may outweigh its benefit, particularly in short-term therapy.[298] The price of one blood gas analysis may exceed the cost of 24 to 48 hours of oxygen therapy. In many cases, pulse oximetry can serve as a cost-effective alternative to arterial blood gas analysis for monitoring oxygen therapy.

Clinical Approach to Oxygen Therapy

The first step before the actual administration of oxygen is to classify each patient into one of two groups: oxygen-sensitive or non–oxygen-sensitive. This is important because the approach to therapy in each group is markedly different. Verification of the presence or absence of oxygen sensitivity can usually be accomplished through a physical examination and review of the patient's medical record.

Non–Oxygen-Sensitive Patients

In the absence of chronic obstructive pulmonary disease (COPD), chronic CO_2 retention, or acute

Box 10-2	AARC Clinical Practice Guideline—Oxygen Therapy in the Acute Care Hospital: Nuts & Bolts

INDICATIONS:	PaO$_2$ <60 mm Hg
	SpO$_2$ <90%
	Acute Potential for Hypoxia
	    Severe Trauma
	    M.I.
	    Postoperative Status

OBJECTIVE:	PaO$_2$ >60 mm Hg SpO$_2$ >90%

COMPLICATIONS:	Acute Hypercapina in COPD
	    PaO$_2$ > or = 60 mm Hg may cause
	Absorption altectasis
	Leukocyte/ciliary depression
	Oxygen toxicity
	    More vulnerable with
	    Paraquat poisoning or Bleomycin Rx
	    FIO$_2$ > or = 0.50 may cause

EQUIPMENT:	Nasal Cannula
	    Flows up to 6 LPM
	    Humidification unnecessary <4 LPM
	Simple Oxygen Mask
	    Flows 5–10 LPM
	    Always >5 LPM to prevent rebreathing
	Partial Rebreathing Mask
	    Flows 6–10 LPM
	    Always >5 LPM to prevent rebreathing
	Non-Rebreathing Mask
	    Flows 10–15 LPM
	Venti-Masks
	    Accurate FIO$_2$ at recommended flows
	    May not meet flow needs with >35% settings

MONITORING:	COPD <2 hrs FIO$_2$ >0.40 <8 hrs FIO$_2$ <0.40 <12 hrs Check system daily Acute M.I. <72 hrs

Reference: Oxygen therapy for adults in the acute care facility—2002 revision and update. AARC Clinical Practice Guideline. Respir. Care 47:717–720, 2002.

Box 10-3	AARC Clinical Practice Guidelines—Oxygen Therapy in Acute Setting Preterms/Neonates: Nuts & Bolts

INDICATIONS:	Hypoxemia
	Acute Potential for Hypoxia
OBJECTIVE:	PaO_2 50–80 mm Hg
	SpO_2 >88%
	Capillary O_2 >40 mm Hg
COMPLICATIONS:	Retinopathy of Prematurity
	Persistent Fetal Circulation
	Irregular breathing if cool flow on trigeminal
	Potential for tracheal ignition during laser bronchoscopy
EQUIPMENT:	Nasal Cannula
	Variable FIO_2 performance
	Humidification not necessary
	Maximum flow <2 LPM
	Use low increment flowmeters (0–200 mL/min)
	Flowrate increments <0.125 LPM
	Simple Oxygen Mask
	Variable FIO_2 performance
	Approximate FIO_2 = 0.35 – 0.50
	Primary use emergency transport
	Poorly tolerated by infants
	Interfere with feeding
	Oxygen hoods
	Fixed FIO_2 performance
	Set air entrainment devices to FIO_2 1.0
	Control FIO_2 with oxygen blenders
	Flow >7 LPM to wash out deadspace
	Maintain temperature to neutral thermal environment
	High flow may produce harmful noise exposure
	Non-isotonic in nebulizers may cause airway hyperactivity
	O_2 Administrative Devices to Avoid
	Incubators
	Primary purpose to control temperature
	High risk of infection if use incubator humidifier
	Partial Rebreathing Masks
	Non-Rebreathing Masks
	Naso-pharyngeal catheters
MONITORING:	Check all equipment at least daily

Reference: Selection of an Oxygen Delivery Device for Neonatal and Pediatric Patients—2002 Revision and Update. AARC Clinical Practice Guideline. Respir. Care, 47:707–716, 2002.

severe asthma,[700] oxygen therapy may be administered without concern for inducing hypoventilation. It has been said that "the brain softens before the lung hardens," in reference to the reluctance of clinicians to administer oxygen for fear of oxygen toxicity. Oxygen therapy must not be withheld in the case of a patient who may be hypoxic.

When PaO_2 falls below 55 mm Hg acutely, short-term memory is altered and euphoria or impaired judgment may be observed.[298] Therefore, in most clinical situations the PaO_2 should be targeted to 60 to 80 mm Hg.

Oxygen-Sensitive Patients

The approach to oxygen therapy in the patient with COPD, acute severe asthma,[700] or chronic hypercapnia is completely different. In these individuals, *caution* is the byword. Excessive oxygen therapy administered to these oxygen-sensitive patients could potentially have fatal consequences. Nevertheless, even in these patients, when hypoxia is suspected, oxygen therapy should never be withheld simply because the patient may be sensitive to oxygen. Correction of hypoxia is always the first priority.

Specifically, the first line of supportive treatment in acute exacerbation of COPD is low FIO_2 therapy. Typically, the patient with COPD in acute respiratory failure has blood gases approximating those shown in Example 10-1.[300]

Example 10-1

Typical Blood Gases during Acute Respiratory Failure in Patients with Chronic Obstructive Pulmonary Disease

pH	7.23–7.39
$PaCO_2$	60–80 mm Hg
PaO_2	~ 40 mm Hg

Despite $PaCO_2$ levels in excess of 60 to 65 mm Hg, many patients with COPD can be treated without mechanical ventilation.[306] In general, mechanical ventilation should not be initiated unless pH falls below 7.20[297,306] and after all else fails.[297,307] The decision to institute mechanical ventilation in COPD is always difficult and requires consideration of a host of variables.

A reasonable target PaO_2 in acute exacerbation of COPD is 60 mm Hg.[308] This level

guards against hypoxia and is unlikely to cause substantial hypercapnia and acidosis.

FIO₂ Selection

A useful guideline for FIO_2 selection in acute exacerbation of COPD is the fact that PaO_2 increases approximately 3 mm Hg for each 0.01 increase in FIO_2.[300,309] Thus, if a patient with COPD is seen in the emergency department during an acute exacerbation with a PaO_2 of 39 mm Hg on FIO_2 of 0.21, the FIO_2 level indicated to achieve a PaO_2 of 60 mm Hg is 0.28. In other words, an FIO_2 increase of 0.07 should increase PaO_2 approximately 21 mm Hg (7×3 mm Hg).

The formula shown in Equation 10-1 may be used to determine the appropriate percentage of oxygen to be applied in acute exacerbation of COPD, assuming a target PaO_2 of 60 mm Hg. Of course, this is just a guideline, and individual cases may vary considerably. It must also be remembered that this guideline **applies only to the patient with COPD in acute exacerbation.** It should also be noted that when in doubt it is probably wise to administer more oxygen rather than less.

Equation 10-1
$$60 \text{ mm Hg} - \text{room air } PaO_2/3 = \text{required } \% \ FIO_2 \text{ increase}$$

Following the initial application of oxygen therapy and after allowing 30 minutes to obtain a steady state, therapy should be titrated to achieve an SpO_2 of 90%. It is noteworthy that arterial oxygen saturation also increases on average 3% to 4% per 0.01 increase in FIO_2 in acute COPD.[300] This substantial increase shows the tremendous value of oxygen therapy in acute COPD. Because these patients are often on the steep portion of the oxyhemoglobin curve, the amount of oxygen actually present in the blood rises sharply with only a small increase in PaO_2.

Progressive Hypercapnia

One must always keep in mind that increases in PaO_2 in patients with COPD may also be accompanied by increases in $PaCO_2$. Although a slight increase in $PaCO_2$ is inconsequential, a large increase with a concomitant acidosis must be avoided. There is increasing evidence, however, that it is not the hypercapnia *per se* that results in deleterious effects[316] but rather the progressive acidemia, muscle weakness, and exhaustion, which must be carefully monitored.

The patient is more likely to have an increase in $PaCO_2$ in response to O_2 administration when initial $PaCO_2$ is greater than 70 mm Hg,[309,700] or when the initial PaO_2 is very low.[310] Also, the clinician should be aware that worsening hypercarbia may be observed several hours after the onset of oxygen therapy.[306]

The increase in $PaCO_2$ also tends to be proportional to the level of FIO_2 delivered. In one study, $PaCO_2$ increased on average 5 mm Hg with administration of FIO_2 0.24 and 8 mm Hg on FIO_2 0.28.[307] In another study, modest FIO_2 levels of 0.35 to 0.40 substantially aggravated hypercapnia.[311] When excessive oxygen therapy appears to be responsible for progressive hypercapnia, FIO_2 should be reduced gradually, because abrupt cessation of oxygen may result in further deterioration of the patient.

The buildup of CO_2 to high levels in the blood gives rise to the syndrome known as *CO_2 narcosis*. This syndrome, which may be a misnomer,[316] is characterized by increasing $PaCO_2$ levels, acidemia, stupor, and coma.[310] Additional clinical signs suggestive of mild-to-moderate hypercarbia include decreased cerebral function, headache, drowsiness, lethargy, and asterixis.[312] See Box 9-3 for a more complete list of the signs and symptoms associated with hypercapnia, although it is difficult to differentiate some of these symptoms from acidemia.

Sometimes, severely hypercapnic patients (i.e., $PaCO_2$ ~ 150 mm Hg) may be relatively asymptomatic. Nevertheless, the clinician must be continuously on guard for any signs or symptoms of hypercapnia and progressive acidosis while administering oxygen to the patient with COPD.

Some authors suggest that high doses of oxygen therapy may be safely administered to patients with COPD if hypercapnia is not present initially.[298,313] In my experience, I have observed increasing $PaCO_2$ levels after oxygen therapy in COPD despite the absence of preexisting hypercarbia.

The phenomenon of normal $PaCO_2$ levels in a patient who actually has chronic hypercapnia could be explained by the observation that

$PaCO_2$ levels in some patients with COPD seem to decrease during acute exacerbation of the disease (see Chapter 14).[10] Thus, when blood gases are first sampled in the hospital, $PaCO_2$ levels could appear lower than their normal baseline. In other words, chronic CO_2 retention may go unrecognized during acute exacerbation because $PaCO_2$ is within the normal range. In any event, it appears prudent to approach oxygen therapy cautiously in *all* patients with COPD, regardless of $PaCO_2$ levels.

Recently, it has been shown that patients with acute, severe asthma often develop acute hypercapnia when 100% oxygen is administered.[700] In addition, they also respond with a decreased peak expiratory flow rate. This is in marked contrast to the response when 0.28 FIO_2 is administered. These patients typically responded with a decreased $PaCO_2$.[700]

The device selected for the administration of oxygen is somewhat a matter of personal preference. High-flow systems such as air-entrainment masks with low FIO_2 levels have the advantage of accurate FIO_2 rates regardless of breathing pattern and are advocated by some as the safest, most effective method to deliver oxygen.[308] However, the patient's comfort and compliance with these devices are not good. In addition, these masks are often unsightly, awkward, and noisy.

Low-flow systems (e.g., nasal cannula) are more often used. They are less obtrusive, quieter, and better tolerated. For more precise FIO_2 control, however, flowmeters marked in flow increments less than 1 L/minute may be required.[314] Furthermore, one must always remember that a nasal cannula is a low-flow system and, as such, may allow considerable FIO_2 variation with changes in ventilatory pattern.

Excessive Oxygen Therapy

Few clinicians feel the fear of oxygen toxicity is greater than the concern for tissue hypoxia.

D.R. Hess, R.B. Kacmarek[305]

Excessive oxygen therapy may produce consequences similar to the symptoms of hypoxia and is also dangerous.[317] The net potential for harm depends on the net interaction of three critical variables: FIO_2, PaO_2, and duration of exposure.

High FIO₂ Levels

High FIO_2 levels (i.e., ≥0.60) for extended periods ultimately cause some cytotoxic and functional damage. In animals, FIO_2 of 1.0 has caused death within 48 to 72 hours due to non-cardiogenic pulmonary edema.[305]

In humans, the precise onset of oxygen toxicity is somewhat controversial.[305] Signs of oxygen toxicity in the form of substernal distress have been observed within 6 hours after the onset of 1.0 FIO_2 administration.[318] In other cases, FIO_2 resulted in inflammatory airway changes and bronchitis within 24 hours.[305] In contrast, no striking effects while breathing 1.0 FIO_2 were observed in postoperative open heart patients after 24 to 48 hours of therapy.[318] Nonetheless, it seems prudent to minimize the exposure time to high levels of FIO_2 in *all* patients.

High FIO_2s also result in the development of oxygen free radicals (superoxide, hydrogen peroxide, hydroxyl ion) that result in structural lung changes.[305] Various drugs and chemicals may enhance this effect. These include the chemotherapeutic agent Bleomycin, the antiarrhythmic agent Amiodarone,[319] and poisons such as paraquat. Indeed, it has been suggested that clinicians target a PaO_2 of only 50 mm Hg and avoid an FIO_2 over 0.4 during the administration of Bleomycin.[305] In contrast, in the severely damaged lung, antioxidants are present that help minimize lung damage despite high FIO_2.[305]

High FIO_2 levels (particularly $FIO_2 = 1.0$) also predispose individuals to the development of *absorption atelectasis*. Gas trapped in an alveolus is absorbed more quickly when the oxygen concentration is high. This is observed even in healthy individuals, who may develop up to a 10% shunt after breathing an FIO_2 of 1.0. Consequently, high FIO_2 levels are particularly worrisome in patients with shunt-producing disease, because they can ill afford a further reduction in gas exchange.

Arguments have been presented that hyperoxemia, even for short periods, is not innocuous and should be avoided. Indeed, hyperoxemia has been associated with worsening oxygen consumption,[348] muscle fatigue, and ventilation-perfusion mismatch. Overall, although the clinical evidence is conflicting, as a general rule most clinicians believe oxygen administration at FIO_2 greater than or equal to 0.60 should be avoided whenever possible for greater than 48 hours.[305]

Nonetheless, whenever oxygen status or cardiopulmonary integrity are in doubt, oxygen should be administered.[305] This is especially true during suctioning, bronchoscopy, transport, periods of instability, and during initiation of mechanical ventilation. Many believe it is also true during mechanical ventilation in ARDS where the fear of high alveolar pressures and volutrauma often supersede the fear of oxygen toxicity.[305]

High PaO₂ Levels

High PaO_2 levels similarly may cause harm to a patient and must be avoided. Notable is the phenomenon of *retrolental fibroplasia*, more recently referred to as diffuse retinopathy of prematurity. In this disorder, high PaO_2 levels in the retinal arteries cause vasoconstriction, which may, in turn, result in permanent blindness. This disorder is primarily a disease of premature infants with poorly developed retinal vessels.

As described previously, in some COPD and asthma patients, high PaO_2 levels may lead to the development of progressive *hypoventilation* and hypercarbia. Occasionally, a dramatic increase in PaO_2 levels in these oxygen-sensitive individuals may result in apnea.[81] Again, despite these caveats, oxygen therapy should never be withheld from *any* patient when the presence of hypoxia is likely.[81,305]

Finally, a PaO_2 greater than 150 mm Hg may cause coronary vasoconstriction and lead to arrhythmias in susceptible individuals with coronary disease.[320,321] In summary, oxygen should always be administered in the lowest dose possible. However, hypoxia, when suspected, must always be treated.

Nothwithstanding the clear focus of this text on insuring sufficient oxygen is administered, a controversial opposing view has been presented in a recent article.[696] John B. Downs, a well-respected critical care physician, purports that our excessive use of oxygen may, indeed, delay appropriate respiratory care. This provocative article is worth reading and challenges many of our long-held notions regarding oxygen therapy.[696]

ON CALL | CASE 10-1 *ABGs and Critical Thinking*

You are the only person available to care for this patient. You must assess the patient/situation and act accordingly.

A patient with a history of 50-pack years of smoking presents with a barrel chest, flattened diaphragms on chest radiography, and pursed lip breathing to the emergency department. He has had a recent upper respiratory infection and is now congested with shortness of breath.

ARTERIAL BLOOD GASES

SaO_2	75%
pH	7.32
$PaCO_2$	65 mm Hg
PaO_2	42 mm Hg
$[HCO_3]$	31 mEq/L
FIO_2	room air

ASSESSMENT

Abnormalities: List abnormal data and other noteworthy information. Classify ABG.

Explanation: List possible diseases, pathology, or other situations that may have led to this patient's condition.

Evaluation: Suggest additional data that would be useful in helping understand the situation or in making a diagnosis.

INTERVENTION

Importance: Prioritize concern(s) of treatment in order of urgency and/or seriousness as you see the overall situation.

Objective: Specifically state the measurable or observable outcomes you would like treatment to accomplish.

Action: Describe your specific plan of action.

MECHANICAL VENTILATION

Introduction

Mechanical ventilation is generally *not* a first-line treatment for oxygenation disturbances. Specifically, mechanical ventilation is reserved for the treatment of *ventilatory* problems, evidenced by an increased $PaCO_2$ and a low pH. Sometimes, however, oxygenation disturbances may be so severe that cardiopulmonary collapse seems eminent or the work of breathing is exhaustive. In these situations, mechanical ventilation may be useful to help the patient to rest and to allow for more effective breathing.

Acute Lung Injury/Acute Respiratory Distress Syndrome

Probably the most common clinical use of mechanical ventilation is in the treatment of acute lung injury (ALI) and the acute respiratory distress syndrome (ARDS). ALI/ARDS may be caused by a direct lung insult (e.g., pneumonia, aspiration) or an indirect lung insult (e.g., transfusion, diffuse inflammatory response). Regardless of the cause, the ultimate result is altered capillary permeability and pulmonary edema.

The American-European Consensus Conference in 1994 defined ARDS using the criteria in Box 10-4. If the oxygenation ratio is 2.0 to

3.0, the patient is classified as having ALI.[322] Based on chest radiography, ALI/ARDS was previously believed to be a diffuse lung disease that impacted the entire lung in a uniform manner. However, it has become increasingly clear with the use of computed tomography that this syndrome affects the microscopic lung in a heterogeneous manner. Some alveolar-capillary units are edematous and collapsed whereas others are normal. The overall lung is functionally small.

The heterogeneous nature of this disorder leads to the overfilling of normal alveoli during traditional mechanical ventilation and volutrauma. Volutrauma is an iatrogenic problem that refers to lung damage similar in nature to

---

Box 10-4   ARDS Definition Criteria

1. Acute onset
2. Bilateral infiltrates
3. No evidence of congestive heart failure (pulmonary wedge pressure <18 mm Hg)
4. Oxygenation ratio <2.0

From Brower, R.G., Matthay, M.A., Morris, A., et al: Ventilation with lower tidal volumes as compared with traditional tidal volumes for acute lung injury and the acute respiratory distress syndrome. N. Eng. J. Med. 342: 1301–1308, 2000.

ARDS but caused by excessive pressure and/or stress in lung units. The injury is sometimes referred to as volume-induced lung injury (VILI) and is likely to occur when plateau pressures measured in the lungs exceed 30 cm H_2O.[305] VILI leads to inflammation, repair, and remodeling of the lung.

It has also been known for years that many patients with ARDS do not die because of pulmonary dysfunction but rather due to the onset of multiple organ dysfunction syndrome (MODS). This syndrome is characterized by tissue injury secondary to inflammatory mediators/cells, bacteremia, and/or tissue hypoxia. Many clinicians currently believe that VILI may facilitate the release of inflammatory mediators and contribute to MODS. The ARDS/Net study discussed in the following section supports this hypothesis.

Acute Respiratory Distress Syndrome/Net

Traditional application of mechanical ventilation in ARDS involved the use of tidal volumes of 10 to 15 mL/kg of body weight. In the ARDS/Net study, it was hypothesized that these high volumes could induce VILI, exacerbate MODS, and contribute to mortality. Therefore, patients in the experimental group were mechanically ventilated with a tidal volume target of 6 mL/kg of ideal body weight with plateau pressures of 30 cm H_2O or less.[323] The intent was to reduce injurious lung stretch and the release of inflammatory mediators. PEEP was applied in the range of 10 to 20 cm H_2O to maintain alveolar recruitment.

The results were striking and, in fact, the ARDS/Net study was prematurely terminated based on the clear superiority of the low tidal volume technique.[323] Application of the ARDS/Net technique resulted in significant decreased mortality (22%) and fewer patient days on the ventilator.[323] These results occurred despite higher FIO_2s and PEEP levels used in the low tidal volume group.

Open Lung Approach

The open lung approach to mechanical ventilation is an alternative to the ARDS/Net approach. In the open lung approach, the focus is on maintaining a low plateau pressure while using pressure controlled ventilation. Alveolar recruitment maneuvers and higher levels of PEEP are used to maximize alveolar recruitment.

Presently, the ARDS/Net approach seems to be gaining increasing popularity. However, the modes and methods of mechanical ventilation continue to evolve, and the specific characteristics of future approaches are certain to change. The myriad details of mechanical ventilation and application of PEEP and positive pressure is beyond the scope of this text.

Permissive Hypercapnia

Application of the open lung approach or the ARDS/Net technique for mechanical ventilation often results in the development or worsening of hypercapnia. It is a common belief, however, that hypercapnia may be acceptable as long as pH can be maintained within an acceptable range. Arterial pH is typically maintained above 7.20 through the use of increased respiratory rates or bicarbonate infusion if necessary.[305]

Notwithstanding, even small increases in $PaCO_2$ will increase cerebral perfusion; therefore, permissive hypercapnia should be avoided when intracranial pressure is increased. Hypercapnia also stimulates ventilation; however, patients are often heavily sedated or paralyzed for controlled ventilation. Also, hypercapnia usually results in an increased cardiac output and pulmonary hypertension, although results may be variable.

Most often, the primary limiting factor in permissive hypercapnia is pH. Gradual pH change is better tolerated than abrupt pH change and younger patients seem to tolerate pH change better than the elderly. Administration of buffers (e.g., sodium bicarbonate) to protect pH is controversial. Sodium bicarbonate is also known to cause intracellular acidosis, which may have adverse effects.

The open lung approach and the ARDS/Net technique represent a radical departure in priorities and focus as compared to traditional mechanical ventilation. Whereas, maintenance of a normal $PaCO_2$ was traditionally considered prerequisite to alveolar pressure, it is considered secondary to alveolar pressure with the newer ventilation strategies. Thus, hypercapnia, although undesirable, represents a trade-off for minimizing alveolar pressure and lung stress exposure.

PaO$_2$ Targets and Permissive Hypoxemia

In the healthy adult lung, PaO$_2$ will exceed 80 mm Hg. Mild hypoxemia (>60 mm Hg) is generally considered acceptable in mild-to-moderate lung disease, particularly when there is concern for VILI or oxygen toxicity. In *severe* lung disease, or during Bleomycin therapy, PaO$_2$ may be consciously allowed to remain as low as 50 mm Hg provided no other serious side effects are manifested.[305] In permissive hypercapnia, PaCO$_2$ may be allowed to increase to 80, perhaps 100, mm Hg in the presence of severe lung disease provided acidosis is not severe.[305] Likewise, mild acidosis may be tolerated during ALI/ARDS, provided pH does not fall below 7.20.[305]

The idea of permissive hypoxemia (i.e., consciously allowing PaO$_2$ to remain at levels below 60 mm Hg) is gaining increased interest with some very prominent physicians.[696,701] As Dr. Downs argues in a compelling manner, there is little evidence to support the idea of maintaining a "normal" PaO$_2$. Indeed, it is his belief that by doing so, we are masking the real pulmonary problems and delaying appropriate treatment.

He argues systematically that oxygen consumption remains normal down to PaO$_2$ <30 mm Hg. He asserts that saturation is surely more important than PaO$_2$, and it is likely that the body could sustain arterial saturations below 50%. If one considers the ability of the body to withstand falls in cardiac output or [Hb] of a similar magnitude, why should the body be in such peril with only a 10% to 15% decline in SpO$_2$ down below 90%?

The editor of *Respiratory Care*, David Pierson, MD, asks a similar question regarding treatment in ARDS.[701] Does it really make a difference if the PaO$_2$ is 50 mm Hg or 100 mm Hg? Perhaps not, and the patient may be paying a great physiological price for us to keep it near 100 mm Hg. These questions are far from resolved and, for now, it is prudent to follow traditional guidelines. Nevertheless, just as permissive hypercapnia would have been unheard of 15 years ago, permissive hypoxemia may be the norm in years to come.

POSITIVE END-EXPIRATORY PRESSURE

Overview

Absolute shunting responds poorly to all of the palliative measures discussed previously. In particular, oxygen therapy is ineffective because the inspired oxygen cannot enter collapsed or fluid-filled alveoli. Furthermore, increasing the inspired oxygen concentration in itself tends to accentuate the capillary shunting process.[324] Because the rudimentary problem in absolute capillary shunting is loss of functional alveoli, effective treatment should aim towards restoring these alveoli to a functional state. The efficacy of PEEP lies in its ability to prevent or reverse alveolar collapse, increase lung volume, and thus reduce the capillary shunt.

PEEP was first used in clinical medicine in approximately 1938 by Alvan Barach.[325] Later, in a classic paper published in 1967, PEEP was described by Ashbaugh and Petty as an effective therapeutic modality for the treatment of ARDS.[294] Previously, PEEP was often characterized as the mainstay or cornerstone in the treatment of ARDS.[335] Although ARDS/Net has changed our focus somewhat, PEEP remains a key component in the treatment of arterial hypoxemia.

A technique with a similar goal to PEEP is known as the alveolar recruitment maneuver (ARM). The intent here is to apply an increased inflation pressure to the lung (typically 30 to 45 cm H$_2$O) and hold it to recruit collapsed alveoli. The maneuver typically lasts for approximately 1 minute, is done periodically, and has been shown to improve gas exchange. One must be cautious to avoid significant decreases in cardiac output during the maneuver.

Despite improvement during and immediately after the maneuver, gas exchange has been shown to deteriorate again within 15 minutes.[347] The use of PEEP in conjunction with ARM helps to avoid de-recruitment or re-collapse of alveoli. This represents one of the prime goals of PEEP in the management of ALI/ARDS.

Definition and Waveforms

PEEP is defined as *a pressure above atmospheric at the airway opening at the end of expiration.*[326]

Most often, PEEP is applied in conjunction with mechanical ventilation. *Continuous positive airway pressure* (CPAP) is a form of PEEP that is applied to spontaneously breathing patients. CPAP may be defined as a system for applying PEEP to spontaneously breathing patients, in which the applied pressure remains positive throughout the breathing cycle.[327] Although it is a spontaneously breathing modality, many ventilators are also capable of providing CPAP.

When the pressure in a PEEP system is allowed to fall below ambient pressure during spontaneous inspiration, the breathing system/mode does not meet the criteria for CPAP. A system that would allow this to occur is sometimes referred to simply as *PEEP with spontaneous breathing* or *expiratory positive airway pressure* (EPAP). It has been shown that EPAP is associated with a greater work of breathing than is CPAP; therefore, PEEP is best applied in the form of CPAP in the spontaneously breathing individual.

Figure 10-5 shows pressure tracings during controlled mechanical ventilation (CMV), CPAP, and PEEP with CMV. An EPAP tracing would be similar to that in Figure 10-5,*B*, with one important difference: during inspiration, the tracing would fall below the zero baseline.

Equipment Systems

Figure 10-6 shows one of the earliest systems used to administer CPAP. In this system, the depth of the underwater seal determines the CPAP level administered to the patient.

When selecting equipment to be used for the administration of PEEP or CPAP, there are several important considerations. First, the PEEP/expiratory valve assembly that is used should provide only minimal resistance to expiratory flow. Valves associated with increased flow resistance increase the mean airway pressure and the risk of complications. Another important consideration related to CPAP equipment is the use of a system that minimizes the work of breathing. It is becoming increasingly clear that deleterious consequences are associated with increased work of breathing.

Basically two types of valves have been used to maintain PEEP within breathing systems: threshold resistors and flow resistors. *Threshold resistors* apply a relatively constant

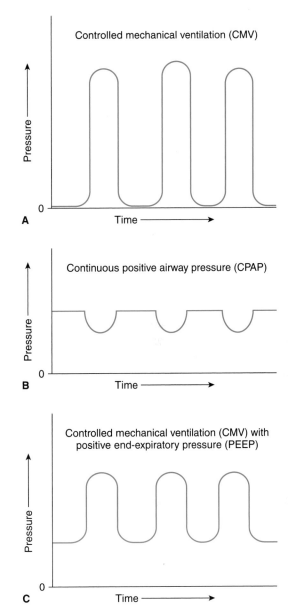

Figure 10-5. **Various modes of ventilation.** Pressure tracings for (**A**) controlled mechanical ventilation; **B**, continuous positive airway pressure; and **C**, controlled mechanical ventilation with positive end-expiratory pressure.

force against expiratory flow and abruptly close when flow stops. *Flow resistors*, on the other hand, do not in themselves maintain positive pressure; rather, they limit expiratory flow to the point that the pressure does not have sufficient time to fall to zero. Threshold resistors

Figure 10-6.   **Continuous positive airway pressure system.** Schematic diagram of system to provide continuous positive airway pressure in a spontaneously breathing person. Airway and alveolar pressures throughout the respiratory cycle are set by submerging the expiratory tube in a water reservoir to achieve the desired amount of PEEP.

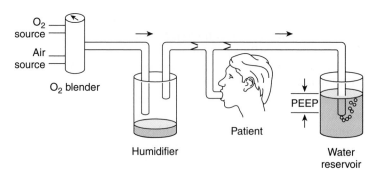

generally are better than flow resistors for the application of PEEP because they have a lower potential for cardiovascular side effects.

Indications

The primary indication for PEEP therapy is the presence of substantial absolute shunting. The classic indication for PEEP is a diagnosis of idiopathic respiratory distress syndrome (IRDS) in newborns or ALI/ARDS in adults. These diseases are associated with progressive, often severe, true capillary shunting that is potentially fatal if left untreated. The use of 10 to 20 cm H_2O of PEEP is used in ARDS to prevent alveolar collapse.

PEEP has been used in many conditions that are not related to increased capillary shunting (e.g., obstructive sleep apnea, neonatal apnea, chest trauma, control of mediastinal bleeding after open heart surgery).[332] Most of these other applications are controversial; however, CPAP therapy is widely accepted in the treatment of obstructive sleep apnea.

It is also known that the insertion of an artificial airway decreases the functional residual capacity (FRC). Therefore, in intubated infants and adults, 3 to 5 cm H_2O of PEEP or CPAP is typically applied.

PEEP has also been applied to various other capillary shunt disorders besides ARDS. CPAP has been applied intermittently and continuously to reverse or minimize the incidence of postoperative atelectasis.[331] The major drawback to this application appears to be its questionable cost-effectiveness.[331]

PEEP is often effective in the treatment of cardiogenic pulmonary edema.[331] PEEP would seem to help these patients in two ways: (1) it tends to reverse the capillary shunt, and (2) the

decreased venous return associated with PEEP (described in the section on complications) may actually enhance cardiac performance.

It is certainly reasonable to attempt a trial of PEEP therapy in most patients with a substantial true capillary shunt. Of course, the potential complications of PEEP must also be considered in this decision. In the patient with absolute shunting who does *not* require ventilatory support, the CPAP mode should be used.

Mechanism of Effectiveness

The effectiveness of PEEP is related to its ability to increase the FRC, recruit alveoli, and improve the ventilation-perfusion match. Figure 10-7 shows how PEEP applied via an endotracheal tube helps to reverse low ventilation-perfusion ratios and capillary shunting.

PEEP may also have a desirable effect through the redistribution of lung water. Several studies suggest that PEEP shifts water from alveoli to the perivascular space, where it does not impair gas exchange.[333,334]

Complications

The two most widely recognized complications of PEEP therapy are decreased cardiac output and pulmonary barotrauma.

Decreased Cardiac Output

Decreased cardiac output is probably the most commonly cited complication of PEEP or CPAP therapy.[335] This side effect is dose-related, and hypovolemic patients are especially susceptible to this problem.[336]

Two mechanisms that have been postulated to explain the PEEP-induced decrease in cardiac output are shown in Figure 10-8. Decreased venous return (see Fig. 10-8,*A*) secondary to

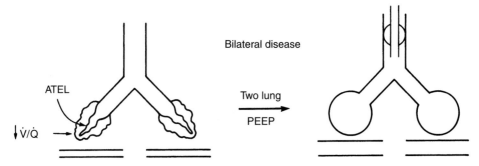

Figure 10-7. **Mechanism of PEEP effectiveness.** Application of PEEP to both lungs through a single-lumen tube in patients with bilateral lung disease usually results in a reversal of low ventilation-to-perfusion relationships and atelectasis in both lungs. (ATEL, atelectasis; $\downarrow\dot{V}/\dot{Q}$ low ventilation-perfusion ratio.)

compression of the great veins that results in a decreased venous return gradient is probably the most important mechanism.[335] In addition, increased pulmonary vascular resistance may cause right ventricular dysfunction due to distention and decreased contractility (see Fig. 10-8,*B*).

Surprisingly, many patients who receive PEEP therapy do not have a decrease in cardiac output. The cardiac effects resulting from a given dose of PEEP depend on the interaction of many different variables, including lung compliance, functional residual capacity (FRC), mean airway pressure, blood volume, and pulmonary wedge pressure. The mechanisms

through which some of these factors may decrease the cardiac output are explored.

Compliance

Presumably, when lung compliance is low, such as in ARDS, pressure in the lungs is poorly transmitted to the intrapleural space, and therefore, cardiac effects are diminished. On the other hand, in an individual with healthy lungs, alveolar pressure is more readily transmitted to the pleural space, and cardiac output is more likely to decrease. Thus, cardiac output is more likely to decrease with application of PEEP in the patient with healthy lungs. One study

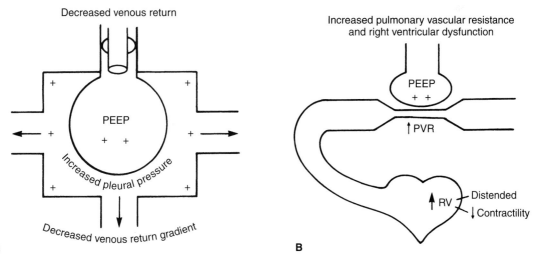

Figure 10-8. **Mechanisms of PEEP-induced decreased cardiac output.** Two of the mechanisms responsible for the decrease in cardiac output associated with PEEP are shown. **A**, Intrathoracic pressure increases as the lung expands. The positive intrathoracic pressure compresses the great veins and decreases the venous return gradient. **B**, PEEP also compresses the pulmonary vasculature which, in turn, distends the right ventricle and decreases contractility.

confirmed that pressure transmission is related to compliance; however, it failed to support the presumption that this in turn leads to hemodynamic consequences.[337]

Functional Residual Capacity

Theoretically, the administration of PEEP does not adversely affect cardiac output unless normal FRC is exceeded. Therefore, administration of PEEP to individuals with below-normal FRC should not substantially decrease cardiac output. Conversely, if PEEP is administered in doses sufficient to increase the FRC above normal limits, depression of cardiac output is likely. Because lung compliance is best at normal FRC, some clinicians had used compliance measurements as an indicator of the ideal PEEP level. If progressive PEEP levels increase compliance, the assumption is that FRC is moving closer to normal. On the other hand, if progressive PEEP levels are associated with a decrease in compliance, the assumption is that the lungs or alveoli are overdistended. However, because it has been demonstrated that ARDS is not homogeneous throughout the lung, this approach to determining ideal PEEP levels may result in VILI.

Furthermore, it has more recently been shown that if PEEP is applied in ARDS to prevent alveolar collapse, compliance may actually decrease despite an improvement in gas exchange.[305] Similarly, because patients with COPD already have an increased FRC, PEEP should be used in this group with extreme caution.

Mean Airway Pressure

Finally, the tendency of PEEP to decrease the cardiac output is directly proportional to the mean airway pressure rather than to the peak airway pressure. For this reason, flow resistors have a greater tendency than threshold resistors to decrease cardiac output because flow resistors maintain a higher mean airway pressure. When high levels of PEEP must be administered, every effort should be made to keep mean airway pressure at the lowest possible level.

Pulmonary Barotrauma

Pulmonary barotrauma (e.g., pneumothorax, subcutaneous emphysema, pneumomediastinum) may occur with the administration of

PEEP. It seems probable that the higher the level of PEEP, the greater is the tendency for barotrauma. Also, as stated previously, barotrauma is more likely when FRC is above normal.

Deterioration of Ventilation-Perfusion Ratio

Occasionally, the administration of PEEP leads to a paradoxical fall in PaO_2. This phenomenon is most likely to occur when PEEP is applied to an individual with unilateral lung disease.[305] Presumably, PEEP preferentially inhibits perfusion to the healthy lung because of the normal compliance. Thus, as shown in Figure 10-9, more blood is routed through the diseased lung with subsequent worsening hypoxemia.

Sophisticated application of PEEP to only the diseased lung has been carried out with apparent success.[339,340] To apply *differential lung* PEEP, a double-lumen tube must be placed in the lungs. Different levels of PEEP can then be applied to each lung as needed. Figure 10-10 shows schematically the application of differential lung PEEP through a double-lumen catheter.

Miscellaneous Complications

The administration of PEEP may lead to neurologic and renal complications. Like any clinical application of positive pressure, PEEP may

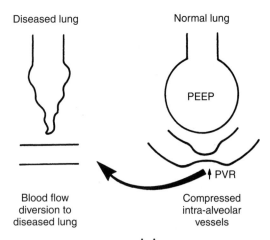

Figure 10-9. Worsening $\dot{V}/\dot{Q}$ with PEEP application. PEEP preferentially inhibits perfusion to the normal lung because of the normal compliance, which leads to increased perfusion of the diseased lung and decreased PaO_2.

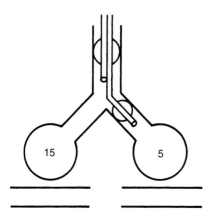

Figure 10-10. **Differential lung PEEP.** By using a double-lumen endotube, different levels of PEEP are applied independently to each lung in proportion to their needs.

increase intracranial pressure and reduce cerebral perfusion pressure.[341] This change may be a serious complication in the patient with neurologic disease.

PEEP may impair renal function due to decreased perfusion or by increasing antidiuretic hormone. Also, an increase in the amount of fluid present in the lungs with PEEP application has also been reported.[342] As described previously, however, PEEP probably improves the *distribution* of lung water from the alveoli to the perivascular space, which actually enhances gas exchange.[333,334]

Clinical Approach

There is no question that PEEP is beneficial in the patient with profound ARDS. PEEP should be applied at the minimum level necessary for adequate gas exchange and to prevent alveolar collapse. This is typically approximately 10 to 20 cm H_2O. PEEP should always be adjusted in small increments and decrements.

During withdrawal, FIO_2 should first be reduced to 0.50, then PEEP should be reduced very gradually to 5 cm H_2O. If SpO_2 decreases when PEEP is decreased, the previous level of PEEP should be re-established. After PEEP is reduced to 5 cm H_2O, FIO_2 can be reduced to 0.40. If the patient is stable at 5 cm H_2O and FIO_2 0.40, mechanical ventilation can be discontinued.

Auto–Positive End-Expiratory Pressure

The phenomenon termed *auto-PEEP* has been found to be very prevalent in mechanically ventilated patients (i.e., 39%).[343,344] In auto-PEEP positive pressure remains in the alveoli at the end of expiration, although it is not reflected on the pressure manometer of the ventilator. This *covert form* of PEEP has also been referred to as inadvertent PEEP, occult PEEP, or pulmonary gas trapping.

Predisposing Factors

It appears that the prolonged expiratory time required by patients with COPD predisposes them to the auto-PEEP effect. Nevertheless, this phenomenon is not exclusive to patients with COPD. It has also been observed in newborns and patients who are on controlled ventilation with high minute volumes.[344,345]

Effects

Auto-PEEP may have deleterious consequences. It may substantially diminish venous return and decrease cardiac output and blood pressure. It can hamper monitoring because it distorts static compliance measured at the bedside. Also, in the presence of auto-PEEP, spontaneous inspiration requires greater effort to decrease alveolar pressure below atmospheric pressure, which is associated with a substantial increase in the work of breathing. Finally, it may increase peak airway pressure and lead to barotrauma.

On the other hand, because auto-PEEP is indeed true PEEP, it may be responsible for improved PaO_2 levels. In this case, a reduction in auto-PEEP may improve the cardiac output but, at the same time, may lead to worsening hypoxemia.

Detection

Because normal passive monitoring of airway pressure does not reflect auto-PEEP, the clinician must actively detect this phenomenon. The following procedure may be used to evaluate a patient for auto-PEEP. At the end of exhalation (immediately before the next ventilator inspiratory phase), the expiratory valve is manually occluded. The pressure manometer

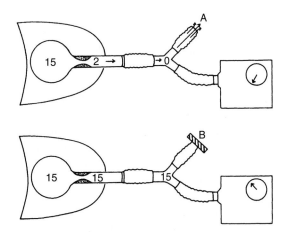

Figure 10-11.   **Detection of auto-PEEP.** The auto-PEEP effect. During mechanical ventilation of a patient with airflow obstruction, expiratory flow is too slow to allow complete deflation of the lung to its normal relaxed state before the ventilator delivers another breath. Slow flow continues until interrupted by the next inflation. Alveolar pressure remains positive at end-exhalation but is not measured by the ventilator manometer located downstream of the site of flow limitation (**A**). Alveolar pressure at end-exhalation can be quantified by stopping flow transiently at the end of the set exhalation period (**B**).

is then observed until pressure equilibrium is established. The pressure equilibrium point reflects the level of auto-PEEP. Respiratory movements by the patient during this measurement distort the readings and nullify the findings.

The phenomenon of auto-PEEP is shown in Figure 10-11. Note that the auto-PEEP effect is not detected at the proximal airway pressure monitor unless the expiratory valve is occluded immediately before the ventilator inspiratory phase.

Measurement of auto-PEEP is often difficult or awkward at the bedside. New ventilation technologies and devices such as the Braschi valve have simplified the process and improved accuracy of measurements.

Management

The first step in the management of auto-PEEP is to evaluate whether it is beneficial or detrimental to the patient. In some cases, it may indeed be beneficial.

There are several ways that auto-PEEP can be decreased when it is considered to be hazardous. Increasing the inspiratory flow rate in patients with COPD has been shown to improve oxygenation and decrease FRC.[328,329] Aggressive bronchodilation helps to control airway resistance. Normalization of the pH in acidemia helps to minimize minute volume requirements (i.e., respiratory compensation for metabolic acidosis increases minute ventilation). Use of lower compressible volume ventilator circuits may also decrease the auto-PEEP effect.[330]

Positive End-Expiratory Pressure on Auto–Positive End-Expiratory Pressure

Interestingly, the application of very low levels of applied external PEEP superimposed on auto-PEEP has been advocated to decrease the work of breathing.[343,346] With only auto-PEEP, the patient must exert a tremendous amount of effort to establish the negative pressure necessary for inspiration. This situation is similar to inspiration with an EPAP system.

The use of PEEP on auto-PEEP tends to minimize the effort required, much as CPAP improves the work of breathing compared with EPAP. Nevertheless, this form of therapy (i.e., PEEP on auto-PEEP) should be applied cautiously. In particular, the untoward effects of excessive PEEP must be avoided. The peak inspiratory pressure may serve as a crude index of appropriate PEEP levels, because the peak pressure should not increase with proper application of PEEP on auto-PEEP.[346]

BODY POSITIONING

Often, a simple change in a patient's body position may substantially alter PaO_2. Despite the wealth of documentation available to support this, little emphasis is usually placed on this subject. Positioning can be a practical, effective clinical tool in PaO_2 management.

Factors in Gas Exchange

At least three factors may alter pulmonary gas exchange when body position is changed.[351] First, a change in cardiac output may occur, with subsequent effects on PaO_2, such as those described in Chapter 9. Second, airway closure may develop or may be accentuated during tidal

ON CALL| CASE 10-2 *ABGs and Critical Thinking*

You are the only person available to care for this patient. You must assess the patient/situation and act accordingly.

A patient is hypotensive and septic in the critical care unit. The following day the patient is on a high-flow aerosol FIO_2 1.0 system and blood gases are drawn. The chest radiograph shows a diffuse white-out and the pulmonary wedge pressure is normal.

ARTERIAL BLOOD GASES

SaO_2	77%
pH	7.20
$PaCO_2$	52 mm Hg
PaO_2	54 mm Hg
$[HCO_3]$	19 mEq/L
FIO_2	1.0

ASSESSMENT

Abnormalities: List abnormal data and other noteworthy information. Classify ABG.

Explanation: List possible diseases, pathology, or other situations that may have led to this patient's condition.

Evaluation: Suggest additional data that would be useful in helping understand the situation or in making a diagnosis.

INTERVENTION

Importance: Prioritize concern(s) of treatment in order of urgency and/or seriousness as you see the overall situation.

Objective: Specifically state the measurable or observable outcomes you would like treatment to accomplish.

Action: Describe your specific plan of action.

---

breathing by assumption of the supine position.[351] Third, gravity alters the distribution of ventilation and perfusion. The net interaction of these effects as well as the effect of body position on the work of breathing determines the optimal position for each patient.

Cardiac Output

One should first consider the effect that a change in body position has on cardiac output because cardiac output is a critical factor in tissue oxygen delivery. Healthy individuals tend to have an increase in cardiac output in the supine position compared with the sitting position. Venous return is enhanced in the supine position because blood does not have to be pumped "uphill" back to the heart.

In the presence of disease, one must carefully consider whether the patient would benefit from more or less venous return. In hypovolemic shock, in which venous return is diminished, the patient will likely have an improved cardiac output when supine. The improvement in cardiac status in the supine position may also be accompanied by an increase in PaO_2.[352]

Congestive heart failure, on the other hand, may be aggravated by assumption of the supine position. In this case, the failing heart is unable to pump the increase in venous return. The supine position may predispose the patient to

a decrease in cardiac output and development or worsening of pulmonary edema. Here, assumption of the sitting position, with the concomitant decrease in venous return and enhanced cardiac performance, may be life-saving. In the presence of cardiovascular disease, the primary goal of positioning the patient is to optimize cardiac function and the patient's comfort.

Airway Closure

In patients likely to have high closing volumes, as described in Chapter 6, (e.g., the elderly, obese patients, smokers), PaO_2 is usually higher in the sitting versus the supine position.[351] The increase in FRC associated with the sitting position is probably the major reason why PaO_2 is improved. This may help to explain why PaO_2 levels observed in patients with cystic fibrosis are slightly higher in the sitting position compared with the supine position.[354]

An additional consideration in patients with COPD or obese patients is the work of breathing associated with body position. In these individuals, the work of breathing may be considerably higher in the supine position due to the difficulty in displacing the abdominal contents with the diaphragm. Thus, when airway closure or chronic obstructive pulmonary disease is suspected, the patient should most often be placed in the sitting position.

Surprisingly, however, some patients with COPD show an improvement in PaO_2 with recumbency.[355]

Gravity

As described in Chapter 6, ventilation and perfusion are generally distributed to the most gravity-dependent areas of the lungs. The application of positive pressure ventilation disrupts this pattern slightly and relatively more ventilation enters the non–gravity-dependent regions. Thus, the ventilation-perfusion match is not quite as good during mechanical ventilation compared with spontaneous breathing.

Clinical Application

Diffuse Lung Disease

In the presence of diffuse lung disease, patients are most often placed in the supine position unless cardiac output or airway closure considerations dictate otherwise. Assumption of the prone position has been shown to substantially increase PaO_2 (approximately 40 mm Hg) in most ALI/ARDS patients, compared with the supine position.[353] Three possible mechanisms for this include: improved $\dot{V}/\dot{Q}$, changes in lung mass and shape, and alterations in chest wall compliance.

Although prone positioning improves oxygenation, it has not been shown to improve survival. Side effects are uncommon but include dislodgment of endotracheal and other tubes or lines. The prone position may also present a considerable problem regarding patient access and care. Thus, although prone positioning is still being implemented in some places and it does indeed increase oxygenation in most cases, enthusiasm for its use seems to be waning.[305]

In patients with diffuse lung disease, there is also some evidence to suggest that lying on the right side may result in a higher PaO_2 than lying on the left side.[356] This may be related to the greater surface area present in the right lung.

Unilateral Lung Disease

In the presence of unilateral lung disease, correct body position may be very beneficial. Patients with unilateral lung disorders should normally be positioned with the healthy lung down.[352,356,357] This is true whether the patient is breathing spontaneously or is being mechanically ventilated.

One study, in which the patient population was small, reported a mean PaO_2 improvement of 121 mm Hg when mechanically ventilated patients with unilateral lung disease were positioned with the diseased lung up versus down.[358] Increased distribution of ventilation and perfusion to normal lung regions theoretically explains this vast improvement in oxygen loading.

Surprisingly, there is some evidence to suggest that, in infants and young children with unilateral lung disease, gas exchange is actually better with the diseased lung down.[359] In addition there have been reports in adults as well where gas exchange improved with the diseased lung down, in particular with pulmonary embolus.[360,361] Further studies are necessary, however, before application of this finding becomes standard clinical practice.

Summary

Patients with abnormal pulmonary status should not be subjected to positioning that could potentially lower their PaO_2 or cardiac output to dangerous levels which could, in turn, compromise tissue oxygenation. Because body position may substantially affect PaO_2, it is wise to record body position at the time of blood gas analysis. The patient's position should be an integral part of the therapeutic plan.

NITRIC OXIDE

Inhaled nitric oxide has also been employed as a therapeutic agent to enhance gas exchange in ALI/ARDS.[350] Nitric oxide is a selective pulmonary vasodilator and small airway dilator.[349] Other pulmonary vasodilators may also cause systemic hypotension which is undesirable. In contrast, the short half-life and rapid absorption by hemoglobin ensures nitric oxide has no systemic effects.

Potential side effects include development of methemoglobinemia or formation of nitric or nitrous acid, although this has not been common. The other significant deterrent to nitric oxide use is cost which is substantial for a patient population with a high mortality.

LONG-TERM OXYGEN THERAPY

Combined results of the Nocturnal Oxygen Therapy Trial (NOTT)[692] and the Medical Research Council Working Party[693] demonstrated that survival in COPD patients was greatest with continuous oxygen use.

The classic indication for long-term oxygen use is the presence of COPD and a PaO_2 less than or equal to 55 mm Hg or SaO_2 less than or equal to 88%. If the PaO_2 is less than or equal to 59 mm Hg, the patient may be eligible if any of the following other criteria are present: (1) hematocrit greater than or equal to 55%, (2) p pulmonale on electrocardiography, or (3) peripheral edema secondary to right-heart failure. This needs to be demonstrated two times in the patient who is medically stable and seated. Desaturation to SaO_2 less than 88% following a 6-minute walk or during sleep also suggests the need for oxygen therapy. It is not uncommon for individuals with COPD to have a 10 mm Hg or more decrease in PaO_2 during sleep.

Continuous long-term oxygen therapy appears to benefit individuals by: (1) increased survival, (2) decreased pulmonary vascular resistance, (3) increased exercise capacity, (4) improved oxygenation during sleep, and (5) increased neuro-psychological performance.

Oxygen therapy should likewise be considered in COPD patients when traveling by airplane. One can expect a 4-mm Hg decrease in PaO_2 for each 1000-ft elevation.[695] Airplanes are required by the Federal Aviation Administration to maintain cabin pressures at least equivalent to 8000-ft elevation.[694] Thus, one might expect PaO_2 to decrease a maximum of 32 mm Hg during flight.

Because long-term hypoxia is tolerated slightly better, these recommendations state that *chronic* oxygen therapy may not be necessary unless PaO_2 is less than 55 mm Hg with the patient in the recumbent position. Oxygen therapy may also be required if PaO_2 falls below 55 mm Hg during sleep or exercise.

EXERCISES

Exercise 10-1 Oxygen Therapy

Fill in the blanks or select the best answer.

1. The first line of treatment for all oxygen-loading disturbances is _____.

2. Tissue hypoxia is likely when (mild/moderate/severe) hypoxemia is present.

3. ACCP recommendations state that oxygen therapy is indicated when PaO_2 is less than _____ mm Hg, or SaO_2 is less than _____%.

4. Oxygen therapy increases (ventilation-perfusion ratios/alveolar oxygen supply).

5. Oxygen therapy is most effective when hypoxemia is caused by (relative/true) shunting.

6. Oxygen therapy can be most precisely delivered with (low-flow/high-flow) administration devices.

7. In an individual with a normal breathing pattern, a nasal cannula set at 1 L/minute delivers an FIO_2 of approximately _____.

8. If the patient's tidal volume is less than normal while breathing via a low-flow oxygen administration system, the FIO_2 is (lower/higher) than Table 10-1 indicates.

9. (High-flow/Low-flow) oxygen administration systems have the most widespread use because of their simplicity and patient comfort.

10. Partial rebreathing masks tend to deliver an FIO_2 of about _____.

Exercise 10-2   Hazards and Guidelines in Oxygen Therapy

Fill in the blanks or select the best answer.

1. When PaO_2 falls below ___ mm Hg acutely, short-term memory is altered and euphoria or impaired judgment may be observed.

2. In general, mechanical ventilation should not be initiated in COPD unless pH falls below _____ and all else fails.

3. A reasonable target PaO_2 in acute exacerbation of COPD is ____ mm Hg.

4. State the three critical variables that determine the potential for physiologic harm when administering oxygen therapy.

5. A PaO_2 of greater than _____ mm Hg may lead to arrhythmias in patients with coronary disease.

6. In most cases, _____ _____ can serve as a cost-effective alternative to blood gases for monitoring oxygen therapy.

7. The first priority in clinical oxygenation is always (minimizing FIO_2/correction of hypoxia).

8. Oxygen therapy must be administered with extreme caution in the presence of (COPD/heart failure).

9. PaO_2 usually increases approximately _____ mm Hg for every 0.01 increase in FIO_2 in acute exacerbation of COPD.

10. The syndrome that may be a misnomer characterized by increasing $PaCO_2$, acidemia, stupor, and coma is known as _____.

Exercise 10-3   General Treatment and Positioning in Oxygen-Loading Problems

Fill in the blanks or select the best answer.

1. State the three primary goals of oxygen therapy.

2. List at least four general types of therapy that can be used in the supportive treatment of oxygen-loading disturbances.

3. State the three factors that may alter PaO_2 when body position is changed.

4. In hypovolemic shock, cardiac output is likely best in the (sitting/supine) position.

5. In acute congestive heart failure, cardiac output is likely best in the (sitting/supine) position.

6. In the elderly or obese patient, PaO_2 is usually highest in the (sitting/supine) position.

7. Adult patients with unilateral lung disease tend to have improved PaO_2 levels when the diseased lung is placed (up/down).

8. Infants with unilateral lung disease may have improved PaO_2 levels when the diseased lung is (up/down).

9. Ventilation/perfusion balance (is/is not) improved during mechanical ventilation compared with spontaneous breathing.

10. Studies have shown that the (supine/prone) position has been associated with a higher PaO_2 level in ARDS.

Exercise 10-4   Oxygen Toxicity/ALI/ARDS

Fill in the blanks or select the best answer.

1. The chemotherapeutic agent _____ may accelerate oxygen toxicity.

2. The anti-arrhythmic agent _____ may contribute to the progression of oxygen toxicity.

3. Poisons such as _____ may also contribute to oxygen toxicity.

4. It has been suggested that clinicians target a PaO_2 of only ___ mm Hg and avoid an FIO_2 over 0.4 during the administration of Bleomycin.

5. ALI and ARDS stand for _____ and _____.

6. ALI is (more/less) severe than ARDS.

7. ARDS affects the lung in a (homogeneous/heterogeneous) manner.

8. It is believed that lung damage tends to occur when the alveolar pressure exceeds ___ cm H_2O.

9. VILI is the symbol for _____ _____ _____ _____.

10. MODS is the symbol for _____ _____ _____ _____.

11. The study that dramatically changed the mechanical ventilation approach to ARDS was called _____.

12. Tidal volumes using the ARDS/Net approach are limited to ____ mL/Kg.

13. Allowing the $PaCO_2$ to increase, as a consequence of ventilating with low tidal volume and alveolar pressures, is referred to as _____ _____.

14. Mortality was significantly (increased/decreased) in ARDS using the ARDS/Net approach.

15. The pH should not be allowed to fall below ____ even with permissive hypercapnia.

Exercise 10-5   PEEP/CPAP

Fill in the blanks or select the best answer.

1. PEEP has often been referred to as the cornerstone in the treatment of the pulmonary disorder called _____.

2. (PEEP/CPAP) is the therapy best suited for the spontaneously breathing patient.

3. (Oxygen/PEEP) therapy is the most effective treatment for absolute shunting.

4. When PEEP applied to a spontaneously breathing patient falls below ambient pressure during inspiration, the system is referred to as (CPAP/EPAP).

5. A (flow/threshold) resistor applies a relatively constant force against expiratory flow and abruptly closes when flow stops.

6. (Continuous/Noncontinuous) flow CPAP systems are associated with the least work of breathing.

7. The use of _____ cm H_2O of PEEP is used in ARDS to prevent alveolar collapse.

8. The use of PEEP (is/is not) effective in the treatment of sleep apnea.

9. PEEP usually (improves/worsens) ventilation-perfusion matching.

10. PEEP most likely has a (beneficial/detrimental) effect on the distribution of lung water.

Exercise 10-6   **Complications of PEEP**

Fill in the blanks or select the best answer.

1. List the two most commonly cited complications associated with PEEP therapy.

2. (Hypervolemic/Hypovolemic) patients are especially susceptible to a decreased cardiac output after the initiation of PEEP.

3. PEEP therapy is most likely to decrease cardiac output when pulmonary compliance is (high/low).

4. PEEP therapy tends to have adverse effects on cardiac output when FRC is (above/below) normal.

5. The tendency of PEEP to decrease cardiac output is directly proportional to the (peak/mean) airway pressure.

6. PEEP therapy may be associated with a fall in arterial PO_2 when administered to an individual with (diffuse/unilateral) lung disease.

7. PEEP devices that create only (flow/threshold) resistance are associated with lower mean airway pressures.

8. The major mechanism responsible for the decrease in cardiac output associated with PEEP is (decreased venous return/right ventricular dysfunction).

9. PEEP may (decrease/increase) intracranial pressure.

10. A specialized form of PEEP used in unilateral lung disorders is _____ lung PEEP.

Exercise 10-7   **Auto-PEEP**

Fill in the blanks or select the best answer.

1. Inadvertent PEEP during mechanical ventilation is referred to as _____.

2. Patients with (COPD/ARDS) are especially susceptible to auto-PEEP.

3. Auto-PEEP is very common during mechanical ventilation at (low/high) minute ventilation.

4. Auto-PEEP (increases/decreases) the work of breathing.

5. Auto-PEEP (is/is not) reflected on the pressure manometer of a ventilator without intervention.

6. Auto-PEEP can be detected by performing an (inspiratory/expiratory) pressure hold.

7. Auto-PEEP can be treated by (increasing/decreasing) ventilator flow rate.

8. (High/Low) compressible ventilator circuits tend to increase auto-PEEP.

9. Low doses of applied PEEP may (increase/decrease) the work of breathing associated with auto-PEEP.

10. Peak pressure on the ventilator (should/should not) increase with proper application of applied PEEP to auto-PEEP.

Internet Work

1. Go to http://www.emedicine.com/radio/Topic770.htm.
   A. Describe the incidence of ARDS in the United States.
   B. List at least five possible etiologies of ARDS.

NBRC Challenge 10

Please select the best answer for the following multiple-choice questions.

1. A known COPD patient arrives in the emergency department in acute exacerbation. Blood gases are drawn and the PaO_2 is 51 mm Hg. Which of the following oxygen set-ups would be most likely to result in a PaO_2 of 60 mm Hg for him?
   A) Simple oxygen mask at 6 LPM
   B) Partial rebreathing oxygen mask at 7 LPM
   C) Vent-mask at FIO_2 0.30
   D) Nasal cannula 1 LPM
   E) Nasal cannula 3 LPM
   (RRT EXAMINATION — NBRC
      MATRIX II,A,1.a.1)

2. In attempting to ventilate an ARDS patient using the ARDS/Net approach, which of the following guidelines would be adhered to?
   I. Tidal volume 6 mL/kg ideal body weight
   II. Maximum alveolar pressure of 30 cm H_2O
   III. PEEP of 5 cm H_2O
   A) I only
   B) II only
   C) I and II only
   D) I and III only
   E) II and III only
   (CRT EXAMINATION — NBRC
      MATRIX III,C,1,d)

3. Which of the following therapies may be beneficial in the patient on a ventilator with cardiogenic pulmonary edema?

   A) PEEP
   B) Nitric oxide
   C) Prone position
   D) Trendelenburg position
   E) Increased fluids intravenously
   (CRT EXAMINATION — NBRC
      MATRIX III,C,2,a)

4. What clinical recommendations could be made for an ARDS patient to improve $\dot{V}/\dot{Q}$ matching?
   I. Decrease alveolar ventilation
   II. Prone positioning
   III. Nitric oxide
   A) I only
   B) II only
   C) I and II only
   D) II and III only
   E) I, II, and III
   (RRT EXAMINATION — NBRC
      MATRIX III,B,4,c)

5. A patient with ALI is being ventilated at an FIO_2 of 0.50 and 10 cm H_2O of PEEP. If oxygenation is quite good, the next move would be to:
   A) discontinue mechanical ventilation.
   B) decrease FIO_2 to 0.35.
   C) decrease PEEP to 5 cm H_2O.
   D) extubate the patient.
   E) change to intermittent mechanical ventilation mode.
   (RRT EXAMINATION — NBRC
      MATRIX III,B,4,a)

11
Hypoxia: Assessment and Intervention

Hypoxia not only breaks the machine, it wrecks the machinery.

T. S. Haldane[376]

Clearly, the process of tissue oxygen delivery is a complex one and unlikely to be easily defined by the measurement of simple parameters.

David R. Dantzker[377]

Outline

OVERVIEW

The prevention, detection, and treatment of hypoxia must be foremost in the minds of clinicians treating cardiopulmonary patients. *The ultimate goal in the management of oxygenation is the prevention of tissue hypoxia.* When hypoxia is present, the goal is immediate recognition and intervention to minimize untoward effects.

There is no single, simple index or way to quickly and accurately assess tissue oxygenation. Rather, tissue oxygenation status is best assessed by systematically analyzing the various components of the oxygenation system and by evaluating related laboratory data. I have divided tissue hypoxic assessment into two phases.

First, as a matter of routine, one should evaluate the three essential components of oxygen supply shown in Box 11-1. The ABCs of tissue oxygen supply are **A**rterial oxygenation assessment, **B**lood hemoglobin concentration, and **C**irculatory status. A deficiency in any one of these components may compromise oxygenation of the tissues.

Although evaluation of oxygen supply components is a logical starting point, in many cases, it is still difficult to conclude whether tissue hypoxia is, indeed, present. Therefore, when more definitive information is needed, the clinician may look to specific indices that suggest oxygenation failure and tissue hypoxia. Potential markers of tissue hypoxia are listed in Box 11-2. These include lactate measurement, indices of mixed venous oxygenation, oxygen uptake and utilization, and gastric mucosal acidosis.

OXYGEN SUPPLY VARIABLES

Each of the oxygen supply variables as shown in Box 11-1 will be described in detail.

Arterial Oxygenation

There are two primary indicators of arterial oxygen supply: PaO_2 and SaO_2. An approximate gauge of SaO_2 is often reflected by pulse oximetry and in this case may be referred to as SpO_2. The student should understand that true SaO_2 can only be measured by CO-oximetry as described later in this chapter and Chapter 15. Nevertheless, SpO_2 provides a crude index of SaO_2 in the absence of abnormal Hb species.

PaO_2

PaO_2 as an Index of Hypoxia

When available, the partial pressure of oxygen in the arterial blood (PaO_2) is a logical starting point in tissue oxygenation assessment. As described in previous chapters, the degree of hypoxemia in a given individual is a simple indicator of the likelihood of hypoxia.

Hypoxia is unlikely in mild hypoxemia, possible in moderate hypoxemia, and likely in severe hypoxemia. In moderate hypoxemia, development of hypoxia depends mainly on the integrity of the cardiovascular system.

These guidelines represent clinical rules of thumb. There are, of course, exceptions to every rule. It has been shown that under certain conditions, hypoxia does not occur despite the presence of severe hypoxemia.[378-380] For example, mountain climbers at the summit of Mt. Everest had PaO_2 levels below 30 mm Hg without apparent adverse consequences.[378] Similarly, patients with congenital heart disease had PaO_2 levels averaging 37 mm Hg without notable physiologic impairment.[380] Furthermore, these patients were capable of some exercise, during which PaO_2 levels decreased further to 28 mm Hg.[380]

Finally, despite the fact that a PaO_2 of less than 20 mm Hg is generally considered to be incompatible with life, 13 of 22 patients in one study recovered without permanent physiologic impairment despite PaO_2 levels of less than 21 mm Hg.[379] Thus, PaO_2 alone, even when extremely low, is inadequate as an index of tissue hypoxia.

Also, one must not rely too heavily on PaO_2 alone because measurements in stable critically ill patients in one study varied as much as 13% from one reading to another.[381] This constitutes an average variance of about 16 mm Hg in PaO_2 measurements without a noticeable change in patient condition.

Prevention of Hypoxemic Hypoxia

The guidelines presented previously, notwithstanding the exceptions, represent a prudent approach to the classification of hypoxemia and the prevention of hypoxia. One must remember that in normal persons, when PaO_2 decreases to about 55 mm Hg, judgment and short-term memory may be impaired, presumably due to hypoxia.[382] Therefore, in all but unusual circumstances, it is unacceptable to allow moderate or severe hypoxemia (i.e., PaO_2 < 60 mm Hg) to persist.[382] This is true even in patients with chronic obstructive pulmonary disease (COPD), because a PaO_2 of 60 mm Hg is not associated with a great risk of increasing hypercarbia.[382]

As described in Chapter 10, there are some circumstances (e.g., paraquat poisoning, ARDS) when moderate degrees of hypoxemia may be considered acceptable or permissive. Indeed, a rebuttal of the traditional approach to treatment of hypoxemia has been presented.[696] Nevertheless, treatment of moderate hypoxemia seems prudent until clear evidence suggests otherwise.

Methods available to treat hypoxemia have been discussed in detail in Chapter 10. Although the PaO_2 is a useful starting point in clinical hypoxic assessment, it is foolhardy to equate a normal PaO_2 with normal tissue oxygenation. The myriad other factors that may influence O_2 transport and internal respiration must also be evaluated.

SaO_2

SaO_2 Determination

The SaO_2 is the percentage of hemoglobin that is carrying oxygen in the arterial blood. It should be remembered that 98% of oxygen is carried in arterial blood combined with Hb. Regarding saturation, it is important for the clinician to note the technique that is being used to determine SaO_2, because the values obtained by different techniques may vary. Saturation may be calculated via a nomogram or measured by oximetry, CO-oximetry, or pulse oximetry.

Calculated SaO_2 Using a Nomogram. Some laboratories use a nomogram to predict the SaO_2, based on the PaO_2 and pH.[383] This calculated SaO_2 does not account for factors other than the pH that may alter HbO_2 affinity. Furthermore, this methodology assumes that no abnormal forms of Hb are present, such as HbCO or MetHb. Obviously, calculated SaO_2 provides little more information than PaO_2 and may sometimes lead to a false sense of security. Some laboratories label calculated saturation as SO_2.

Oximetry. SaO_2 may be measured more accurately via oximetry. Oximeters are two-wavelength spectrophotometers. The specific technique underlying two-wavelength oximetry is discussed in Chapter 15.

It is important to understand two essential points when SaO_2 is measured with the two-wavelength method. First, when only two wavelengths are used, abnormal forms of Hb such as HbCO and MetHb cannot be detected.[383] Second, SaO_2 measured in this way is the percentage of HbO_2 *compared with the sum of HbO_2 and desaturated Hb only*. Because this measurement does *not* include abnormal forms of Hb, it is sometimes referred to as *functional SaO_2*.[383] Functional SaO_2 is the percentage of HbO_2 compared with the quantity of Hb *capable* of carrying O_2. MetHb and HbCO are not capable of carrying O_2; therefore, they are not specifically considered in this measurement.

Pulse oximetry, as described subsequently, is used routinely to evaluate oxygen saturation. Since pulse oximeters use only two wavelengths, they may likewise provide incorrect information when substantial MetHb or HbCO is present. It is imperative that we always keep these important issues in mind and do not routinely assume a normal pulse oximeter reading always indicates adequate oxygen saturation.

CO-oximetry. Functional SaO_2, as described previously, is in contrast with SaO_2 measurement using a CO-oximeter. As the name implies, this instrument can measure HbCO% in addition to the SaO_2. Also, methemoglobin levels may be measured as a percentage of total Hb with this unit.[384]

In CO-oximeter measurements, *all* forms of Hb are included in the calculation of the total Hb concentration. Thus, with this instrument, SaO_2 is the percentage of HbO_2 compared with *all forms of Hb (including abnormal forms of Hb)*. SaO_2 measured in this way is sometimes referred to as *fractional SaO_2*, which may be substantially different from functional SaO_2 in certain situations.

In review, the percentage of HbO_2 compared with the sum of Hb and HbO_2 is called functional SaO_2; the percentage of HbO_2 compared with *all* forms of Hb is called fractional SaO_2.

Pulse Oximetry. The saturation as measured by pulse oximetry (SpO_2) is a functional SaO_2 measurement as described earlier. As a two-wavelength device, the pulse oximeter cannot distinguish between HbO_2 and HbCO; therefore, SpO_2 is equal to the sum of HbO_2 and HbCO percentages.[385]

Other factors that have been thought to alter pulse oximetry readings include hypothermia, dark fingernail polish, vasoconstriction associated with shock, and infusion of dyes.[386] Interestingly, SpO_2 readings may be slightly higher if the finger being used for the test is elevated, presumably because of changes in venous congestion.[387] Newer pulse oximeter technology tends to eliminate many potential measurement errors (see Chapter 15).

SaO_2 as an Index of Hypoxia

SaO_2 is a better indicator of arterial oxygen content than is the PaO_2. Approximately 98% of blood oxygen is carried in the combined state (e.g., HbO_2); therefore, SaO_2 more accurately reflects the quantity of oxygen in the blood than the PaO_2. Clinically, as long as SaO_2 exceeds 90%, most clinicians are confident that the patient is not hypoxic. Usually a red flag is raised, however, when SaO_2 falls below 90%.

Furthermore, with the advent of routine SpO_2, understanding of the oxyhemoglobin curve assumes greater clinical importance. Important relationships between PO_2 and SO_2 must be committed to memory (i.e., PO_2 of 60 mm Hg = SO_2 of 90%; PO_2 of 40 mm Hg = SO_2 of 75%). The clinician must be able to mentally equate and interchange these two important parameters of oxygenation.

The PO_2–SO_2 relationships described earlier hold true given normal oxyhemoglobin affinity. A change in this relationship (e.g., PO_2 = 60 mm Hg; SO_2 = 80%) is indicative of a change in Hb–O_2 affinity (i.e., shift in oxyhemoglobin curve) that may be clinically important to recognize. For example, in the presence of alkalemia and hypocarbia, SpO_2 may remain above 90% even when PaO_2 is much lower than 60 mm Hg.

There is sometimes concern that a left-shifted oxyhemoglobin dissociation curve may cause tissue hypoxia because the hemoglobin will not release oxygen to the tissues. This phenomenon alone, especially in chronic conditions, is probably unlikely to cause tissue hypoxia as a patient with a P_{50} of 11 mm Hg did not appear to show any evidence of hypoxia.[436]

Finally, the relative *insensitivity* of SaO_2 must also be recognized. Although SaO_2 is a superior index of quantitative oxygen content in the blood, it is inferior to PaO_2 as a sensitive index of pulmonary deterioration, mild hypoxemia, and/or hyperoxemia. Because the normal individual has an SaO_2 on the flat portion of the oxyhemoglobin dissociation curve, relatively large changes in PaO_2 result in minimal or no change in SaO_2.

SpO_2 and Abnormal Hb Species

As described earlier, SpO_2 measures functional saturation, not fractional saturation. Thus, abnormal Hb species (e.g., HbCO, MetHb) are not reflected. HbCO is recorded as HbO_2 because only two wavelengths of light are being measured. This could lead to a false sense of security regarding the patient with significant levels of abnormal Hb species. If, for example, an individual has an HbCO level of 20% and a fractional HbO_2 level of 70%, SpO_2 will read approximately 90%.

Thus, pulse oximetry may be misleading in the patient with recent exposure to carbon monoxide. With increased methemoglobinemia, SpO_2 readings tend to migrate toward 85%. As always, one cannot depend too heavily on any single technology as a replacement for thorough clinical evaluation.

Although pulse oximetry has some shortcomings as a true measure of oxygen saturation, it is useful particularly as a monitor of *desaturation*. In other words, when there is a fall in oxygen saturation from previous levels, it will usually be reflected. For this reason, pulse oximetry is an excellent method to *monitor* oxygen status on a real-time basis.

Maintenance of an Adequate SaO_2

In summary, SaO_2 values may vary substantially depending on the technique of measurement. The clinician must understand the method being used and its implications regarding patient management. When abnormal forms of Hb are suspected, SaO_2 should always be measured by using CO-oximetry.

When fractional SaO_2 is low, as determined by CO-oximetry, therapy is focused on decreasing the amount of any abnormal Hb species present in the blood and increasing blood oxygen content to satisfactory levels.

High levels of HbCO are treated with fraction of inspired oxygen (FIO_2) of 1.0 and, when available, hyperbaric oxygen. The half-life of HbCO is approximately 5 hours on room air. Thus, it takes the body about 5 hours to eliminate 50% of HbCO while breathing room air. Breathing 100% O_2 decreases the half-life to about 1 hour. Furthermore, the high levels of inspired oxygen maximally saturate available Hb and enhance dissolved O_2 concentration. In the case of very high MetHb levels, methylene blue is often useful to accelerate the reduction of MetHb to Hb.

In most clinical situations, conventional wisdom is simply to maintain the fractional SaO_2 above 90% to 92%. This usually equates to a $PaO_2 > 60$ mm Hg. When SaO_2 falls below this point, however, immediate action is usually indicated to restore SaO_2 to safer levels. One must remember that below 90% saturation, SaO_2 will fall precipitously with further PaO_2 reductions. Although this approach has been recently challenged,[696] presently it is probably best to adhere to conventional wisdom.

Blood Hemoglobin Concentration

Anemia

Not only is the SaO_2 important in tissue oxygenation, but the absolute quantity of hemoglobin present in the patient must be adequate to carry and deliver oxygen throughout the body. The normal red blood cell concentration (abbreviated [RBC]) is 5 million/mm³ (±700,000) for men and 4.5 million/mm³ (±500,000) for women. The normal Hb concentration (abbreviated [Hb]) is 15 g% (15 g/100 mL of blood) in men and 13 to 14 g% in women.

A reduction in the amount of circulating RBCs or Hb is termed *anemia*. In general, the classic criterion for an individual to be considered anemic is if [RBC] is less than 4 million/mm³ or if [Hb] is less than 12.5 g%.[702] Actual normal values vary with age and sex. Anemia may greatly diminish the ability of the blood to transport oxygen because hemoglobin is responsible for approximately 98% of oxygen transport.

When blood is centrifuged or allowed to stand, it separates into two layers: (1) a layer of *formed elements* that includes RBCs, white blood cells (WBCs), and platelets; and (2) a layer of straw-colored fluid called *plasma*. The percentage of formed elements by volume

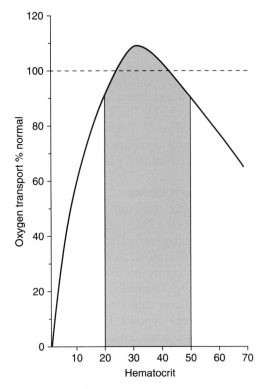

Figure 11-1. **Hematocrit and oxygen transport.**

is known as the *hematocrit* (Hct). Hematocrit is normally approximately 47% in men and approximately 42% in women. Because the RBCs make up the major portion of the hematocrit, it is also a useful indicator of anemia.

In a sense, hematocrit is a double-edged sword. If Hct is extremely low, arterial oxygen content and oxygen transport will be compromised. Conversely, when Hct is excessive, blood viscosity is increased and again, oxygen transport may be diminished due to a fall in cardiac output (Fig. 11-1). The optimal clinical Hct is likewise controversial and, in different patient populations, has been shown to be as low as 30% or as high as 45%.[437]

Laboratory Diagnosis of Anemia

When anemia is observed, the cause should be investigated. A thorough discussion of the various types of anemia and differential diagnosis is beyond the scope of this book; however, some fundamentals and terminology involved in anemia are reviewed.

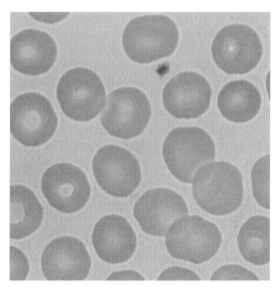

Figure 11-2.   **Mature erythrocytes, peripheral blood (×1000, Wright's stain).**

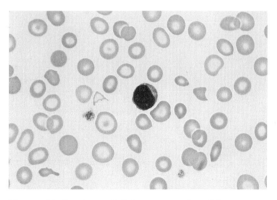

Figure 11-4.   **Iron deficiency anemia with hypochromia and microcytosis.** Note the presence of many small (microcytic) cells and the decreased amount of hemoglobin pigment (hypochromia) within the cells.

Anemia is generally classified and diagnosed based on the characteristics of the RBCs observed and the number of immature RBCs seen. In particular, the size, shape, and amount of Hb have diagnostic significance.

Mean Corpuscular Volume

Normal RBCs are, for the most part, approximately 7 µm in diameter. Figure 11-2 shows a normal RBC film magnified 1000 times. *Anisocytosis* is said to exist when there are abnormal variations in cell size (Fig. 11-3).

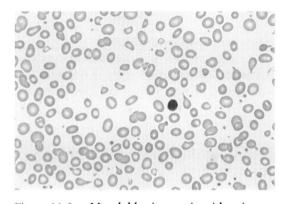

Figure 11-3.   **Megaloblastic anemia with anisocytosis and macrocytosis.** Abnormal variation in cell size (anisocytosis) is evident. Large, nucleated, oval-shaped megaloblasts can also be seen.

The presence of great numbers of large (>10 µm) RBCs is called *macrocytosis*. This condition is also seen in Figure 11-3. Conversely, the presence of great numbers of small (<5 µm) RBCs is called *microcytosis* (Fig. 11-4).

Cell size is measured in the clinical laboratory using the *mean corpuscular volume (MCV) index*. Normal MCV is 90 (±8) femptoliters (fL).[388] Decreased [Hb] associated with an MCV less than 82 fL is called *microcytic anemia*; decreased [Hb] associated with an MCV greater than 98 fL is called *macrocytic anemia*.

Red Blood Cell Shape

Abnormalities in the shape of RBCs are called *poikilocytosis*. An example of a cell with an abnormal shape is the *megaloblast*. These cells are large (11 to 20 µm), nucleated RBCs that are oval and slightly irregular in shape (see Fig. 11-3). Megaloblasts are found in anemia due to vitamin B_{12} deficiency (i.e., pernicious anemia) or in folic acid deficiency.

Immature Red Blood Cells

The presence of large numbers of immature RBCs in the blood suggests that anemia may be due to acute blood loss. Under normal conditions, between 0.5% and 1.5% of RBCs are in the immature form known as *reticulocytes* (Fig. 11-5).[389] The presence of increased reticulocytes in the blood is called *reticulocytosis*.

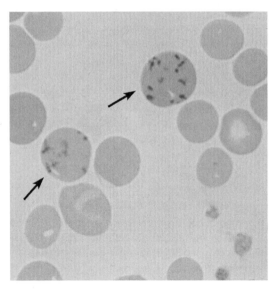

Figure 11-5. **Reticulocyte(s), peripheral blood** (×1000, new methylene blue stain).

Reticulocytosis leads to rapid oxygen consumption in acquired blood samples and may lower blood PaO_2 if not measured promptly. Another type of immature RBC, the *normoblast*, is not normally found in the blood but may be observed in anemia secondary to acute blood loss. A normoblast is a nucleated RBC similar in size to a normal RBC.

Mean Corpuscular Hemoglobin Concentration

The percentage of the RBC volume occupied by Hb is another useful diagnostic aid in anemia. Normally, approximately one-third of the RBC consists of Hb. The clinical laboratory test used to evaluate RBC [Hb] is the *mean corpuscular hemoglobin concentration* (*MCHC*). Normal MCHC is $34 \pm 2\%$[388] and is called *normochromia*. *Hyperchromia* (MCHC >36%) is rare; however, *hypochromia* (MCHC

<32%) is seen commonly in iron deficiency anemia (see Fig. 11-4).

Summary

Table 11-1 compares MCV and MCHC. Table 11-2 summarizes many of the terms used in describing RBCs when diagnosing anemia. Common types of anemia associated with each laboratory finding are also shown in Box 11-3.

Types of Anemia

Some of the more common types of anemia are briefly discussed here to acquaint the reader with the variety of potential anemic mechanisms (see Table 11-2). The presence of anemia means either (1) that there is a decrease in the production of RBCs or hemoglobin or (2) that RBCs or Hb is being lost or destroyed at an accelerated rate.

Decreased production may be due to a problem at the production site (i.e., bone marrow) or to a deficiency in one of the necessary constituents for RBC/Hb production. On the other hand, accelerated loss or destruction may be due to excessive rupture (hemolysis) of RBCs or to excessive blood loss.

Bone Marrow Failure

Abnormal development (aplasia) of the bone marrow may occur without apparent cause, but more commonly this condition follows exposure to some chemical or physical agent. Chemical agents known to be associated with *aplastic anemia* include the drug chloramphenicol, insecticides such as DDT, and arsenic. Physical causes include excessive exposure to radiation.

Inadequate Hemoglobin Synthesis

The most common problem in Hb synthesis is iron deficiency. Iron supply is normally not a problem, because iron is recycled following

Table 11-1. RED BLOOD CELL INDICES

Mean Corpuscular Volume (MCV)	Mean Corpuscular Hemoglobin Concentration (MCHC)
Measurement of average size or volume of individual RBCs	Measurement of average [Hb] in 100 mL of packed RBCs
Normal value: 90 ± 8 fL	Normal value: 34 ± 2%
MCV <82 fL indicates microcytosis	MCHC <32% indicates hypochromia
MCV >98 fL indicates macrocytosis	MCHC >36% indicates hyperchromia

Table 11-2. Erythrocyte Abnormalities

Terminology	Description	Types of Anemia
Anisocytes	Abnormal variations in cell size	Nonspecific
Hypochromia	Pale cells due to decreased [Hb] within cell	Iron deficiency
Macrocytes	Large cells greater than 10 μ	Pernicious anemia and folic acid deficiency
Megaloblasts	Large, oval, irregular, nucleated cells	Pernicious anemia and folic acid deficiency
Microcytes	Small cells less than 5 μ	Iron deficiency, thalassemia
Normoblasts	Immature, nucleated red blood cells of normal size	Acute blood loss
Poikilocytes	Abnormal variations in cell shape	Nonspecific
Reticulocytes	Immature red blood cells containing a network of granules or filaments	Acute blood loss
Sickle cells	Crescent or sickle-shaped cells	Sickle cell anemia

the destruction of old RBCs. However, when iron is lost from the body, as in hemorrhage, or when additional iron is required, such as in pregnancy, it may be in short supply for Hb production.

Probably the most common cause of *iron deficiency anemia* is chronic blood loss. It may also be seen in infants or in mothers during pregnancy. An interesting diagnostic characteristic observed in some individuals with iron deficiency is *pagophagia*.[438] Pagophagia is a type of "pica" or craving for unusual substances. Pagophagia is a strong craving for ice and is the most common type of pica seen in iron deficiency anemia. Pica occurs in up to 58% of patients with iron deficiency.[438]

In recent years, severe iron deficiency has become relatively uncommon. Nevertheless, mild iron deficiency is still far too common and can have damaging long-term consequences.[439]

| **Box 11-3** | Common Types of Anemia |

Small Red Blood Cells (Microcytic)
   Iron deficiency (chronic hemorrhage)
   Thalassemia
Large Red Blood Cells (Macrocytic)
   Folic acid deficiency
   Vitamin B$_{12}$ deficiency (pernicious anemia)
Normal-sized Red Blood Cells (Normocytic)
   Hemolytic
   Aplastic
   Acute hemorrhagic

Thus, we must continue to be vigilant in its identification and prevention.

Production of Hb may be abnormal in a genetic disorder called *thalassemia*. Thalassemia, also known as *Cooley's anemia* or *Mediterranean disease*, may manifest itself in one of two forms: *thalassemia major* is a severe form of the disease that may be associated with severe anemia; *thalassemia minor* is a milder form.

Inadequate production of Hb is associated with hypochromia and the presence of small RBCs (microcytosis).

Inadequate Red Blood Cell Formation

Production of RBCs depends on an adequate supply of folic acid, vitamin B$_{12}$, and the hormone erythropoietin. Folic acid is plentiful in green leafy vegetables. Alcohol, however, interferes with the metabolism of folic acid. Therefore, poor diet or alcoholism may lead to *folic acid deficiency*.

Vitamin B$_{12}$, sometimes referred to as *extrinsic factor*, is normally absorbed in the stomach. This absorption is facilitated through a substance that has been labeled *intrinsic factor*. Individuals lacking in this intrinsic factor may develop anemia due to vitamin B$_{12}$ deficiency. Anemia that develops by this mechanism is known as *pernicious anemia*.

Anemia is also common in chronic renal failure and is due at least in part to decreased erythropoietin. Some loss of RBCs into the urine may also occur due to increased permeability of the diseased glomerulus.

Anemia due to folic acid or vitamin B_{12} deficiency leads to a high number of large RBCs (i.e., macrocytosis). In addition, megaloblasts may be observed in the blood of these individuals.

Red Blood Cell Loss/Hemolysis

Immediately after acute blood loss, [RBC] may be normal. Soon after, however, fluid enters the blood from the interstitial space and thus leads to anemia.

Hemolysis is usually the result of the presence of toxins in the blood. Toxins may originate from infectious processes or may directly enter the blood, such as in poisonous snakebites. Many chemical agents may be associated with hemolysis. Finally, chronic hemolysis with acute exacerbation may occur in disorders such as sickle-cell disease (see Chapter 7) or thalassemia.

The pain rate (episodes per year) is a useful measure of the severity of sickle cell disease.[440] Treatment, which has been discussed briefly in Chapter 7, may include bone marrow transplant, or more commonly, administration of pharmacological agents (e.g., hydroxyurea) aimed at increasing the amount of fetal Hb (HbF).[441] Increases in HbF have an ameliorating effect on the disease and symptoms. Many of these chemotherapeutic agents, however, may cause adverse effects and drugs with less potential of side effects (e.g., butyrate) continue to be explored.[441]

Reticulocyte levels typically are increased in conditions associated with hemolysis or blood loss. In most long-term hemolytic anemias, reticulocytes exceed 5%.[390] When evaluating the reticulocyte levels, however, one must keep in mind that reticulocytes are usually expressed as a percentage of total RBCs.

It is probably better to think in terms of the actual count of reticulocytes rather than the percentage. The normal actual count of reticulocytes is about 50,000 cells/mm^3 or 1% of [RBC]. If [RBC] decreases from 5 million to 2.5 million/mm^3, and the reticulocyte count remains constant (i.e., 50,000 cells), the percentage of reticulocytes would be 2%. If the *actual* reticulocyte count is not considered, this could be wrongly interpreted as an increase in RBC production.

The presence of normoblasts in the blood is abnormal and a sign of accelerated RBC production. Anemia secondary to the loss of RBCs is typically normocytic in laboratory analysis.

Anemia and Hypoxia

Surprisingly, mild anemia (i.e., [Hb] 10 g%) usually will *not* result in hypoxia. The large reserve of O_2 normally present in the blood and the body's compensatory mechanisms both tend to ensure adequate tissue oxygenation. As discussed previously, usually only about 25% of the oxygen in arterial blood is extracted by the tissues; therefore, mild anemia does not substantially affect tissue O_2 supply.

Furthermore, the body responds to anemia by increasing cardiac output and increasing 2,3-diphosphoglycerate (DPG) levels. In healthy individuals, mild, acute normovolemic anemia is compensated for by increases in cardiac output up to 50%.[391] Within 2 weeks the cardiac output returns to preanemic levels, with an increase in DPG accounting for the compensation. Thus, the major compensatory mechanism in *acute* anemia is an increased cardiac output, whereas in *chronic* conditions, increases in DPG prevail.

In moderate to severe anemia (i.e., [Hb] = 6 to 9 g%) hypoxia may occur, depending on the cardiac reserve and the acuteness of onset. Anemic hypoxia in all likelihood will be seen when [Hb] falls below 6 g% and the capabilities of compensatory mechanisms are exceeded.[392]

Blood Transfusions

Blood transfusion is the treatment of choice for severe anemia; however, this therapy may be associated with substantial risk. Some adverse effect to blood transfusion may occur in as many as 20% of recipients.[442] Immune side effects are seen in approximately 3% of all transfusions.[393] Typically these are mild allergic reactions, although potentially fatal hemolytic reactions are observed in approximately one of 6000 transfusions.[393]

In addition, anaphylactic reactions may occur, and not infrequently patients contract post-transfusion hepatitis.[393] Finally, blood is a complex substance and may carry with it additional risk factors not yet clearly identified. The acquired immunodeficiency syndrome has been a painful lesson in this regard.

The ideal hematocrit and [Hb] in critically ill patients are also a matter of some controversy. Certainly, Hct need not be within the normal range in order to ensure adequate oxygenation. Optimal levels are probably somewhere between 30% and 45% depending on the individual's particular pathology.[394,437] There is some evidence to suggest that the optimal hematocrit in critically ill patients is about 33% (see Fig. 11-1), because further increases do not result in increased cellular O_2 availability.[395] Obviously, low Hct levels are associated with decreased ability of the blood to carry oxygen. In contrast, high Hct levels increase blood viscosity and thereby dampen cardiac output.

A [Hb] blood transfusion trigger of less than 7.0 g/dL has been recommended and is probably a useful guideline.[444] Nevertheless, at high altitude, or for patients with brain injury, a much higher trigger (e.g., 10 g/dL) is probably appropriate.[443]

Circulatory Status

Cardiac Output

The cardiovascular system is the core of the human oxygenation system. The *cardiac minute output* (abbreviated Q̇ or sometimes CO) is the volume of blood ejected from the left side of the heart each minute. Cardiac output is a crucial index concerning tissue oxygenation. Cardiac output is approximately 5 L/min in normal individuals. The *cardiac index* (CI) relates cardiac output to body size and expresses cardiac output as liters per minute per body surface area in square meters (m^2). Thus, the cardiac index should be the same in all individuals regardless of size or weight. The normal cardiac index is 3.5 ± 0.7 L/min/m^2.

Measurement

The cardiac output can be measured easily by thermodilution technique or can be calculated using the Fick equation if a pulmonary artery (Swan-Ganz) catheter is in place. Placement of a pulmonary artery catheter is an invasive procedure with potentially serious complications. Therefore, insertion of these catheters is usually restricted to critically ill patients in the intensive care unit who require precise monitoring of fluid balance and function of the left side of the heart.

In recent years, noninvasive cardiac output monitors have become available that facilitate measurement of cardiac output in the absence of a Swan-Ganz catheter.[445] These devices, which make use of the Fick equation, have been shown to be reasonably accurate in clinical situations.

Clinical Assessment

Notwithstanding, in many clinical situations, cardiac output must be assessed indirectly. This assessment is accomplished through evaluation of a host of clinical signs and symptoms. Urine output, neurologic status, blood pressure, pulse, capillary refill (i.e., the speed at which color returns to the skin after it is depressed), cyanosis, and warmth of extremities all provide clues about the adequacy of circulation. Although all these indicators provide useful information, they cannot replace actual measurement of cardiac output when it is in serious question.

Even when cardiac output is measured, however, complete cardiovascular assessment must include sequential evaluation of the three basic components of the cardiovascular system: (1) the pump (heart), (2) the fluid (blood), and (3) the tubules (blood vessels). The interaction of these three components determines the important cardiovascular parameters of cardiac output and arterial blood pressure. Furthermore, this chronologic assessment aids in determining the root cause of any cardiovascular disturbance.

Shock

Shock is a state of collapse of the cardiovascular system usually associated with a loss of arterial blood pressure. The signs and symptoms of shock are a result of inadequate perfusion to a particular organ or may be due to the compensatory response of the central nervous system to the shock state. The sympathetic portion of the autonomic nervous system is typically stimulated in shock, resulting in the release of epinephrine and norepinephrine. These substances, in turn, lead to an increased heart rate and constriction of peripheral blood vessels, which represents an attempt of the body to preserve cardiac output and arterial blood pressure.

Clinical Symptoms

Restlessness, anxiety, or alteration in consciousness may be early signs of shock caused by decreased cerebral perfusion. Cyanosis, decreased urine output, and lactic acidosis may likewise suggest poor perfusion status. Rapid breathing and respiratory alkalosis are often observed with shock, presumably as a secondary response to hypoperfusion mediated through the peripheral chemoreceptors or as a result of high $\dot{V}/\dot{Q}$ in the lungs.

Vasoconstriction secondary to the release of norepinephrine and, to a lesser extent, epinephrine may also lead to cold, pale extremities. Sympathetic stimulation of the sweat glands in conjunction with the peripheral vasoconstriction tends to make the skin appear cold and clammy.

Etiology

Shock may occur due to failure of the heart as a pump; failure to maintain an adequate blood volume, as in hemorrhage; or failure of the blood vessels to maintain adequate muscular tone, as in vasodilation with subsequent loss of pressure. Systematic evaluation of the cardiovascular system in shock should proceed by individually assessing each of these three components.

Pump Effectiveness

Cardiac output is the product of heart rate and stroke volume. Thus, pump effectiveness depends on the frequency of beats (heart rate) and the volume of blood ejected with each beat (stroke volume).

Heart Rate and Stroke Volume. Normal heart rate is approximately 70 beats per minute. Slower rates tend to reduce cardiac output unless they are accompanied by a concurrent increase in stroke volume. Well-trained athletes often manifest bradycardia (decreased heart rate) but maintain a normal cardiac output. In this case, cardiac output remains normal because of the enhanced stroke volume performance of the conditioned heart muscle.

Conversely, high cardiac rates tend to increase cardiac output. When the heart rate increases to approximately 2 to $2\frac{1}{2}$ times normal, however, cardiac output tends to drop. This occurs because the rapid heart rate does not allow for appropriate filling of the heart between beats. Therefore, cardiac output actually decreases in severe tachycardia due to the simultaneous fall in stroke volume.

Congestive Heart Failure. Pump effectiveness may be diminished acutely when heart muscle is not adequately perfused or oxygenated, as in *myocardial infarction* (heart attack). A similar situation may occur in chronic hypertension where the heart is faced with relentless pumping against substantial resistance. When the heart is unable to pump the blood within it, congestion of blood occurs in the heart; thus, the name *congestive heart failure* (CHF). CHF may be the result of a faulty heart valve, inadequate oxygenation of heart muscle (e.g., in myocardial infarction), fluid overload of the heart, or prolonged stress on the heart from pumping against high resistance (e.g., in chronic hypertension).

When CHF originates from the left side of the heart, congestion also accumulates in the lungs (i.e., pulmonary edema). Symptoms of acute left-sided heart failure include edema, jugular vein distention, hypoxemia, shortness of breath, abnormal heart sounds, and fine crackles in the lung fields. The diagnosis is confirmed when the chest radiograph shows increased hilar markings and lung fluid. Also, hemodynamic measurements typically display high pressures in the heart.

Optimal management of severe left-sided heart failure often includes insertion of a Swan-Ganz catheter in the pulmonary artery. Presence of this catheter allows for monitoring of the pulmonary wedge pressure, as described later. Pulmonary wedge pressure is an excellent index of the function of the left side of the heart and congestive heart failure. Furthermore, it is a very useful index to follow in fluid management and the *treatment* of left-sided heart failure.

Cardiogenic Shock. Cardiovascular collapse due to failure of the heart as a pump is called *cardiogenic shock*, because its origin is the

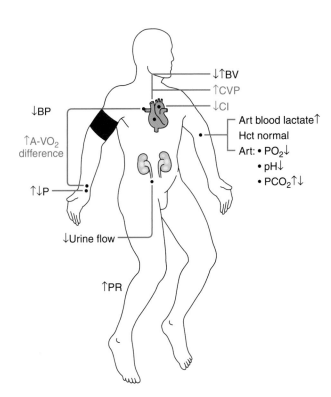

Figure 11-6.   **Cardiogenic shock.** The principal hemodynamic and metabolic abnormalities seen in cardiogenic shock.

heart itself. Figure 11-6 shows some of the principal hemodynamic and metabolic changes that are associated with cardiogenic shock.

Blood Volume

The output of the heart as a pump can never exceed its input; thus, cardiac output volume cannot exceed venous return volume. *Venous return* is the amount of blood returning to the right side of the heart. Inadequate venous return, regardless of cause, results in a decreased cardiac output. The loss of 20% of total blood volume may reduce arterial pressure by 15% and cardiac output by 41%.[446]

Hypovolemia. A decrease in blood volume is called *hypovolemia*. Hypovolemia may be *absolute*, such as in the case of hemorrhage with the actual loss of blood; alternatively, hypovolemia may be *relative*, as in the case of systemic vasodilation and pooling of blood in the extremities. Relative hypovolemia also may result from loss of intravascular fluid to the interstitial space, which can occur in burn injuries. Regardless of whether hypovolemia is relative or absolute, fluids must be administered in sufficient quantities to reverse the

hypovolemia and maintain an adequate cardiac output.

When a central venous pressure line is in place, low central venous pressure readings are a good indication of hypovolemia. In the absence of invasive monitoring, however, the patient should be evaluated for clinical signs of hypovolemia. These include dried mucous membranes, tachycardia, postural hypotension (falling arterial pressure upon assumption of the standing position), high specific gravity of the urine, and poor skin turgor.

Hypovolemic Shock. Cardiovascular collapse secondary to inadequate blood volume is termed *hypovolemic shock*. When the shock is due to actual internal or external bleeding, it may also be termed *hemorrhagic shock*. Hemorrhagic shock is commonly observed following trauma or surgery. Figure 11-7 shows some of the principal hemodynamic and metabolic changes seen in hypovolemic or hemorrhagic shock.

The long-term intensive care unit (ICU) population often requires transfusion due to the excessive loss of blood used for laboratory diagnosis. In one example, 85% of all patients

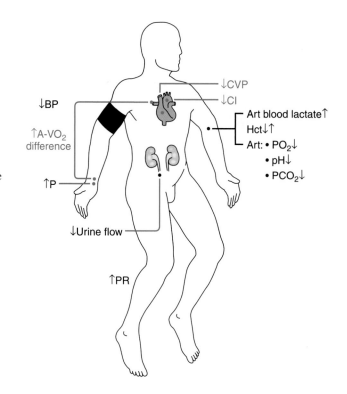

Figure 11-7. Hypovolemic shock. The principal hemodynamic and metabolic abnormalities seen in hypovolemic or traumatic shock.

who were in ICU for more than 7 days required blood transfusions.[453] Therefore, decreasing phlebotomy blood loss is an important goal in ICU patient management.

Vascular Tone

Maintenance of arterial blood pressure and cardiovascular integrity requires the presence of some muscle tone (vasoconstriction) in the peripheral circulation. If all peripheral arterioles were to dilate simultaneously, arterial pressure would fall to dangerous levels.[396] Vascular tone throughout the body is an important factor that affects blood pressure, heart work, and the allocation of perfusion. The muscular tone of peripheral vessels must be carefully controlled to minimize cardiac stress while providing optimal cardiac output, blood pressure, and cellular perfusion.

Neurogenic Shock. There are several types of shock in which there is a loss of vascular tone with a subsequent decrease in blood pressure. In *neurogenic shock*, nervous system control of vascular tone is lost and may result in profound vasodilation. This may occur after an injury such as a fractured spine or after cardiac arrest.

Psychogenic shock (fainting) is a similar albeit less serious phenomenon in which transient vasodilation results from an emotional stimulus or because of extreme heat or exhaustion.

Septic Shock. Profound vasodilation may also result from a chemical origin. This may be secondary to the presence of some toxin in the blood, as in *septic shock*, or to administration of a foreign substance into the body, with a subsequent severe allergic reaction. Septic shock is a condition caused by infection or an inflammatory reaction in the blood. In septic shock, cardiac output is usually quite high. Nevertheless, blood pressure may still be low and tissue perfusion may not be adequate because of the profound vasodilation. The principal hemodynamic and metabolic changes seen in septic shock are shown in Figure 11-8. It is becoming increasingly clear that increases in cardiac output are not always distributed ideally throughout the body and that the distribution of blood may be a critical, yet often neglected variable.

Anaphylactic Shock. When severe vasodilation is secondary to an allergic reaction, the condition is termed *anaphylactic shock*. Anaphylactic shock is mediated by the release

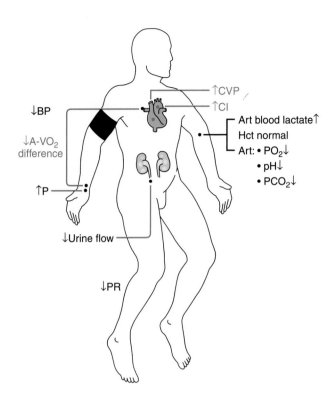

↑CVP

↑CI

↓BP

↓A-VO$_2$
difference

↑P

↓Urine flow

↓PR

Art blood lactate↑
Hct normal
Art: • PO$_2$↓
      • pH↓
      • PCO$_2$↓

Figure 11-8. **Septic shock.** The principal hemodynamic and metabolic abnormalities seen in hyperdynamic septic shock.

of histamine, which is a potent vasodilator. Anaphylaxis may be responsible for as many as 500 deaths each year.[447]

Even when anaphylaxis is anticipated and rapidly treated by experienced personnel, severe reactions may not respond. The treatment of choice in anaphylactic shock is the administration of epinephrine (a sympathomimetic drug) to maintain cardiac output and increase vascular tone. It is also probably best to hospitalize all patients with serious anaphylaxis for 24 hours because relapses may occur.[447]

Summary

It is evident that the presence of shock or a decrease in cardiac output may originate from the heart, the blood, or the tone of the peripheral blood vessels. Clinical evaluation of the cardiovascular system requires that each of these three components be considered as a possible source of cardiovascular disturbance.

Hemodynamic Monitoring

As alluded to previously, it is common to perform hemodynamic monitoring in the critical care setting, particularly in the management of congestive heart failure. Therefore, the clinician should be familiar with some of the basic terminology, techniques, and values used in hemodynamic evaluation. Just as the term implies, *hemodynamic* refers to *blood movement* and to the various pressures generated throughout the cardiovascular system because of this movement.

Arterial Blood Pressure

Historically, arterial blood pressure has been the clinician's primary hemodynamic measurement. In the past, priority was placed on the maintenance of arterial blood pressure. Drugs were liberally administered to ensure that arterial blood pressure remained at a satisfactory level. Unfortunately, cardiac output was sometimes adversely affected by efforts that were focused solely on the blood pressure. It is now recognized that the maintenance of cardiac output is of greater importance than the maintenance of the blood pressure *per se.*

Arterial blood pressure is usually measured indirectly using a blood pressure cuff and pressure gauge (sphygmomanometer). When continuous monitoring of arterial blood pressure is desirable, insertion of an arterial line may be useful. Newer, noninvasive devices are also available for continuous monitoring.

Upon insertion, an arterial line allows for (1) continuous monitoring of blood pressure, (2) arterial blood gas sampling, and (3) more precise measurement of arterial blood pressure than possible with indirect assessment. Although useful, arterial blood pressure monitoring provides only limited information about overall cardiovascular status. Furthermore, it is an invasive monitor that increases the risk of infection.

Central Venous Pressure

A *central venous pressure* (CVP) line is a more sophisticated form of hemodynamic assessment. A CVP line is a catheter placed in a peripheral vein and threaded into the superior vena cava or the right atrium of the heart. Thus, the CVP reflects the right atrial pressure (RAP). Normal CVP is 2 to 10 mm Hg. A high CVP (>20 mm Hg) suggests congestive heart failure or fluid overload with subsequent backup of fluid in the heart. An extremely low CVP, on the other hand, may indicate hypovolemia.

Pulmonary Artery Pressure

Pulmonary Artery Catheter. A more accurate technique with which to evaluate hemodynamic status is the Swan-Ganz pulmonary artery catheter. An illustration of a pulmonary artery catheter is shown in Figure 11-9. This multilumen catheter is inserted similarly to the CVP catheter. Insertion differs, however, in that the catheter actually passes through the right side of the heart and into the pulmonary circulation. Figure 11-10 shows how the catheter moves through the heart and the corresponding pressure tracings that are normally found as it passes through the heart.

Pulmonary Artery Catheter Insertion. Movement of the catheter through the heart is accomplished by inflating a small balloon on the catheter tip, which allows the catheter to float through the heart chambers. Thus, the pulmonary artery catheter is often referred to as a balloon flotation catheter. As illustrated in Figure 11-10, the catheter is actually inserted until it wedges in a pulmonary artery, whereupon the balloon is deflated.

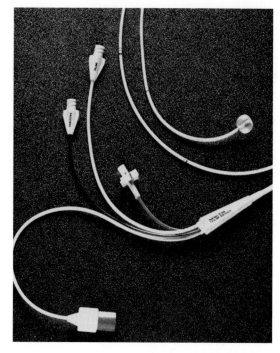

Figure 11-9.   **Pulmonary artery catheter.**

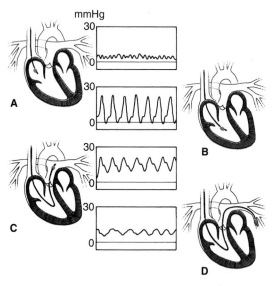

Figure 11-10.   **Pulmonary catheter insertion.** Insertion of a Swan-Ganz balloon flotation catheter into the pulmonary artery with accompanying pressure tracings at each step. **A,** Right atrium. **B,** Right ventricle. **C,** Pulmonary artery. **D,** Pulmonary artery "wedge" position.

While the balloon is deflated, the pressure measured through the catheter is the *pulmonary artery pressure* (PAP) (see Fig. 11-10,C). Normal PAP is 25 mm Hg systolic and 10 mm Hg diastolic. Increases in pulmonary vascular resistance (PVR), such as may occur with pulmonary emboli or severe hypoxemia or acidemia, are reflected by an increase in PAP. Pulmonary vascular resistance may also increase with positive end-expiratory pressure (PEEP) therapy. Left-sided heart failure also increases the PAP.

Pulmonary Wedge Pressure

Technique. Insertion of a Swan-Ganz catheter also allows for measurement of the *pulmonary wedge pressure* (PWP). PWP is the pressure obtained when the balloon on the catheter is inflated and forward blood flow cannot proceed past the catheter tip. Therefore, the pressure being measured is actually a measure of backpressure from the left side of the heart. In most clinical situations, PWP closely parallels the left ventricular end-diastolic filling pressure (LVEDP), which is very informative regarding function of the left side of the heart. Normal PWP is approximately 5 to 12 mm Hg.[397,398]

Increased Pulmonary Wedge Pressure. The concept of *preload* refers to the filling volume within the ventricles of the heart before contraction. Clinically, the pressure within the ventricles (rather than the volume) before contraction is used as an indicator of preload. Pressure is used because it is easier to measure than volume and because normally there is a good relationship between preload pressure and volume. The CVP is an indicator of right ventricular preload, whereas the PWP is an index of left ventricular preload.

In contrast to preload, the concept of *afterload* refers to the resistance or impedance that the heart must pump against. Diastolic blood pressure and vascular resistance contribute to the afterload. High pulmonary vascular resistance contributes to a high afterload for the right side of the heart. Similarly, arterial hypertension suggests increased afterload for the left side of the heart. High afterload contributes to increased heart work. (The pulmonary artery catheter, however, is used primarily to evaluate preload.)

Starling's curve shows that normally the heart muscle increases its force of contraction in response to an increase in preload. Therefore, as preload increases, myocardial performance and cardiac output likewise increase. When pulmonary wedge pressure exceeds 18 to 20 mm Hg, however, the left ventricle is unable to handle the increased filling pressure, and left-sided heart failure ensues.[399]

At this point, therapeutic measures must be undertaken to reduce the pressure. Therapy in CHF typically includes digitalis to improve the force of ventricular contraction and furosemide (Lasix) to reduce the filling pressure of the heart. These measures allow the heart to function more effectively and thereby reduce the buildup of pulmonary edema.

Thus, PWP serves as an excellent means to monitor left-sided heart function or failure. It has been shown that PWP is a more accurate indicator of left-sided heart failure than is CVP.[399]

Pulmonary Artery Catheter and Differential Diagnosis

When the Swan-Ganz catheter is properly positioned, both CVP readings and PWP readings can be obtained through different ports in the catheter. The availability of both measurements allows for further clarification of the cardiovascular status. For example, *cardiogenic shock* can be differentiated from *hypovolemic shock*. Shock of cardiac origin is associated with an increased PWP, whereas hypovolemic shock shows a relatively normal PWP and a low CVP.

Various different hemodynamic values either can be directly measured or can be calculated with a pulmonary artery catheter in place. Table 11-3 gives normal ranges for various hemodynamic measurements and calculations. Table 11-4 lists typical hemodynamic and metabolic findings observed in various types of shock.

The PWP is especially useful in differentiating cardiogenic from noncardiogenic pulmonary edema. *Cardiogenic pulmonary edema* is associated with an increased PWP. Figure 11-11 illustrates the various hemodynamic changes associated with cardiogenic shock and CHF. Conversely, if the pulmonary edema is

Table 11-3. NORMAL RANGES OF
HEMODYNAMIC VALUES

Pressures	Normal Range
Central venous pressure (CVP)	2–10 mm Hg
Right ventricle	
Systolic	15–30 mm Hg
Diastolic	0–5 mm Hg
Pulmonary artery	
Systolic	15–30 mm Hg
Diastolic	5–12 mm Hg
Mean	11–18 mm Hg
Pulmonary wedge	5–12 mm Hg
Hemodynamics	
Cardiac output	4.4–8.9 L/min
Cardiac index	3.5 ± 0.7 L/min/m^3
Stroke volume	60–129 mL/beat
Stroke volume index	46 ± 3/beat/m^3
Pulmonary vascular resistance	70 ± 20 dyn/sec/cm^{-5}
Arteriovenous O_2 difference	4.0 ± 0.6 mL/100 mL

Modified from Cherniak, R.M., and Cherniak, L.:
Respiration in Health and Disease, 3rd ed. Philadelphia,
W. B. Saunders, 1983, p. 59.

noncardiogenic (e.g., acute respiratory distress syndrome [ARDS]), then the PWP is relatively normal. Characteristics of these two entities are compared in Table 11-5.

Pulmonary Artery Diastolic Pressure

It is noteworthy that the pulmonary artery diastolic pressure is close to the PWP in the absence of pulmonary disease (i.e., normal PVR). Thus, if there is some technical reason why PWP readings cannot be obtained (e.g., cannot get catheter to wedge), diastolic pulmonary artery pressure readings could be substituted in the patient with *normal pulmonary status*. On the other hand, the presence of increased pulmonary vascular resistance is characterized by an increased PAP with no increase in PWP. This could be the result of a pulmonary embolus or of pulmonary vasoconstriction secondary to severe hypoxemia or acidemia.

Cardiac Output/P$\bar{v}O_2$

Catheters equipped with thermistors (temperature sensors) near their tips permit easy determination of cardiac output via the thermodilution technique. Furthermore, mixed venous blood gas samples can be acquired through these catheters. Mixed venous gases can provide still more information regarding the status of tissue oxygenation.

Some pulmonary artery catheters can also measure mixed venous oxygen saturation continuously; others are equipped with cardiac pacemakers. The use of pulmonary artery catheters in the critical care setting remains somewhat controversial due to the lack of data on mortality and complications. Nevertheless, most believe the development of pulmonary artery catheters has been a valuable breakthrough in critical care medicine.

Left Atrial Pressure

In some institutions, a catheter may be placed directly into the left atrium to monitor left ventricular function. Normal values for left atrial

Table 11-4. HEMODYNAMIC AND METABOLIC DIFFERENCES IN VARIOUS TYPES OF SHOCK

Type of Shock	Arterial Blood Pressure	Pulse Rate	PWP/ CVP	Cardiac Index	Urine Flow	Response to Volume Load	PaO$_2$	C (a–$\bar{v}$)O$_2$	Aterial Blood Lactate
Hypovolemic	↓†	↑‡	↓	↓	↓	↑	↓	↑	↑
Cardiogenic	↓	↑ or ↓	↑	↓	↓	↓	↓	↑	↑
Neurogenic	↓	↑	↓	↓	↓	↓	↓	↑	↑
Septic (hyperdynamic)	↓	↑	↑	↑	↓	↓	↓	↓	↑

†↓ = decreased.
‡↑ = increased.
From Sabiston, D.C., Jr.: Davis-Christopher Textbook of Surgery, 11th ed. Philadelphia, W. B. Saunders, 1977, p. 73.

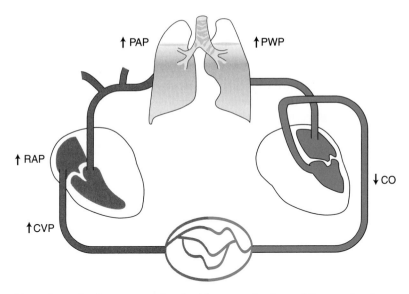

Figure 11-11.   **Hemodynamic changes associated with congestive heart failure and pulmonary edema.**
CVP, central venous pressure; RAP, right atrial pressure; PAP, pulmonary artery pressure; PWP, pulmonary
artery wedge pressure; CO, cardiac output.

pressure are essentially the same as for PWP. Obviously, this is a more direct measurement and may be more accurate; however, it is unclear whether this degree of precision is really necessary. Certainly Swan-Ganz catheters are more widely used and accepted.

Treatment

A detailed discussion of treatment of cardiovascular disorders is beyond the scope of this text. Nevertheless, a brief description of some of the fundamentals of treatment of cardiovascular disorders is appropriate. Two major aspects of treatment are considered: (1) optimization of venous return, and (2) drug intervention.

Optimization of Venous Return

Venous return is most readily manipulated via intravenous infusions or alteration of body position. Venous return should be enhanced in noncardiogenic shock by elevating the feet and increasing the volume of intravenous therapy. A fluid challenge of 50 to 200 mL until PWP increases by at least 3 mm Hg may be a useful approach to the treatment of relative hypovolemia.[10]

Conversely, venous return should be *decreased* in the treatment of cardiogenic shock and heart failure. This can be accomplished by having the patient assume a sitting position and by positive pressure breathing, administration of diuretics, and/or fluid restriction.

Table 11-5.   CATEGORIES OF PULMONARY EDEMA

Feature	Cardiogenic	Noncardiogenic
Major etiologies	Left ventricular failure, Mitral stenosis	ARDS†
Pulmonary wedge pressure	Increased	Normal
Pulmonary capillary permeability	Normal	Increased
Protein content of edema fluid	Low	High

†ARDS = acute respiratory distress syndrome.
From Weinberger, S.E.: Principles of Pulmonary Medicine. Philadelphia, W. B. Saunders, 1986, p. 301.

Precise regulation of fluids may require insertion of a pulmonary artery catheter.

Drug Intervention

In a very simplistic approach, cardiovascular drugs generally affect one of the following: heart rate (chronotropic effect), arrhythmia (abnormal heart beat) control, vascular tone, or the force of cardiac contraction (i.e., ejection volume). A general pharmacology text or publication should be consulted for a more detailed, current review.

KEY INDICATORS OF HYPOXIA

Lactate

The cells have a remarkable ability to withstand challenges in oxygen supply. Indeed, it requires only a PO_2 of 1 mm Hg to maintain cellular respiration at maximal levels.[437] The immediate response of the cell to hypoxia is the onset of anaerobic (without O_2) metabolism. The two major anaerobic pathways are glycolysis and the creatine kinase reaction.

In glycolysis, pyruvate becomes the terminal electron acceptor; in the process, pyruvate is reduced to lactate and lactic acid accumulates. The excess lactic acid in the blood may serve as an indirect measure of hypoxia. Because lactic acid is almost completely dissociated at the physiologic pH of the blood, the lactate anion is measured as an index of lactic acid in the blood (blood lactate concentration). At rest, normal blood lactate concentration is 0.9 to 1.9 mM/L.[400] In milligram per deciliter units, normal blood lactate concentration is 8 to 17 mg/dL (conversion factor is 9 × mM/L = mg/dL). In the past, lactate measurements were of little use because the laboratory turnaround time was nearly 2 hours. Presently, lactate can be measured within 90 seconds, which makes it considerably more useful.[459]

Often, a patient with marginal oxygenation status will not have a lactate level on the laboratory report but will have an unexplained metabolic acidosis. The combination of metabolic acidosis and marginal oxygenation status, and especially when the cardiac output is in question, is highly suggestive of tissue hypoxia and lactic acidosis.

Mortality

Elevated blood lactate concentration (*hyperlactatemia*) is most often the result of tissue hypoxia. In addition, the severity of hyperlactatemia correlates with mortality in lactic acidosis and shock and, as such, is a useful prognostic index.[401,402] In particular, there is a striking increase in mortality as lactate increases above 2.5 mM/L[403]; thus, lactate values greater than this should be clearly considered clinically significant. Furthermore, when blood lactate concentration increases to a level greater than 8 mM/L and remains there for more than 2 hours, mortality increases to 90%.[401]

Sensitivity

Although blood lactate elevation is usually observed in severe shock, lactate is not a highly sensitive indicator of hypoxia.[400,404,405] This is because lactic acid levels do not rise linearly with progressive hypoxia; rather, they rise rapidly in the first few minutes of hypoxia, with production falling off as energy stores are depleted.[406] Blood lactate levels may also be 10 times higher inside the cell than in the blood immediately outside the cell where it is typically measured.[405] Indeed, in animal models, lactate doesn't increase until perfusion is restored.[436] Obviously, lactate may be a late marker of tissue hypoxia.

Furthermore, the normal liver takes up excess lactate quickly in the presence of normal perfusion.[407] In addition, it is generally assumed that the ability of the liver to remove lactate is several-fold greater than the ability of the tissues to produce it.[437] Therefore, elevated blood lactate levels are transient unless circulatory failure or liver impairment is also present.[405]

Variations in blood lactate measurements also may occur related to the site of measurement. Arterial blood is better suited than peripheral venous blood as an indicator of generalized hypoxia because arterial blood is representative of the whole body. Venous blood sampled from a pulmonary artery catheter or a central venous catheter (not peripheral venous blood), however, yields lactate concentrations essentially equivalent to those in arterial blood.[402] In clinical practice, a reasonable expectation is that [HCO$_3$] should decrease approximately 1 mEq/L for every 1 mEq/L of lactate accumulation.[436] One mEq/L is equal to one mM/L in univalent ions.

Specificity and the Lactate/Pyruvate Ratio

Another major drawback of blood lactate as an indicator of hypoxia is its *lack of specificity*.[405] An increase in lactate levels may occur in two ways. First, increased lactate is associated with any rise in blood pyruvate (e.g., infusion of pyruvate, glucose, or bicarbonate). Second, blood lactate levels may increase independent of pyruvate, as in hypoxia, liver disease, or during exercise.

The lactate/pyruvate (L/P) ratio is useful for differentiating lactate elevations that are due to *primary hyperlactatemia* (e.g., hypoxia) from elevations that are simply due to increased metabolism of pyruvate *(secondary hyperlactatemia)*. When the L/P ratio is normal (i.e., 10:1), the elevation in lactate level is due to secondary hyperlactatemia.

An L/P ratio in excess of 10:1 is called *primary hyperlactatemia* or "excess lactate." Primary hyperlactatemia is most commonly the result of hypoxia; however, other causes have been identified, including liver disease, leukemia, beta-adrenergic drugs,[408] and congenital defects.[409]

Creatine Kinase Reaction

In some organs (e.g., heart, brain, muscle), the creatine kinase reaction provides an anaerobic alternative to glycolysis.[410] In this reaction, stored phosphocreatine transfers a high-energy phosphate bond to adenosine diphosphate (ADP), converting it to adenosine triphosphate (ATP). This anaerobic pathway actually consumes hydrogen ions, in direct contrast to glycolysis, which produces lactic acid. This metabolic pathway is limited, however, by the supply of phosphocreatine.

Cyanide in Smoke Inhalation

The importance of recognition of HbCO in smoke inhalation victims has been described earlier. In evaluating internal respiration, it is important to recognize that the presence of hydrogen cyanide is also a major concern in many cases of smoke inhalation.[460,461] Residential fires may produce cyanide toxicity, which leads to problems with cellular use of oxygen.

In addition, cyanide toxicity is difficult to recognize because cyanide disappears relatively quickly from the blood. Diagnosis is further complicated because laboratory measurement of cyanide may take up to 5 hours.[460]

Increased lactate in victims of smoke inhalation and in the absence of high HbCO levels may suggest cyanide toxicity. Indeed, lactate has been shown to correlate better with cyanide levels than HbCO levels in some cases. Early recognition of cyanide toxicity is important because the patient can be treated with mechanical ventilation, FIO$_2$ 1.0, and nitrites. Nitrites facilitate the formation of methemoglobin, which, in turn, rapidly absorbs cyanide.[461]

Summary

Based on the complex interrelationships in anaerobic metabolism, it is not surprising that clinical studies have often failed to show a good correlation between decreased oxygen transport or low mixed venous oxygen levels and the onset of increased blood lactate levels.[411] On new frontiers, magnetic resonance spectroscopy (MRS) is a technique that holds great promise for measuring intracellular metabolic activity and variables such as phosphocreatine levels and pH.[412]

Although measurement of blood lactate provides us with valuable information regarding hypoxia and prognosis, it is not a sufficiently sensitive or specific index of hypoxia when used alone.

Mixed Venous Oxygenation Indices
Measurement

Mixed venous blood must be distinguished from peripheral venous blood. Blood gases from peripheral venous blood provide us with limited information because they reflect only local conditions. Conversely, mixed venous gases provide us with a more global picture of oxygenation because mixed venous blood is an average of all venous blood returning to the heart.

Table 11-6.   NORMAL MIXED VENOUS
             BLOOD VALUES

$P\bar{v}O_2$	35–45 mm Hg
$S\bar{v}O_2$	75%
$C\bar{v}O_2$	15 vol%
pH	7.38
$P\bar{v}CO_2$	46–48 mm Hg

Unfortunately, mixed venous blood samples are available only when the patient has a pulmonary artery catheter in place. Furthermore, the catheter must be in the proper position if samples are to truly represent mixed venous blood. Normal values for mixed venous blood are shown in Table 11-6.

Mixed Venous Oxygen Saturation

The oxygen saturation of mixed venous blood ($S\bar{v}O_2$) can be measured using a single blood sample or can be monitored continuously using a fiber-optic catheter. Continuous monitoring of $S\bar{v}O_2$ provides a useful way to monitor circulatory changes, because $S\bar{v}O_2$ usually decreases with deterioration of cardiovascular status. In addition, cardiovascular drugs or PEEP therapy may be titrated to optimal dosage through continuous $S\bar{v}O_2$ monitoring.[413] In general, an increase in $S\bar{v}O_2$ is a positive response, whereas a decrease is undesirable. Figure 11-12 illustrates several conditions that may result in a decreased $S\bar{v}O_2$.

Mixed Venous Oxygen Partial Pressure

Mixed venous PO_2 and, to a lesser extent, $S\bar{v}O_2$ have been advocated as useful indicators of hypoxia. The value of mixed venous blood in the assessment of hypoxia lies in the fact that it is a reflection of the *interaction* of the pulmonary and cardiovascular systems. The oxygenation status of arterial blood, on the other hand, is primarily a reflection of only the pulmonary system. Arterial blood provides information regarding *oxygen supply* to the tissues, whereas mixed venous blood provides information regarding the balance of *oxygen supply and demand*.

Mixed venous PO_2 has received considerable attention as an index of hypoxia because it seems to represent the *average end-capillary oxygen-driving pressure*. It is also well known that the body attempts to maintain the end-capillary PO_2 in a variety of hypoxic threats, presumably in an attempt to preserve tissue oxygenation.[414] Mixed venous PO_2 has been purported to be the best single index of tissue hypoxia,[415,416] although other reports dispute this claim.[410,417] A major shortcoming of mixed venous oxygen values is that venous blood is heterogeneous and mixed venous samples depend on the distribution of the cardiac output.

Although it is now clear that mixed venous PO_2 is not always a reliable indicator of

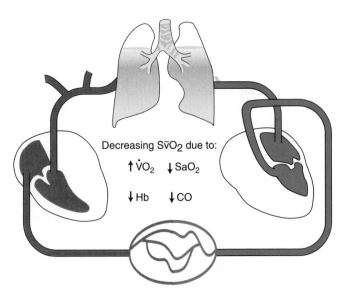

Figure 11-12.   **Causes of decreased $S\bar{v}O_2$.** Potential sources of decreased $S\bar{v}O_2$ include increased oxygen consumption ($\dot{V}O_2$), decreased arterial oxygen saturation (SaO_2), anemia (decreased Hb), and decreased cardiac output (CO).

Decreasing $S\bar{v}O_2$ due to:

↑$\dot{V}O_2$ ↓SaO_2

↓Hb   ↓CO

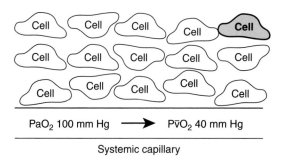

Figure 11-13.   **Normal precapillary and post-capillary PO_2.**

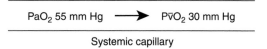

Figure 11-15.   **Moderate hypoxemia without an increased cardiac output.**

hypoxia or cardiac output,[418] it is important to understand why it was initially considered to be the ideal hypoxic index. Whether a given cell in the body receives sufficient oxygen to meet metabolic requirements depends essentially on two factors: (1) the driving pressure propelling oxygen from the capillaries to the cells, and (2) the distance of the cell from the capillary itself.

Driving Pressure

Figure 11-13 illustrates the average normal precapillary and post-capillary PO_2. As the blood traverses the normal (average) capillary, the PaO_2 decreases from approximately 100 to 40 mm Hg. The driving pressure that moves oxygen from the capillaries to the tissues is the difference between the capillary PO_2 and the cellular PO_2. Therefore, the oxygen-driving pressure is lowest at the end of the capillary.

Distance of the Cell from the Capillary

Also, the pressure of oxygen (PO_2) tends to be lowest in those cells that are farthest away from the capillary. Thus, in the theoretical model shown in Figure 11-13, the specific cell that would have the lowest PO_2 would be the cell in the upper right-hand corner.

If we further assume that this cell is just barely oxygenated at normal $P\bar{v}O_2$, it follows that any decrease in $P\bar{v}O_2$ will prohibit oxygenation of this cell and thus lead to hypoxia. If $P\bar{v}O_2$ continues to fall, more and more cells are affected and hypoxia increases in severity. Therefore, as a general guide, hypoxia is probable when $P\bar{v}O_2$ is less than 35 mm Hg.[415]

Clinical Oxygenation Disturbances and $P\bar{v}O_2$

Hypoxemia

The body responds to moderate hypoxemia by increasing cardiac output and thus by maintaining $P\bar{v}O_2$ (Fig. 11-14). Thus, tissue oxygenation ($P\bar{v}O_2$) is preserved despite the fall in oxygen content. The increased cardiac output allows the blood to traverse the capillary more quickly and minimizes the decrease in PO_2. In patients unable to increase cardiac output, $P\bar{v}O_2$ may decrease (Fig. 11-15).

Decreased Cardiac Output and Anemia

In circulatory shock, PaO_2 remains relatively normal; however, $P\bar{v}O_2$ decreases (Fig. 11-16). A similar relationship between PaO_2 and $P\bar{v}O_2$ is observed in hypoxia due to severe anemia or carbon monoxide poisoning.

High $P\bar{v}O_2$ and Hypoxia

In septic shock, hypoxia is not due to the oxygen-driving pressure; rather, it is the result of shunting of blood past the tissues or of cellular metabolic dysfunction. Thus, $P\bar{v}O_2$ in this disorder may actually be increased although the patient still has hypoxia (Fig. 11-17). Interestingly, however, short-term instability

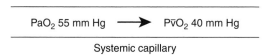

Figure 11-14.   **Moderate hypoxemia with an increased cardiac output.**

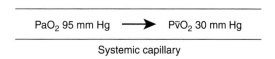

Figure 11-16.   **Circulatory shock.**

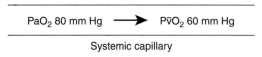

Systemic capillary

Figure 11-17.   **Septic shock.**

may still be recognized in these individuals by acute declines in mixed venous oxygenation from baseline.[454]

A similar paradoxical increase in $P\bar{v}O_2$ is also seen in cyanide poisoning, again because of the inability of the cell to utilize oxygen. $P\bar{v}O_2$ has also been shown to be misleading in various conditions associated with supply-dependent oxygen consumption to be described in the following section.

Clinical Application

In summary, the theory behind changes in mixed venous oxygenation is very useful to understand. Changes in mixed venous oxygen saturation should essentially parallel changes in mixed venous PO_2. Nevertheless, changes in mixed venous oxygenation must always be treated with some degree of suspicion since it is a composite measurement from all organs and tissues. Indeed, some have speculated that a decline in mixed venous PO_2 may be interpreted

as a good sign indicating a return of local vascular control.[437] Notwithstanding, clinical studies seem to indicate that a mixed venous PO_2 less than 28 mm Hg is associated with a poor prognosis.[437]

In clinical practice, saturation is most often monitored because this value can be routinely monitored with a special Swan-Ganz catheter in place. Monitoring of $S\bar{v}O_2$ is especially useful when trending patients. Abrupt changes certainly suggest a more thorough evaluation of the cardiopulmonary system.

Oxygen Uptake and Utilization
Normal Oxygen Uptake

Oxygen uptake by the tissues normally remains relatively constant despite variations in O_2 transport (O_2 delivery), because oxygen transport usually far exceeds tissue O_2 requirements. If O_2 transport decreases substantially, however, a critical point is eventually reached at which O_2 transport is insufficient to meet tissue demands. Below this *critical oxygen delivery point*, hypoxia develops and the accumulation of lactic acid is likely. This is called *physiologic oxygen supply dependency* and can be demonstrated in all people.

The critical O_2 delivery point has been shown to be about 8 to 10 mL/kg/min in critically

---

ON CALL | CASE 11-1 *ABGs and Critical Thinking*

You are the only person available to care for this patient. You must assess the patient/situation and act accordingly.

A 43-year-old female patient with severe cardiogenic pulmonary edema is being mechanically ventilated with 10 cm H_2O PEEP. Despite being on FIO_2 0.70, her PaO_2 is only 65 mm Hg and her mixed venous PO_2 is 35 mm Hg. The PEEP is increased to 15 cm H_2O and arterial and mixed venous blood gases are drawn 30 minutes later.

BLOOD GASES

SaO_2	93%
pH	7.36
$PaCO_2$	38 mm Hg
PaO_2	74 mm Hg
[HCO_3]	22 mEq/L
FIO_2	0.70
$P\bar{v}O_2$	27 mm Hg

ASSESSMENT

Abnormalities: List abnormal data and other noteworthy information. Classify ABG.

Explanation: List possible diseases, pathology, or other situations that may have led to this patient's condition.

Evaluation: Suggest additional data that would be useful in helping understand the situation or in making a diagnosis.

INTERVENTION

Importance: Prioritize concern(s) of treatment in order of urgency and/or seriousness as you see the overall situation.

Objective: Specifically state the measurable or observable outcomes you would like treatment to accomplish.

Action: Describe your specific plan of action.

ill patients.[419,420] In a normal 70-kg individual, this would correspond to an O_2 transport of approximately 550 to 700 mL O_2/min. When O_2 transport falls below this level, tissue hypoxia should be assumed. It has been shown that when oxygen transport falls below 8 mL/kg/min, blood lactate greatly increases and survival is poor.[420] Oxygen transport may indeed be one of the most sensitive indicators of hypoxia at our disposal, although further study of this notion is necessary.

Thus, maintenance of O_2 transport in excess of the critical delivery point is crucial in the management of critically ill patients. This is particularly true when PEEP is being used because PEEP may be associated with a fall in O_2 transport despite improvement in PaO_2.

The clinician should also be aware of those conditions that may increase O_2 consumption and elevate the critical oxygen delivery point. These conditions include shivering, convulsions, sepsis, and fever. A higher minimum level of O_2 delivery is indicated in these circumstances.

Normal Supply-Independent Oxygen Uptake

As described in the previous section, attainment of O_2 transport levels markedly higher than the critical delivery point is probably not necessary because this does not lead to greater oxygen use. Thus, maintenance of *normal* O_2 transport is probably not an appropriate or necessary clinical goal.

Another way of describing the relationship between O_2 transport and uptake is to say that above the critical O_2 delivery point, there is a plateau in O_2 uptake. Above the critical point, O_2 uptake is independent of O_2 transport. The tissues apparently have no need for an additional supply of O_2.

Covert Hypoxia

It has been observed that O_2 uptake may increase with O_2 transport in some individuals with septic shock,[421] ARDS,[422] acute liver failure,[423] congestive heart failure,[424] COPD,[425] increased pulmonary vascular resistance,[426] and respiratory failure in general.[427] This phenomenon has also been described as *pathological oxygen supply dependency*.

In other words, O_2 uptake does not plateau as in normal individuals; rather, it increases as

O_2 transport increases even beyond normal levels. The presumed reason for this deviation from the norm is that there is some form of O_2 debt present in these individuals[428] and that even with normal O_2 transport, they may be hypoxic. This *covert (or occult) hypoxia* presumably is due to a derangement in internal respiration. The term *covert hypoxia* should be used with great caution, however, because the reason for this increased O_2 consumption is unclear—it could be due simply to an aberration in metabolism. Nevertheless, it could also represent a need for life-sustaining O_2.

Figure 11-18 depicts graphically the normal relationship between O_2 transport and uptake (see Fig. 11-18, *solid line*). The normal critical O_2 delivery point (see Fig. 11-18, *solid circle*) is approximately 8 mL/kg/min. Note that, normally, higher levels of O_2 transport have no effect on O_2 uptake. In so-called covert hypoxia, there continues to be increased O_2 uptake with progressive increases in O_2 transport.

The exact mechanism responsible for covert hypoxia is not known. It has been postulated that the hypoxia and lactic acidosis associated with septic shock are due to some derangement of O_2 use in the cell.[429] Some studies, however,

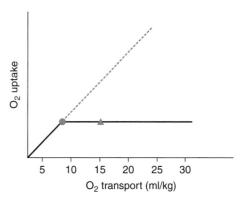

Figure 11-18. Covert hypoxia. In normal humans, oxygen consumption decreases when oxygen delivery falls below the critical point. However, increases in oxygen delivery above the critical O_2 delivery point do not ordinarily increase oxygen uptake. In covert hypoxia, progressive increases in oxygen delivery result in progressive increases in oxygen uptake.

suggest that a decline in nutrient blood flow rather than cellular dysfunction is the predominant mechanism.[421,429] Microemboli and release of various vasoactive substances have been shown in supply-dependent oxygen uptake and could explain the mechanism responsible for the circulatory disturbance and the so-called covert hypoxia.

Vasodilator Effects

Prostacyclin is a potent vasodilator that also tends to increase O_2 transport and prevent formation of microemboli in the systemic capillaries.[428] Administration of prostacyclin to critically ill patients may help to identify individuals with covert hypoxia, because these patients show an increase in O_2 uptake after the administration of this drug.[428] Administration of dobutamine has been associated with similar effects.[430]

Prognosis

Patients whose O_2 uptake increases in response to increased O_2 transport and tissue perfusion are more likely to die.[428] Use of prostacyclin or a similar drug may therefore help the clinician to recognize the presence of covert hypoxia and to provide a prognostic indicator. Perhaps in the future this drug or a similar vasodilator will prove to be beneficial in the management of covert hypoxia.

Recognition of supply-dependent O_2 uptake may be important in the approach to management of the critically ill. First, the notion that tissue oxygenation is always acceptable when O_2 transport is in the acceptable range must be re-evaluated. Some patients may benefit from further increases in O_2 transport beyond normal. In addition, understanding that the condition of an individual with covert hypoxia is probably in a downward spiral suggests that aggressive attempts to maintain oxygenation may be warranted.

Pathological Supply Dependency
Controversy

This concept of pathological supply dependency is very controversial. Some studies have demonstrated very beneficial positive outcomes by increasing oxygen transport in these patients,[448,449] whereas other investigators[451,452] have shown that the phenomenon is due to some artifact. The apparent increase in oxygen consumption may be due to a drug effect (i.e., prostacyclin), temperature variances,[450] or, as many believe, it is simply a mathematical error due to the method of calculation.[451,452]

Multiple Organ Dysfunction Syndrome

The same pathologic entities that manifest supply-dependent O_2 uptake (septic shock, ARDS, COPD) are often associated with the disorder known as *multiple organ dysfunction syndrome* (MODS). This phenomenon is often observed in critically ill patients in whom several organ systems fail (e.g., respiratory, renal, hepatic, circulatory, central nervous system). Multiple organ failure is the most common cause of death in patients with ARDS.

It is unclear whether multiple organ dysfunction syndrome is caused by hypoxia or by some other mechanism. Although earlier the presence of hypoxia was considered to be unlikely, the discovery of covert hypoxia suggests that hypoxia may indeed be present in these individuals and may be responsible to a great extent for the deterioration often observed.[431] In particular, death from septic shock seems to be related more to persistent peripheral vascular changes than to cardiac output problems.[432]

Summary

Studies have shown a poor correlation between $P\bar{v}O_2$ and other measures of hypoxia such as lactic acid and oxygen consumption.[433] Despite its theoretical attractiveness, $P\bar{v}O_2$ has not proved to be the "perfect" index of hypoxia. As stated previously, *there is no perfect index of hypoxia.*

Notwithstanding, $P\bar{v}O_2$ and lactate are useful variables to follow in the critically ill patient with potential hypoxia. Changes in $P\bar{v}O_2$ provide valuable information regarding changes in the patient's cardiovascular status and are particularly useful in understanding concurrent changes in PaO_2.[410] From a practical standpoint, venous oxygenation values are relatively sensitive indicators of the oxygenation disturbances that accompany routine bedside procedures such as endotracheal suctioning[434] and positioning of the patient.[435]

ON CALL | CASE 11-2 *ABGs and Critical Thinking*

You are the only person available to care for this patient. You must assess the patient/situation and act accordingly.

A patient with sepsis and ARDS is in the critical care unit.

BLOOD GASES

SaO_2	91%
pH	7.25
$PaCO_2$	42 mm Hg
PaO_2	68 mm Hg
$[HCO_3]$	16 mEq/L
FIO_2	0.60
$P\bar{v}O_2$	47 mm Hg
Lactate	9 mEq/L

ASSESSMENT

Abnormalities: List abnormal data and other noteworthy information. Classify ABG.

Explanation: List possible diseases, pathology, or other situations that may have led to this patient's condition.

INTERVENTION

Importance: Prioritize concern(s) of treatment in order of urgency and/or seriousness as you see the overall situation.

Objective: Specifically state the measurable or observable outcomes you would like treatment to accomplish.

Gastric Tonometry

Gastric tonometry is a relatively new technique for evaluating tissue oxygenation and hypoxia. It is well known that when the body has a limited supply of oxygen, blood will be distributed to the vital organs (e.g., heart, brain, kidneys) at the expense of the gastrointestinal tract and less vulnerable organs. Therefore, the gut should be one of the first organs to be affected by a hypoxic crisis.[455] Furthermore, the unique microvasculature of the gut make it especially sensitive to local hypoxia.[459]

Tonometry is a technique that makes use of the principle that fluid or air in contact with tissue can be used to estimate conditions within the tissue. With gastric tonometry, air or fluid, within a special nasogastric tube is equilibrated with the gastric mucosa. Following equilibration, the PCO_2 is measured from this air or fluid. The $[HCO_3]$ from a concurrent arterial blood gas is then used to calculate the local tissue pH.[459] The technique is also of interest since it is essentially a *noninvasive* measure of tissue oxygen status.

Measuring gut pH is also useful as poor perfusion of the gut may causes life-threatening stress bleeding and release of toxins into the bloodstream. Gastric tonometry has been shown to be a sensitive and reproducible method for evaluation of blood flow to the gut.[456,457] Gastric pH has also been shown to correlate with mortality in critically ill patients.[458] Despite these promising results, further studies are needed to demonstrate its safety and value.

Vital Organ Function

In the face of hypoxic threats, the body tries to maintain oxygenation of the vital organs such as the brain and the heart. It follows that if compensatory mechanisms are effective, normal organ function is preserved. Therefore, the monitoring of vital organ function is another useful tool in oxygenation assessment. Unfortunately, organ failure may occur rather abruptly and without warning. Thus, we finish where we began, in the realization that there is no single, simple, accurate index of the adequacy of tissue oxygenation.

EXERCISES

Exercise 11-1   Hypoxic Assessment

Fill in the blanks or select the best answer.

1. State the three main components (ABCs) to be evaluated in oxygen supply assessment.

2. The ultimate goal in the management of oxygenation is the prevention of (hypoxemia/hypoxia).

3. There (is/is not) a simple, single index of hypoxia.

4. The best place to begin in hypoxic assessment is _____ _____.

5. PaO_2 less than 45 mm Hg is (usually/always) associated with hypoxia.

6. PaO_2 (is/is not) a highly stable measurement in critically ill patients.

7. In general, PaO_2 should be maintained above _____ mm Hg in most clinical situations.

8. Normal PaO_2 (ensures/does not ensure) adequate tissue oxygenation.

9. Judgment and short-term memory are usually impaired in normal individuals when PaO_2 falls below _____ mm Hg.

10. In moderate hypoxemia, the development of hypoxia depends mainly on the integrity of the _____.

Exercise 11-2 SaO_2

Fill in the blanks or select the best answer.

1. Calculated SaO_2 (is/is not) an accurate, reliable way to measure SaO_2.

2. Oximeters that use two wavelengths to measure SaO_2 (do/do not) measure the quantity of MetHb present.

3. SaO_2 determined by two-wavelength oximetry measures (fractional/functional) saturation.

4. The concentration of HbCO (is/is not) directly measured with functional saturation.

5. The CO-oximeter measures (functional/fractional) SaO_2.

6. All forms of Hb are included in the calculation of total Hb in the measurement of (fractional/functional) SaO_2.

7. Pulse oximeters measure (functional/fractional) SaO_2.

8. Pulse oximeters are most useful for (trending of/accurate measure of) SaO_2.

9. SaO_2 measurements by two-wavelength oximetry and by CO-oximetry (are/are not) always identical.

10. Pulse oximeters use (two-/four-) wavelength oximetry.

Exercise 11-3 **Laboratory Diagnosis of Anemia**

Fill in the blanks or select the best answer.

1. State the normal [RBC] and [Hb] in the blood.

2. A reduction in the number of circulating RBCs or [Hb] is called _____.

3. The percentage of formed elements in the blood is called _____.

4. When there are abnormal variations in cell size, _____ is said to be present.

5. The presence of many cells larger than 10 μm in diameter is called _____.

6. Cell size is indicated by the (MCHC/MCV).

7. Abnormality in the shapes of RBCs is called _____.

8. Normally, there are 1.0% to 1.5% immature RBCs present in the blood, which are called _____.

9. Normal MCHC is _____%.

10. Iron deficiency anemia is typically associated with (hyperchromia/normochromia/hypochromia).

Exercise 11-4 **Types of Anemia and Treatment**

Fill in the blanks or select the best answer.

1. Inability of the bone marrow to produce RBCs secondary to exposure to some chemical or physical agent is called _____ anemia.

2. Chronic blood loss may lead to a form of anemia associated with microcytosis and hypochromia that is called _____ anemia.

3. A genetic disorder that may hamper Hb production and lead to anemia is called _____.

4. State the three substances besides Fe needed for normal RBC production.

5. Individuals unable to absorb vitamin B_{12} owing to the absence of intrinsic factor may have _____ anemia.

6. The presence of megaloblasts and macrocytosis is common in (Cooley's anemia/folic acid deficiency).

7. The major compensatory mechanism in acute anemia is _____, whereas the major compensatory mechanism in chronic anemia is _____.

8. The optimal Hct may be anywhere from ____% to ____%.

9. Snake venoms may lead to _____ anemia.

10. Mediterranean disease is another name for _____.

Exercise 11-5 Cardiovascular System/Shock

Fill in the blanks or select the best answer.

1. The volume of blood ejected from the left side of the heart each minute is called the _____.

2. The symbol for cardiac minute output is _____.

3. When cardiac output is adjusted for body size by dividing it by body surface area, the resultant value is called the _____.

4. State two methods that can be used to measure cardiac output invasively.

5. There (is/is not) a technique to measure cardiac output noninvasively.

6. List at least five ways in which cardiac output can be assessed indirectly.

7. List the three basic components of the cardiovascular system.

8. Collapse of the cardiovascular system associated with a decrease in blood pressure is called _____.

9. In shock, stimulation of the sympathetic nervous system leads to (vasodilation/vasoconstriction).

10. List at least five signs and symptoms that are associated with shock.

Exercise 11-6 Types of Shock

Fill in the blanks or select the best answer.

1. Write the formula for cardiac output.

2. Cardiac output generally (increases/decreases) with slight decrease in heart rate.

3. Cardiac output generally (increases/decreases) with a slight increase in heart rate and (increases/decreases) with extreme increases in heart rate.

4. Cardiovascular collapse due to failure of the heart as a pump is called _____ shock.

5. A decrease in blood volume is called _____.

6. A useful indicator of hypovolemia is a (low/high) CVP.

7. Jugular vein distention, hypoxemia, fine crackles in the lungs, and abnormal heart sounds are found in the cardiovascular problem known as _____.

8. Cardiovascular collapse secondary to inadequate blood volume is called _____ shock.

9. In _____ shock, cardiac output is usually high and profound vasodilation and blood infection are present.

10. Shock secondary to a profound allergic reaction and vasodilation is called _____ shock.

Exercise 11-7   **Hemodynamic Monitoring**

Fill in the blanks or select the best answer.

1. Central venous pressure (CVP) is measured in the _____.

2. Normal CVP is _____ mm Hg.

3. A high CVP suggests (heart failure/hypovolemia).

4. The balloon-tipped, multilumen catheter that is inserted into the pulmonary artery for hemodynamic monitoring is called the _____.

5. Normal PAP is _____ mm Hg.

6. PWP is normally about _____ mm Hg.

7. A PWP of 25 mm Hg suggests (left-sided heart failure/pulmonary emboli).

8. Pulmonary edema associated with a PWP of 10 mm Hg is consistent with the diagnosis of (congestive heart failure/ARDS).

9. In the patient with normal pulmonary vascular resistance, a reasonable substitute for the PWP, when there is a technical problem in trying to get the catheter to wedge, is the (diastolic/systolic) PAP.

Exercise 11-8   **Cardiovascular Treatment**

Fill in the blanks or select the best answer.

1. In the presence of left-sided heart failure and acute pulmonary edema, the patient usually benefits from assumption of the (feet-up/sitting) position.

2. In the presence of blood loss and shock, the patient usually benefits by assumption of the (feet-up/sitting) position.

3. Positive pressure breathing is usually (beneficial/detrimental) in hypovolemic shock; it is usually (beneficial/detrimental) in cardiogenic shock.

4. A drug that increases heart rate is said to have a positive (chronotropic/inotropic) effect.

Exercise 11-9   **Blood Lactate**

Fill in the blanks or select the best answer.

1. Anaerobic metabolism leads to an excess of _____ acid.

2. The _____ anion is measured as a reflection of lactic acid levels.

3. Normal blood lactate in mM/L is _____.

4. Blood lactate concentration in mg/dL is approximately _____ times higher than lactate concentration in mM/L.

5. Hyperlactatemia (correlates/does not correlate) with mortality.

6. Normally, the (kidney/liver) takes up lactate from the blood (slowly/quickly).

7. Blood lactate (is/is not) a sensitive indicator of hypoxia.

8. The normal blood lactate/pyruvate ratio is _____.

9. In hypoxia, the blood lactate/pyruvate ratio is (normal/increased/decreased).

10. Blood lactate (is/is not) a highly specific indicator of hypoxia.

Exercise 11-10   Mixed Venous Oxygenation Indices

Fill in the blanks or select the best answer.

1. Mixed venous blood can be obtained only when a _____ is in place.

2. Normal $S\bar{v}O_2$ is _____%.

3. A fiber-optic catheter can be used to measure ($S\bar{v}O_2$/$P\bar{v}O_2$).

4. As a general guide, hypoxia is likely when $P\bar{v}O_2$ is less than _____ mm Hg.

5. $S\bar{v}O_2$ and $P\bar{v}O_2$ are affected by (pulmonary changes only/cardiovascular changes only/both pulmonary and cardiovascular changes).

6. A PaO_2 of 55 mm Hg and a $P\bar{v}O_2$ of 40 mm Hg are indicative of (increased/decreased) cardiac output.

7. A PaO_2 of 95 mm Hg and a $P\bar{v}O_2$ of 25 mm Hg are indicative of (decreased/increased) cardiac output.

8. Severe anemia or carboxyhemoglobinemia results in a relatively (low/high/normal) PaO_2 and a (low/high/normal) $P\bar{v}O_2$.

9. $P\bar{v}O_2$ levels may be surprisingly (high/low) in septic shock.

10. Low levels of $P\bar{v}O_2$ (usually/always) indicate hypoxia.

Exercise 11-11   Oxygen Uptake/Utilization

Fill in the blanks or select the best answer.

1. In healthy individuals, a slight increase or decrease in O_2 transport (is/is not) associated with a similar change in O_2 consumption.

2. The point at which O_2 transport is inadequate to meet tissue O_2 demands is called the _____.

3. The critical oxygen delivery point in critically ill patients is about _____ mL/kg/min.

4. Maintenance of *normal* values of O_2 transport in critically ill patients is usually (necessary/unnecessary).

5. In septic shock, ARDS, and acute liver failure, it has been shown that O_2 uptake (is always constant/may be increased) when O_2 transport increases even beyond normal levels.

6. The presence of hypoxia despite apparently normal O_2 transport is called _____ hypoxia.

7. Patients who display covert hypoxia have a (good/poor) prognosis.

8. Covert hypoxia may be responsible for a common cause of death in ARDS due to _____.

9. A potent vasodilator that may be useful in demonstrating covert hypoxia is _____.

10. In normal persons, O_2 uptake is (increased/unchanged) with an increase in O_2 transport beyond normal; in individuals with septic shock, O_2 uptake (may be increased/is unchanged) with an increase in O_2 transport beyond normal.

11. The apparent (physiologic/pathologic) oxygen supply dependency may simply be due to a mathematical error.

Exercise 11-12 | Internet Work

1. Go to internet site: http://www.mtsinai.org/pulmonary/books/physiology/chap6_1.htm.

   A. List 3 to 5 clues suggesting tissue hypoxia.

   B. Determine which patient has the lowest CaO_2 in clinical problem 2.

NBRC Challenge 11

Please select the best answer for the following multiple-choice questions.

1. Given the following, which diagnosis is most likely?
   CVP = 1 mm Hg   PWP = 5 mm Hg
   BP = 90/P
   A) Cardiogenic shock
   B) ARDS
   C) Hypovolemic shock
   D) Left heart failure
   E) Mitral valve failure
   (RRT EXAMINATION — NBRC MATRIX I,B,9,e)

2. Which of the following techniques or measurements might assist in determining if a patient has tissue hypoxia?
   A) Blood pyruvate
   B) Tensilon test
   C) Gastric tonometry
   D) Blood chloride levels
   E) Serum magnesium
   (RRT EXAMINATION — NBRC MATRIX I,A,1,i)

3. Given the following, which diagnosis is most likely?:
   CVP = 15 mm Hg PWP = 25 mm Hg
   BP = 90/P
   A) Cardiogenic shock
   B) ARDS
   C) Hypovolemic shock

D) Septic shock
E) Anaphylactic shock
(RRT EXAMINATION — NBRC MATRIX I,B,10,e)

4. A patient with left heart failure is admitted to the critical care unit on FIO_2 0.60 via face mask. The patient should be placed in the _____ position.
   A) sitting
   B) Trendelenburg
   C) prone
   D) supine
   E) reverse Trendelenburg
   (RRT EXAMINATION — NBRC MATRIX III,B,1,d)

5. An abrupt decrease in cardiac output might be identified by evaluating:
   I. SpO_2.
   II. [Hb].
   III. $C(a-\bar{v})O_2$.
   IV. $S\bar{v}O_2$.
   A) I and II only
   B) I and III only
   C) I and IV only
   D) II and IV only
   E) III and IV only
   (CRT EXAMINATION — NBRC MATRIX III,D,2)

Clinical Acid Base

Chapter 12

Regulation of Acids, Bases, and Electrolytes

Regulation of Volatile Acid (Ventilation)...
One might guess that respiration would increase whenever cells of the body use more O_2 and form more CO_2 and would decrease whenever they need less O_2 and form less CO_2. This, indeed, is the case.

Julius H. Comroe[81]

Regulation of Fixed Acids, Bases, and Electrolytes...
It cannot be stated too often that neither the water, nor the electrolytes, nor the acid-base balance may be studied individually because of the strong interaction between them.

Gosta Rooth[462]

Outline

OVERVIEW

The prominent roles of the lungs and the kidneys in acid-base homeostasis were described in Chapter 8. In this chapter, we take a more in-depth look at precisely how the lungs and the kidneys perform these functions. Regarding the regulation of volatile acid, some of the major factors that control and regulate ventilation in health and disease are reviewed.

This is followed by a review of kidney (renal) function. Processes used by the kidneys to excrete wastes and to maintain fluid and electrolyte balance are examined. In particular, sodium regulation and its effect on blood bicarbonate are explored.

The effects of certain therapeutic interventions, such as diuretics and steroids, are also considered. In addition, the value of the serum electrolyte profile in evaluating acid-base disturbances is discussed.

REGULATION OF VENTILATION

As described earlier, the volume of carbon dioxide (and, therefore, volatile acid) excretion varies directly with the quantity of alveolar ventilation. The amount of alveolar ventilation, in turn, depends on the mechanisms responsible for the *control and regulation of ventilation*. Thus, a brief review of the major factors that regulate ventilation in health and disease is in order.

The control of ventilation is a complex physiologic process. The major factors that play a role in the regulation of ventilation are shown in Figure 12-1. The primary respiratory center (generator) is located in the medulla of the brain (*medullary center*). Output of the medullary center is influenced by several other centers in the brain that affect respiration. The *apneustic* and *pneumotaxic centers* in the pons tend to modify the ventilatory pattern, and the *cerebral cortex* may participate in voluntary input into the system.

Reflexes and chemoreceptors serve to measure the output of the system and provide feedback loops back to the medulla. As such, reflexes and chemoreceptors play a vital role in the regulation of ventilation. Although a detailed analysis of all the factors that mediate ventilation is beyond the scope of this text, a basic review of the chemoreceptors and a few prominent reflexes is important to understand arterial blood gas application.

Chemoreceptors

The chemoreceptors are probably the single most important mechanism by which ventilation is regulated. Two basic groups of chemoreceptors influence ventilation: (1) the *central chemoreceptors*, located within the central nervous system; and (2) the *peripheral chemoreceptors*, located within the cardiovascular system.

Central Chemoreceptors

Location and Response
The central chemoreceptors are chemosensitive areas located on the medulla of the brain. These chemoreceptors in the medulla should not be confused with the *medullary respiratory center*, because they are distinctly separate entities. *The chemoreceptors are bathed in cerebrospinal fluid*

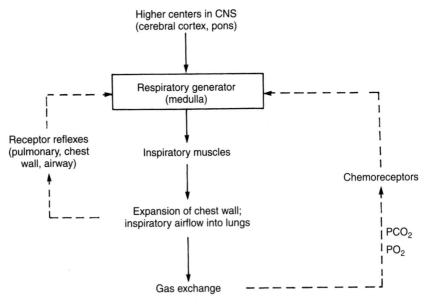

Figure 12-1.   Regulation of ventilation. Organization of the respiratory control system. The dashed lines show feedback loops affecting the respiratory generator.

(CSF) and respond directly to the pH of the cerebrospinal fluid. When the hydrogen ion concentration of the CSF increases (i.e., pH decreases), an increase in ventilation is triggered. Conversely, when the pH of the CSF increases, the ventilatory drive and the volume of ventilation are diminished. The central chemoreceptors do *not* respond to oxygen levels in the blood.

Blood-Brain Barrier

The CSF is separated from the blood by the *blood-brain barrier*, which is readily permeable to gases but relatively impermeable to ions. Gases equilibrate quickly across the blood-brain barrier. Some ions, such as bicarbonate, may tend to equilibrate across the barrier, but the exchange process is active transport rather than simple diffusion. The active transport of ions across the blood-brain barrier may take a considerable time (i.e., hours to days)[81] compared with the immediate diffusion of gases.

Thus, when the $PaCO_2$ increases, PCO_2 in the CSF immediately follows suit. This, in turn, lowers the pH of the CSF, and the ventilatory drive is augmented within minutes. In metabolic acidosis, however, the bicarbonate ion is transported slowly out of the CSF. Therefore, it takes longer for the pH of the CSF to decrease, and consequently the ventilatory response is delayed.

Cheyne-Stokes Ventilation

It is noteworthy that even with respiratory (i.e., PCO_2) gas changes, there is some delay from the time when the alveolar PCO_2 changes until this change is reflected in the CSF. This time delay explains why the ventilatory response to increased or decreased alveolar PCO_2, although highly sensitive, is not instantaneous. Furthermore, if circulation is impaired, such as in congestive heart failure, this delay may be exaggerated because it takes longer for blood from the lungs to reach the medulla. In theory, this circulatory delay may explain the Cheyne-Stokes breathing that is sometimes observed in congestive heart failure.

Cheyne-Stokes breathing is a recurrent pattern of ventilation characterized by a progressive rise and fall of tidal volume (Fig. 12-2). A period of apnea may sometimes occur between cycles. The related alveolar and central chemoreceptor PCO_2 levels at different points in the breathing cycle are also shown in Figure 12-2.

Peripheral Chemoreceptors

Location

The second group of chemosensitive cells (chemoreceptors) that affects ventilation is located adjacent to the walls of certain arterial blood vessels. These peripheral chemoreceptors are located in two distinct anatomic areas: the carotid and aortic bodies.

The *carotid bodies* are a group of cells located near the bifurcation of the common carotid artery into the internal and external carotid arteries. They appear as small, pink nodules, approximately 3 to 5 mm in diameter.[81] The *aortic bodies* are located within the arch of the aorta.

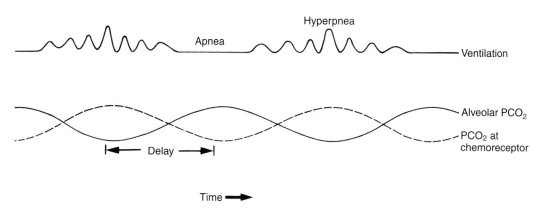

Figure 12-2. Cheyne-Stokes breathing. Cheyne-Stokes breathing, showing a cyclic pattern of ventilation. In patients with a prolonged circulation time, the delay between the signal to the central chemoreceptor (PCO_2 at the chemoreceptor) and ventilatory output (reflected by alveolar PCO_2) is shown.

The two sets of cells, which are referred to collectively as the *peripheral chemoreceptors*, serve to chemically monitor the blood passing by them. To perform this function, the peripheral chemoreceptors receive a relatively large blood flow in proportion to their size.

Responsiveness

Unlike the central chemoreceptors, the peripheral chemoreceptors respond to several different blood gas stimuli: the PaO_2, arterial pH, and $PaCO_2$. In addition, when blood flow past the peripheral chemoreceptors is diminished (e.g., in shock), an increase in ventilation is also stimulated. The peripheral chemoreceptors generally do not respond to anemia (e.g., methemoglobinemia, HbCO poisoning), although there is some response when anemia is severe. Interestingly, the peripheral chemoreceptors stimulate severe hyperpnea (increased tidal volume) in cyanide poisoning.[81]

PaCO₂/pH

Although both the peripheral and central chemoreceptors respond to increased $PaCO_2$ and decreased pH, they are not equally sensitive to these stimuli. Specifically, a relatively *large* increase in $PaCO_2$ or a decrease in pH (e.g., $PaCO_2$ increase = 10 mm Hg; pH decrease = 0.1)[81] is necessary before a notable increase in ventilation will be triggered via the peripheral chemoreceptors. Conversely, the central chemoreceptors respond to very *slight* changes in $PaCO_2$. In a normal young man, minute ventilation increases approximately 2.5 L with only a 1-mm Hg increase in $PaCO_2$.[81]

PaO₂

The response of the peripheral chemoreceptors to a low PaO_2 sets them apart from the central chemoreceptors and is their most important mechanism clinically. Even in normal humans, *some*, albeit few, impulses are sent to the brain from the peripheral chemoreceptors stimulating ventilation. $PaCO_2$ and the central chemoreceptors are the primary mechanisms of ventilatory control during normal ventilation.

Regulation of ventilation in pulmonary disease is often in marked contrast. Here, the peripheral chemoreceptors often play the dominant role in determining the ventilatory pattern.

The number of peripheral chemoreceptor impulses sent to the brain to stimulate ventilation in hypoxemia may increase greatly. Initially, ventilatory impulses increase only slightly as PaO_2 falls slightly below the normal range. When PaO_2 falls *below* 60 mm Hg, however, there is a *dramatic increase in impulse production and ventilation.*

Not only do the peripheral chemoreceptors greatly stimulate ventilation when PaO_2 falls below this critical point; they also stimulate the cardiovascular system. Clinically, this is manifested by a rise in heart rate and arterial blood pressure. Restoration of PaO_2 to normal, however, allows ventilation, heart rate, and blood pressure to return to normal levels.

Chemoreceptor Interactions

The breathing pattern observed at any given time is the net result of the integration of various different inputs. As stated earlier, messages may originate from brain centers, chemoreceptors, reflexes, or even voluntary commands. Notwithstanding, the chemoreceptors are often the most dominant forces that control ventilation. In some situations, the peripheral and central chemoreceptors work together for a potentiated response. In other circumstances, they tend to antagonize each other and blunt individual responses. A few examples of chemoreceptor interactions follow.

Normal Ventilation

The regulation of ventilation in normal individuals is primarily under the control of the central chemoreceptors; however, as previously mentioned, the peripheral chemoreceptors send weak messages to the brain to ventilate and have some, albeit small, influence on the ventilatory pattern. Thus, the ventilatory pattern is the net result of the integration of the two sets of chemoreceptors.

Acute Hypoxemia

In the presence of disease, the peripheral chemoreceptors may take the dominant role in the regulation of ventilation. For example, in acute, severe hypoxemia, the peripheral chemoreceptors send a powerful message to the brain to increase ventilation and generally will override the central chemoreceptors.

Subsequently, the increased ventilation that accompanies severe, acute hypoxemia lowers $PaCO_2$. The decreased $PaCO_2$, in turn, has the effect of making the CSF alkalotic and depressing ventilation via the central chemoreceptors.

Thus, in acute hypoxemia, two conflicting messages are sent to the brain. The severe hypoxemia requires an increase in ventilation via the peripheral chemoreceptors, whereas the low $PaCO_2$ depresses the central chemoreceptors. Because the number of impulses resulting from severe hypoxemia is large and the decrease in impulses resulting from the falling $PaCO_2$ is small, the individual will display a *net increase* in ventilation. It is important to recognize, however, that the central chemoreceptors tend slightly to blunt the hyperventilation.

Chronic Hypoxemia

In chronic hypoxemia, $PaCO_2$ also remains low. After a few hours, however, the pH of the CSF, made alkalotic by the hypocarbia, begins to return to normal as bicarbonate ions are actively transported out of the blood-brain barrier. When the pH of the CSF returns to normal, it no longer depresses ventilation via the central chemoreceptors. At this point, the individual actually begins to hyperventilate to a greater degree. It is, in fact, well known that the ventilatory response to chronic hypoxemia is greater than the ventilatory response to acute hypoxemia because of this mechanism.[81] Again, the ventilatory pattern at any point in time depends on the *interaction* of the chemoreceptors.

Progressive Pulmonary Deterioration

Lung diseases, such as emphysema, chronic bronchitis, and chronic asthma, are often grouped into a single category called chronic obstructive lung disease (COLD), chronic obstructive pulmonary disease (COPD), or chronic airflow obstruction (CAO). A common denominator of these diseases is that they may lead to a progressive inability of the lungs to normally exchange gases and maintain ventilation.

Normal Lung Function

The effects of progressive pulmonary deterioration on the chemoreceptors and blood $PaCO_2$ and PaO_2 levels are shown in Table 12-1. Normal lung function is associated with normal blood gases and ventilation is primarily under the control of the central chemoreceptors.

Mild Disease

The initial blood gas abnormality associated with mild pulmonary disease is mild hypoxemia with a normal $PaCO_2$ (see Table 12-1). In this early stage, the increase in peripheral chemoreceptor stimulation is so minute that it is not clinically detectable. The central chemoreceptors maintain primary control over ventilation.

Moderate Disease

As deterioration in external respiration continues, PaO_2 continues to decline. At a PaO_2 level of approximately 60 mm Hg (although there may be considerable individual variation with regard to the specific PaO_2 when this occurs), a dramatic increase in peripheral chemoreceptor

Table 12-1. REGULATION OF VENTILATION AND BLOOD GASES IN PROGRESSIVE PULMONARY DISEASE

		Progressive Disease		
	Normal	Mild	Moderate	Severe
Blood gases				
PaO_2	100 mm Hg	65 mm Hg	55 mm Hg	50 mm Hg
$PaCO_2$	40 mm Hg	40 mm Hg	34 mm Hg	50 mm Hg
Central chemoreceptors	++++	++++	++	+
Peripheral chemoreceptors	+	++	+++	++++
Control	C	C	P	P

C = central chemoreceptors.
P = peripheral chemoreceptors.

stimulation is seen, and the peripheral chemo-receptors assume primary control of ventilation. The strong peripheral chemoreceptor drive usually results in an increase in alveolar ventilation and a fall in the $PaCO_2$ (see Table 12-1).

It is important to note that, during this phase, the cardiovascular system is also required to increase the heart rate and to elevate the blood pressure. From a teleologic perspective, because O_2 levels are falling to a critical point on the oxyhemoglobin curve, the cardiovascular system appears to be trying to ensure sufficient tissue O_2 delivery.

Severe Disease

If external respiration continues to deteriorate, CO_2 excretion is ultimately impaired and $PaCO_2$ levels begin to increase. Furthermore, PaO_2 levels continue to fall (see Table 12-1). Indeed, the *classic* definition of acute respiratory failure is a $PaCO_2$ greater than 50 mm Hg and/or a PaO_2 less than 50 mm Hg.

The same pattern of progressive pulmonary deterioration can also occur over a short time (days or hours) in acute pulmonary disease. This pattern may be observed in pneumonia, postoperative respiratory failure, or acute asthma. It is always important to identify patients with moderate impairment (i.e., moderate disease as described in Table 12-1), because further deterioration leads to hypercarbia. The classic example of this is the patient in status asthmaticus (sustained unresponsive asthma) whose condition deteriorates progressively over a period of days, leading ultimately to exhaustion and to the abrupt onset of respiratory acidemia.

In patients with severe chronic lung disease, administration of oxygen may lead to progressive hypercapnia and occasionally even to apnea. For years, it was believed that this occurred because these patients were breathing exclusively in response to the so-called hypoxic drive of the peripheral chemoreceptors. It was assumed that the central chemoreceptors had become dulled because of the chronic hypercarbia; it followed, then, that oxygen therapy increased the PaO_2 and knocked out the drive to breathe.

Other studies have shown that the worsening hypercarbia associated with oxygen therapy in these patients is more likely a result of ventilation-perfusion alterations than a result of a decrease in ventilatory drive.[463] Furthermore, the Haldane effect (release of CO_2 from Hb into the blood in the presence of increased oxygen) may be responsible for some of the ensuing hypercarbia.[464] The precise mechanism responsible for this hypoventilation remains a controversial issue and multiple factors may be influencing ventilation simultaneously. Regardless of the exact mechanism, worsening hypercarbia must be recognized as a possible consequence of oxygen therapy in chronic lung disease.

Reflexes

At least six different reflexes have been described in relation to the regulation of ventilation.[81] The precise role of many of these reflexes must still be defined. Nevertheless, two reflexes may be useful in helping the clinician to understand the origin of respiratory alkalosis in certain pulmonary conditions.

Hering-Breuer Reflex

The *Hering-Breuer reflex*, or stretch reflex, is probably the most widely known of the reflexes involved in the regulation of ventilation. This reflex appears to regulate tidal volume and respiratory rate to minimize the muscular work of breathing.

The Hering-Breuer reflex is not usually active during normal breathing. Rather, it is activated when the lung is overinflated or underinflated. The Hering-Breuer reflex is often described as two separate reflexes: an *inflation reflex*, which inhibits inspiration, and a *deflation reflex*, which stimulates inspiration when the lung volume is low.

The deflation reflex may be responsible, at least in part, for the hyperventilation observed in restrictive lung diseases. The ventilatory pattern commonly observed in these patients is characterized by a rapid respiratory rate and a low tidal volume. This pattern, although beneficial in terms of the work of breathing, may lead to respiratory alkalosis.

J Receptors

The *juxtapulmonary capillary receptors* (*J receptors*) are located in the interstitial tissue of the alveolar-capillary membrane. It is believed that these receptors are stimulated by an increased thickness of the alveolar-capillary membrane. Stimulation of these receptors could then explain the tachypnea and hyperventilation seen with pulmonary edema, congestion, or fibrosis. Certainly alveolar hyperventilation is common in these conditions.

RENAL FUNCTION

The renal system has essentially three primary functions. First, the kidneys are responsible for excreting nonvolatile waste products, including fixed acids. Second, the kidneys are responsible for the regulation of blood volume. Third, the kidneys must regulate blood concentrations of various electrolytes (e.g., HCO_3^-) and other blood constituents.

Macroscopic Anatomy and Physiology

The gross anatomy of the kidney is shown in Figure 12-3. Each of the two kidneys consists of an outer cortex and an inner medulla. Urine formed in the functional units of the kidney gathers in the renal pelvis and then flows through the ureters down to the urinary bladder, where it is stored. Ultimately, urine is excreted through the urethra.

Microscopic Anatomy and Physiology

The functional unit of the kidney is the *nephron*. Each kidney contains approximately 1 million nephrons. A schematic drawing of the functional nephron is shown in Figure 12-4. Blood enters the nephron through the *afferent arteriole*, which in turn enters an enclosed capsule. This capsule, called *Bowman's capsule*, is actually the first portion of the renal tubular system.

Encased within the capsule, the afferent arteriole branches into a capillary network and then leaves Bowman's capsule through the *efferent arteriole*. The capillary tuft or network within the capsule is called the *glomerulus*. The capillaries that make up the glomerulus are very porous, and much of the plasma is filtered into Bowman's capsule. The fluid that accumulates within the capsule is called the *glomerular filtrate*, which begins its journey through the nephron.

The tubule that the glomerular filtrate passes through immediately upon leaving Bowman's capsule is called the *proximal tubule*, because it is close (proximal) to the capsule. Actually, this tubule follows a very convoluted path, and it is sometimes referred to as the *proximal*

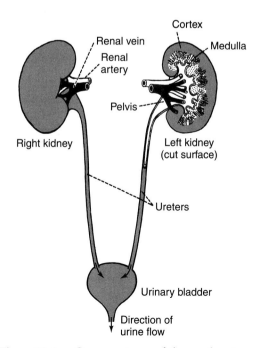

Figure 12-3.   **Gross anatomy of the renal system.**

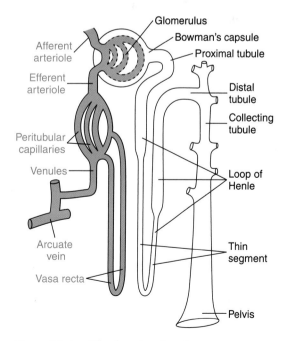

Figure 12-4.   **The functional nephron.**

convoluted tubule. The glomerular filtrate then travels through the *loop of Henle*, the *distal convoluted tubule*, and, ultimately, the *collecting duct*. The fluid that accumulates in the collecting duct is essentially urine, which then flows to the renal pelvis en route to be excreted.

Urine Formation

Three processes are involved in the formation of urine: (1) glomerular filtration, (2) tubular reabsorption, and (3) tubular secretion. Through these processes, the kidney can accomplish its functions, which are described at the beginning of this section.

Glomerular Filtration

The glomerulus functions as a semi-permeable membrane that allows for the diffusion of fluid similar in ionic concentration to plasma into the filtrate. Cells and proteins do not normally pass through the glomerulus into the filtrate. In fact, *proteinuria* (protein in the urine) and *hematuria* (blood in the urine) may be important findings that suggest renal disease.

The volume of glomerular filtrate formed depends on the volume of renal perfusion. Normally, the kidneys receive approximately 20% of the cardiac output. The amount of this volume that is filtered out into the glomerular filtrate is also large. A volume roughly equivalent to the entire extracellular fluid volume (i.e., 15 L) passes through the glomeruli every 2 hours.[465] In the patient with reduced volume and metabolic alkalosis, glomerular filtration is likewise reduced. This perpetuates the syndrome of metabolic alkalosis as excess [HCO_3] cannot be excreted.[480] Thus, correction of metabolic alkalosis is dependent on adequate renal perfusion and glomerular filtration.

Any drug that increases cardiac output (e.g., epinephrine, digitalis) or preferentially increases renal perfusion (e.g., aminophylline) tends to increase urine formation. A *diuretic* is any substance that increases urine flow. Therefore, in a broad sense, these drugs may be considered to be mild diuretics, although they are not generally administered primarily for this purpose. An increase in the amount of urine excreted is called *polyuria*; a decreased urine output is called *oliguria*.

Tubular Reabsorption

Approximately 99% of all the fluid that passes into the glomerular filtrate is reabsorbed. As the filtrate passes through the nephron, various electrolytes and substances are reabsorbed in proportion to the body's needs. As shown in Figure 12-4, a rich supply of capillaries (i.e., peritubular capillaries and vasa recta) is immediately adjacent to the renal tubules that facilitate reabsorption of many of these electrolytes back into the bloodstream.

Tubular Secretion

The cells that line the renal tubules are also capable of secreting certain electrolytes into the filtrate in exchange for the reabsorption of other electrolytes that the body seeks to recapture. This process of exchanging one electrolyte for another in the filtrate is called *tubular secretion*.

BODY FLUIDS AND ELECTROLYTES

Fluid Compartments

Approximately 60% of the body's weight is made up of water. This water is separated by membranes into various body fluid compartments (Fig. 12-5). As further shown in Figure 12-6, approximately two-thirds of the water (approximately 65%) is located in the *intracellular* fluid space, or within cells. The remaining

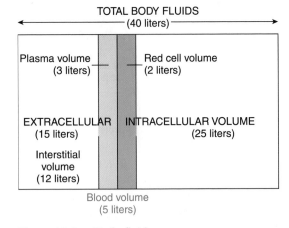

Figure 12-5. **Body fluid compartments.** Diagrammatic representation of the body fluids, showing the extracellular fluid volume, intracellular fluid volume, blood volume, and total body fluids.

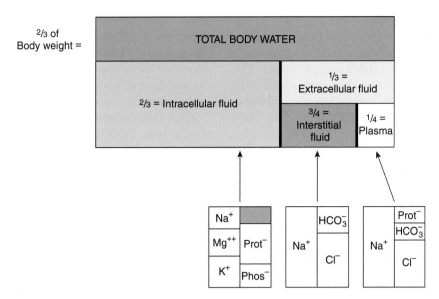

Figure 12-6.   **Composition of body fluid compartments.** Percentage of total body water and approximate electrolyte composition of various compartments is shown.

35% exists in the *extracellular* fluid compartment or outside the cells.

The body fluids can also be categorized concerning whether they exist within the vascular system (i.e., *intravascular* fluid or blood volume) or outside it (i.e., *extravascular* fluid). The portion of the extracellular fluid that exists within the vascular space is the *plasma*. If plasma is allowed to coagulate and the coagulated fluid is centrifuged, the clear fluid that remains is called *serum*.

The portion of the extracellular fluid that exists outside the vascular space is also called the *interstitial* fluid, because it lies in the spaces between the various cells throughout the body. As graphically shown in Figures 12-5 and 12-6, most of the extracellular fluid consists of interstitial fluid.

Electrolytes

Two types of chemical substances are found in body water: non-electrolytes and electrolytes. *Non-electrolytes* are uncharged substances that remain intact. Urea, creatinine, and glucose are examples of non-electrolytes. *Electrolytes*, on the other hand, dissociate and carry electrical charges. Electrolytes that carry a positive charge are called *cations*; those that carry a negative charge are called *anions*.

Electrolyte Distribution

Each of the body fluid compartments contains electrolytes. However, each compartment has its own unique electrolyte composition. Often there may be a striking contrast from one compartment to another in electrolyte concentration, as shown in Figures 12-6 and 12-7. For example, potassium is the most abundant intracellular cation, with a concentration of approximately 141 mEq/L. In sharp contrast, the potassium concentration in the plasma is only approximately 4 mEq/L.

Similarly, the major intracellular anion is phosphate, with a concentration of approximately 75 mEq/L; on the other hand, the plasma

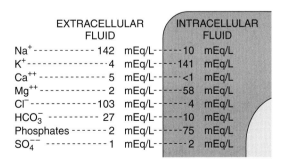

	EXTRACELLULAR FLUID		INTRACELLULAR FLUID
Na$^+$	142	mEq/L	10 mEq/L
K$^+$	4	mEq/L	141 mEq/L
Ca^{++}	5	mEq/L	<1 mEq/L
Mg^{++}	2	mEq/L	58 mEq/L
Cl$^-$	103	mEq/L	4 mEq/L
HCO$_3^-$	27	mEq/L	10 mEq/L
Phosphates	2	mEq/L	75 mEq/L
SO$_4^{--}$	1	mEq/L	2 mEq/L

Figure 12-7.   **Intracellular versus extracellular electrolyte composition.**

phosphate level is near 2 mEq/L. Clearly, the concentration of an electrolyte in one compartment does not always mirror the concentration of that electrolyte in other compartments. The values for intracellular electrolytes shown in Figure 12-7 are only approximate; actual intracellular electrolyte concentrations may vary substantially from one type of cell to another.

Plasma Electrolytes

Clinical measurements of electrolyte concentrations are most often made from intravascular fluid samples—specifically, the plasma or serum. The plasma closely reflects the electrolyte composition of the entire extracellular fluid compartment; however, it does *not* reflect the intracellular fluid composition.

Major Plasma Cations

As shown in Table 12-2, there are essentially four important cations in the plasma: sodium (Na^+), potassium (K^+), calcium (Ca^{2+}), and magnesium (Mg^{2+}). In general, the kidney more precisely regulates the concentrations of cations than anions, because even small abnormalities in the concentrations of most cations have adverse effects on the patient. In contrast, small abnormalities in the concentrations of most anions are usually inconsequential.

Sodium

As shown in Table 12-2, sodium (Na^+) is the most abundant extracellular cation, with a concentration of 142 mEq/L. As such, Na^+ regulation is related intimately to osmosis and fluid balance. Generally speaking, body water

Table 12-2.   PLASMA ELECTROLYTES

Cation Charges	(mEq/L)	Anion Charges	(mEq/L)
Na^+	142	Cl^-	103
K^+	4	HCO_3^-	27
Ca^{2+}	5	HPO_4^{2-}	2
Mg^{2+}	2	SO_4^{2-}	1
Others (trace Elements)	1	Organic acids$^-$	5
		Protein$^-$	16
	154		154

From Tietz, N.W.: Fundamentals of Clinical Chemistry, 3rd ed. Philadelphia, W. B. Saunders, 1987.

tends to follow Na^+. Therefore, excessive loss of Na^+ into the urine is associated with polyuria and potentially with hypovolemia. Most diuretics inhibit Na^+ reabsorption in the nephron, thus causing diuresis by allowing Na^+ to be excreted in the urine.

High concentrations of sodium seen in the plasma (e.g., Na > 158 mEq/L) generally indicate a water or volume deficit. This is sometimes referred to as an extracellular volume contraction that may lead to metabolic alkalosis as the kidneys attempt to retain sodium bicarbonate. Conversely, low sodium concentrations (Na < 120 mEq/L) indicate water excess and may cause what is referred to as a dilution acidosis. Severe hyponatremia may also be caused by the administration of diuretics, especially thiazides.[469] Insuring a normal sodium concentration is critical to maintenance of fluid and acid-base balance.

Potassium

In contrast to Na^+, the normal plasma concentration of K^+ is within the range of 3.5 to 5 mEq/L. Potassium must be precisely maintained within this narrow range in the extracellular fluid or serious adverse consequences may occur. In particular, K^+ is closely related to neuromuscular activity.

Both plasma *hypokalemia* (i.e., low [K^+]) or plasma *hyperkalemia* (i.e., increased [K^+]) may lead to abnormalities in muscle contractility and life-threatening arrhythmias. Because the normal plasma concentration of this cation is so low, there is very little margin for deviation without untoward effects.

Potassium imbalances are also associated with abnormal ECG tracings. The characteristic ECG changes associated with both hypokalemia and hyperkalemia are shown in Figure 12-8; however, ECG changes may not be seen in mild imbalances. Knowledge and recognition of these abnormal tracings may be useful in helping to identify serious potassium disturbances.

Serious hyperkalemia is most often due to renal failure or metabolic acidosis. In contrast, hypokalemia, which is probably the most common electrolyte disturbance, may be caused by diuretics, steroids, or beta agonist drugs.[478] Hypokalemia may also be associated with muscle weakness or cramps. Severe hypokalemia

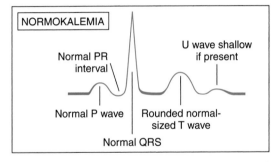

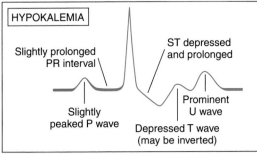

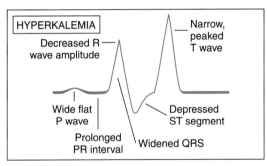

Figure 12-8. **ECG changes seen in potassium imbalances.**

(K < 3.0) has been implicated as a potential cause of ventricular arrhythmias and cardiac arrest.[478,479]

Calcium

Calcium is important to the body for several reasons. It is important in the initiation of muscular contraction and in maintaining normal neuromuscular irritability. Calcium is also essential for normal blood coagulation and for maintaining normal structural integrity of bones and teeth.

Calcium is normally present in approximately equal amounts as ionized Ca^{2+} and un-ionized Ca. Alkalemia decreases the concentration of ionized Ca^{2+}, which results in increased neuromuscular irritability and possible tetany.

Magnesium

The magnesium cation is predominantly an intracellular cation. It is involved in many enzyme reactions within the body and plays a role in neuromuscular functions. It is also important in normal central nervous system function.

SODIUM REGULATION IN THE KIDNEY

Sodium regulation by the kidney is intimately related to acid-base balance. A complex inter-relationship is involved in the renal regulation of blood $[Na^+]$, $[HCO_3^-]$, $[K^+]$, and $[H^+]$. For this reason, the specific chemical mechanisms related to Na^+ reabsorption from the glomerular filtrate are reviewed here. These same mechanisms also help to explain renal regulation of the other important acid-base electrolytes.

Chemical Mechanisms

Most of the Na^+ that enters the glomerular filtrate is recaptured by the renal tubular cells by two different chemical mechanisms: the NaCl mechanism and the $NaHCO_3$ mechanism.

NaCl Mechanism

Ions that move across cell membranes may do so by diffusion or by active transport. *Diffusion* is a passive process by which molecules move from a high concentration to a low concentration. In contrast, *active transport* requires the expenditure of cellular energy to move a substance across a membrane, often against a concentration gradient. Much of the electrolyte reabsorption and secretion that occurs in the nephron is through active transport.

The NaCl mechanism of Na^+ reabsorption is shown in Figure 12-9. The Na^+ cation is actively transported from the glomerular filtrate into the renal tubular cell. To maintain electroneutrality, the Cl^- anion passively accompanies Na^+. Both Na^+ and Cl^- are then transported from the renal tubular cell to the extracellular fluid immediately outside the renal tubular cells and ultimately to the plasma.

Thus, each time this complete reaction takes place, both a Na^+ cation and a Cl^- anion are recaptured from the glomerular filtrate back into the extracellular fluid (blood). All through

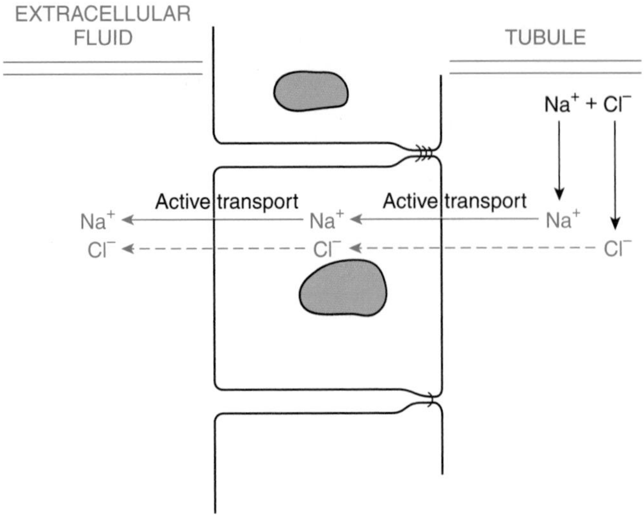

EXTRACELLULAR FLUID

TUBULE

Figure 12-9. **Sodium reabsorption via the NaCl mechanism.** Sodium is actively transported from the filtrate to the renal tubular cell and then to the extracellular fluid and blood. Chloride passively accompanies sodium to maintain electroneutrality.

the renal tubule (i.e., proximal tubule, loop of Henle, distal tubule) Na reabsorption occurs via this mechanism.

NaHCO₃ Mechanism

The other reaction by which Na^+ is recaptured from the filtrate is slightly more complex. In this reaction, an H^+ ion is secreted from the renal tubular cell by active transport into the filtrate in exchange for Na^+ cation, which enters the renal cell as shown in Figure 12-10. Hydrogen ions are made available within the renal tubular cells through the hydrolysis reaction.

Carbonic anhydrase, the enzyme that accelerates the hydrolysis reaction, is available within the renal cells.

After the Na^+ enters the renal cell from the filtrate, it is then actively transported to the extracellular fluid. In the NaCl mechanism described earlier, Cl^- was available inside the renal cell to accompany the Na^+ into the extracellular fluid. In this reaction, the anion HCO_3^-, which was generated via the hydrolysis reaction, accompanies the Na^+ into the extracellular fluid.

As shown in Figure 12-10, the H^+ secreted into the filtrate fuels the hydrolysis reaction

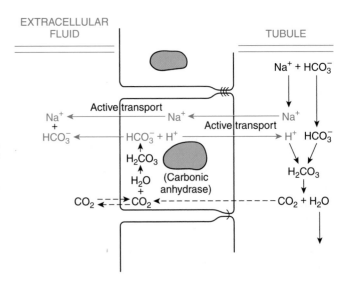

Figure 12-10. **Sodium reabsorption via H^+ secretion and the NaHCO₃ reaction.** Hydrogen ions, available through the hydrolysis reaction, are secreted into the filtrate in exchange for sodium. The sodium is then transported from the renal cell to the extracellular fluid and ultimately to the plasma. Bicarbonate, also available from the hydrolysis reaction, accompanies sodium into the extracellular fluid to maintain electroneutrality.

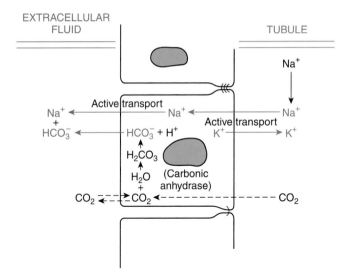

Figure 12-11. **Sodium reabsorption via K+ secretion and the NaHCO₃ reaction.** Potassium ions are secreted into the filtrate in exchange for sodium. The sodium is then transported from the renal cell to the extracellular fluid and ultimately to the plasma. Bicarbonate accompanies sodium into the extracellular fluid to maintain electroneutrality.

and leads to increased dissolved CO_2. The increased dissolved CO_2, in turn, diffuses from the filtrate into the renal cell to fuel the hydrolysis reaction in the intracellular space. It has been postulated that carbonic anhydrase is also available along the border of the renal cell to accelerate the hydrolysis reaction within the filtrate.

There is another important variation of the $NaHCO_3$ reaction. In some cases, a K^+ cation rather than an H^+ ion is secreted into the filtrate in exchange for the Na^+ cation (Fig. 12-11). In fact, because most K^+ that enters the filtrate in the glomerulus is totally reabsorbed in the proximal tubule, it is only through this $NaHCO_3$ reaction in the distal tubule that excess K^+ can be excreted.

The renal cells can selectively secrete K^+ or H^+ into the glomerular filtrate, depending on the body's needs. For example, in the presence of alkalemia, H^+ ions are retained because of their relative shortage. This, in turn, leads to selective K^+ loss and, potentially, to hypokalemia. Thus, *alkalemia tends to cause hypokalemia.*

Abnormalities in potassium concentration have a similar effect. Intracellular hypokalemia (low $[K^+]$) results in increased H^+ secretion. This condition is often difficult to recognize because measurements of serum potassium may be normal even when intracellular potassium is depleted.

Regardless of whether an H^+ ion or a K^+ cation is secreted, each time the $NaHCO_3$

reaction is used to reabsorb Na^+, an HCO_3^- anion enters the extracellular fluid. It follows that any condition that increases this reaction may cause metabolic alkalosis (i.e., increased blood $[HCO_3^-]$). Conversely, any condition that decreases this reaction tends to cause metabolic acidosis (i.e., decreased blood $[HCO_3^-]$).

Renin-Angiotensin System

One of the primary ways that the body regulates sodium reabsorption and ensures an adequate blood volume and renal perfusion is through the *renin-angiotensin-aldosterone system.* An integral part of this system is a group of cells in the walls of the afferent arterioles immediately adjacent to the glomerulus, which have the ability to detect decreased renal perfusion. These cells, because they lie close to the glomeruli, are called the *juxtaglomerular* cells. When blood flow through the renal arterioles is decreased, the juxtaglomerular cells secrete renin into the bloodstream.

Immediately after renin enters the bloodstream, it reacts with angiotensinogen in the plasma and forms the substance *angiotensin I* (Fig. 12-12). Within minutes, angiotensin I is converted to *angiotensin II* by an enzyme present in the lungs. Angiotensin II has effects that tend to elevate blood pressure and increase renal perfusion.

Angiotensin II causes systemic vasoconstriction, which in turn increases the blood pressure.

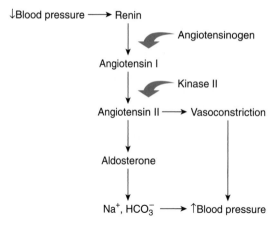

Figure 12-12. **The renin-angiotensin-aldosterone mechanism.**

Table 12-3. SITE AND MECHANISM OF SODIUM REABSORPTION

Mechanism	Site in Tubule			
	Proximal	*Loop*	*Distal*	*% Total*
% Total reabsorption as NaCl	47	25	8	80
% Total reabsorption as NaHCO$_3$	18	—	2	20
% Total reabsorption	65	25	10	100

Modified from Frazier, H.S., and Yager, H.: The clinical use of diuretics (Pt. I). N. Engl. J. Med., *288*: 246, 1973; Frazier, H.S., and Yager, H.: The clinical use of diuretics (Pt. II). N. Engl. J. Med., *288*: 455, 1973.

Angiotensin II also stimulates increased production of the hormone *aldosterone* by the adrenal cortex. Aldosterone, in turn, stimulates NaHCO$_3$ reabsorption in the distal tubule of the nephron. Because water reabsorption follows Na reabsorption, blood volume increases and perfusion to the kidney should also improve. Some physiologic results of aldosterone secretion are shown in Figure 12-13.

Total Sodium Reabsorption

In Table 12-3, total Na$^+$ reabsorption is broken down according to its site in the tubule, and the respective percentages reabsorbed by each of the two mechanisms are shown.[466,467] Note that most Na$^+$ is reabsorbed in the proximal tubule (65%), approximately 25% in the loop, and only 10% in the distal tubule. Also note that 80% of total Na$^+$ reabsorption is in the

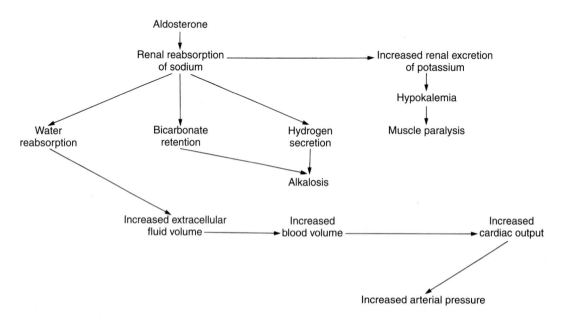

Figure 12-13. **Physiologic results of aldosterone secretion.**

form of NaCl; only 20% normally is reabsorbed as $NaHCO_3$.

Regulation of [HCO_3]

The $NaHCO_3$ reaction is also the mechanism by which tubular reabsorption of the HCO_3^- anion is accomplished. Technically speaking, HCO_3^- is not reabsorbed; rather, it is reclaimed, because it must be transformed into dissolved CO_2 before it can cross from the filtrate into the renal tubular cells. Table 12-3 shows that 90% of HCO_3 reabsorption occurs in the proximal tubule.[466] The final 10% is reabsorbed in the distal tubule.

Because HCO_3^- is actually generated in this reaction, any increase in this reaction will elevate blood [HCO_3^-]. At least three factors are known to stimulate HCO_3^- production[468]: (1) increased blood PCO_2 stimulates increased bicarbonate reabsorption as an acid-base compensatory mechanism; (2) low serum potassium stimulates bicarbonate reabsorption and tends to cause metabolic alkalosis; and (3) decreased blood volume stimulates bicarbonate reabsorption through the renin-angiotensin mechanism.

Diuretics

Diuretics (drugs which can increase the urine output) commonly have important effects on acid-base balance. The specific effect of a given diuretic depends on its mechanism of action. From an acid-base perspective, diuretics that interfere with Na reabsorption can be classified as (1) those that interfere with NaCl reabsorption and (2) those that interfere with $NaHCO_3$ reabsorption.

Interference with NaCl Reabsorption

Most of the commonly used diuretics act by this mechanism. These include thiazide (e.g., Diuril, Hydrodiuril) and loop diuretics such as furosemide (Lasix) and ethacrynic acid (Edecrin). Thiazide diuretics interfere with Na^+ reabsorption in the distal tubule. Because the amount of Na^+ reabsorption in the distal tubule is not large (see Table 12-3), thiazides are not particularly potent. Loop diuretics, as their name implies, act in the loop of Henle and are much stronger diuretics.

Both types of diuretics (i.e., thiazides, loop diuretics) may lead to the development of metabolic alkalosis and hypokalemia. However, it is not the diuretic itself that causes these effects. Rather, these effects are mediated through the renin-angiotensin system because of the loss of Na^+ and decreased renal perfusion. It is, in fact, the compensatory response to the loss of fluid imposed by the diuretic that leads to high aldosterone levels and excessive $NaHCO_3$ reabsorption. The magnitude of the aldosterone response is related directly to the strength of the diuretic and to the degree of concomitant renal hypoperfusion.

Interference with NaHCO$_3$ Reabsorption

A few types of diuretics interfere directly with $NaHCO_3$ reabsorption. These diuretics include carbonic anhydrase inhibitors, such as acetazolamide (Diamox), and drugs that compete with aldosterone for distal tubule chemical sites such as spironolactone (Aldactone). In contrast to NaCl-inhibiting diuretics, these diuretics tend to cause metabolic acidosis because they inhibit $NaHCO_3$ reabsorption. Aldactone also tends to cause hyperkalemia, because the $NaHCO_3$ absorption mechanism per se is blocked. Diamox, on the other hand, may actually increase potassium excretion because it only inhibits the formation and availability of H^+ ions via the hydrolysis reaction.

Diuretics that interfere with $NaHCO_3$ reabsorption are the diuretics of choice in the patient with metabolic alkalosis. However, these diuretics generally are not very potent and, when given alone, are often inadequate to obtain satisfactory levels of diuresis.

Hyperaldosteronism

Normally, some aldosterone circulates in the bloodstream; however, when aldosterone levels are excessive (i.e., hyperaldosteronism), $NaHCO_3$ reabsorption (and H^+ excretion) is also excessive, and metabolic alkalosis results. Hyperaldosteronism likewise tends to cause hypokalemia. The administration of diuretics that interfere with NaCl reabsorption may cause the triad of hyperaldosteronism, hypokalemia, and metabolic alkalosis.

Secondary Hyperaldosteronism

Hyperaldosteronism that occurs as a result of the renin-angiotensin system (e.g., diuretic- or hypoperfusion-induced), is termed *secondary hyperaldosteronism*, because the high aldosterone levels are secondary to the decreased renal perfusion.

Chemically, aldosterone is classified as a *mineralocorticoid*. Therefore, high aldosterone levels are also sometimes referred to as *mineralocorticoid excess*. The term *secondary mineralocorticoid excess* is analogous to secondary hyperaldosteronism.

Primary Hyperaldosteronism

High aldosterone levels may also be the result of some abnormality in adrenal cortex secretion such as an adrenocortical tumor or Cushing's syndrome. This form of aldosteronism is called *primary hyperaldosteronism*. Primary hyperaldosteronism may cause metabolic alkalosis.

Steroids (glucocorticoids), which are commonly administered therapeutically, are chemically similar to the mineralocorticoids and have similar properties. Thus, *steroids in relatively large doses* may cause metabolic alkalosis. Surprisingly, licorice also has a similar chemical component. In relatively high doses, licorice may also lead to metabolic alkalosis.

URINARY BUFFERS AND H⁺ EXCRETION

The excretion of fixed acids (e.g., phosphoric, sulfuric, hydrochloric acid) by the kidney depends on the availability of the urinary buffers. Secretion of H^+ ions into the filtrate occurs only until the pH falls to approximately 4.5. Therefore, it is important that the tubular fluid can accept a large number of hydrogen ions without allowing the pH to fall to this point. This process is accomplished in health and disease through the urinary buffers.

There are three important urinary buffers: *bicarbonate, ammonia,* and *phosphate.* The buffering of H^+ ions in the tubule by the bicarbonate buffer system has been illustrated in Figure 12-10. The other two urinary buffers are briefly described here.

Ammonia

As shown in Figure 12-14, ammonia (NH_3) is generated in the renal tubule cells from glutamine and other amino acids. Being a gas, ammonia then diffuses into the tubular fluid where it can combine with an H^+ ion and minimize the fall in pH. The new substance formed, ammonium (NH_4^+), cannot diffuse back into the tubule cell because it is ionized. Hence, ammonium (and an H^+ ion) is excreted in the urine.

The conjugate bases associated with the accumulation of fixed acids (e.g., Cl^-) can be excreted with any cation (e.g., Na^+, K^+). In normal individuals, most of the H^+ ions associated with fixed acid excretion are disposed of by NH_3. Furthermore, in the presence of acidemia, there is increased ammonia production and H^+ excretion. The kidney can increase

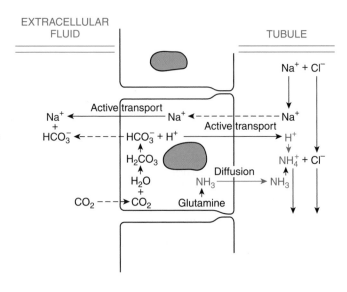

Figure 12-14. Ammonia and urinary buffering. Ammonia is generated in the renal tubule cell and then diffuses into the filtrate. Within the filtrate, ammonia combines with a H⁺ and forms ammonium. Ammonium is excreted in the urine.

ON CALL | CASE 12-1 *ABGs and Critical Thinking*

You are the only person available to care for this patient. You must assess the patient/situation and act accordingly.

A 54-year-old man with CHF is being chronically treated with digitalis and thiazide diuretics. He arrives in the emergency department complaining of weakness, lethargy, and muscle cramps. ECG demonstrates an inverted T wave and a prominent U wave. Blood gases and electrolytes are drawn.

ARTERIAL BLOOD GASES

SaO_2	97
pH	7.54
$PaCO_2$	48 mm Hg
PaO_2	91 mm Hg
$[HCO_3]$	40 mEq/L
FIO_2	0.21
Na	133 mEq/L

CO_2	42 mEq/L
Cl	79 mEq/L
K	2.6 mEq/L

ASSESSMENT

Abnormalities: List abnormal data and other noteworthy information. Classify ABG.
Explanation: List possible diseases, pathology, or other situations which may have led to this patient's condition.

INTERVENTION

Importance: Prioritize concern(s) of treatment in order of urgency and/or seriousness as you see the overall situation.
Objective: Describe the specific goal or target of treatment.

acid excretion by as much as fourfold by this mechanism.[480]

Phosphate

The other major buffer in the filtrate is phosphate. As shown in Figure 12-15, $Na^{++} + HPO_4^{++}$, which is present in the filtrate, can exchange an Na^+ for an H^+ ion from the renal tubular cell, as described earlier in the $NaHCO_3$ mechanism for reabsorption of Na. The H^+ that enters the filtrate can immediately combine with HPO_4^{2-} to form $H_2PO_4^-$. Therefore, the phosphate buffer also facilitates increased H^+ excretion. Acidemia increases phosphate excretion and thereby enhances the ability of the kidneys to excrete H^+.

PLASMA pH AND [K$^+$]

The clinician should also be aware of the important relationship between the pH of the plasma and the potassium ion concentration of the plasma ($[K^+]$). In acidemia, for example, the plasma $[K^+]$ usually increases. Conversely, in respiratory or metabolic alkalemia, the plasma $[K^+]$ decreases.

Apparently, when plasma H^+ levels are high, some of the excess H^+ is actively transported to the intracellular space (Fig. 12-16,*A*). This may represent an attempt by the body to spread out the H^+ load to a larger fluid space, perhaps as an intracellular-extracellular fluid buffer mechanism. In any event, in exchange for the H^+ that enters the cells, K^+ is released to the

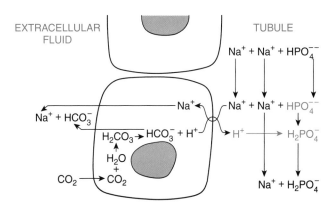

Figure 12-15. **Phosphate and urinary buffering.** Phosphate in the filtrate can accept an H^+ and minimize the fall in pH.

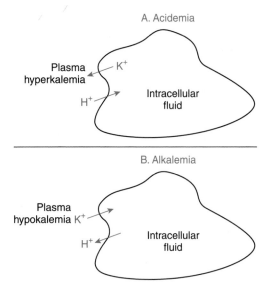

Figure 12-16. **pH and plasma potassium.**
A, Plasma acidemia tends to cause hyperkalemia as hydrogen ions from the plasma exchange with potassium ions from the intracellular fluid. **B,** Plasma alkalemia tends to cause plasma hypokalemia as potassium ions from the plasma move into the intracellular fluid in exchange for hydrogen ions.

plasma. Plasma potassium rises approximately 0.5 mEq/L for every 0.1 decrease in pH.[470]

In organic acidemia (e.g., lactic acidosis, ketoacidosis), the inverse relationship between pH of the plasma and [K+] does not always hold true.[471–473] The reasons for this are unclear but perhaps they are related to the fact that organic acidosis typically originates in the intracellular fluid.

In alkalemia, the exchange of hydrogen ions and potassium ions is in the opposite direction (see Fig. 12-16,B). Hydrogen ions leave the intra-cellular space to replenish the deficiency in the plasma space.[474] Conversely, potassium ions enter the cells in exchange for hydrogen ions. Thus, alkalemia leads to plasma hypokalemia because of the migration of potassium to the intracellular space.

LAW OF ELECTRONEUTRALITY

Principle of Electroneutrality

The *law of electroneutrality* states that in a volume of fluid, the total positive charges of the cations are equal to the total negative charges of the anions. Thus, in units of milliequivalents per liter, the concentration of cations is equal to the concentration of anions in any specific fluid compartment. Table 12-2 demonstrates that the total concentration of cations in the plasma (154 mEq/L) is equal to the total concentration of anions in the plasma (154 mEq/L). Thus, the law of electroneutrality is maintained.

As stated earlier in this chapter, the kidneys more precisely control the concentration of plasma cations than anions. This probably occurs because alterations in major cations are generally more detrimental. Conversely, the concentration of the most abundant anion, chloride, can change appreciably with almost no clinical consequences.

Thus, the body allows the concentration of chloride to vary in a somewhat passive manner. The serum chloride concentration generally varies in response to the need for electroneutrality. For example, if the body has lost another anion (e.g., bicarbonate) and has a total anion deficiency, the chloride concentration increases.

Hypochloremic Metabolic Alkalosis

The law of electroneutrality helps to explain the inverse relationship between chloride and bicarbonate anions in metabolic alkalosis. If the total cation concentration is normal, an increase in bicarbonate (i.e., metabolic alkalosis) is always associated with *hypochloremia* (i.e., decreased chloride), which must inevitably occur if electroneutrality is to be maintained. Patients with chronic obstructive pulmonary disease and chronic hypercarbia often selectively retain the base bicarbonate in order to normalize pH. These patients also manifest hypochloremia to maintain electroneutrality.

The phrase *hypochloremic metabolic alkalosis* is sometimes used to refer to metabolic alkalosis that *originated* as a result of a loss of chloride (e.g., due to diuretics, loss of gastrointestinal secretions). This terminology is not recommended here, however, because metabolic alkalosis of *any* origin is likely to be associated with a low serum chloride (i.e., hypochloremia) regardless of the mechanism of its origin.

Anion Gap

The anion gap is an index that can be used to aid in the diagnosis of metabolic acidosis. Figure 12-17,A shows the balance between sodium, which is the major cation, and chloride

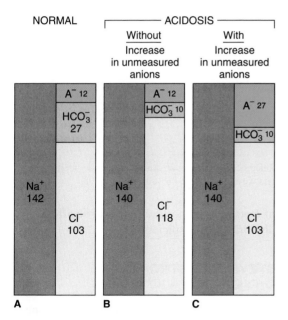

Figure 12-17. The anion gap and metabolic acidosis. A, The normal anion gap. **B,** Normal anion gap in metabolic acidosis due to loss of base, so-called hyperchloremic metabolic acidosis. **C,** Increased anion gap in metabolic acidosis due to increased fixed acid.

and bicarbonate, which are the two most abundant (major) anions. The mathematical difference between sodium (Na+) and the sum of chloride and bicarbonate (HCO$_3^-$ and Cl−) represents the *anion gap* (A−), or unmeasured anions.

Because total CO$_2$ rather than bicarbonate is often reported with serum electrolytes, it is acceptable to substitute total CO$_2$ for bicarbonate in the anion gap formula, as shown in Equation 12-1. The normal anion gap, which is calculated in Equation 12-1, is approximately 12 mEq/L (see Fig. 12-17,*A*). The normal anion gap range is 12 to 14 mEq/L. An increased anion gap usually represents an increase in blood fixed acids. A low anion gap is uncommon, although it may be observed as a result of hypoalbuminemia.

Equation 12-1

$$[Na^+] - ([Cl^-] + [TCO_2]) = A^-$$
$$142 - (103 + 27) = 12$$

Hyperchloremic Metabolic Acidosis

Metabolic acidosis (i.e., decreased [HCO$_3^-$]) may be caused by a loss of base such as

bicarbonate from the body, or it may be caused by the accumulation of some fixed acid. Based on the law of electroneutrality, if excessive bicarbonate were to be lost from the body (e.g., renal tubular disease, diarrhea), the chloride concentration would have to increase to maintain sufficient anions for electroneutrality. Thus, *metabolic acidosis caused by a loss of base* is often called *hyperchloremic metabolic acidosis*, because it is typically associated with hyperchloremia.

Figure 12-17,*B* shows that, in metabolic acidosis caused by the loss of base (i.e., hyperchloremic metabolic acidosis), the anion gap is *normal*. Because the chloride anion (a measured anion) increases to replace the bicarbonate anion, the number of *unmeasured* anions remains constant.

High Anion Gap Acidosis

Metabolic acidosis (i.e., decreased [HCO$_3$]) is more commonly due to the abnormal accumulation of fixed acids (e.g., lactic acid, keto acids). Referring back to Table 12-2, it can be seen that the *unmeasured anions* that make up the anion gap include anions from fixed acids (e.g., lactate, sulfate, phosphate). Therefore, when there is excessive accumulation of these acids, the anion gap increases.

In the presence of increased fixed acids in the blood, the bicarbonate concentration decreases due to buffering. Thus, in the presence of increased fixed acids, plasma bicarbonate decreases but chloride does not increase. Rather, the increase in anions necessary for electroneutrality occurs in the unmeasured anions. Figure 12-17,*C* shows the electrolyte pattern that is seen with metabolic acidosis secondary to increased accumulation of fixed acids.

Summary

The anion gap is a useful index for differentiating the general causes of metabolic acidosis. When metabolic acidosis is caused by a loss of base (so-called hyperchloremic metabolic acidosis), the anion gap is normal. Conversely, when increased fixed acids are present in the blood, the anion gap increases.

Notwithstanding, the anion gap is not a particularly sensitive index, and mild A− elevations (e.g., to 14–16 mEq/L) may be seen in some conditions other than metabolic acidosis. In particular, alkalosis and hyperalbuminemia tend to increase the anion gap. Nevertheless, an anion gap above 16 mEq/L strongly suggests increased fixed acids in the blood. Furthermore, the higher the anion gap, the greater is the likelihood of increased fixed acids and metabolic acidemia. Therefore, the anion gap is a useful diagnostic index in the assessment and the differential diagnosis of metabolic acidosis.

Hypoalbuminemia and the Anion Gap

As mentioned previously, the protein concentration has a significant impact on the anion gap. The most abundant protein is albumin, therefore the clinician should realize that changes in albumin will substantially change the anion gap. Normal albumin is approximately 4.4 g/dL in the blood.

For every 0.4 g/dL drop in albumin, the anion gap will decrease 1 mEq/L.[481] Because hypoalbuminemia is quite common in the critical care setting, the normals for anion gap should be adjusted for each patient accordingly as shown in Table 12-4. Using Table 12-4 will help identify those patients with increased fixed acids that may go unrecognized. Again, increased fixed acid is the most common cause

Table 12-4.   ANION GAP ADJUSTED FOR HYPOALBUMINEMIA

Albumin (g/dL)	Maximum A$^-$ (mEq/L)
4.4	16
4.0	15
3.6	14
3.2	13
2.8	12

Reference: Figge, J. et al: Anion gap and hypoalbuminemia. Crit. Care Med. 26:1807–1810, 1998.

of metabolic acidosis and should be afforded a high index of suspicion.

STEWART'S STRONG ION DIFFERENCE

In 1981, Peter Stewart advocated a new approach to acid-base diagnosis[475] that continues to be espoused by some clinicians.[477] Through a series of complex mathematical calculations, Stewart concluded that there are only three independent variables that determine pH. The three independent variables are PCO_2, the strong ion difference (SID), and total concentration of the nonvolatile weak acids $[A_{TOT}]$. The strong ion difference can be calculated as SID = ([Na] + [K] + Ca^{2+} + Mg^{2+} + [other strong

---

ON CALL | CASE 12-2 *ABGs and Critical Thinking*

You are the only person available to care for this patient. You must assess the patient/situation and act accordingly.

A 62-year-old man with a history of chronic anemia arrives in the emergency department short of breath. Blood gases and electrolytes are drawn.

ARTERIAL BLOOD GASES

SaO$_2$	97
pH	7.22
PaCO$_2$	20 mm Hg
PaO$_2$	84 mm Hg
[HCO$_3$]	8 mEq/L
FIO$_2$	0.21
Na	135 mEq/L
CO$_2$	10 mEq/L
Cl	109 mEq/L

K	5.2 mEq/L
Albumin	3.2 g/dL

ASSESSMENT

Abnormalities: List abnormal data and other noteworthy information. Classify ABG.

Explanation: List possible diseases, pathology, or other situations which may have led to this patient's condition.

Evaluation: Suggest additional data which would be useful in helping understand the situation or in making a diagnosis.

INTERVENTION

Importance: Prioritize concern(s) of treatment in order of urgency and/or seriousness as you see the overall situation.

anions]).[477] Stewart advocates disregarding [HCO_3] because it is a *dependent* variable and not one of the three key independent variables.

Despite the precision of this approach, its *cumbersome* and technical nature make it difficult to understand and apply in clinical practice.[476] Notwithstanding, I believe its focus on [Na], [Cl], and [protein] is of great value in understanding how changes in these values impact acid-base and fluid balance. In particular, careful analysis of electrolytes and protein can assist in understanding the nature of extracellular fluid contraction alkalosis, dilution acidosis, and protein disturbances.

EXERCISES

Exercise 12-1 Regulation of Ventilation

Fill in the blanks or select the best answer.

1. The primary respiratory center (generator) located in the central nervous system is in the _____.

2. The central chemoreceptors respond directly to the pH of the (blood/CSF).

3. The blood-brain barrier is readily permeable to (ions/gases) but is relatively impermeable to (ions/gases).

4. The circulatory delay has been suggested to explain the breathing pattern sometimes observed in congestive heart failure called _____ respiration.

5. The peripheral chemoreceptors are located in two distinct anatomic areas: the _____ and _____ bodies.

6. Designate which of the following may stimulate the peripheral chemoreceptors:
   a. Mild anemia
   b. Hypoxemia
   c. Cyanide poisoning
   d. Hypercarbia ($PaCO_2$ 70 mm Hg)
   e. Cardiogenic shock
   f. pH 7.32

7. The (central/peripheral) chemoreceptors respond to low oxygen levels in the blood.

8. When PaO_2 falls below _____ mm Hg, there is a dramatic increase in impulse production and ventilation.

9. The regulation of ventilation in healthy individuals is primarily under the control of the (central/peripheral) chemoreceptors.

10. In acute hypoxemia, the central chemoreceptors are (stimulated/depressed).

11. The ventilatory response to chronic hypoxemia is (less/greater) than the ventilatory response to acute hypoxemia.

12. The initial blood gas abnormality associated with mild pulmonary disease is mild (hypoxemia/hypercarbia).

13. In severe pulmonary disease, blood gases typically show (hypocarbia/hypercarbia).

14. Administration of oxygen to individuals with chronic pulmonary disease may result in progressive (hypercarbia/hypocarbia).

15. The (J receptor/Hering-Breuer) reflex is located in the interstitial tissue of the alveolar-capillary membrane.

Exercise 12-2	**Renal Function**

Fill in the blanks or select the best answer.

1. Each of the two kidneys consists of an outer _____ and an inner _____.

2. Urine gathers in the renal pelvis and then flows through the _____ down to the urinary bladder, where it is stored.

3. The functional unit of the kidney is the _____.

4. The capillary network within Bowman's capsule is called the _____.

5. Blood enters the nephron through the (afferent/efferent) arteriole.

6. The tubule that the glomerular filtrate passes through immediately after leaving Bowman's capsule is called the _____ _____ _____.

7. Cells and proteins (can/cannot) normally pass through the glomerulus into the filtrate.

8. Decreased urine output is called _____.

9. The process of exchanging one electrolyte for another in the filtrate is called tubular (absorption/secretion).

10. The fluid that accumulates within Bowman's capsule is called the _____.

Exercise 12-3	**Body Fluids and Electrolytes**

Fill in the blanks or select the best answer.

1. Most body water is located in the (extracellular/intracellular) fluid space.

2. Fluid within the vascular system is called the _____ fluid.

3. If plasma is allowed to coagulate and the coagulated fluid is centrifuged, the clear fluid that remains is called _____.

4. The portion of the extracellular fluid that exists outside the vascular space is called the _____ fluid.

5. Glucose is an example of a/an (electrolyte/non-electrolyte).

6. Electrolytes that carry a positive charge are called (cations/anions).

7. (Sodium/potassium) is the most abundant intracellular cation.

8. List the four major cations in the plasma with their normal concentrations.

9. The most abundant extracellular cation is (potassium/sodium).

10. (Na^+/K^+) is intimately related to osmosis and fluid balance.

Chemical Mechanisms of Sodium Reabsorption and the Renin-Angiotensin System

Fill in the blanks or select the best answer.

1. State the two different chemical mechanisms by which Na^+ is reabsorbed from the glomerular filtrate.

2. To maintain electroneutrality, the anion _____ passively accompanies Na^+ from the filtrate to the renal tubular cell in the NaCl mechanism.

3. State the two possible cations that can be secreted into the filtrate in exchange for a Na^+ in the $NaHCO_3$ reaction.

4. Carbonic anhydrase (is/is not) present in the renal tubular cells.

5. Hydrogen ions available to be secreted in the $NaHCO_3$ reaction are produced as a result of the (NaCl/hydrolysis) reaction.

6. In the presence of alkalemia, (H^+/K^+) is selectively secreted in the $NaHCO_3$ reaction and (H^+/K^+) is retained.

7. The group of cells that are located in the walls of the afferent arterioles of the nephrons immediately adjacent to the glomerulus and that have the ability to detect decreased renal perfusion are called the _____ cells.

8. The juxtaglomerular cells secrete (angiotensin/renin) into the bloodstream.

9. Angiotensin II stimulates the production of _____ from the adrenal cortex.

10. Aldosterone stimulates (NaCl/$NaHCO_3$) reabsorption.

Total Sodium Reabsorption and Diuretics

Fill in the blanks or select the best answer.

1. Most Na^+ is reabsorbed in the (proximal/distal) tubule.

2. Normally, (20%/80%) of Na^+ reabsorption is in the form of NaCl.

3. Na^+ reabsorption in the distal tubule is primarily in the form of (NaCl/$NaHCO_3$).

4. Technically speaking, HCO_3 is (reabsorbed/reclaimed) from the filtrate.

5. About 90% of bicarbonate reabsorption occurs in the (proximal/distal) tubule.

6. Most of the commonly used diuretics interfere with (NaCl/$NaHCO_3$) reabsorption.

7. (Thiazide/Loop) diuretics are quite potent.

8. Loop and thiazide diuretics may lead to the development of metabolic (acidosis/alkalosis) and (hypokalemia/hyperkalemia).

9. The metabolic alkalosis seen with administration of loop diuretics (is/is not) due to an aldosterone response.

10. The diuretic of choice in metabolic alkalosis is (thiazide/acetazolamide).

| Exercise 12-6 | **Hyperaldosteronism, Urinary Buffers, and Potassium** |

Fill in the blanks or select the best answer.

1. Hyperaldosteronism leads to metabolic (acidosis/alkalosis).

2. Hyperaldosteronism leads to (increased/decreased) H^+ excretion and (hyperkalemia/hypokalemia).

3. Hyperaldosteronism that occurs as a result of the renin-angiotensin system (e.g., diuretic- or hypoperfusion-induced) is called (primary/secondary) hyperaldosteronism.

4. Aldosterone is classified chemically as a (mineralocorticoid/glucocorticoid).

5. Cushing's syndrome is an example of (primary/secondary) hyperaldosteronism.

6. Steroids administered therapeutically are classified chemically as (glucocorticoids/mineralocorticoids).

7. Secretion of H^+ ions into the filtrate occurs only until the pH of the filtrate falls to approximately _____.

8. Name the three urinary H^+ buffer systems.

9. In acidemia, the serum $[K^+]$ usually (increases/decreases).

10. The increased K^+ observed in the plasma in acidemia originates from the (interstitial/intracellular) space.

| Exercise 12-7 | **Law of Electroneutrality, Anion Gap, and Stewart's Strong Ion Difference** |

Fill in the blanks or select the best answer.

1. Because of the law of electroneutrality, metabolic alkalosis is usually associated with (hypochloremia/hyperchloremia).

2. The anion gap is an index that can be used to help to determine the cause of metabolic (alkalosis/acidosis).

3. Write the formula for calculation of the anion gap using serum electrolytes.

4. The normal anion gap range is about _____ mEq/L.

5. Metabolic acidosis with a normal A^- is called (hypochloremic/hyperchloremic) metabolic acidosis.

6. In the presence of increased fixed acids in the blood, the anion gap (increases/decreases).

Calculate the anion gap, given the following electrolytes, and indicate whether the metabolic acidosis is due to increased fixed acids or to a decreased base (assume normal albumin).

	Na^+	Cl^-	TCO_2
7.	140	98	14
8.	142	105	15
9.	135	115	10
10.	134	102	17

11. Low albumin tends to (increase/decrease) the anion gap.

12. According to Stewart's strong ion difference, [HCO_3] is a/an (dependent/independent) acid-base variable.

13. State the three independent variables in Stewart's strong ion difference approach to acid-base analysis.

Exercise 12-8 Internet Work

1. Search the internet for Stewart's Strong ION Difference. Suggested site: http://ccforum.com/content/4/1/6.
   A. List the body's strong ions.
   B. State the purported advantage of using Stewart's strong ion difference.

2. Search the internet for "increased anion gap metabolic acidosis."
   A. What does the acronym "MUDPILES" stand for?

NBRC Challenge 12

Please select the best answer for the following multiple-choice questions.

1. A blood gas on a patient reveals a primary metabolic acidosis. One of the first tests you would consider to determine the primary diagnosis would be:
   A) chest radiograph.
   B) pulmonary function studies.
   C) serum electrolytes.
   D) 12 lead ECG.
   E) fluid I&0.
   (RRT-CSE EXAMINATION — NBRC
      MATRIX I,A,1,c)

2. Following administration of KCl I.V. for a patient with metabolic alkalosis, the serum potassium level is 4.0 mEq/L. You would recommend:
   A) increasing the dosage of potassium chloride.
   B) calculation of the anion gap.
   C) obtaining a chest radiograph.
   D) holding the administration of KCl.
   E) obtaining an ECG.
   (RRT EXAMINATION — NBRC
      MATRIX III,A,1,g)

3. An ECG tracing of a patient with chronic renal failure manifests a prolonged PR interval, a widened QRS, and a narrow peaked T wave. It would be important to evaluate:

A) the patient's anion gap.
B) serum potassium.
C) PaO_2.
D) $PaCO_2$.
E) [Hb].
(RRT EXAMINATION — NBRC
   MATRIX I,A,2,a)

4. In critically ill patients, the anion gap should be interpreted in light of the _____ level.
   A) albumin
   B) hemoglobin
   C) magnesium
   D) ionized calcium
   E) non-ionized calcium
   (RRT EXAMINATION — NBRC
      MATRIX III,A,1,g)

5. After administration of FIO_2 1.0, the patient's anion gap moves from 23 to 12 mEq/L, one can conclude the patient most likely:
   A) had ketoacidosis.
   B) was hypokalemic.
   C) had lactic acidosis.
   D) had hyperchloremic acidosis.
   E) had cyanide toxicity.
   (RRT-CSE EXAMINATION — NBRC
      MATRIX III,B,1,h)

13
Differential Diagnosis of Acid-Base Disturbances

...it should be emphasized that a given set of acid-base values is never diagnostic of a particular acid-base disorder, but rather consistent with a wide range of acid-base abnormalities.

J.A. Kraut and N.E. Madias[540]

For each class of disorders (i.e., metabolic acidosis, respiratory alkalosis, etc.), a wide range of possibilities exists ... When the diagnosis is not immediately apparent from the history or clinical setting, however, laboratory data can be extremely helpful.

Jordan J. Cohen and
Jerome P. Kassirer[483]

As with all acid-base disorders, analysis of arterial blood gas samples and serum electrolytes provide the quantitative basis for diagnosis and treatment.

Erik Swenson[484]

The value of establishing a diagnosis is to provide a logical basis for treatment and prognosis.

Clayton L. Thomas[482]

Outline

INTRODUCTION

A systematic method for classification of acid-base status, based on the arterial blood gas report, was described in Chapter 2, and limits, rules, and steps in classification were clearly delineated. Application of these principles leads to consistent results regardless of the background of the interpreter. In fact, these limits and steps can be programmed into a computer that will provide reproducible classifications.

There is no question that blood gas classification is useful in the clinical assessment of acid-base status. It is an excellent way to summarize the blood gas report and to focus attention on important problem areas. However, many acid-base disorders go unrecognized if *only* the blood gas report is considered. Furthermore, general acid-base diagnoses such as metabolic acidosis or respiratory alkalosis do not provide a great deal of information about the underlying disorder. Optimal patient treatment and follow-up requires a more specific, in-depth, understanding of the nature of the problem.

Complete Picture

Just as the PaO_2 is only one piece in the puzzle of tissue oxygenation, the blood gas is similarly only one piece in the puzzle of acid-base balance. All laboratory tests should be interpreted within the context of the patient as a whole. The effective clinician considers more than numbers from a solitary test. The conglomerate of pre-existing disease, knowledge of physiology and pathology, effects of therapeutic interventions, and integration of historical data must all be considered. The ability to integrate these myriad considerations is indeed the *art* of acid-base diagnosis.

Classification versus Diagnosis

The clinician must keep in mind that when the terms *acidosis* or *alkalosis* are applied to a patient, they reflect a pathologic acid-base process, and not simply an isolated laboratory finding. It is technically incorrect to state that the patient has a metabolic acidosis simply because the bicarbonate or base excess on the blood gas report is low. A low base excess represents a laboratory measurement (laboratory metabolic acidosis) and not necessarily an abnormal patient process (i.e., perhaps it is due to compensation). Thus, the clinician must seek additional evidence that supports the presence of a *primary* abnormal acid-base process.

Support Information

Additional information that must be used to supplement and modify blood gas findings includes drug therapy, vital signs, chest radiograph, electrocardiography, pulmonary function studies, and physical assessment. Assessment of various blood tests is also important. Measurement of electrolytes, blood glucose, blood urea nitrogen (BUN), creatinine, red blood cell count, and white blood cell count provides valuable insight into the patient's acid-base status, particularly in the critical care setting. Indeed, many blood gas machines now include many of these measurements along with blood gases.

Definitive Acid-Base Diagnosis
General versus Definitive Diagnosis

An acid-base diagnosis based on blood gas classification alone lacks specificity. Even after complete acid-base assessment, a diagnosis of respiratory acidosis or metabolic acidosis is a *general* acid-base diagnosis. A general acid-base diagnosis does not reveal the patient's underlying disease or problem.

Examples of more definitive acid-base diagnoses are *lactic metabolic acidosis secondary to hypoxia* or *respiratory alkalosis secondary to hypoxemia*. Compared with a general acid-base diagnosis, a definitive diagnosis provides the clinician with a much clearer understanding of the acid-base pathophysiology. Furthermore, depiction of the specific root problem in a given acid-base disturbance is a prerequisite to optimal treatment and therapy.

Thus, the clinician should not conclude acid-base assessment with only a blood gas classification or a general acid-base diagnosis (e.g., respiratory acidosis, metabolic alkalosis). A more descriptive etiology (i.e., definitive diagnosis) must be determined after careful analysis of physical findings, symptoms, history, and supplemental laboratory data. Furthermore, identification of the specific acid or base that has caused the disturbance (e.g., increased carbonic acid, increased lactic acid, loss of bicarbonate) also helps to clarify thinking and understanding.

Common Causes of General Disturbances

In this chapter, some of the more common causes of respiratory and metabolic acid-base disturbances are briefly discussed. The novice clinician is encouraged to review this information before he or she attempts to make a definitive acid-base diagnosis at the bedside. A diligent attempt has been made to include all the common causes of these general acid-base disorders and some causes that are less common. Obviously, it is impossible to list every possible cause.

In general, the boxes have been constructed as functional groupings of acid-base disorders. Problems with similar mechanisms (e.g., neuromuscular problems) have been clustered together rather than trying to list every specific disease that could cause a particular type of acid-base disorder.

It is noteworthy that often more than one root problem is responsible for a general acid-base diagnosis. A patient may have metabolic alkalosis due to a combination of factors. For example, it is not uncommon for a patient to be receiving both diuretics and steroids and, in addition, to manifest hypokalemia. In this case, three different underlying factors could be contributing to a metabolic alkalosis. Therefore, it is advisable to review and consider *all* possibilities, even if one mechanism is already evident.

RESPIRATORY ACIDOSIS

Respiratory acidosis may result from a variety of acute and chronic causes. It threatens acid-base balance through the accumulation of carbonic acid. Furthermore, it compromises oxygenation via decreased alveolar delivery and hypoxemia.

Physiologic Response to Respiratory Acidosis (Hypercapnia)

The clinical manifestations of acute hypercapnia are predominantly neurologic.[485] Symptoms may vary from anxiety and irritability to lethargy and somnolence. Pulmonary symptoms may include dyspnea and distress. Stupor and coma appear to be rare but may occur when $PaCO_2$ exceeds 70 mm Hg.[485]

It is also important to remember that hypercapnia causes increased cerebral perfusion and intracranial pressure. Indeed, during acute hypercapnia, cerebral blood flow may more than double while, conversely, it will decrease by more than 50% when $PaCO_2$ falls by about 10 mm Hg.[496] This may be especially important in the patient with CNS trauma or following CNS surgery where low intracranial pressure is a goal in patient treatment. In chronic hypercapnia, cerebral blood flow is normal and responsiveness to changes in $PaCO_2$ is reduced. It appears that interstitial acidosis is really the primary regulator of cerebral dilation and perfusion.[497]

Cardiovascular effects in mild to moderate hypercapnia typically include an increased cardiac output and tachycardia mediated through an adrenergic response. On clinical examination, the skin may be flushed and warm. The patient may also be diaphoretic and demonstrate a bounding pulse. In *severe hypercapnia*, hypotension and/or arrhythmia may occur as a direct effect of $PaCO_2$ on the myocardium and vasculature.[485]

Physiologic changes may be more related to concurrent acidemia and hypoxia than hypercapnia. Certainly there is a less dramatic response when hypercapnia develops slowly. The somewhat innocuous nature of hypercapnia has lead to the therapeutic approach of "permissive hypercapnia"[498] where hypercapnia is tolerated in an effort to avoid excessive alveolar volume and pressure (see Chapter 10). Many believe that substantial hypercapnia is likely associated with very few adverse effects.[498]

Common Causes of Respiratory Acidosis

As discussed previously, it is important to identify the underlying cause of the acid-base disorder to optimize management. Some common causes of respiratory acidosis are shown in Box 13-1.

Some may find it easier to think of the potential *origins* of the various fundamental acid-base disturbances. For example, as shown in Figure 13-1, eight common sources of primary respiratory acidosis are: the lungs (e.g., chronic obstructive pulmonary disease [COPD]), drugs (e.g., anesthetics/narcotics), mechanical ventilation (e.g., iatrogenic hypoventilation), muscle fatigue (e.g., status asthmaticus), central nervous system (CNS; e.g., central alveolar hypoventilation), neuromuscular junction

Box 13-1	Causes of Respiratory Acidosis

Chronic obstructive pulmonary disease (COPD)
Oxygen excess in COPD
Drugs
   Barbiturates
   Anesthetics
   Narcotics
   Sedatives
Extreme ventilation-perfusion mismatch
Exhaustion
Neuromuscular disorders
   Poliomyelitis
   Amyotrophic lateral sclerosis
   Guillain-Barré syndrome
   Electrolyte deficiencies (K^+, PO_4^-)
   Myasthenia gravis
Iatrogenic respiratory acidosis
Neurologic disorders
Excessive CO_2 production
   Total parenteral nutrition
   Sepsis
   Severe burns
   $NaHCO_3$ administration

(e.g., Guillain-Barré syndrome), increased metabolism in cells/tissues (e.g., burn patients), and oxygen excess depressing ventilatory drive (e.g., in COPD).

Chronic Obstructive Pulmonary Disease

The most common cause of *chronic* respiratory acidosis is COPD. Emphysema, chronic bronchitis, and asthma are the major subgroups of COPD. COPD is characterized by progressive airway disease that leads to gas trapping, uneven distribution of ventilation, hypoxemia, and, ultimately, in severe disease, respiratory acidosis.

The patient with COPD is readily recognized on physical examination by the presence of a barrel chest, adventitious (abnormal) breath sounds, labored breathing, and forced expiration. Hyperaeration and flattened diaphragm are present on the chest radiograph. Pulmonary function studies show a diminished forced expiratory flow (FEF) in the mid-expiratory flow in moderate disease, progressing to a decreased forced expiratory volume in 1 second (FEV_1) in more severe disease.

Chronic respiratory acidosis is only seen in approximately 25% to 33% of patients with significant chronic airflow obstruction.[499] Chronic hypercapnia appears to be a mechanism whereby some patients avoid excessive respiratory muscle fatigue. Indeed, because of the hypercapnia, these patients can eliminate CO_2 with far less ventilatory effort.[499,500]

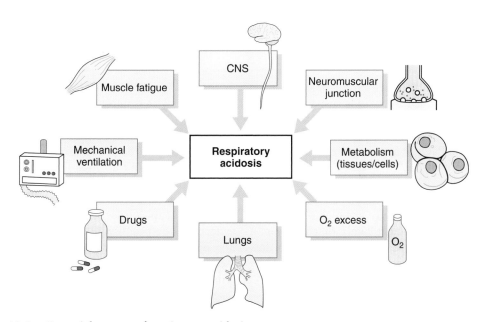

Figure 13-1.   Potential sources of respiratory acidosis.

Therefore, hypercapnia appears to be a useful strategy for avoiding inspiratory muscle overloading and failure.[499] Notwithstanding, due to their limited ventilatory reserve, acute pneumonia can and frequently does lead to a superimposed *acute* ventilatory failure in these individuals.[501]

Oxygen Excess in Chronic Obstructive Pulmonary Disease

As described previously, *chronic respiratory acidosis* is common in end-stage COPD. In addition, when high concentrations of oxygen are administered to patients with end-stage COPD (especially those with hypercarbia), they may manifest an acute rise in $PaCO_2$ levels above their chronically elevated baseline $PaCO_2$. This acute respiratory acidosis is most apt to occur when $PaCO_2$ levels are very high and/or when PaO_2 levels are very low at the time when the oxygen is administered.[486,487] Actually, baseline hypoxia and acidosis are better predictors of those patients likely to have worsening respiratory acidosis than baseline $PaCO_2$.[485]

Even slight elevations in FIO_2 may cause this effect.[488,489] The acute hypercarbia may be progressive and may occasionally result in respiratory arrest. The rise in $PaCO_2$ may be caused by obliteration of the hypoxic drive of the peripheral chemoreceptors; however, some evidence suggests that it is due primarily to a worsening of ventilation-perfusion matching.[490] In all likelihood, it is a multi-factorial response.

Regardless of the potential for acute respiratory acidosis, when *hypoxia* is suspected, oxygen must be administered in doses sufficient to relieve it. The target of oxygen therapy in COPD is typically a PaO_2 of approximately 60 mm Hg, although not higher.[486,491] When acute respiratory acidosis is observed in a patient with COPD who has a PaO_2 level greater than 60 mm Hg, the FIO_2 may be excessive. The higher the PaO_2 and FIO_2 level, the more likely that the respiratory acidosis is at least in part related to the oxygen therapy.

A trial of decreased FIO_2 followed by arterial blood gases should reveal whether excess oxygen was in fact the cause of the acute respiratory acidosis. If $PaCO_2$ improves at a lower FIO_2, it is logical to assume that oxygen therapy was excessive.

Interestingly, oxygen therapy may worsen hypercapnia in other chronic disorders as well. Although the mechanism is unclear, these include patients with neuromuscular disease, asthma, diaphragmatic dysfunction, or obesity hypoventilation syndrome.[485]

Drugs

Depressant drugs such as morphine may diminish respiratory drive,[492] with resultant hypercarbia and acidosis. The response of a given patient depends on the individual, the drug, and the dosage. Barbiturates, anesthetics, narcotics, and sedatives may cause this effect. Narcotic overdose characteristically manifests itself in a slow respiratory rate in the spontaneously breathing patient.

Individuals with COPD are particularly vulnerable to the respiratory effects of sedatives and narcotics and may exhibit further CO_2 retention even at normal dosages. Although the usual setting for drug-induced hypoventilation is the emergency room, respiratory acidosis secondary to drug effects may also be seen in the postoperative or critical care milieu.

Neuromuscular blocking agents may also be used to control ventilation in the ICU. This is particularly true with many of the new ventilatory techniques such as inverse I:E ratios and "permissive hypercapnia," which may render the patient uncomfortable or anxious. Barring the obvious problem of potential ventilator disconnect, one must be careful to avoid paralysis without adequate sedation. The terror of conscious paralysis is unthinkable.

Extreme Ventilation-Perfusion Mismatch

As stated earlier, the mechanism that ultimately leads to respiratory acidosis in COPD is most likely deterioration in the ventilation-perfusion match. Regardless of the disease, whenever gas exchange capabilities of the lung become extremely compromised, the ability of the lungs to excrete CO_2 may become impaired. This may occur in severe lung cancer, pneumonia, or any other severe pulmonary parenchymal disease. In summary, *any acute or chronic disease that results in severe lung damage may ultimately lead to respiratory acidosis.*

Exhaustion

Acute respiratory acidosis may likewise occur as a result of simple exhaustion due to excessive work of breathing over an extended period. This mechanism may explain the sudden onset of respiratory acidosis that has been observed in patients with status asthmaticus after a sustained period of laborious breathing.

In progressive pulmonary disease of any origin, there appears to be some point at which the work of breathing is so great that adequate ventilation can no longer be maintained. The patient may respond to this scenario with progressive hypercapnia or even with respiratory arrest due to extreme fatigue. Mechanical ventilation is indicated at this point "to give the patient a rest."

There is also some evidence to suggest that the onset of exhaustion is related to the degree of lactic acidosis that develops as a result of the extreme workload.[447]

Neuromuscular Disorders

Neuromuscular Disease

Diseases that affect the neuromuscular junction or the function of the respiratory muscles themselves may progress to hypoventilation and respiratory acidosis. Some of the more common disorders that may affect neuromuscular integrity include myasthenia gravis, poliomyelitis, amyotrophic lateral sclerosis, and the Guillain-Barré syndrome.

Guillain-Barré syndrome is characterized by loss of reflexes and symmetric paralysis, typically beginning in the legs, with eventual nearly complete or complete recovery.[502] Acute Guillain-Barré usually begins with fine paresthesias in the toes or fingertips, followed within days by leg weakness that makes walking and climbing stairs difficult. Weakness usually ascends and pain is common. Approximately two-thirds of cases follow an infection. Increased protein in the cerebrospinal fluid is a valuable diagnostic marker. Patients with very low (i.e., < 18 mL/kg) or rapidly declining vital capacities should be transferred and observed in ICU.

The trend of neuromuscular dysfunction on ventilation can be observed at the bedside through serial measurements of vital capacity. A falling vital capacity may indicate progressive hypoventilation and perhaps the onset of respiratory acidosis. Figure 13-2 designates suggested clinical management of the Guillain-Barré syndrome based on progressive deterioration of the vital capacity.

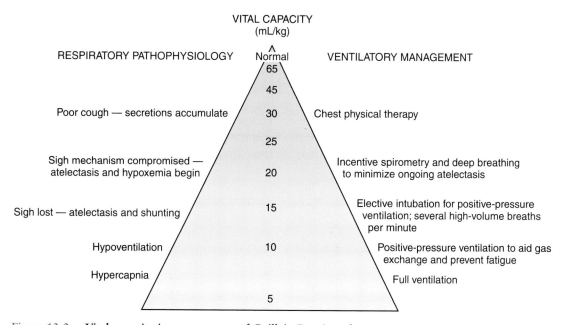

Figure 13-2. **Vital capacity in management of Guillain-Barré syndrome.**

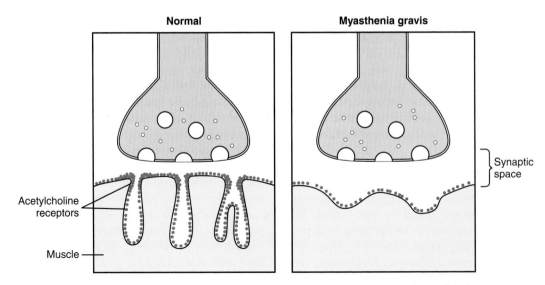

Figure 13-3.   **Neuromuscular junction in myasthenia gravis.** (Note the decreased acetylcholine receptors and the widened synaptic space.)

Myasthenia gravis affects approximately 25,000 people each year in the United States. The basic abnormality in myasthenia gravis is a decrease in the number of acetylcholine receptors in the neuromuscular junction.[503] Figure 13-3 illustrates the decreased number of acetylcholine receptors and the widened synaptic space in myasthenia gravis as compared to the normal neuromuscular junction. The clinical result of this disease is neuromuscular weakness and fatigue.

Electrolyte Deficiencies

Hypokalemia, a common electrolyte disorder in the critical care setting, is also associated with muscle weakness and even paralysis. The clinician must be particularly alert to this problem when trying to wean patients from mechanical ventilation. The presence of hypokalemia may result in unsuccessful weaning attempts. Low phosphate levels, although less common, may similarly impede normal neuromuscular control.

Iatrogenic Respiratory Acidosis

During mechanical ventilation, some aspects of the ventilatory pattern (e.g., tidal volume, respiratory rate) may not be under the direct control of the patient; rather, they are a product of the machine settings. This is particularly true in the apneic or paralyzed patient in whom the rate and volume of ventilation is exclusively a result of the ventilator settings. Thus, especially in the patient on mechanical ventilation, there is always the possibility of therapy-induced (iatrogenic) respiratory acidosis.

Inappropriately low ventilator settings for tidal volume or respiratory rate results in an elevated $PaCO_2$ and a blood gas classification of respiratory acidosis. Thus, insufficient mechanical ventilation may induce respiratory acidosis, particularly when drugs have been administered to facilitate control of the patient's ventilation.

Subsequent manipulation of ventilatory settings corrects only the *iatrogenic respiratory acidosis*. These ventilator changes cannot, of course, correct the underlying condition (e.g., respiratory acidosis secondary to CNS depression) that was responsible for the initiation of mechanical ventilation in the first place.

Permissive Hypercapnia

In most applications of mechanical ventilation, the goal is to normalize $PaCO_2$. Notwithstanding, in contrast to traditional mechanical ventilation, it is now common in acute lung injury and acute respiratory distress syndrome (and some other disorders) to allow respiratory acidosis to develop in an effort to avoid excessive alveolar pressure or volume. This so-called permissive hypercapnia is considered to be potentially less harmful than using higher lung inflation pressures to ensure a normal $PaCO_2$. Nevertheless, severe hypercapnia should still be avoided, even in this population, and even mild hypercapnia may be harmful if there is concern regarding excessive cerebral perfusion or when there is substantial acidemia.

Neurologic Disorders

Neurologic disease or trauma (including spinal cord injury) may also lead to hypoventilation and respiratory acidosis. The mechanism by which this effect occurs is via depression or malfunction of the respiratory centers or an increased intracranial pressure. Similarly, CNS dysfunction is probably responsible for the respiratory acidosis that commonly follows cerebral hypoxia and cardiac arrest.

The CNS is also responsible for the respiratory acidosis that occurs during sleep in patients with *central sleep apnea*. In addition, central mechanisms may play a role in the chronic respiratory acidosis associated with obesity that is known as the *Pickwickian syndrome*. Finally, *Ondine's curse*, a condition characterized by unexplained hypoventilation, most likely has a neurologic origin.

Excessive CO₂ Production

As described in Chapter 8 in the section on CO_2 homeostasis, the $PaCO_2$ depends not only on the quantity of CO_2 leaving the blood (i.e., $\dot{V}A$), but also on metabolism and CO_2 production ($\dot{V}CO_2$). The significance and effects of CO_2 production on ventilation and acid-base status in critically ill patients have only recently been appreciated. Carbon dioxide production depends on both the type and the quantity of metabolism.

Type of Metabolism

The Respiratory Quotient and CO₂ Production. As described in Chapter 7, the respiratory quotient (RQ) relates CO_2 production to oxygen consumption ($\dot{V}CO_2/\dot{V}O_2$). The numeric value of the RQ, in turn, depends on the type of body fuel being metabolized. Fat metabolism for example, results in less CO_2

production (RQ of 0.7) than carbohydrate metabolism (RQ of 1.0).

Total Parenteral Nutrition and the Respiratory Quotient. Total parenteral nutrition (TPN) is a nutritional support formula administered intravenously to critically ill patients to avoid the adverse effects of malnutrition.[493] TPN consists of a mixture of glucose and amino acids. As such, TPN is high in carbohydrates and increases the RQ and the production of CO_2 after administration. In the patient unable to meet the increased ventilatory requirement necessary to excrete this additional CO_2, respiratory acidosis may ensue.

Specifically, acute respiratory acidosis has been observed in patients with chronic lung disease in response to the administration of TPN.[494] This effect may occur both in nonintubated patients and in patients on mechanical ventilation.[494,495] During mechanical ventilation, the risk of TPN-induced respiratory acidosis is reduced if the minute volume of the ventilator is increased just before TPN administration.[495]

In addition, the development of hypercapnia has been reported in two young patients without COPD during weaning from mechanical ventilation while receiving TPN.[338] Furthermore, when the number of carbohydrate calories given to these patients was decreased, CO_2 production likewise dropped, and the respiratory acidosis was corrected.[338] In summary, a high RQ may contribute to the onset or maintenance of respiratory acidosis.

Quantity of Metabolism: Thermic Effect

Just as a high RQ can increase CO_2 production, a general increase in the quantity of energy metabolism (*thermic effect*), such as may occur with fever, will also increase CO_2 production and may contribute to respiratory acidosis.

Malignant hyperthermia (MH) is an inherited condition in which some medications (especially anesthetics) trigger sustained skeletal muscle contraction and hypermetabolism.[504] Symptoms include rapid, acute severe respiratory acidosis; hyperthermia; ventricular dysrhythmias; hyperkalemia; and muscular rigidity.[505] The clinical course of the disorder is short, usually 1 to 3 days. Untreated, MH may have a 70% mortality.[504] Treatment includes termination of the triggering agent, and control of pH, temperature, and potassium.[505]

Patients with severe burns also have an increase in total body metabolism secondary to tissue destruction and the reparative process. This response is greater than the hypermetabolism seen in sepsis or other forms of trauma. The magnitude and duration of the metabolic response parallel burn severity with metabolism doubling in a 60% total body burn.[506]

Other causes of hypermetabolism include sepsis, fever, thyrotoxicosis, and trauma.[485] In fever, CO_2 production will increase approximately 13% for each degree centigrade elevation in body temperature. TPN is associated not only with a high RQ; it also has a thermic effect secondary to the protein component of the solution.[550] Consequently, TPN tends to increase CO_2 production through changes in both the type and quantity of metabolism.[550]

Indeed the thermic effect appears to have an even stronger impact on CO_2 production than the type of substrate used for metabolism. The administration of excess calories will also lead to increased CO_2 production through lipogenesis, which has an RQ of nearly 8.0.[507]

Thus, the number of calories, the percentage of carbohydrate, and the nature of the patient's illness must all be considered regarding the CO_2 production load. In contrast, CO_2 production may sometimes be reduced by decreased glucose intake, cooling, or paralyzing the patient.[498]

Sodium Bicarbonate Administration

Administration of sodium bicarbonate ($NaHCO_3$) intravenously also increases blood CO_2 levels via the hydrolysis reaction. In spontaneously breathing individuals who are capable of increasing alveolar ventilation, this excess CO_2 is immediately excreted. However, in the patient unable to excrete the additional blood CO_2 (e.g., because of neurologic disease or controlled mechanical ventilation), hypercarbia and acute respiratory acidosis develop.[365]

Severe hypercapnia and respiratory acidosis of mixed venous blood has been shown to accompany resuscitation during cardiac arrest.[567] It is presumed that these mixed venous gases reflect tissue conditions. The administration of $NaHCO_3$ in this setting may further elevate the tissue PCO_2 and thus exacerbate the tissue acidosis. This issue is discussed in greater detail in Chapter 14 in the section on treatment of metabolic acidosis.

RESPIRATORY ALKALOSIS

Respiratory alkalosis, like respiratory acidosis, may result from a variety of acute and chronic causes. It disrupts acid-base balance by depleting the normal blood stores of carbonic acid. Respiratory alkalosis is a very common acid-base disorder.

Physiologic Response to Respiratory Alkalosis (Hypocapnia)

Patients with respiratory alkalosis often present with dyspnea and chest pain or tightness.[512] In addition to renal compensation (i.e., decreased [HCO_3]) for respiratory alkalosis, hypocapnia will decrease cerebral blood flow, alter some electrolyte concentrations, and increase the production of lactic acid.

Regarding potassium, there is an initial abrupt onset of hyperkalemia. This is rapidly followed by the development of hypokalemia.[508] Typically, serum potassium will decrease 0.3 mEq/L for each 0.1 unit increase in pH.[508] Occasionally, electrolyte disturbances will be associated with muscle spasm. In addition, respiratory alkalosis increases production and decreases the clearance of lactic acid; however, the increase in lactic acid levels is only modest.[508]

Neurologic Response

Hypocarbia has been associated with painful tingling in the hands and feet and numbness and sweating of the hands. Dizziness is also sometimes observed. Typically, these symptoms require $PaCO_2$ to decline approximately 20 mm Hg. As described previously, decreased cerebral perfusion has also been associated with hypocarbia; however, this effect appears to be mediated by acidosis.

Cardiovascular Response

Cardiovascular effects of hypocarbia include peripheral vascular constriction, tachycardia, and increased cardiac output. Hypocarbia may also decrease coronary blood flow and potentially induce arrhythmias. The patient may sometimes complain of palpitations, chest pain, or tightness.

Overall Appearance

In patients admitted to the emergency department, one hospital found the most common presenting complaints with substantial hypocapnia were dyspnea (61%), chest pain or tightness (43%), paresthesias (35%), panic (30%), dizziness (13%), palpitations (13%), and muscle spasm (9%).[512] Finally, acute respiratory alkalosis may be associated with nausea, vomiting, or changes in gastrointestinal motility.[508]

Common Causes of Respiratory Alkalosis

Although mild hypocapnia may be seen in females and children younger than the age of 3 years, most often respiratory alkalosis is not normal. Some of the most common causes of respiratory alkalosis are shown in Box 13-2. Six possible *origins* of primary respiratory alkalosis are shown in Figure 13-4. These include the lungs (e.g., pulmonary fibrosis), drugs (e.g., salicylate toxicity), mechanical ventilation, the CNS (e.g., tumor), the cardiovascular system (e.g. cardiogenic shock), and thoracic cage abnormalities (e.g., scoliosis).

Box 13-2	Causes of Respiratory Alkalosis

Hypoxemia (moderate to severe)
Overzealous mechanical ventilation
Restrictive lung disorders
    Fibrosis
    Ascites
    Scoliosis and thoracic cage deformities
    Third trimester of pregnancy
    Pneumonia
    Acute respiratory distress syndrome
    Congestive heart failure
    Emboli in pulmonary circulation
Neurologic origin
    Fever
    Anxiety
    Cerebrospinal fluid acidosis
    Trauma
    Severe pain
Shock/decreased cardiac output

Hypoxemia

Hypoxemia is one of the most common and important causes of *hyperventilation* and *respiratory alkalosis*. Moderate hypoxemia ($PaO_2 < 60$ mm Hg) stimulates the peripheral chemoreceptors causing increased alveolar ventilation and respiratory alkalosis. For this reason,

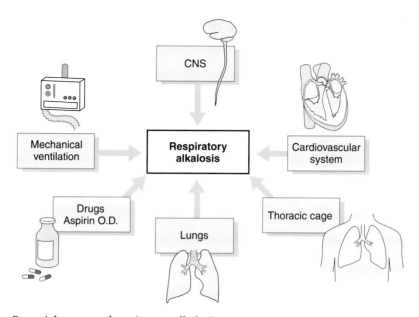

Figure 13-4. **Potential sources of respiratory alkalosis.**

whenever a PaO$_2$ less than 60 mm Hg is seen in conjunction with respiratory alkalosis, a cause-and-effect relationship should be presumed. Normalization of the PaO$_2$ is often all that is necessary to restore a normal PaCO$_2$. In some patients, multiple mechanisms will be present. Therefore, when normalization of PaO$_2$ fails to correct respiratory alkalosis, other underlying causes should be sought (see Box 13-2).

Overzealous Mechanical Ventilation

The application of mechanical ventilation may lead to iatrogenic respiratory alkalosis.[509] Respiratory alkalosis may be the result of an excessive tidal volume or respiratory rate setting. At times, hyperventilation to a PaCO$_2$ of 25 to 30 mm Hg is used therapeutically to decrease intracranial pressure in head trauma or CNS disorders.

Restrictive Lung Disease

When expansion of the lungs, thoracic cage, or alveoli is restricted, certain reflexes are activated (e.g., Hering-Breuer, J receptors) that stimulate hyperventilation and respiratory alkalosis (see Chapter 12). The various disorders shown under restrictive lung disease in Box 13-2 all have in common some restriction of lung or alveolar expansion.

The Hering-Breuer reflex may play a role in the hyperventilation of thoracic cage problems. The hyperventilation of ascites (accumulation of fluid in the peritoneal cavity), thoracic cage deformities, and the third trimester of pregnancy could be, at least in part, a reflex reaction to the mechanical restriction of inspiration.

It is known, however, that the respiratory alkalosis of pregnancy is also related to the hormone progesterone, which stimulates ventilation.[510] During pregnancy, especially the third trimester, PaCO$_2$ is usually approximately 28 to 32 mm Hg.[510] Furthermore, most women also experience dyspnea even in the first two trimesters of pregnancy.[508]

The exact role of the J receptor reflex has not been clarified. These receptors, situated within the alveolar-capillary membrane, have been postulated to respond to thickening of or edema within the alveolar-capillary membrane. This is a feasible explanation for the hyperventilation commonly noted in various disorders that may affect the alveolar-capillary membrane, including congestive heart failure, acute respiratory distress syndrome, fibrosis, pneumonia, and pulmonary emboli.

Neurologic Disorders

There are a variety of conditions that may cause respiratory alkalosis via the central nervous system stimulation. These conditions include chemical stimuli, acidosis of the cerebrospinal fluid, and physical and emotional stimuli.

Chemical Stimuli

Infection/Toxins. Although some neurologic disturbances cause respiratory acidosis, many neurologic problems may result in hyperventilation. The respiratory alkalosis may be chemically induced by an infectious condition such as meningitis or septicemia. Presumably, the infection produces a chemical that crosses the blood-brain barrier and stimulates the central chemoreceptors. The accumulation of other chemicals or toxins may similarly stimulate hyperventilation. In hepatic (i.e., liver) encephalopathy, for example, ammonia accumulates in the blood and stimulates ventilation via the CNS.

Salicylates

Salicylates (e.g., aspirin) in large doses also stimulate the respiratory centers and cause hyperventilation. Therefore, a respiratory alkalosis usually accompanies salicylate poisoning or overdose. For unknown reasons, adults seem to display respiratory alkalosis as the dominating acid-base disturbance in salicylate intoxication, whereas children more often have metabolic acidosis due to the accumulation of salicylic acid as the dominant disturbance.

Acidosis of the Cerebrospinal Fluid

Acidosis of the cerebrospinal fluid (CSF) leads to hyperventilation through stimulation of the central chemoreceptors. The change in pH of the CSF most often parallels the change in pH of arterial blood. However, because of the relative impermeability to ions of the blood-brain barrier, occasionally a change in pH in the blood is not immediately reflected in the CSF.

CSF acidosis without blood acidemia is likely to occur (1) after the correction of blood acidemia with bicarbonate, (2) following descent from acclimatization to a high altitude, or (3) during weaning from mechanical ventilation when a patient has had sustained hyperventilation while on the ventilator. Although these situations are not seen frequently, the clinician should always keep these possibilities in mind when hyperventilation cannot be easily explained.

Physical/Emotional Stimuli

In addition to chemical stimuli, the respiratory centers may be stimulated by physical changes in the CNS. Physical changes may result from CNS trauma with resultant increased intracranial pressure, or from a disease process such as a CNS tumor. Fever is also known to be associated with hyperventilation.

Emotional stimuli may likewise lead to substantial hyperventilation during extreme stress or severe pain. It is not uncommon for patients to present with respiratory alkalosis in the emergency room or physician's office due to hysteria, panic, or anxiety.

The term "hyperventilation syndrome" was first used in 1938 to describe patients who presented with hypocapnia and anxiety.[511] Hyperventilation syndrome is purported to affect nearly 10% of the population.[508] It affects predominantly females and occurs most often in the third or fourth decade of life.[508] One must be careful, however, to rule out a compensatory response to other acid-base disturbances such as ketoacidosis or myocardial infarction.[512]

Shock/Decreased Cardiac Output

Finally, shock and decreased perfusion may lead to respiratory alkalosis. It is not uncommon to see patients in profound hypotension and low cardiac output states manifesting substantial arterial hyperventilation. The hyperventilation is probably due in part to peripheral chemoreceptor stimulation secondary to diminished perfusion.

Perhaps more importantly, the low cardiac output contributes to arterial hyperventilation by another mechanism. The fall in pulmonary perfusion associated with this state may lead to a *relative hyperventilation* of the lungs due to many high alveolar $\dot{V}/\dot{Q}$ units and despite normal minute ventilation. In contrast to the *arterial*

respiratory alkalosis, however, it is likely that these individuals have *high venous PCO_2* levels and tissue respiratory acidosis. As described in detail in Chapter 14 in the section on the venous paradox, arterial blood gases may reflect poorly the overall acid-base status in these patients.

METABOLIC ACIDOSIS

Metabolic acidosis occurs in a variety of diseases and even during normal heavy exercise.

Physiologic Response to Metabolic Acidosis

Probably the most serious consequences of metabolic acidosis are on the cardiovascular system. Metabolic acidosis directly suppresses myocardial contractility and vascular smooth muscle. This, in turn, may lead to a decreased cardiac output and blood pressure. Concurrent sympathetic nervous system stimulation may somewhat counteract the direct effects of acidosis on the cardiovascular system when metabolic acidosis is mild.

Metabolic acidosis may also result in hyperkalemia as potassium migrates from the intracellular space to the plasma (see Chapter 12) in exchange for hydrogen ions. This effect is most prominent in non-organic types of acidosis.

Finally, as previously described, respiratory acid-base compensation will lead to hyperventilation and often dyspnea. Similarly, when possible, renal compensation will include increased acid excretion and bicarbonate absorption. In metabolic acidosis of non-renal origin, the kidney can increase hydrogen ion excretion three- to fourfold.[484]

Common Causes of Metabolic Acidosis

Respiratory acid-base disturbances always reflect a change in blood volatile acid concentration, specifically carbonic acid. Clinical metabolic acidosis, on the other hand, may be the result of either *the accumulation of some fixed acid in the blood* or *the loss of normal blood base*.

After a general acid-base diagnosis of metabolic acidosis (primary) has been established, the patient's biochemical profile should be evaluated. Typically, the biochemical profile consists of electrolyte concentrations (Na$^+$, K$^+$, Cl$^-$, and HCO$_3^-$ or total CO$_2$), blood glucose, and an index of renal function (BUN or creatinine).

Using the electrolytes from the biochemical profile, the first step in determining a specific acid-base diagnosis is calculation of the anion gap [Na − (TCO$_2$ + Cl) = A$^-$]. The anion gap (A$^-$) is helpful particularly in the diagnosis of metabolic acidosis because it allows us to differentiate conditions associated with increased fixed acids in the blood from conditions associated with the loss of blood base.

As described in Chapter 12, when the anion gap exceeds 16 mEq/L, an increase in blood fixed acids is highly probable. Furthermore, the higher the anion gap, the greater is the confidence in this conclusion. Conversely, when the anion gap is normal (i.e., 12 to 14 mEq/L), a loss of blood base is more likely the cause of the metabolic acidosis. Like all laboratory data, marginal findings indicate the need for a more comprehensive evaluation of the patient and his or her overall status. In addition, we must always be cognizant of the effect of albumin concentrations on the anion gap (hypoalbuminemia decreases the anion gap) especially in critical care. The anion gap may be corrected for albumin levels as described in Chapter 12.

The potential causes of metabolic acidosis can thus be separated into two groups: (1) those associated with the accumulation of fixed acids and therefore with a high anion gap, and (2) those associated with the loss of base and

a normal anion gap. Again, it is sometimes useful to think of the various potential sources of general acid-base disturbances. Figure 13-5 illustrates common sources of high anion gap metabolic acidosis. High anion gap acidosis may occur as a result of: toxins (e.g., methanol poisoning), the kidneys (e.g., azotemic renal failure), metabolism (e.g., lactic acidosis/ketoacidosis), or, less commonly, the liver (e.g., cirrhosis).

High Anion Gap Metabolic Acidosis

Box 13-3 lists the most common causes of high anion gap metabolic acidosis and the specific acids that tend to accumulate with each disorder. Other data reported on the biochemical profile (e.g., BUN, glucose) and the oxygenation indices on the blood gas report are useful in making a definitive acid-base diagnosis. Probably the three most common types of metabolic acidosis are ketoacidosis, azotemic renal failure, and lactic acidosis.

Toxins

Aspirin Overdose. Salicylate toxicity may follow aspirin overdose, ingestion of oil of wintergreen (methyl salicylate), or ingestion of other salicylate products. It should be noted that one teaspoon of oil of wintergreen is equivalent to approximately 21 regular strength aspirin tablets.[513] The high anion gap acidosis is a result of the accumulation of salicylic acid, lactic acid, and ketoacids. Salicylate toxicity is most

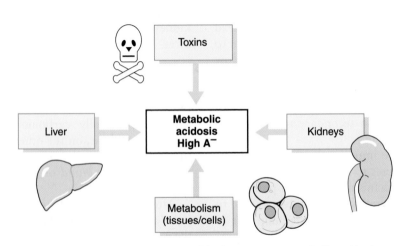

Figure 13-5.   **Potential sources of high anion gap metabolic acidosis.**

Box 13-3	Causes of High Anion Gap Metabolic Acidosis	

Etiology	Accumulated Acid(s)
Toxins	
Aspirin overdose	Salicylic, lactic, ketoacids
Wood alcohol (methanol)	Formic, lactic
Ethylene glycol	Glycolic, oxalic, lactic
Paraldehyde	Formic, lactic
Toluene	Benzoic
Azotemic renal failure	Phosphoric, sulfuric
Lactic acidosis	Lactic
Hypoxia	
Ethanol	
Liver failure	
Poisonings (e.g., methanol)	
Ketoacidosis	Acetoacetic, beta-hydroxybutyric
Starvation	
Alcoholic	
Diabetic	

often seen in children less than 1 year old but is also relatively common in adults.

Early clinical manifestations of salicylate toxicity include hyperventilation, mild confusion, tinnitus, and decreased auditory acuity. These mild symptoms can rapidly progress to seizures, coma, and death.[513] The presence of fever is a particularly ominous sign.[513]

The metabolic acidosis of salicylate poisoning is usually accompanied by a primary respiratory alkalosis, particularly in adults.[515] Frequently in adults, the pH is near 7.40 or slightly alkaline despite an anion gap near 20 mEq/L.[513] Salicylate poisoning may be confused with ketoacidosis because the acid-base and clinical picture is similar in both problems (i.e., hyperglycemia, ketosis). The diagnosis can be confirmed, however, based on a history of salicylate ingestion and high blood salicylate concentration, usually greater than 30 mg/dL; however, it may be much higher.[516] The clinician should also be aware that salicylate levels may continue to increase following admission especially with ingestion of enteric coated aspirin.[513] For this reason, serial salicylate levels are imperative.

Poisons/Drug Effects

Wood Alcohol (Methanol). Ingestion of wood alcohol leads to inebriation and metabolic acidosis. It is also characterized by engorged retinal vessels and blurred vision. There may be a profound elevation of the anion gap. This type of poisoning is most likely to be seen in the alcoholic.

Ethylene Glycol. Ethylene glycol is the active ingredient of antifreeze. It has a sweet, pleasant taste, and it may be accidentally ingested by children because of its taste and appearance (i.e., color). Ethylene glycol has euphoric effects and may be substituted for ethanol by alcoholics or ingested in an attempt at suicide. Ethylene glycol ingestion causes an estimated 60 deaths each year; as little as 100 mL may be lethal.[517] Notwithstanding, with early diagnosis and effective treatment, mortality is close to zero.[514]

The clinical features of ethylene glycol ingestion occur in three distinct phases.[518] Within 30 minutes to 12 hours, neurologic symptoms are observed (e.g., hallucinations, stupor, coma). In 12 to 24 hours, cardiovascular complications may occur (e.g., heart failure, arrhythmia). Finally, the breakdown of ethylene glycol results in oxalic acid, which crystallizes in the kidney. Thus, acute renal failure constitutes the third stage of toxicity.

Treatment of ethylene glycol poisoning focuses on preventing its metabolism and on facilitating its excretion. Because it helps to prevent the metabolism of ethylene glycol, ethanol is usually administered intravenously. The drug 4-methylpyrazole has been reported to be even more effective than alcohol in this regard, however it is very expensive[514,519] at approximately $4000/case.[514] Hemodialysis is also recommended to facilitate the removal of ethylene glycol.[518]

Paraldehyde. Paraldehyde (Paral) is a sedative/hypnotic drug sometimes used during delirium tremens in alcoholics or as an analgesic in obstetrics. Paraldehyde intoxication may cause high anion gap metabolic acidosis.

Toluene. Toluene is the active ingredient in transmission fluid and paint thinner. Social abuse of this drug has been reported. Sniffing or inhaling toluene may cause lightheadedness and euphoria and may lead to high anion gap acidosis.[520]

Azotemic Renal Failure

Many different types of renal disease may be seen clinically. Renal failure associated with a high anion gap and the inability to excrete fixed acids is called *azotemic renal failure.* Other types of renal disease may be associated with a normal anion gap acidosis (e.g., renal tubular acidosis) secondary to the loss of blood base (see discussion of normal anion gap acidosis later in this chapter). The specific acids that accumulate in azotemic renal failure are phosphoric and sulfuric acid.

Azotemia. *Azotemia* is the accumulation of nitrogenous wastes in the blood from protein metabolism. The specific blood values that are elevated in azotemia are BUN and creatinine.

Blood Urea Nitrogen. Normal BUN is less than 23 mg/dL. The BUN in a given patient depends on the balance between the amount of urea being produced and the amount being excreted. Urea production depends on the quantity of protein metabolism, and urea excretion depends on renal function. In addition to impaired renal function, certain drugs and upper gastrointestinal bleeding may also elevate the BUN.

Creatinine. Normal blood creatinine is 0.5 to 1.5 mg/dL. Creatinine formation is determined only by body muscle mass and is therefore relatively constant. Creatinine excretion is determined by renal function. Because creatinine is less affected by diet, it is a more reliable indicator of renal function than is BUN.

Azotemia and Decreased pH. The pH typically does not begin to decrease until azotemia is fairly substantial (e.g., BUN > 40 mg/dL and creatinine > 4 mg/dL).[521]

Etiology. Azotemic renal failure may be due to the nephrotoxic effects of certain drugs (e.g., antibiotics) or heavy metals. Alternatively, azotemic renal failure may be caused by poor renal perfusion and ischemia or hypertension. *Prerenal azotemia* is a condition in which azotemia is due to inadequate renal perfusion. In prerenal azotemia, restoration of adequate renal perfusion corrects the azotemia. More severe or protracted renal hypoperfusion may cause *acute tubular necrosis* and dysfunction. This true form of acute renal failure cannot be reversed immediately by restoration of normal renal perfusion.

Clinical Picture. Azotemic renal failure may be acute or chronic. The clinical course of acute renal failure is characterized by an oliguric phase followed by a polyuric phase. Because erythropoietin is produced in the kidneys, anemia is common in renal disease, especially chronic renal failure. The anemia is typically normochromic and normocytic. In addition, the anemia is remarkably asymptomatic even at hematocrit levels of 15% to 20%.[523] Therefore, transfusions are generally withheld until the patient is symptomatic.[523]

Uremia is a toxic clinical condition associated with azotemia and renal failure. Uremia affects a variety of body systems and causes a host of symptoms (e.g., somnolence, depression, nausea and vomiting, and circulatory disturbances).

Lactic Acidosis

Lactic acidosis is probably the most common cause of high anion gap acidosis. As such, it should be afforded a high index of suspicion. As described in Chapter 11, lactic acid concentration is reflected by measurement of the lactate concentration in the blood. Blood lactate measurement may not be routinely included on the biochemical profile; therefore, the diagnosis of lactic acidosis is often made after other causes of high anion gap acidosis have been ruled out. However, lactic acidosis can be confirmed by actually measuring blood lactate concentration.

Normal blood lactate levels are about 1.8 mM/L (18 mg/dL). Slight elevations in blood lactate concentration, up to about 3 mM/L, are fairly common (e.g. stress, respiratory alkalosis) and generally are not associated with acidemia.[521] Further elevations, however, tend to lower the pH. Typically, in lactic acidosis, blood lactate exceeds 5 to 7 mM/L and may be three or four times higher.[484,521] Lactic acidosis is most often due to tissue hypoxia. However, several other causes have been reported.

Hypoxia. The assessment of hypoxia has been described in detail in Chapter 11. Hypoxia may be secondary to anemia, cardiovascular failure, or pulmonary decompensation. Indices of oxygen supply and indicators of tissue hypoxia (PaO_2, SaO_2, [Hb], $P\bar{v}O_2$, $S\bar{v}O_2$, cardiac output) are particularly useful in this evaluation.

Lactic acidosis has been reported immediately after grand mal seizures (pH of 7.14).[484,524]

In blood gases performed 60 minutes later, however, the pH had returned to normal.[524]

Other Causes. Causes of lactic acidosis not related to tissue hypoxia include excessive ethanol intake, methanol ingestion, leukemia, neoplasms, drugs,[525] and congenital heart defects.[526] Also, when pH falls below 7.10, regardless of the initial cause, lactic acid begins to accumulate.[523]

Any condition that elevates pyruvate (e.g., intravenous glucose administration) causes a rise in blood lactate levels. These conditions are known collectively as *secondary hyperlactatemia* (see Chapter 11).

In the presence of oxygen, the liver rapidly converts lactate in the blood back to glucose or CO_2 and, in the process, produces bicarbonate in the blood. Both acute and chronic hepatic insufficiency can, therefore, lead to lactic acidosis.[527]

Ketoacidosis

When glucose is unavailable within the body's cells, fat is metabolized at an accelerated rate. Fat metabolism, in turn, leads to the accumulation of acetoacetic and beta-hydroxybutyric acid. These two acids are known collectively as ketoacids; their increased production may lead to *ketoacidosis* with a high anion gap.

The anions associated with these acids are acetoacetate and beta-hydroxybutyrate. A small portion of acetoacetate is converted to *acetone*. Acetone is responsible for the characteristic fruity odor of the patient's breath in ketoacidosis. Acetone, acetoacetate, and beta-hydroxybutyrate are known collectively as ketone bodies. Their accumulation in the blood is referred to as *ketosis*. Ketosis and ketoacidosis may be seen in starvation, alcoholism, and diabetes mellitus.

Starvation. Ketosis may occur if carbohydrates are severely restricted in the diet. Ketoacidosis generally is not severe unless glucose stores are severely depleted, such as in starvation. Fortunately, starvation is rare in the United States, although it may be seen in conditions such as anorexia nervosa.

Alcoholic Ketoacidosis. Alcoholics may present in the emergency room with a normal or slightly elevated blood glucose (i.e., <250 mg/dL) and ketoacidosis. Interestingly, when acetoacetate levels are measured in the blood, they are not elevated. In alcoholic ketoacidosis, the primary acid disturbance is elevation of beta-hydroxybutyric acid and this is not reflected by the routine Acetest (measurement of acetoacetate). The Acetest is a qualitative Na nitroprusside reaction in which acetoacetate bodies manifest a purple color.[519]

Dextrose and water is the treatment of choice in alcoholic ketoacidosis.[523,528] Dextrose converts beta-hydroxybutyrate into acetoacetate and serves as a source of carbohydrate.

Diabetes Mellitus. The Greek term *diabetes*, which means *passing through*, is used to describe those diseases characterized by excessive urination. The term *mellitus* means *sweet*, which is in contrast to the term *insipidus*, which means *uninteresting* or *insipid*. In acute diabetes mellitus, there is increased urination, and the urine is sweet due to high levels of glucose (*glycosuria*). Early physicians tasted the urine in order to differentiate this disorder from diabetes insipidus, a very different pathologic condition in which urination is also excessive but the urine is not sweet.

Pathology. The common pathologic defect in patients with diabetes mellitus is insulin deficiency. Insulin is necessary to transport glucose from the extracellular fluid to the intracellular fluid. When insulin is not available, glucose levels rise in the plasma (*hyperglycemia*) and fat metabolism increases with resultant ketoacidosis. Adult-onset (type II) diabetics produce insulin but their cells are unable to use it fully.

The high levels of plasma glucose, in turn, lead to increased urine output (*hyperosmolar diuresis*) in an effort to maintain blood osmolarity. The loss of fluids may also lead to dehydration. In addition, the compensatory response to acidemia results in a characteristic deep, gasping type of ventilation called *Kussmaul's breathing*.

Laboratory Findings. The average plasma glucose level in diabetic ketoacidosis is approximately 500 mg/dL.[518] The severity of the hyperglycemia depends primarily on the degree of volume depletion from the diuresis and vomiting that is often present. There are increased levels of blood ketones, which are shown by a positive Acetest. Hyperkalemia secondary to acidemia is also common. The urine shows increased levels of glucose (glycosuria) and ketones (ketonuria).

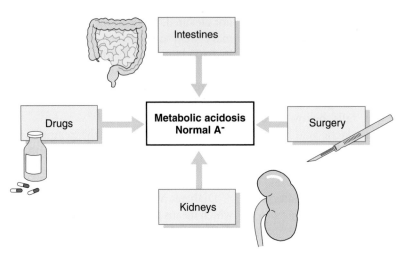

Figure 13-6. Potential sources of normal anion gap metabolic acidosis.

Normal Anion Gap Metabolic Acidosis

Normal anion gap acidosis (i.e., hyperchloremic metabolic acidosis) is due to the loss of base. The two major organs usually responsible for the body losing or excreting bases are the kidneys and the intestine (Fig. 13-6). The intestinal secretions are very high in bicarbonate concentration. Thus, in the differential diagnosis of normal anion gap acidosis, it is wise to suspect a loss of intestinal secretions (e.g., diarrhea) or bicarbonate excretion via the kidneys (e.g., renal tubular acidosis). Other causes may include drugs (e.g., carbonic anhydrase inhibitors) or intestinal surgical procedures (e.g., ileostomy). A variety of potential causes of normal anion gap metabolic acidosis are shown in Box 13-4.

Box 13-4   Causes of Normal Anion Gap Metabolic Acidosis

Renal tubular acidosis
Enteric drainage tubes
Diarrhea
Urinary diversion
Carbonic anhydrase inhibitors
Early renal disease
Dilution acidosis
Biliary or pancreatic fistulas
Acidifying salts
Sulfur, hydrogen sulfide, drugs
Eucapnic ventilation posthypocapnia

Renal Tubular Acidosis

Description. Renal function may be impaired secondary to diminished *glomerular* filtration or renal *tubular* dysfunction. Azotemic renal failure (i.e., associated with a high anion gap and high BUN and creatinine levels) is due to diminished glomerular function. When renal acidosis is caused specifically by the failure of the renal tubules to absorb bicarbonate, it is termed *renal tubular acidosis* (RTA). From an acid-base perspective, azotemic renal failure is due to the accumulation of acids, whereas RTA is due to a loss of base (i.e., HCO_3^-). In contrast to azotemic renal failure, glomerular filtration is typically adequate in RTA, and therefore azotemia is mild or absent. In addition, the plasma bicarbonate in RTA is usually only mildly decreased and is most often greater than 15 mEq/L.[484]

Urine pH. The compensatory response of the kidney to acidemia is acidification (i.e., excretion of H^+ ions) of the urine. In hydrogen ion excess, H^+ ions are secreted into the filtrate, and urine pH is typically quite low (pH $\cong$ 4.50). In RTA, urine pH is inappropriately high (pH of 6.00 to 7.00) despite blood acidemia. This is a result of the increased bicarbonate content of the urine.

Other Findings. Other findings in RTA include hypokalemia, hypophosphatemia, and nephrocalcinosis. Nephrocalcinosis is the deposit of calcium phosphate in the renal tubules. Serum chloride characteristically is between 110 and 120 mEq/L (i.e., hyperchloremic metabolic acidosis).

Causes. RTA may be a component of an inherited defect (e.g., Lowe syndrome, Fanconi syndrome). Alternatively, it may be drug-induced (e.g., outdated tetracycline, sulfonamides) or a result of some metabolic disorder (e.g., vitamin D deficiency, secondary hyperparathyroidism).

Enteric Drainage Tubes

The bicarbonate concentration of secretions in the small intestine is higher than in plasma (e.g., 70 mEq/L in the small intestine versus 24 mEq/L in arterial blood).[529] The pancreas, biliary tree, and duodenal glands all produce and secrete alkaline secretions. Therefore, surgical conditions that necessitate enteric drainage tubes may lead to a loss of bicarbonate. In particular, ileostomy may be complicated by a high volume of fluid and electrolyte loss.

Diarrhea

Diarrhea is probably the most common cause of hyperchloremic metabolic acidosis in the intensive care unit.[484] The mechanism of metabolic acidosis in diarrhea is exactly the same as in excessive drainage through enteric tubes. Large quantities of base are excreted along with fluid and electrolytes in the stool. The prototype of metabolic acidosis associated with diarrhea is seen in cholera, in which stool volume can exceed 15 L/day. Severe hyperchloremic metabolic acidosis may also occur. Hypovolemia and hypokalemia resulting from the excessive loss of intestinal secretions are also critical problems in severe diarrhea. Laxative abuse should also be suspected in the patient with unexplained hyperchloremic metabolic acidosis.[484]

Urinary Diversion

In certain urinary disorders (e.g., tumors, congenital anomalies), the ureters may be surgically diverted to the intestine to allow for urine excretion (*uretero-enterostomy*). Uretero-enterostomy may be associated with severe hyperchloremic metabolic acidosis. *Uretero-ileostomy* appears to cause fewer acid-base and electrolyte problems than *uretero-sigmoidostomy*.[516]

Carbonic Anhydrase Inhibitors

Chronic administration of drugs that act by inhibition of carbonic anhydrase almost invariably leads to *mild metabolic acidosis.*[529] Carbonic anhydrase is, of course, important in the renal tubular cells in order to facilitate $NaHCO_3$ reabsorption. When carbonic anhydrase–inhibiting agents are administered, the effect on renal tubules is similar to that of RTA, in that bicarbonate is poorly reabsorbed and is therefore excreted in the urine.

Acetazolamide (Diamox) is a carbonic anhydrase inhibitor that is used sometimes as a diuretic. This drug may, in fact, be the diuretic of choice in metabolic alkalemia because of its tendency to promote bicarbonate excretion. Acetazolamide is not often used alone for diuresis, however, because it is only a moderately potent diuretic. Administration of this drug may lead to metabolic acidosis, particularly in patients with renal failure.

Mafenide acetate (Sulfamylon acetate cream), also a carbonic anhydrase inhibitor, is a broad-spectrum bacteriostatic agent that may be applied topically in the treatment of burns. Sulfamylon is absorbed easily through heat-damaged skin, and repeated use may result in metabolic acidosis.

Early Renal Disease

Azotemic acidosis may accompany end-stage renal disease; in *early* renal disease (e.g., interstitial nephropathy, diabetic nephropathy), hyperchloremic metabolic acidosis may be seen.[515] This disturbance is probably related to the diminished ability of renal cells to secrete ammonia, a major urinary buffer. Because ammonia accounts for more than 50% of buffering, its absence greatly limits hydrogen ion excretion and HCO_3^- reabsorption.

Dilution Acidosis

Sudden, rapid infusion of a sodium chloride solution may dilute the blood sufficiently to lead to metabolic acidosis. *Dilution acidosis* due to expansion of the fluid space has caused hyperchloremic metabolic acidosis in children.[529] In contrast, dilution acidosis is rare in adults.

Biliary or Pancreatic Fistulas

A *fistula* is an abnormal connection from a normal cavity or tube to another cavity or free surface. Fistulas may be congenital or may be caused by trauma, abscess, or inflammation.

Fistulas can develop in the gastrointestinal system from the biliary tree or the pancreas directly to the intestine and thus lead to the loss of pancreatic secretions or bile. The bicarbonate concentration of bile may be 60 mEq/L and as high as 100 mEq/L in pancreatic secretions.[529] Obviously, a large loss of these secretions may lead to hyperchloremic metabolic acidosis.

Acidifying Salts

Acidifying salts (e.g., ammonium chloride, HCl, arginine hydrochloride) that are sometimes used in the treatment of severe alkalemia have the potential to cause normal anion gap acidosis. Ammonium chloride intoxication has a similar effect.

Sulfur, Hydrogen Sulfide, Drugs

Elemental sulfur and hydrogen sulfide have been implicated as unusual causes of normal anion gap acidosis.[529] Other uncommon causes of metabolic acidosis include intravenous tetracycline and carbenicillin; however, the mechanism responsible for the acidosis is unclear.[529]

Eucapnic Ventilation Posthypocapnia

Eucapnia is the presence of normal amounts of CO_2 (i.e., $PaCO_2$ 35 to 45 mm Hg) in the blood. Hypocarbia, is the presence of low levels of CO_2 in the blood (i.e., $PaCO_2 < 35$ mm Hg).

In patients with sustained hypocarbia (e.g., during mechanical ventilation or during prolonged hyperventilation associated with asthma), the base bicarbonate is excreted by the kidneys as a compensatory mechanism. If hypocarbia is quickly corrected to eucapnic ventilation (normal $PaCO_2$), the blood gas may appear as a hyperchloremic metabolic acidosis. This acid-base condition has been commonly observed in patients with severe, acute asthma.[530]

It may be argued that the resultant metabolic acidosis is not a true acidosis at all, because it really originates from a compensatory mechanism. Nevertheless, at a given point in time, the blood gas appears as a primary metabolic acidosis, and this must be recognized. The issue is not whether this abnormality should be called a metabolic acidosis; rather, it is important that the chain of events that has caused this problem is understood.

METABOLIC ALKALOSIS

Metabolic alkalosis is very common in acute illness.[480] In a study of more than 13,000 hospitalized patients, metabolic alkalosis was the most frequent acid-base disturbance encountered and was present in more than half of all patients with abnormal acid-base status.[531] Furthermore, more than half of the surgical

---

ON CALL | CASE 13-1 *ABGs and Critical Thinking*

You are the only person available to care for this patient. You must assess the patient/situation and act accordingly.

A 50-year-old woman arrives in the emergency department after ingesting an unknown quantity of enteric-coated aspirin. She appears relatively normal. Blood gases and electrolytes are drawn.

Cl	104 mEq/L
K	5.2 mEq/L
Salicylate level	22 mg/dL

ASSESSMENT

Abnormalities: List abnormal data and other noteworthy information. Classify ABG.

Explanation: List possible diseases, pathology, or other situations that may have led to this patient's condition.

INTERVENTION

Importance: Prioritize concern(s) of treatment in order of urgency and/or seriousness as you see the overall situation.

ARTERIAL BLOOD GASES

SaO_2	97
pH	7.42
$PaCO_2$	22 mm Hg
PaO_2	114 mm Hg
$[HCO_3]$	14 mEq/L
FIO_2	0.35
Na	142 mEq/L
CO_2	15 mEq/L

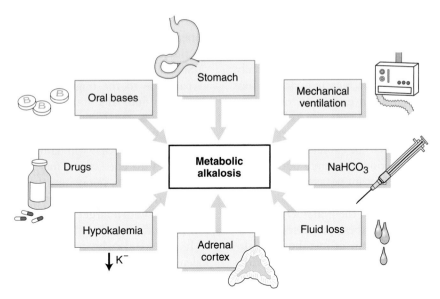

Figure 13-7.   **Potential sources of metabolic alkalosis.**

patients who have blood gas determinations are likely to be alkalemic at some point during their hospitalizations.[532]

Physiologic Response to Metabolic Alkalosis

Metabolic alkalosis may have serious consequences in the central nervous and cardiovascular systems. Mild-to-moderate metabolic alkalosis may cause lethargy and confusion, whereas severe alkalemia may lead to seizures and/or coma. Neuromuscular irritability may cause spasm, twitching, or tetany. Depressed myocardial contractility and arrhythmias may occur. Severe alkalemia has been associated with increased mortality and should be avoided.

Common Causes of Metabolic Alkalosis

Metabolic alkalosis may be caused by an abnormal loss of fixed acid from the body or by the abnormal accumulation or production of blood base. Most often, a loss of acid (e.g., renal H^+ excretion, loss of HCl from the stomach) is accompanied by concurrent production of blood bicarbonate.

The more common origins of metabolic alkalosis are shown in Figure 13-7. Drugs may be responsible (e.g., diuretics, steroids), or the administration of excessive sodium bicarbonate or oral bases. Loss of gastric secretions (e.g., vomiting), or excessive mechanical ventilation

of the patient with chronic respiratory acidosis (e.g., posthypercapnic respiratory acidosis) may also be causative. In addition, the excessive fluid loss and hypokalemia from any cause will stimulate bicarbonate retention. Finally, excessive secretion of the adrenal cortex (e.g., hyperaldosteronism) will also result in renal retention of bicarbonate.

Unlike metabolic acidosis, the potential causes of metabolic alkalosis may be listed in a single box (Box 13-5).

Box 13-5   Causes of Metabolic Alkalosis

Hypokalemia
Ingestion of large amounts of alkali or licorice
Gastric fluid loss
  Vomiting
  Nasogastric drainage
Hyperaldosteronism secondary to nonadrenal factors
  Bartter's syndrome
  Inadequate renal perfusion
  Diuretics (inhibiting NaCl reabsorption)
Bicarbonate administration
  Sodium bicarbonate overcorrection
  Blood transfusions
Adrenocortical hypersecretion (e.g., tumor)
Steroids
Eucapnic ventilation posthypercapnia

Hypokalemia

Metabolic Alkalosis–Hypokalemia Syndrome

In the presence of an intracellular potassium deficit, the renal tubular cells preferentially, although not exclusively, secrete hydrogen ions (acid) into the urine in exchange for sodium (see Chapter 12). In addition, the kidneys cannot conserve potassium. Therefore, some potassium continues to be excreted in the urine even with the depletion of normal body stores. Furthermore, when serum potassium levels are low or when alkalemia is present, total bicarbonate reabsorption via the $NaHCO_3$ reaction is stimulated.[533] All of these processes together tend to foster a syndrome of metabolic alkalosis and hypokalemia. Hypokalemia causes metabolic alkalosis and metabolic alkalosis tends to perpetuate hypokalemia.

Incidence of Hypokalemia

Hypokalemia is common in hospitalized patients. Many pharmacologic agents may cause an increased loss of potassium into the urine and, thus, hypokalemia. These agents include NaCl-inhibiting diuretics and steroids. Inhaled beta 2 agonists can also cause significant hypokalemia.[541]

It is noteworthy that any condition that results in loss of fluids and volume contraction may lower serum potassium. Thus, loss of gastrointestinal secretions may lead to hypokalemia (e.g., vomiting, nasogastric suction, biliary fistulas).

Serum Potassium

The serum potassium concentration is not a particularly sensitive indicator of the total potassium content in the blood. The percentage of total blood potassium in the intracellular fluid (i.e., 98%) far exceeds its percentage in the plasma (2%). Fortunately, serum hypokalemia *usually* reflects total body potassium deficits. However, the *degree* of serum hypokalemia does not reflect accurately the magnitude of the total body potassium deficiency. Therefore, plasma or serum $[K^+]$ must be interpreted carefully.

The assessment of potassium status is further clouded by the intracellular-extracellular shifts in potassium that accompany changes in pH and the administration of catecholamines. As described in Chapter 12, serum potassium levels tend to vary inversely with pH. Indeed, serum potassium levels may increase with acidemia despite a moderate total potassium deficit.

Similarly, serum hypokalemia in alkalemia is in part due to the migration of extracellular potassium into the intracellular fluid space. Nevertheless, regarding acid-base balance, the clinician must be sure that there is not a true potassium deficit that will hamper the ability of the kidney to correct the metabolic alkalosis. As a general rule, potassium should be administered *slowly* when the patient manifests a low serum $[K^+]$ with a target serum potassium in the low normal range.

It should also be remembered that hypokalemia tends to cause muscle weakness and may impair a marginal patient's ability to ventilate adequately. Furthermore, extracellular potassium ion concentration is the single most important determinant of myocardial membrane stability.[541]

Ingestion of Large Amounts of Alkali or Licorice

Alkali Loading

The kidney readily excretes single doses of alkali, which may transiently elevate blood bases. When *large* amounts of base are administered over a long period, however, renal excretion may be unable to keep pace with the alkali load. This is particularly true in patients with low extracellular fluid volumes or impaired renal function.[529]

The *milk-alkali syndrome* is an example of this phenomenon. This syndrome is sometimes seen in patients with peptic ulcer disease who ingest large quantities of milk and absorbable alkaline medications during a sustained period. The syndrome consists of metabolic alkalosis, hypercalcemia, and renal impairment.[529]

Ingestion by infants of large quantities of bicarbonate or soy-protein formula has similarly resulted in metabolic alkalosis due to ingestion of excessive base. These conditions can be readily recognized by a history of ingestion of large quantities of base and the presence of alkaline urine.[529]

Excessive Licorice Ingestion

The agent glycyrrhizic acid, which is present in licorice, certain medicines, candies, and chewing tobacco, is similar structurally and chemically to aldosterone.[529] Therefore, when ingested in large quantities (e.g., 20 to 40 g of licorice),[523] it has effects similar to those of hyperaldosteronism and may lead to metabolic alkalosis. Recently, it has been argued that glycyrrhizic acid may not actually be the active ingredient that causes metabolic alkalosis.[542] Nevertheless, it still appears that licorice does indeed cause metabolic alkalosis.

Gastric Fluid Loss

The loss of large quantities of gastric secretions is probably the most common cause of *severe* metabolic alkalosis (i.e., plasma [HCO_3] 50 to 60 mEq/L).[529] A large volume of gastric secretions may be lost by severe and prolonged vomiting or in the presence of nasogastric suctioning.

Mechanism of Alkalosis

Loss of Acid. Gastric secretions are very acidic. They contain hydrochloric acid (HCl), and the pH may be close to 1.0 (i.e., [H^+] of 100 mEq/L). When the HCl in these secretions is lost, new HCl must be generated by the cells in the gastric mucosa. The chemical process by which this occurs is shown in Figure 13-8.

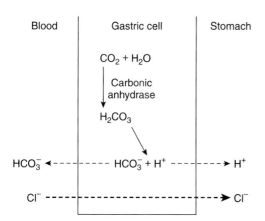

Figure 13-8.   Production of HCl in gastric cells. Hydrogen ions generated in the gastric cells via the hydrolysis reaction are secreted into the stomach with chloride. The bicarbonate produced via the hydrolysis reaction enters the blood in exchange for the chloride.

The presence of carbonic anhydrase in the gastric cells facilitates the hydrolysis reaction. In turn, the hydrogen ion generated via the hydrolysis reaction is secreted into the stomach along with chloride from the blood. In exchange for the chloride anion that has left the blood, the bicarbonate anion, present in the gastric cells from the hydrolysis reaction, enters the blood. Thus, the regeneration of HCl tends to cause metabolic alkalosis by *increasing blood bicarbonate.*

Loss of Fluid and Electrolytes. The loss of gastric secretions may lead to hypovolemia and stimulation of aldosterone. The effect of increased aldosterone is, as discussed earlier, stimulation of $NaHCO_3$ reabsorption in renal tubules accompanied by increased potassium secretion.

Other electrolytes are also lost with the gastric secretions. Sodium is often slightly depleted, and potassium and chloride may be substantially depleted. The potassium concentration of gastric secretions is approximately 20 mEq/L.[529] The anion gap may be elevated owing to contraction of the extracellular fluid space, which causes an increased protein concentration.[534]

Chloride Replacement

Administration of chloride permits gradual correction of the alkalemia. The presence of chloride facilitates increased renal NaCl retention and, therefore, a diminished need for renal $NaHCO_3$ retention and hydrogen ion secretion.

Hyperaldosteronism Secondary to Nonadrenal Factors

Secondary hyperaldosteronism is the condition of increased blood aldosterone levels secondary to some stimuli outside the adrenal gland itself. Typically, secondary hyperaldosteronism is due to increased renin-angiotensin activity triggered by diminished renal perfusion (see Chapter 12). Conditions and drugs that may lead to secondary hyperaldosteronism include Bartter's syndrome, inadequate renal perfusion, and diuretics.

Bartter's Syndrome

Bartter's syndrome is a relatively rare disorder that can cause hyperaldosteronism secondary to high levels of renin. The hyperaldosteronism, in turn, leads to hypokalemia and metabolic alkalosis. Arterial blood pressure is typically normal or low. The unique component of this disease is hyperplasia (i.e., excess proliferation of normal cells) of the juxtaglomerular cells.

Gitelman syndrome, which is even more rare, is a similar disorder that is typically seen in late childhood or early adulthood.[480]

Inadequate Renal Perfusion

When perfusion to the kidney is diminished, the renin-angiotensin system is activated, and metabolic alkalosis may develop. Conditions that decrease cardiac output, blood volume, or selective renal perfusion may have this effect. Cardiac output may be low in diseases such as congestive heart failure. Low functional blood volume (hypovolemia) may accompany dehydration or migration of fluid to the interstitial space. A selective decrease in renal perfusion may occur in renal artery stenosis or in renal disease secondary to hypertension.

Diuretics

Most diuretics facilitate urinary excretion of NaCl by impeding its reabsorption in the renal tubules. The transient blood volume loss may lead to secondary hyperaldosteronism, hypokalemia, and metabolic alkalosis. Generally, the more potent the diuretic, the greater is its potential to cause metabolic alkalosis.

Bicarbonate Administration

Sodium Bicarbonate Overcorrection

Sodium bicarbonate ($NaHCO_3$) is sometimes used in the treatment of metabolic acidemia. Presently, the use of sodium bicarbonate in some types of metabolic acidosis (e.g., lactic acidosis during cardiac arrest) is controversial. (This controversy is addressed in Chapter 14 regarding treatment of acid-base disorders.) Nevertheless, sodium bicarbonate continues to be the treatment of choice for metabolic acidosis, and the development of metabolic alkalosis secondary to overcorrection is not uncommon.

Overcorrection of metabolic acidosis occurs frequently for two reasons. First, the appropriate dose of sodium bicarbonate that should be administered in a given situation is not clear-cut;

it depends on the patient's total extracellular fluid volume as well as on the rate and type of abnormal acid production. Second, there is an elevation of bicarbonate produced within the body (*endogenous production*) during liver metabolism of the conjugate bases in lactic and ketoacidosis. Lactate can be broken down only in the presence of a sufficient quantity of oxygen.

The breakdown of anions, such as lactate, citrate, and acetate, generates blood bicarbonate. In fact, lactate was used in the past for the treatment of metabolic acidosis due to its ability to generate blood bicarbonate.

Blood Transfusions

During storage of blood, the pH tends to decrease.[535,536] Indeed, administration of massive blood transfusions over a short period may cause a transient metabolic acidosis that clears up rather quickly.[535] More important, metabolism of citrate, the anticoagulant most commonly used for storage of blood, leads to the gradual onset of metabolic alkalosis after massive transfusions. Metabolic alkalosis tends to peak about 24 hours after transfusion.[535]

A unit of whole blood contains approximately 17 mEq of citrate, whereas a unit of packed cells contains only 5 mEq.[515] For each mole of citrate metabolized, 3 moles of bicarbonate are produced.[537] Thus, the potential for citrated blood transfusions to cause metabolic alkalosis is apparent. It is important to recognize metabolic alkalosis resulting from massive blood transfusions in the critical care setting, because this condition has been reported to complicate weaning from mechanical ventilation.[538]

Adrenocortical Hypersecretion

Excessive secretion of aldosterone directly by the adrenal cortex leads to metabolic alkalosis through renal potassium excretion and bicarbonate retention. This mechanism is often referred to as *primary hyperaldosteronism* or primary mineralocorticoid excess. It is most often due to a tumor of the adrenal cortex (aldosteronoma). In primary hyperaldosteronism, aldosterone secretion cannot be suppressed by volume expansion.

ON CALL | CASE 13-2 *ABGs and Critical Thinking*

You are the only person available to care for this patient. You must assess the patient/situation and act accordingly.

A 55-year-old man arrives in the emergency department comatose following severe sustained vomiting. Blood gases and electrolytes are drawn.

ARTERIAL BLOOD GASES

SaO_2	86%
pH	7.62
$PaCO_2$	56 mm Hg
PaO_2	54 mm Hg
$[HCO_3]$	52 mEq/L
FIO_2	0.21
Na	135 mEq/L
CO_2	54 mEq/L

Cl	61 mEq/L
K	2.2 mEq/L

ASSESSMENT

Abnormalities: List abnormal data and other noteworthy information. Classify ABG.

Explanation: List possible diseases, pathology, or other situations that may have led to this patient's condition.

INTERVENTION

Importance: Prioritize concern(s) of treatment in order of urgency and/or seriousness as you see the overall situation.

Steroids

Glucocorticoids, commonly called steroids, have a large and varied application in medicine. The chemical structure of glucocorticoids is very similar to that of mineralocorticoids such as aldosterone; as a result, glucocorticoids show similar properties. Therefore, steroid therapy, especially in large doses, may cause metabolic alkalosis.

Eucapnic Ventilation Posthypercapnia

Chronic hypercapnia is associated with renal bicarbonate retention as a compensatory mechanism. In chronic hypercapnia, if $PaCO_2$ is decreased abruptly toward normal laboratory values (which may occur during mechanical ventilation), the blood gas picture may appear as metabolic alkalosis.

Although in a sense this is not a true primary metabolic alkalosis, an understanding of its origin is nevertheless important. This is especially true because adequate chloride intake is essential for its correction. Furthermore, the high incidence of posthypercapneic metabolic alkalosis (40% in one study[539]) makes it an important consideration in acid-base assessment in critical care.

EXERCISES

Exercise 13-1	**Respiratory Acidosis**

Fill in the blanks or select the best answer.

1. Respiratory acidosis threatens acid-base balance through the (accumulation/loss) of carbonic acid.

2. The most common cause of *chronic* respiratory acidosis is _____.

3. The presence of a barrel chest, adventitious (abnormal) breath sounds, labored breathing, and forced expiration suggests that the patient has _____.

4. When a patient with COPD is likely to be hypoxic, oxygen therapy (should/should not) be withheld because of the risk of acute respiratory acidosis.

5. Individuals with COPD (are/are not) particularly vulnerable to the respiratory effects of sedatives and narcotics.

6. Exhaustion may explain the sudden onset of respiratory acidosis that has been observed in patients with _____ after a sustained period of laborious breathing.

7. The progress of neuromuscular function can be monitored at the bedside through serial measurements of (blood gases/vital capacity).

8. (Hyperkalemia/Hypokalemia), a common electrolyte disorder in the critical care setting, is associated with muscle weakness and even paralysis.

9. Fat metabolism results in (less/more) CO_2 production than carbohydrate metabolism.

10. Administration of sodium bicarbonate ($NaHCO_3$) intravenously also (decreases/increases) CO_2 production via the hydrolysis reaction.

11. The thermic effect is a change in the (type/quantity) of metabolism.

12. Total parenteral nutrition is generally associated with a/an (increased/decreased) need for ventilation.

13. Central mechanisms may play a role in the chronic respiratory acidosis observed in obese individuals, which is called the _____ syndrome.

14. A condition characterized by unexplained hypoventilation is sometimes referred to as _____ curse.

15. List eight major causes of respiratory acidosis.

Respiratory Alkalosis

Fill in the blanks or select the best answer.

1. Respiratory alkalosis disrupts acid-base balance by (increasing/depleting) blood carbonic acid.

2. The single most common and important cause of hyperventilation and respiratory alkalosis is _____.

3. The (Hering-Breuer/J-receptor) reflex is also known as the stretch reflex.

4. The (Hering-Breuer/J-receptor) reflex provides a feasible explanation for the hyperventilation commonly noted in various disorders that may have an impact on the alveolar-capillary membrane.

5. Ammonia may (stimulate/depress) ventilation.

6. CSF (alkalosis/acidosis) stimulates hyperventilation.

7. (Increased/Decreased) perfusion of the peripheral chemoreceptors may also lead to respiratory alkalosis.

8. In adults, (respiratory alkalosis/metabolic acidosis) appears to be the dominating acid-base disturbance in salicylate intoxication.

9. Individuals with severe shock and arterial respiratory alkalosis probably have venous respiratory (alkalosis/acidosis).

10. List the five major general causes of respiratory alkalosis.

High Anion Gap Metabolic Acidosis: Toxins and Azotemic Renal Failure

Fill in the blanks or select the best answer.

1. When the anion gap exceeds 16 mEq/L, (decrease in base/increase in fixed acids) in the blood is highly probable.

2. The metabolic acidosis of _____ intoxication is usually accompanied by a primary respiratory alkalosis.

3. Symptoms from ingestion of _____ include engorged retinal vessels and blurred vision.

4. The active ingredient in antifreeze is _____.

5. The active ingredient in transmission fluid and paint thinner is _____.

6. Renal failure associated with a high anion gap and the inability to excrete fixed acids is called (renal tubular acidosis/azotemic renal failure).

7. The specific blood values that are elevated in azotemia are the _____ and _____.

8. _____ azotemia is a condition in which azotemia is due to inadequate renal perfusion.

9. The toxic clinical picture associated with azotemia and renal failure is called

   _____.

10. The pH typically does not begin to decrease until azotemia is fairly substantial and creatinine exceeds at least _____ mg/dL.

Fill in the blanks or select the best answer.

1. Lactic acidosis is probably the most (common/uncommon) cause of high anion gap metabolic acidosis.

2. Both acute and chronic (hepatic/renal) insufficiency may lead to lactic acidosis.

3. Fat metabolism leads to the accumulation of which two ketoacids?

4. _____ is responsible for the characteristic fruity odor of the patient's breath in ketoacidosis.

5. Acetone, acetoacetate, and beta-hydroxybutyrate are known as the _____ bodies.

6. State three conditions that may cause ketoacidosis.

7. The _____ is a qualitative Na nitroprusside reaction in which acetoacetate bodies manifest a purple color.

8. Diabetes (insipidus/mellitus) is associated with (hypoglycemia/hyperglycemia).

9. _____ must be present to transport glucose from the extracellular fluid to the intracellular fluid.

10. Diabetes mellitus is associated with (hypoglycemia/hyperglycemia).

11. (Edema/Dehydration) is common in diabetic ketoacidosis.

12. The average plasma glucose level in diabetic ketoacidosis is approximately (200/500) mg/dL.

13. The compensatory response to ketoacidosis results in a characteristic deep, gasping type of ventilation known as _____ breathing.

14. The increased glucose in the urine associated with diabetic acidosis is called _____.

15. State the four major causes of high anion gap metabolic acidosis.

Fill in the blanks or select the best answer.

1. Normal anion gap acidosis is also called (hypochloremic/hyperchloremic) metabolic acidosis.

2. State the two major organs capable of losing/excreting base from the body.

3. When renal acidosis is caused specifically by the failure of the renal tubules to absorb bicarbonate, it is called _____.

4. In renal tubular acidosis, urine pH is surprisingly (high/low).

5. Surgical conditions that necessitate (gastric/enteric) drainage tubes may lead to a loss of bicarbonate.

6. Metabolic acidosis may result from excessive (vomiting/diarrhea).

7. (Acetazolamide/Furosemide) may lead to metabolic acidosis.

8. Dilution acidosis is most common in (adults/children).

9. The bicarbonate concentration of bile and pancreatic juice is very (low/high).

10. State 11 major causes of normal anion gap acidosis.

Exercise 13-6   Metabolic Alkalosis

Fill in the blanks or select the best answer.

1. The kidneys (can/cannot) conserve potassium.

2. Most potassium is in the (intracellular/extracellular) fluid.

3. Probably the most common cause of metabolic alkalosis is (gastric fluid loss/primary hyperaldosteronism).

4. In the generation of gastric HCl, an (H^+ ion/HCO_3^- anion) enters the blood.

5. Hyperplasia of the juxtaglomerular cells is associated with _____ syndrome.

6. The immediate response to blood transfusion may be metabolic (acidosis/alkalosis), whereas the delayed response may be metabolic (acidosis/alkalosis).

7. Excessive secretion of aldosterone by the adrenal cortex (e.g., tumor) that leads to metabolic alkalosis is called (primary/secondary) hyperaldosteronism.

8. Steroids commonly used therapeutically in medicine are (mineralocorticoids/glucocorticoids).

9. Metabolism of citrate or lactate leads to metabolic (acidosis/alkalosis).

10. State eight major causes of metabolic alkalosis.

Exercise 13-7   Internet Work

1. Search the Internet for "acid base cases" and bring in five cases for classroom discussion.

2. Find cases with the five types of acid-base disturbances: respiratory acidosis, respiratory alkalosis, high anion gap metabolic acidosis, hyperchloremic metabolic acidosis, and metabolic alkalosis.

NBRC Challenge 13

Please select the best answer for the following multiple-choice questions.

1. A hypokalemic, CHF patient with a pH of 7.54 is in need of a diuretic. Which of the following would you recommend?
   A) Lasix
   B) Hydrodiuril
   C) Diamox
   D) Mannitol
   E) Edecrin
   (CSE-RRT EXAMINATION — NBRC MATRIX III,D,13)

2. A patient is in profound cardiogenic shock. A blood gas is drawn and the $PaCO_2$ is 25 mm Hg. What would you conclude regarding the status of the tissues?
   A) Tissues are most likely alkalotic.
   B) Tissues are well oxygenated.
   C) Tissues are likely acidotic.
   D) Tissue pH is probably near normal.
   E) Tissues are not undergoing anaerobic metabolism.
   (RRT EXAMINATION — NBRC MATRIX I,B,9,c)

3. A patient has a lactate level of 8 mM/L, an anion gap of 24 mEq/L, a blood glucose of 123 mg/dL, a BUN of 21 mg/dL, and no evidence of poisoning or salicylate toxicity. What information may be useful in making a diagnosis?
   A) [Hb]
   B) [Ca^{++}]
   C) [Na^+]
   D) [Cl^-]
   E) [Mg^+]
   (CRT EXAMINATION — NBRC MATRIX I,A,1,c)

4. A known COPD patient is admitted with an acute exacerbation. He is placed on a 2 LPM nasal cannula and given a narcotic to calm him and blood gases and electrolytes are drawn. What would you recommend at this time?
   A) Include a lactate measurement.
   B) Include a glucose measurement.
   C) Include a magnesium measurement.
   D) Discontinue the oxygen until the blood gas is done.
   E) Discontinue the narcotic.
   (CSE-RRT EXAMINATION — NBRC MATRIX III,D,13)

5. A patient has a primary metabolic acidosis and an anion gap of 25 mEq/L. What laboratory information would you find useful?
   I. Blood glucose
   II. BUN
   III. Lactate
   IV. Urinary Cl
   A) I and II only
   B) I and III only
   C) II and IV only
   D) I, II, and III only
   E) II, III, and IV only
   (NBRC RRT — CSE MATRIX I,A,2.a)

14

Mixed Acid-Base Disturbances and Treatment

One must develop a clear understanding of the pathophysiologic principles which underlie simple disorders before a comfortable approach to diagnosis and therapy of mixed disorders can be developed.

Robert G. Narins, Michael Emmett[515]

The principal reason that one seeks an accurate assessment of acid-base equilibrium is to obtain an appropriate guide to therapy.

Jordan J. Cohen, Jerome P. Kassirer[483]

Outline

OVERVIEW

Three final aspects of clinical acid-base management are explored in this chapter. First, some of the major diseases and factors that tend to complicate the interpretation of clinical acid-base data are discussed. These factors include chronic lung disease, chronic renal disease, and therapeutic intervention. Blood gas and acid-base interpretation under these circumstances often requires special attention and skill.

Second, methods that can be used to differentiate *simple* (single) acid-base problems from *mixed* (complicated, multiple) acid-base disturbances are reviewed. In particular, the acid-base map and rules of thumb for compensation of

simple acid-base disturbances are described. In addition, common settings and clues that may suggest a mixed acid-base disturbance are presented.

The final portion of this chapter deals with the supportive treatment of the four general acid-base disorders: respiratory acidosis, respiratory alkalosis, metabolic acidosis, and metabolic alkalosis. General guidelines are presented regarding the management of these generic disorders.

In addition, *venous paradox* during cardiopulmonary resuscitation or severe shock is described under metabolic acidosis. This phenomenon has important implications regarding blood gas interpretation as well as the most appropriate use of $NaHCO_3$ therapy.

FACTORS THAT MAY COMPLICATE CLINICAL ACID-BASE DATA

Respiratory/Renal Pathology

The primary organ systems involved in the maintenance of acid-base balance are the respiratory and renal systems. Disease, and in particular chronic disease, in either of these body systems can directly impair acid-base conditions or hamper the ability of the affected organ system to compensate for another acid-base disturbance. Thus, blood gas and acid-base interpretation in these chronic diseases requires special attention and understanding.

Chronic Obstructive Pulmonary Disease

Chronic obstructive pulmonary disease (COPD) is the classic example of a chronic respiratory disease. The typical acid-base picture in COPD is well known to most clinicians. Although respiratory alkalosis may possibly be seen at an early stage of the disease and in acute asthma, the characteristic picture in long-standing, severe, pulmonary disease is hypercapnia (e.g., $PaCO_2$ > 50 mm Hg) with metabolic compensation (increased [BE], [HCO_3]). Example 14-1 shows typical blood gases in long-standing COPD.

Example 14-1
Typical End-Stage COPD Blood Gases
pH	7.38
$PaCO_2$	55 mm Hg
[BE]	5 mEq/L
[HCO_3]	31 mEq/L
PaO_2	55 mm Hg

The pH is often within the normal range (i.e., completely compensated) and may even be on the alkalotic side of the normal range.[10] This finding is not consistent with rules that apply to compensation (i.e., overcompensation should not occur), however, and may be related to a mild concurrent primary metabolic alkalosis. The administration of steroids and diuretics with concomitant hypochloremia or hypokalemia is common in severe COPD.

Arterial blood gases are critical in the diagnosis and management of acute exacerbations of COPD. Nevertheless, blood gases in this group are often confusing and complex. Furthermore, they may be misleading if they are not clearly understood. Abnormal baseline values, unpredictable acute ventilatory changes, and the potential coexistence of lactic acidosis may all interact in a complex manner. The result may be misleading data when a single blood gas is considered in isolation. Some examples are given of how this result may occur.

Relative Hyperventilation

It is not uncommon for a patient with COPD to lower $PaCO_2$ in response to acute hypoxemia arising from an acute lung infection. Superimposing this acute change on the chronic (normal hypercapnic baseline) values shown in Example 14-1 results in blood gases approximating those shown in Example 14-2.

Example 14-2
Relative Hyperventilation in COPD
pH	7.52
$PaCO_2$	40 mm Hg
[BE]	5 mEq/L
[HCO_3]	31 mEq/L
PaO_2	52 mm Hg

Similar results could occur if a patient with COPD were placed on a mechanical ventilator and ventilated to a $PaCO_2$ of 40 mm Hg. Classification of this blood gas in isolation could result in the diagnosis of metabolic alkalosis. The underlying cause is, in fact, eucapnic (normal $PaCO_2$) ventilation posthypercapnia.

Treatment for simple metabolic alkalemia here, however, would be inappropriate; optimal management requires an understanding of the disease process and the likely chain of events that have led to this point. It is probably more desirable to return this patient's $PaCO_2$ to their baseline level.

Relative Hyperventilation with Lactic Acidosis

Another important consideration in the patient with COPD is the potential for hypoxia and lactic acidosis. Individuals with COPD often have increased heart rates and elevated arterial blood pressure under chronic normal conditions to maintain adequate tissue oxygenation. In addition, right-sided heart failure is common in COPD secondary to increased pulmonary vascular resistance. When the acute stress of pneumonia and increasing hypoxemia is superimposed on an already compromised cardiovascular system, hypoxia may develop.

If lactic acidosis compounds the blood gas shown in Example 14-2, the result may appear as shown in Example 14-3. The net effect of these interactions is a relatively normal blood gas acid-base picture despite a severely compromised patient. Thus, *serial* blood gas measurements and other clinical findings are essential in understanding the significance of any isolated blood gas report.

Example 14-3
Relative Hyperventilation with Lactic Acidosis in COPD

pH	7.38
$PaCO_2$	40 mm Hg
[BE]	1 mEq/L
[HCO_3]	24 mEq/L
PaO_2	44 mm Hg

Acute Hypercapnia

Many patients with severe COPD respond paradoxically to acute hypoxemia or oxygen therapy in that their $PaCO_2$ increases instead of decreases. Reasons for this are unclear but are most likely related to worsening ventilation-perfusion mismatch and exhaustion secondary to the work of breathing. In addition, as described previously, excessive oxygen therapy may similarly precipitate acute hypercarbia. This affect has also recently been shown to occur during acute asthma exacerbations and the administration of FIO_2 1.0.[700] Excessive oxygen therapy may also be recognized by the concurrent presence of a PaO_2 in excess of 60 mm Hg. When acute hypercapnia is superimposed on typical COPD chronic blood gases, the result may appear as shown in Example 14-4.

Example 14-4
Acute Hypercapnia in COPD

pH	7.30
$PaCO_2$	75 mm Hg
[BE]	8 mEq/L
[HCO_3]	33 mEq/L
PaO_2	48 mm Hg

This particular blood gas picture is a common finding in acute exacerbation of COPD in the emergency department. The hallmark to recognition of this situation (acute exacerbation of COPD) is the surprisingly normal pH despite severe hypercapnia.

Patients with COPD who present with blood gas results such as those shown in Example 14-4 can often be treated successfully with low concentrations of oxygen therapy, noninvasive ventilation, and bronchial hygiene.[543,544] Thus, mechanical ventilation, with related discomfort and the potential for complications, can often be avoided. Furthermore, a blood gas such as this may be the first clue that the patient has COPD. This finding, in turn, alerts the clinician to the potential for increasing hypercapnia with excessive oxygen therapy. Therefore, recognition of this situation may have great clinical importance.

Acute Hypercapnia with Lactic Acidosis

If lactic acidosis develops coincidentally with the acute hypoventilation shown in Example 14-4 (not an unlikely situation), COPD blood gases may appear as shown in Example 14-5.

Example 14-5
Acute Hypercapnia with Lactic Acidosis in COPD

pH	7.20
$PaCO_2$	75 mm Hg
[BE]	−2 mEq/L
[HCO_3]	28 mEq/L
PaO_2	44 mm Hg

When considered in isolation, this blood gas appears to show an acute hypoventilation (respiratory acidosis). Actually, this individual has two primary acid-base problems: respiratory acidosis and metabolic acidosis. Rather than immediately starting mechanical ventilation, a short, carefully controlled (and monitored) trial of oxygen therapy might mitigate gas exchange problems and obviate the need for mechanical ventilation. If this is unsuccessful, noninvasive ventilation should be attempted prior to full-blown mechanical ventilation.

Again, interpretation and treatment must be tailored to the specific case. These various examples have been provided to emphasize the complexity and the need for careful *serial* analysis of blood gases in COPD.

Chronic Renal Failure

Just as COPD can distort blood gas values, renal failure or disease may affect baseline data. These disorders impair the renal ability to manipulate and control bicarbonate concentration and various electrolytes and body fluids. In severe stages of disease, metabolic acidosis with acidemia may be present. The presence of chronic renal disease must be considered when arterial blood gases and acid-base status are evaluated.

Therapeutic Intervention

Therapy given to a patient may sometimes distort the blood gas findings and may complicate the interpretation. The administration of diuretics, steroids, electrolytes, oxygen, bicarbonate, or mechanical ventilation may cause primary acid-base disturbances or may alter compensatory patterns. These factors must all be considered carefully during acid-base diagnosis, particularly in the critical care setting.

A specific area of application where blood gases may be measured frequently is during mechanical ventilation. The clinician must realize, however, that mechanical ventilation, by its very objective, controls at least a portion of ventilation in a set pattern. Therefore, compensation for metabolic acid-base disturbances cannot occur in *exactly* the same manner as it would in the patient who breathes spontaneously.

Example 14-6
Metabolic Acidosis During Mechanical Ventilation

pH	7.44
$PaCO_2$	18 mm Hg
[BE]	–12 mEq/L
[HCO_3]	12 mEq/L
PaO_2	64 mm Hg

Example 14-6 shows blood gases that may be seen during mechanical ventilation in a patient with a metabolic acidosis. Note that this blood gas in isolation appears to be a completely compensated respiratory alkalosis. Actually, this patient has only a metabolic acidosis. Nevertheless, the rapid respiratory rate

generated as a compensatory mechanism to the acidosis, in conjunction with the delivery of large tidal volumes via mechanical ventilation, has caused the apparent alkalosis. It would be inappropriate, however, to attempt to treat the respiratory alkalosis. The only true primary acid-base problem in this patient is metabolic acidosis. Mechanical ventilation has created the false impression of respiratory alkalosis.

If this same degree of metabolic acidosis developed in this individual during spontaneous breathing (i.e., not during mechanical ventilation), the blood gas picture might more closely resemble Example 14-7. Thus, the potential impact of respiratory assistance on the blood gas findings can be appreciated. The clinician must be mindful of the mode of mechanical ventilation and whether it may influence blood gas patterns.

Example 14-7
Metabolic Acidosis During Spontaneous Breathing

pH	7.32
$PaCO_2$	25 mm Hg
[BE]	–10 mEq/L
[HCO_3]	13 mEq/L
PaO_2	64 mm Hg

The potential for mechanical ventilation to camouflage acid-base events has been described. Similarly, many of the other therapeutic measures mentioned earlier can lead to iatrogenic acid-base disturbances. Arterial blood gases and acid-base disturbances must always be interpreted within the context of therapeutic measures and long-standing pulmonary or renal disease.

MIXED ACID-BASE DISTURBANCES

Definition

The natural tendency of the body to compensate for primary acid-base disturbances was discussed in Chapter 8. Because of this natural phenomenon, whenever opposing respiratory and metabolic conditions were present, compensation was assumed. Although this initial assumption is logical, it may be incorrect. It is not uncommon to have *two opposing primary* acid-base disturbances that give the surface appearance of simple compensation. The coexistence of two primary acid-base disturbances is called a *mixed* acid-base disturbance.

Recognition of Mixed Disturbances

Acid-Base Map

How can simple compensation be differentiated from a mixed acid-base disturbance? Probably the most useful aid in this regard is the *acid-base map* that is shown in Figure 14-1. The labeled areas encompass with 95% confidence the range of pH, $PaCO_2$, and bicarbonate that one would expect to find in patients who have only one *simple* acid-base disturbance. Separate bands are also given for both acute and chronic acid-base problems.

When a patient's values fall outside these bands, it is very unlikely that the patient has just one disturbance. On the other hand, when a patient's values fall within one of these bands it does not ensure that the patient has a single acid-base disturbance, it simply means that the data are compatible with this conclusion.

Figure 14-2 shows how the acid-base map can be used by simply aligning the two adjacent sides of a piece of paper with the patient's respective $PaCO_2$ (horizontal axis) and pH (vertical axis). The corner point of the paper represents where the values intersect on the map. The data in Figure 14-2,*A* are consistent with chronic simple respiratory acidosis. Remember, this does

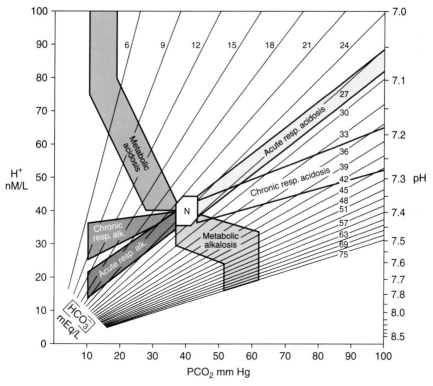

Figure 14-1. **Acid-base map.** *N* indicates the area of normal values. The numbered diagonal lines give the bicarbonate concentrations in milliequivalents per liter. The confidence bands for the expected range of values of the six common acid-base disturbances are illustrated. The map has several potential uses. First, it can serve in place of a pocket calculator and allow the clinician to check, for example, if a patient's reported venous serum bicarbonate concentration is in accord with the measured values for the PCO_2 and pH of his or her arterial blood. Second, it may provide assistance in distinguishing between compensatory responses and mixed disturbances. If the point corresponding to a patient's values falls outside the 95% confidence bands, it is likely that a mixed disturbance exists. The reverse is not necessarily true, however. A point falling within a confidence band does not necessarily mean the presence of a single disorder, because there are several ways to arrive at the same point. Finally, sequential plotting of a patient's values for several hours to days may greatly simplify the understanding and management of complex acid-base disturbances.

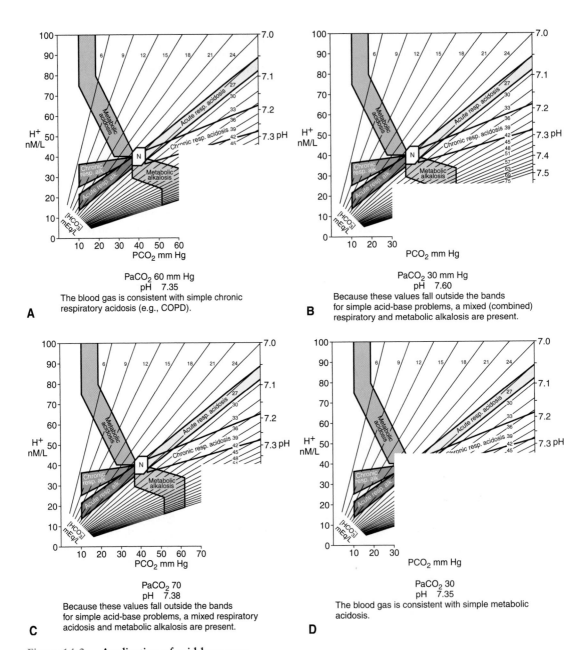

A
PaCO₂ 60 mm Hg
pH   7.35
The blood gas is consistent with simple chronic
respiratory acidosis (e.g., COPD).

B
PaCO₂ 30 mm Hg
pH   7.60
Because these values fall outside the bands
for simple acid-base problems, a mixed (combined)
respiratory and metabolic alkalosis are present.

C
PaCO₂ 70
pH   7.38
Because these values fall outside the bands
for simple acid-base problems, a mixed respiratory
acidosis and metabolic alkalosis are present.

D
PaCO₂ 30
pH   7.35
The blood gas is consistent with simple metabolic
acidosis.

Figure 14-2.   **Application of acid-base map.**

not mean that the elevated bicarbonate cannot
be due to a primary problem, but only that the
data are consistent with usual compensation
for chronic respiratory acidosis.

Figure 14-2,*B* does not fall within any band,
therefore the clinician can be relatively certain
that there are two separate, primary, acid-base
disturbances (respiratory alkalosis and metabolic
alkalosis). Figure 14-2,*C* similarly represents two

primary acid-base disturbances, although in this
case they are in opposite directions (i.e., respiratory acidosis and metabolic alkalosis). Without
an acid-base map, one might assume that these
blood gas results are due to complete compensation. Finally, Figure 14-2,*D* is consistent with
a simple metabolic acidosis.

The acid-base map is a simple, useful tool for
the evaluation of mixed acid-base disturbances.

Pocket versions of this map are available for use at the bedside.

Compensatory Patterns

The degree of compensation observed in the four simple primary acid-base disturbances, although quite similar, is not identical. For reasons that are unclear, some types of acid-base problems (e.g., metabolic alkalosis) result in more complete compensation than others. Nevertheless, in the absence of an acid-base map, it is useful to have some idea of the typical compensatory patterns that should accompany the four simple acid-base disturbances. This can help the clinician to evaluate the appropriateness of the degree of compensation observed in a given individual.

Respiratory Acidosis

The pH falls approximately 0.06 unit for an acute 10-mm Hg increase in $PaCO_2$. After maximal renal compensation, the change in pH associated with an increase of 10 mm Hg in $PaCO_2$ is approximately 0.03 unit. Thus, the pH returns approximately 50% of the way back toward normal after maximal compensation.

Table 14-1 shows the typical compensatory response to respiratory acidosis. This table shows that when the $PaCO_2$ increases to 70 mm Hg acutely, the pH drops immediately to approximately 7.22 (0.06 decrease/10 mm Hg $PaCO_2$ increase). The immediate increase in bicarbonate is a result of the hydrolysis effect that was

discussed in Chapter 8 and it does not represent renal compensation.

After maximal renal compensation (several days later), however, the pH returns approximately halfway back to normal (i.e., 7.31). Thus, complete compensation (i.e., pH in normal range) is not usually seen when respiratory acidosis is quite severe. Complete compensation for respiratory acidosis occurs only when the respiratory acidosis is not severe (i.e., $PaCO_2 <$ 60 mm Hg). In addition, because the mechanism of renal compensation for respiratory acidosis is bicarbonate retention, the chloride anion is typically low to preserve electroneutrality.

Respiratory Alkalosis

Compensation for respiratory alkalosis is similar in magnitude to compensation for respiratory acidosis. In general, the pH should return at least halfway back toward normal. Again, an example is shown in Table 14-1. Surprisingly, however, when the respiratory alkalosis persists for weeks, the pH may actually return completely to normal in some cases.[515] Renal compensation for respiratory alkalosis requires the excretion of bicarbonate; therefore, hyperchloremia often develops to preserve electroneutrality.

Metabolic Acidosis

The major portion of the ventilatory response to metabolic acidosis usually begins quickly; however, the maximal compensatory response

Table 14-1. Compensatory Patterns

Primary Insult	Hypothetical Cases (initial $PaCO_2$ = 40 mm Hg, [HCO_3^-] = 24 mEq/L)	
	Initial Effects	Chronic Response (Several Days)
Metabolic Acidosis ↓[HCO_3^-] to 15 mEq/L	$PaCO_2$ = 40 mm Hg pH = 7.20*	$PaCO_2$ = 30 mm Hg pH = 7.30
Metabolic Alkalosis ↑[HCO_3^-] to 40 mEq/L	$PaCO_2$ = 40 mm Hg pH = 7.62*	$PaCO_2$ = 51 mm Hg pH = 7.51
Respiratory Acidosis ↑$PaCO_2$ to 70 mm Hg	[HCO_3^-] increases to 27 mEq/L pH = 7.22	[HCO_3^-] = 33 mEq/L pH = 7.31
Respiratory Alkalosis ↓$PaCO_2$ to 20 mm Hg	[HCO_3^-] decreases to 20 mEq/L pH = 7.60	[HCO_3^-] = 15 mEq/L pH = 7.50

*In comparing metabolic acidosis and alkalosis, note that to produce the same acute change in pH (~0.2 unit), a much larger change in [HCO_3^-] is necessary in metabolic alkalosis (ΔHCO_3^- = 16 mEq/L) than in metabolic acidosis (ΔHCO_3^- = 9 mEq/L).

Modified from Kokko, J.P., and Tennen, R.L.: Fluids and Electrolytes, Philadelphia, W. B. Saunders, 1986, p. 386.

may take up to 24 hours.[545, 546] When metabolic acidosis develops in the plasma, it takes some time for the pH to fall in the cerebrospinal fluid owing to the limited permeability of ions across the blood-brain barrier. Lactic acidosis, however, may actually develop within the brain cells, and it is therefore associated with a more rapid ventilatory response.[515]

A very useful rule of thumb when an acid-base map is not at hand is that after maximal compensation, the $PaCO_2$ generally approximates the last two digits of the pH.[515] Thus, in simple chronic metabolic acidosis with a pH of 7.30, the $PaCO_2$ is usually approximately 30 mm Hg (see Table 14-1).

Metabolic Alkalosis

The respiratory compensatory response to metabolic alkalosis is hypoventilation with retention of carbonic acid. It has long been assumed, however, that this response was limited by the onset of hypoxemia. Therefore, it is often stated that compensation for metabolic alkalosis will not allow the $PaCO_2$ to exceed 55 to 60 mm Hg.[515]

More recent reviews have shown that hypoventilation is not limited by hypoxemia.[547] Progressive, linear hypoventilation accompanies progressive, simple, metabolic alkalosis when it is not associated with other acid-base problems.[547] As shown in Table 14-1, compensation may sometimes also allow the pH to return halfway back to normal; however, a lesser compensatory response is more common.

Summary

In the absence of an acid-base map, it is useful to know that maximal compensation for most simple acid-base disturbances is approximately 50%. Compensation for respiratory alkalosis is usually slightly greater than this, whereas compensation for metabolic alkalosis is usually slightly less. Knowledge of compensatory patterns can alert the clinician to the presence of a mixed disturbance even when an acid-base map is not available.

Alerts to Mixed Disturbances

Mixed acid-base disturbances are far from uncommon in the hospital setting. When primary

---

Box 14-1 Alerts to Mixed Acid-Base Disturbances

Absence of compensation
Long-standing pulmonary or renal disease
Excessive compensation
Respiratory assistance
Temporal inconsistencies
Settings conducive to mixed disturbances

---

acid-base problems are camouflaged in mixed disturbances, they may easily be missed. In this setting, covert acid-base problems are untreated and are likely to lead to progressive deterioration. Furthermore, even use of the acid-base map does not identify those mixed disturbances that result in blood gas data that coincide with findings that normally accompany simple disturbances.

Therefore, the clinician must look for clues that suggest the presence of multiple (mixed) acid-base disorders. Box 14-1 suggests some situations that should alert the clinician to the likelihood of a mixed acid-base disturbance.

Absence of Compensation

Compensation is the normal response of the body to a primary acid-base problem. When compensation is absent, given sufficient time for its development, suspicion should be aroused. This may, in fact, be the first clue that the organ system that should be compensating (i.e., lungs, kidneys) is itself impaired.

In one report, the absence of compensation in ketoacidosis of diabetes mellitus served to alert the clinicians to the presence of a primary respiratory problem.[548] The patients who did not compensate (display hypocapnia) had occult mucous plugging of major bronchi.[548] After this problem was corrected, these individuals responded appropriately.

Long-Standing Pulmonary or Renal Disease

When chronic pulmonary or renal disease is present, the body should not be expected to compensate normally for other primary disturbances. In addition, diseases of these systems in and of themselves are often associated with chronically abnormal blood gases and simple acid-base disorders. Thus, the abnormal baseline values in these individuals must be appreciated. Furthermore, the ability of these systems to respond to other acid-base insults is compromised.

Excessive Compensation

It has been shown that maximal compensation for simple acid-base disorders is rarely complete, particularly when the primary acid-base insult is substantial. The appearance of complete compensation for a relatively severe acid-base problem should be viewed with skepticism. For example, the likelihood of complete compensation in chronic respiratory acidosis is less than 15% when $PaCO_2$ exceeds 60 mm Hg.[549] Furthermore, the likelihood is less than 1% when the chronic $PaCO_2$ exceeds 70 mm Hg.[549] The presence of complete compensation in fairly substantial acid-base alterations more than likely represents a mixed acid-base disturbance.

Respiratory Assistance

When ventilation is being assisted artificially (e.g., mechanical ventilation), the rate and volume of ventilation are not exclusively under the patient's control. Therefore, these situations complicate acid-base analysis and often appear as mixed, albeit partially iatrogenic, disturbances.

Temporal Inconsistencies

Maximal renal compensation takes 2 to 3 days. When maximal compensation appears to have occurred almost instantaneously, the explanation is more likely to be a mixed acid-base disturbance. Also, as described previously, the absence of compensation despite sufficient elapsed time should also arouse suspicion. Previous blood gas findings should always be taken into account when interpreting current information.

Settings Conducive to Mixed Disturbances

Various clinical settings are commonly associated with mixed acid-base disturbances (Box 14-2). The effective diagnostician is continually on the alert for clues that may unveil or further clarify pathologic disturbances. A barrel chest, an elevated blood sugar, hypokalemia, or hypoxemia, for example, may be the first clues to an unidentified acid-base problem. The message

| **Box 14-2** | Common Settings of Mixed Acid-Base Disorders |

METABOLIC ACIDOSIS/
RESPIRATORY ACIDOSIS

    Cardiopulmonary arrest
    Severe pulmonary edema
    Poisonings

METABOLIC ACIDOSIS/
RESPIRATORY ALKALOSIS

    Salicylate intoxication
    Sepsis
    Severe liver disease

METABOLIC ACIDOSIS/
METABOLIC ALKALOSIS

    Renal failure with vomiting
    Alcoholic ketoacidosis with vomiting

METABOLIC ALKALOSIS/
RESPIRATORY ACIDOSIS

    COPD with vomiting or diuretics

METABOLIC ALKALOSIS/
RESPIRATORY ALKALOSIS

    Critically ill patients
    Severe liver disease with vomiting

From Kokko, J.P., and Tannen, R.L.: Fluids and Electrolytes, Philadelphia, W. B. Saunders, 1986, p. 392.

here is not new. Laboratory data cannot be interpreted in a vacuum. All available information must be assimilated into a meaningful whole.

ACID-BASE TREATMENT

Overview

Clearly, the work and time committed to the pursuit of an accurate acid-base diagnosis will have been in vain if the treatment is inappropriate. Effective treatment must be aimed at specific objectives. The development of these objectives is predicated on the determination of potentially reversible problems. The potential for success with a given therapy must be weighed judiciously against concomitant risks and the urgency of action required. The questions of whether to treat and how best to treat a problem are often complex and are

ON CALL | CASE 14-1 *ABGs and Critical Thinking*

You are the only person available to care for this patient. You must assess the patient/situation and act accordingly.

A 56-year-old woman with long-standing COPD and CHF presents to the emergency department with dyspnea and weakness. She has been taking digitalis and Lasix for control of her CHF and corticosteroids for her long-standing COPD.

ARTERIAL BLOOD GASES

SaO_2	87%
pH	7.45
$PaCO_2$	68 mm Hg
PaO_2	54 mm Hg
$[HCO_3]$	45 mEq/L
FIO_2	0.21
Na	140 mEq/L
CO_2	48 mEq/L
Cl	70 mEq/L
K	3.1 mEq/L

ASSESSMENT

Abnormalities: List abnormal data and other noteworthy information. Classify ABG.

Explanation: List possible diseases, pathology, or other situations that may have led to this patient's condition.

Evaluation: Suggest additional data that would be useful in helping understand the situation or in making a diagnosis.

INTERVENTION

Importance: Prioritize concern(s) of treatment in order of urgency and/or seriousness as you see the overall situation.

Objective: Specifically state the measurable or observable outcomes you would like treatment to accomplish.

Action: Describe your specific plan of action.

complicated by many variables. One goal in this chapter is to provide the clinician with basic guidelines that may improve the quality of these therapeutic decisions.

Supportive versus Corrective Treatment

The general thrust of therapeutic endeavors may be in one of two possible directions. *Supportive* or palliative treatment focuses on the preservation of an acceptable pH and on the prevention of life-threatening changes in pH.

Corrective treatment, on the other hand, aims to actively reverse the underlying acid-base disorder and thus to preclude any further acid-base deviation. In the case of drug-induced hypoventilation, this would include flumazenil for benzodiazepines and naloxone for narcotics. Nevertheless, the broad and diverse nature of corrective treatment prohibits a detailed review of this topic in this text. Rather, basic principles in the application of supportive treatment are explored.

Focus of Supportive Treatment

When considering supportive treatment, it is wise to remember that normalization of the pH is usually the primary objective of intervention

(notable exception ARDS). Clinicians are occasionally distracted from this theme when base excess, bicarbonate, or $PaCO_2$ are significantly abnormal. Erroneously, therapy may be directed primarily toward normalization of these other indices. Although these indices may provide guidelines for treatment, therapy should not be focused primarily on these lesser sub-indices of acid-base status. Rather, *the primary focus of supportive acid-base treatment must be on the pH.*

In Example 14-8, supportive treatment is not indicated. Although the $PaCO_2$ is significantly elevated, the pH, which is more important from an acid-base standpoint, is within acceptable limits. In this example, treatment should be focused on correction rather than on support. The clinician should attempt to identify fully the underlying cause and to initiate corrective action when possible.

Example 14-8

pH	7.35
$PaCO_2$	60 mm Hg
[BE]	5 mEq/L

A similar distraction often occurs when the [BE] is very low. Example 14-9 depicts a situation in which the [BE] is −13 mEq/L. However, to correct the metabolic acidosis in this example would likely put the patient into alkalemia. Appropriate therapy would include identification and correction of the underlying acid-base defect. Supportive therapy is not indicated because the pH is in the normal range.

Example 14-9

pH	7.38
PaCO$_2$	20 mm Hg
[BE]	−13 mEq/L

Regarding treatment, it also should be emphasized that therapy should be focused only on *primary* acid base problems (e.g., true respiratory acidosis, true metabolic alkalosis). Secondary changes in acid-base parameters are compensatory by definition and reverse themselves in the absence of primary problems. For example, a laboratory metabolic acidosis (e.g., [HCO$_3$] 19 mEq/L) may be compensatory and, as such, may not need to be treated.

Information has been provided in this chapter and in this text to aid the clinician in verifying the presence of primary acid-base disturbances and in identifying their origin. Also, regarding treatment, intervention should be considered for *all* primary disturbances, even when these disturbances are relatively minor. Optimal patient treatment should not await a crisis.

In very unusual situations, *therapeutic compensation* may be indicated. For example, if metabolic acidemia during mechanical ventilation is resulting in severe strain on the respiratory system in order to maintain compensation, it is probably in the patient's best interest to provide iatrogenic hyperventilation that may diminish work and may further normalize the pH. The clinician must keep in mind, however, that therapeutic compensation should be reserved only for exceptional and often dire circumstances. The main objective is to treat the primary acid-base problem.

Respiratory Acidosis

Spontaneous Breathing

General Guidelines

Respiratory acidemia is often called ventilatory failure.[10] This term is attractive when considering treatment because it emphasizes the specific defect, that is, a failure of the lungs to adequately excrete CO$_2$ through ventilation. When spontaneous breathing cannot preclude significant respiratory acidemia, mechanical ventilation is likely indicated.

In acute respiratory acidemia, the severity of the acidemia is in all likelihood a more sensitive indicator of the need for mechanical ventilation than is the severity of the hypercarbia. Some have suggested that mechanical ventilation be considered when pH falls below 7.25 or hypercapnia exceeds PaCO$_2$ of 80 mm Hg,[485] although this is currently controversial.[498] Thus, it is a reasonable guide to seriously *consider* mechanical ventilation when the pH is less than 7.25 in respiratory acidemia. The presence of progressive respiratory acidemia, regardless of the specific pH level, is often a stronger indication of the need for mechanical ventilation than is an isolated pH measurement.[551]

Obviously, anything that might diminish muscle strength should be avoided in primary respiratory acidosis. Thus, hypokalemia and hypophosphatemia should be corrected in the patient with respiratory acidosis. Also, in some cases (e.g. obesity hypoventilation syndrome, COPD), respiratory stimulants or progesterone[510] may be effective.

Guidelines in Chronic CO$_2$ Retention

Although acute respiratory acidemia with a pH of less than 7.25 may suggest the need for mechanical ventilation, there are exceptions. The most notable of these is the acute exacerbation of COPD associated with chronic hypercarbia. Initiation of mechanical ventilation is often riddled with complications in patients with COPD.[552] They are difficult to wean, and iatrogenic pulmonary infection is common.

In further support of withholding mechanical ventilation, many patients with COPD in acute pulmonary exacerbation manifest improved acid-base status after the administration of a controlled low concentration of O$_2$ (i.e., FIO$_2$ 0.24 to 0.40). Administration of low doses of O$_2$ in COPD is sometimes referred to as *low-flow O$_2$ therapy*.

Low-flow O$_2$ therapy is a more appropriate therapeutic starting point than expensive and invasive mechanical ventilation.[553,554]

Low-flow O_2 may be effective despite high initial $PaCO_2$ (e.g., $PaCO_2 > 65$ mm Hg). The patient must be monitored continuously with this therapy, however, and if hypercapnia increases or acidemia is not relieved with this conservative management, noninvasive ventilation or intubation and mechanical ventilation may still be required.

Noninvasive pressure support ventilation has been shown to be a good alternative to mechanical ventilation in some patient populations.[558] Noninvasive ventilation (Nasal mask ventilation with Positive Pressure Ventilation) has also been shown to be a very effective method to treat patients with chronic hypoventilation syndromes[556] and COPD.[557]

In recent years, it has been suggested that, in some patients, hypercapnia may actually be viewed as a desirable patient response. For example, it may represent decreased ventilatory work (rather than exhaustion or fatigue) and a positive adaptation in COPD.[499,500] Some have even gone so far as to suggest that administration of oxygen with subsequent worsening hypoxemia may actually enhance survival in COPD.[555]

Likewise, with the advent of permissive hypercapnia, hypoventilation may be viewed as clearly more desirable than high lung inflation pressures and volutrauma in acute lung injury/acute respiratory distress syndrome (ALI/ARDS) during mechanical ventilation. The decision to intubate and initiate mechanical ventilation in the patient with COPD is never easy. All subjective and objective information should be incorporated into the analysis of the problem.

Mechanical Ventilation

Teaching the fundamentals of ventilator care to medical house staff is the most challenging aspect that I acknowledge in their ICU curriculum.

R.D. Hubmayer[562]

General Guidelines

The patient already receiving mechanical ventilation constitutes a special diagnostic and therapeutic situation. During the application of mechanical ventilation, the mode and settings on the mechanical ventilator play a role in determining minute ventilation and alveolar ventilation. It therefore follows that respiratory acidosis in this group may be, in a sense, iatrogenic, that is, caused by treatment (e.g., ventilator settings). Indeed, we have discussed earlier the use of permissive hypercapnia as a therapeutic strategy in ALI/ARDS.

In the patient in whom we choose to correct respiratory acidosis, the ventilator settings may need to be adjusted. The $PaCO_2$ level can be lowered by increasing alveolar ventilation. Alveolar ventilation, in turn, may be increased during mechanical ventilation by three possible methods: increased tidal volume, increased respiratory rate, or decreased mechanical deadspace. The specific changes to make will depend on the ventilator mode as well as the therapeutic objectives and priorities.

Decreasing V̇CO₂

Finally, in some cases of respiratory acidosis, it may be more desirable to attempt to decrease CO_2 production rather than to increase alveolar ventilation.[494] The CO_2 production can be retarded by altering nutrition (e.g., discontinue total parenteral nutrition and reduce the respiratory quotient) or by decreasing the work of breathing (e.g., paralysis).

Guidelines in Chronic CO₂ Retention

Normally, the goal of mechanical ventilation is to restore normal eucapnic ventilation (i.e., $PaCO_2$ 35 to 45 mm Hg) and normal pH. In patients with COPD and chronic hypercapnia, however, the goal is to carefully return the arterial PCO_2 to the chronic normal level for that patient.

Large, abrupt decreases in arterial PCO_2 in the patient with chronic CO_2 retention should be avoided because this reduction may potentially lead to cerebral alkalosis, vasoconstriction, and ischemia.[560] In addition, generalized seizures, decreased cardiac output, or cardiac arrhythmias may occur. Arterial PCO_2 should be lowered slowly and progressively in these patients. In the past, some authors had suggested rates as low as 10 mm Hg per hour,[561] although this would seem hard to achieve in the clinical setting.

Again, the target of arterial PCO_2 reduction in the patient with chronic CO_2 retention is the patient's chronic normal value. When patients with COPD and chronic hypercarbia are mechanically ventilated to eucapnic ventilation (i.e., laboratory normal arterial PCO_2 35 to 45 mm Hg) for sustained periods (i.e., 2 to 3 days), the kidneys excrete the excess bicarbonate that is normally present in the blood. When weaning from mechanical ventilation is then attempted through trials of spontaneous breathing, arterial PCO_2 increases to chronic normal levels and acute uncompensated respiratory acidemia appears. The result is an additional obstacle to successful weaning in patients for whom weaning is already very difficult.

Respiratory Alkalosis
Spontaneous Breathing

As discussed in Chapter 13, the most common cause of respiratory alkalemia is moderate-to-severe hypoxemia. Although listed as a potential underlying cause of respiratory alkalemia, hypoxemia is not truly a root problem because it is a nonspecific symptom of some other cardiopulmonary pathology. Thus, in a very practical sense, the prevention of hypoxemia may be considered as supportive treatment of respiratory alkalemia.

In general, ventilation is increased greatly when PaO_2 falls below approximately 60 mm Hg. Thus, a good starting point in the supportive management of respiratory alkalemia is to ensure that PaO_2 is equal to or exceeds 60 mm Hg. This, of course, normally equates to an SpO_2 of 90%. Of course, a PaO_2 of 60 mm Hg should not be exceeded in the patient with COPD.

Some patients who present with respiratory alkalemia do not have hypoxemia or their respiratory alkalemia fails to improve after the restoration of a normal PaO_2. In these cases, further clarification of the underlying problem is necessary to determine the best course of treatment.

For example, acute anxiety may be accompanied by respiratory alkalemia, paresthesias, and dizziness. Here, simple rebreathing into a bag or tubing may alleviate the respiratory alkalemia and may diminish symptoms. Some patients with chronic hyperventilation verging on panic seem to benefit from breathing

exercises or diaphragmatic retraining.[559,563] Nevertheless, in severe hysteria or pain, pharmacologic sedation or analgesia may be necessary. Most often, supportive treatment of respiratory alkalemia is minimal. Identification and treatment of the underlying cause (corrective treatment) is usually the primary focus of attention in this acid-base disorder.

Mechanical Ventilation

Severe respiratory alkalemia may occur during mechanical ventilation and may diminish cerebral perfusion.[564] This may lead to shock, seizures, and coma.[564] Thus, severe respiratory alkalemia must be avoided during mechanical ventilation.

In the patient with increased intracranial pressure (ICP), hyperventilation is sometimes maintained therapeutically to lower ICP. Nevertheless, ideally the $PaCO_2$ should probably not be allowed to fall below 30 mm Hg,[508] and it should only be used for the short term as prolonged hyperventilation may be associated with cerebral vasoconstriction and ischemia.[565]

Respiratory alkalemia with associated hypocarbia is most often the result of increased alveolar ventilation ($\dot{V}_A$). Therefore, treatment of respiratory alkalemia during mechanical ventilation is accomplished by reducing $\dot{V}_A$. There are three general approaches to reducing $\dot{V}_A$: by the reduction of tidal volume, the addition of mechanical deadspace, or the reduction of the respiratory rate. Sometimes, it is necessary to administer drugs or to change the mode of mechanical ventilation to achieve better control of alveolar ventilation. An important concern regarding the use of muscle relaxants is the potential for extreme patient anxiety. Extreme anxiety is particularly likely when the administration of muscle relaxants is not accompanied by the administration of sedatives or analgesics. Finally, whenever muscle relaxants are administered, the effects of the drug should be explained fully to the patient in advance.

Notwithstanding the preceding caveats, there are times when controlled ventilation via the administration of skeletal muscle relaxants or sedatives is indicated. To allow a patient in severe distress with extreme work of breathing and borderline hypoxia to breathe rapidly and, paradoxically, ineffectively is certainly not optimal patient treatment.

Metabolic Acidosis

The need for therapeutic intervention in metabolic acidemia is gauged primarily by the severity of the acidemia. Mild-to-moderate metabolic acidemia (pH > 7.10) is usually best left untreated with supportive measures.[484] Currently, many would make an argument for rarely using buffer treatments to support the pH in acute metabolic acidosis.[484]

A major problem with traditional therapy for metabolic acidosis (i.e., intravenous sodium bicarbonate) is that therapy simply corrects the acidosis of the extracellular fluid and may, in fact, acutely worsen the intracellular acidosis. It is becoming increasingly clear that many critical organs (e.g., heart, brain, liver, respiratory muscles) have a remarkable intrinsic ability to defend against intracellular acidosis.

Therefore, treatment of the underlying disease and renal physiologic replenishment of depleted bicarbonate most often negate the need for supportive treatment. Occasionally, therapeutic intervention may be necessary to treat moderate acidemia if the patient is in a precarious clinical state with cardiovascular instability or if compensatory work of breathing is exhaustive.[484]

Historically, lactate was a drug used to counteract metabolic acidemia. After administration, lactate is converted to bicarbonate through the process of oxidation. However, lactate is relatively ineffective in the absence of oxygen, and even in its presence, the full alkalizing effect may take 1 or 2 hours to achieve. For these reasons, lactate is a poor alkalizing agent and is almost never used presently. Citrate, which has a similar alkalizing mode of action, is also poorly suited for the clinical treatment of acidemia.

Sodium Bicarbonate Administration

Indications

In the past, intravenous sodium bicarbonate has been the drug most often used for the treatment of severe metabolic acidosis in critical care and during cardiopulmonary resuscitation (CPR). Presently, there is strong evidence to avoid the use of sodium bicarbonate in acute conditions unless there is a need to assist toxin excretion (e.g., salicylate or phenobarbital toxicity) or combat life-threatening hyperkalemia.[484] Administration of sodium bicarbonate should probably not be considered in metabolic acidosis unless pH is less than 7.10 and even then it may not be beneficial.[484] Indeed, in the most severe cases of metabolic acidosis (e.g., lactic, ketoacidosis), alkalizing agents have shown the least efficacy.[484]

Administration of *oral* bicarbonate may be useful in chronic metabolic acidosis. In cases of chronic renal failure it may increase exercise tolerance, prevent growth retardation, and reduce protein wasting and osteoporosis.[484]

Dosage

Equation 14-1 shows the traditional method for calculating the intravenous bicarbonate dose in those rare cases where it may be necessary. Nevertheless, all formulas are estimates because dynamic physiologic acid-base changes continue during the therapeutic period, and different types of metabolic acidosis (e.g., lactic acidosis, poisonings) respond to varying degrees. After administration of the initial dose, blood gases should be analyzed and any additional bicarbonate therapy should be guided based on these results.

Equation 14-1

$$[BE] \times 0.3 \times \text{weight in kg}/2 = HCO_3^- \text{ dose}$$

Cardiac Arrest and Sodium Bicarbonate Therapy

Venous Paradox

Sodium bicarbonate has generally not been shown to improve survival in cardiac arrest, and it is not recommended for routine initial cardiac arrest management by the American Heart Association (AHA).[703] Sodium bicarbonate appears to correct extracellular fluid acidosis at the expense of intracellular acidosis. It does not appear to reduce and may in fact exacerbate intramyocardial acidosis.

In addition, there is considerable evidence that hypertonic buffer solutions may compromise cardiac resuscitation by reducing coronary perfusion pressure.[566] The importance of coronary perfusion pressure in successful resuscitation has been widely acknowledged.

Studies have shown that during cardiopulmonary resuscitation, central venous PCO_2

(average of 54 mm Hg) is about 34 mm Hg higher than the arterial PCO_2 (average of 21 mm Hg).[567] Furthermore, central venous pH had an average of 7.15, whereas arterial pH had an average of 7.41.[567] This phenomenon of venous acidosis with arterial alkalosis has been called the *venous paradox*. These findings are in sharp contrast to the normal difference between arterial and venous PCO_2 of approximately 7 mm Hg and the normal difference in pH of only about 0.02.

Probably the most effective method to combat the metabolic acidosis during cardiac arrest is with hyperventilation and vigorous cardiac compression.[575]

Value of Arterial Blood Gases in Cardiopulmonary Resuscitation

These findings strongly suggest that during cardiopulmonary resuscitation (CPR), severe venous hypercapnia and acidosis often coexist with simultaneous arterial hypocapnia and alkalosis.[567] It follows then that arterial blood gases generally fail to reflect systemic tissue acid-base status and are poorly suited for monitoring systemic acid-base conditions.[567] This is probably true both during CPR and during other low cardiac output states.

Thus, the value of arterial blood gases in CPR is cloudy. Mixed venous gases probably provide a better indication of tissue acid-base status. Nevertheless, some measure of arterial oxygenation may still be important in the assessment of the adequacy of tissue oxygen delivery.[568]

Arterial PCO_2 is typically quite low during CPR,[567] which is probably related to the relative hyperventilation of the lung secondary to the poor perfusion and decreased cardiac output.[569]

The venous hypercapnia, on the other hand, is undoubtedly associated with an extremely high tissue intracellular PCO_2. It is known that during anaerobic metabolism, cellular PCO_2 increases more rapidly than in the blood. This finding is particularly worrisome because an intramyocardial PCO_2 in excess of 475 mm Hg contributes to *electromechanical dissociation*. Electromechanical dissociation occurs when the electrical activity of the heart continues but the mechanical pump does not function.

Complications of Sodium Bicarbonate Therapy

Intracellular Hypercapnia, Cerebrospinal Fluid Acidosis, and Coma

The administration of $NaHCO_3$ will result in a further increase in intracellular and cerebrospinal PCO_2 as it is produced via hydrolysis. Because CO_2 is more permeable through cell membranes and the blood-brain barrier than are bicarbonate ions, the immediate consequence of sodium bicarbonate therapy is a paradoxic intracellular acidosis and rise in cerebrospinal fluid PCO_2.[570] Several detrimental consequences associated with CPR have been attributed to this effect. Specifically, rapid administration of excessive amounts of bicarbonate may precipitate coma or arrhythmia.[571]

Bicarbonate Overcorrection Alkalosis

There are also other complications associated with sodium bicarbonate administration. Iatrogenic alkalemia after bicarbonate therapy is relatively common. This may occur by two mechanisms. First, hyperventilation may persist or even increase due to continued cerebrospinal fluid acidosis despite correction of plasma acidemia. Second, as the body metabolizes anions associated with organic acidosis (e.g., lactate, acetoacetate, 3-hydroxybutyrate), endogenous bicarbonate is produced. The triad of endogenous bicarbonate, exogenous bicarbonate, and persistent hyperventilation may thus lead to significant alkalemia.

Hypokalemia

Acidemia is associated with the migration of potassium (K^+) from the intracellular fluid to the plasma. During bicarbonate therapy, a rapid elevation of pH may result in serious hypokalemia as K^+ returns to the intracellular space. This is particularly of concern during digitalis therapy, because hypokalemia may predispose to digitalis toxicity and arrhythmia. When hypokalemia is present with severe acidemia, bicarbonate must be administered with extreme caution.

Fluid Overload

Another potential complication of bicarbonate therapy is the precipitation of fluid overload or hypernatremia. Because sodium bicarbonate is dispensed as a hypertonic solution, fluid overload may occur in the patient who is sensitive to fluid. For example, this may be of considerable concern in the patient with congestive heart failure. Even more important is the high risk of intra-cranial hemorrhage associated with the administration of sodium bicarbonate in neonates. Special precautions should be followed when sodium bicarbonate is used in neonates.

Arterial Hypercapnia

There is an immediate increase in plasma dissolved CO_2 after the administration of bicarbonate. In most cases, this additional CO_2 is excreted rapidly through increased $\dot{V}_A$; however, in the patient who is unable to increase $\dot{V}_A$ (e.g., neurologic disorder, controlled ventilation), arterial PCO_2 may increase appreciably.[365]

Alternatives to Sodium Bicarbonate Therapy

Tris-hydroxymethyl-aminomethane (THAM) has been suggested as being a superior alkalizing agent to bicarbonate with less potential for complications and increased therapeutic effectiveness. These claims are based on the following purported advantages: the intracellular buffering capability of THAM, the absence of sodium, and the ability to buffer carbonic acid. In early studies, THAM was shown to be a more effective buffer than sodium bicarbonate

in correcting acidosis in the cerebrospinal fluid and intracellular compartment.[573] It has been later shown, however, that neither carbon dioxide–producing or carbon dioxide–consuming buffers improved intracellular myocardial acidosis or resuscitatibility[574]; therefore, the use of THAM is not recommended.

It has also been argued that the effect of introduction of carbon dioxide from buffer therapy is relatively small and that the endogenous carbon dioxide production may be of much greater significance.[574]

Furthermore, THAM is not without complications; it may cause spasm, phlebitis, or thrombosis at the site of administration because of its alkaline pH. Moreover, THAM is stored in a powder form and must be mixed immediately before being administered to a patient. This procedure may delay and complicate administration during cardiac arrests or other emergencies.

Carbicarb, a 1:1 mixture of disodium carbonate and sodium bicarbonate has also been purported to be more beneficial than sodium bicarbonate in hypoxic lactic acidosis.[576] Notwithstanding, Carbicarb has not been shown to be more effective in follow-up studies.[484]

The most disturbing aspect of the use of alkalinizing agents for the treatment of metabolic acidosis is the observation that re-oxygenation

---

ON CALL | CASE 14-2 *ABGs and Critical Thinking*

You are the only person available to care for this patient. You must assess the patient/situation and act accordingly.

A patient with chronic renal failure is admitted to the hospital.

ARTERIAL BLOOD GASES

SaO_2	91%
pH	7.18
$PaCO_2$	21 mm Hg
PaO_2	78 mm Hg
$[HCO_3]$	8 mEq/L
FIO_2	0.21
Na	142 mEq/L
CO_2	15 mEq/L
Cl	101 mEq/L
K	6.7 mEq/L

ASSESSMENT

Abnormalities: List abnormal data and other noteworthy information. Classify ABG.

Explanation: List possible diseases, pathology, or other situations that may have led to this patient's condition.

Evaluation: Suggest additional data that would be useful in helping understand the situation or in making a diagnosis.

INTERVENTION

Importance: Prioritize concern(s) of treatment in order of urgency and/or seriousness as you see the overall situation.

of hypoxic cells is associated with increased cell death when the pH is normal or alkaline. Indeed, this seems to indicate that acidosis may have a protective effect.[484] Nevertheless, it is premature to assume that this is undoubtedly true until further evidence is acquired. For now, we must continue to attempt to maintain what we feel is a minimally acceptable pH, keeping in mind the clearly controversial role of buffer therapy.

The attempt to restore homeostasis in the presence of an acid-base disturbance is not a precise science when it comes to the metabolic component.

J. Morfei[477]

Metabolic Alkalosis

Metabolic alkalosis is one of the most common simple acid-base disturbances in the critical care environment. In one report, more than half of surgical patients who had blood gas determinations were reported to be alkalemic at some point during their hospitalization.[577] Several authors have suggested that metabolic alkalosis accounts for about one-third of all acid-base disturbances.[480]

Metabolic alkalosis may be associated with CNS dysfunction and hypokalemia, which may lead to serious arrhythmia. Moreover, severe alkalemia (pH > 7.55) has been associated with a steep increase in mortality.[579] A mortality rate of 41% has been reported for pH values in excess of 7.55 and 80% mortality may be associated with values greater than 7.64.[578] Timely management of metabolic alkalemia may minimize the incidence and severity of these untoward effects. Furthermore, in patients with mixed respiratory acidosis and metabolic alkalosis, correction of the alkalosis may reduce hypercapnia.[583]

Mild-to-Moderate Metabolic Alkalosis

There are three important elements in the successful management of mild-to-moderate metabolic alkalemia: potassium replacement, chloride replacement, and fluid volume replacement. Indeed, diminished intravascular volume and hypokalemia have been purported to be responsible for the maintenance of 95% of cases of metabolic alkalosis.[581] Control of these three ingredients can likewise prevent the

onset of metabolic alkalosis in patients prone to its development (e.g., receiving loop diuretics, gastric fluid loss).

The drugs cimetidine or ranitidine may be useful in patients at risk for metabolic alkalosis secondary to stomach drainage because they reduce gastric fluid secretion and acid loss.[529] Likewise, potassium-sparing diuretics may be useful to avoid renal loss of potassium.

Potassium

Mechanism of Potassium Loss. Patients with metabolic alkalosis often also present with hypokalemia. The hypokalemia may be due to the mechanism responsible for the alkalosis (e.g., renal $NaHCO_3$ reabsorption, loss of gastric contents) or it may develop as the kidney attempts to compensate for alkalemia. In alkalemia, the renal tubular cells selectively secrete potassium into the urine while retaining hydrogen ions.

Failure to correct potassium deficits will perpetuate the alkalemia or increase its severity. Furthermore, low body potassium may lead to other adverse effects, such as arrhythmias in the patient receiving digitalis.

Potassium Deficit. In general, the severity of the potassium deficit is proportional to the severity of the metabolic alkalosis.[529] Moderate metabolic alkalosis (plasma bicarbonate 30 to 40 mEq/L) is accompanied typically by potassium deficits of 200 to 500 mEq.[529] In severe metabolic alkalosis (i.e., plasma bicarbonate of 40 to 60 mEq/L), the deficit may be as high as 1000 mEq.[529] Replenishment of these deficits can be in the range of 100 to 150 mEq/day for several days in moderate alkalosis and may increase to 200 to 300 mEq/day in the most severe cases.[529]

Potassium Objective. KCl is most often indicated in metabolic alkalemia in doses sufficient to replace body potassium stores, while avoiding plasma hyperkalemia. A reasonable clinical target is a low normal serum potassium ([K^+] 3.5 to 4.0 mEq/L). Maintenance of higher levels may result in dangerously high levels of serum potassium after the pH returns to normal, because potassium moves from the intracellular fluid to the plasma as the pH is decreased.

Serum Potassium. One must always keep in mind that potassium is measured in the extracellular fluid. Extracellular potassium levels may not always precisely reflect total body potassium, because most potassium resides in the intracellular space. Furthermore, in the presence of alkalemia, potassium migrates from the plasma to the intracellular fluid. This is an important reason why therapy should be targeted for a *low normal* serum potassium. A low normal target also seems reasonable because most people actually have serum potassium concentrations toward the upper limits of normal (4.0 to 4.7 mEq/L).[580]

The relatively low serum concentration also dictates that potassium be administered slowly. Slow administration allows the potassium to move gradually to the intracellular space and helps to avoid dangerous variations in extracellular fluid concentrations. Relatively minor changes in serum potassium may be very detrimental. For example, hyperkalemia of 6.0 may lead to serious consequences, and values of 6.5 may likely cause potentially fatal arrhythmias. In summary, potassium replacement is critical in the management of metabolic alkalosis; nevertheless, it must be accomplished slowly, carefully, and systematically.

Chloride and Fluid Volume Replacement

Ninety percent of metabolic alkalosis seen clinically is associated with depletion of chloride.[582] This may result from diuretic therapy or from a loss of excessive gastric fluid. Blood bicarbonate is generated in these circumstances as the kidney attempts to correct fluid volume deficiencies. Correction of alkalemia here can only occur if sufficient fluid volume and NaCl are available to the kidneys.

The amount of NaCl that is necessary depends on the degree of fluid volume depletion. The amount can be evaluated through central venous pressure measurements or, in the absence of a central venous pressure line, through clinical assessment. It is not uncommon for patients with excessive gastric fluid loss to need several liters of fluid replacement.

Some patients have inadequate NaCl and fluid perfusing the kidneys, despite abundant body stores (e.g., congestive heart failure, ascites). Sodium chloride and fluid therapy in these patients would be totally inappropriate.[533] A diuretic that selectively depresses bicarbonate

reabsorption, such as acetazolamide (Diamox), is often beneficial in these patients.

In summary, treatment of mild-to-moderate metabolic alkalosis requires appropriate replacement of potassium, chloride, and body fluids. In selected cases, acetazolamide may be useful, and cimetidine may be used in a preventative fashion.

Severe Metabolic Alkalemia

As mentioned earlier, severe metabolic alkalemia (pH > 7.55) has been associated with a steep rise in mortality. Patients with a pH between 7.60 and 7.64 had a mortality of 65%, whereas a higher pH was associated with even a higher mortality (i.e., 90%).[579] Acute severe alkalemia often reduces cerebral blood flow and may cause seizures and coma.[533]

The treatment described earlier for metabolic alkalosis (i.e., potassium chloride and fluid replacement) is a slow process dependent on renal mechanisms that may require several days. In severe metabolic alkalemia, more aggressive therapy may be indicated to restore the pH to safe levels.

Administration of dilute hydrochloric acid into a central vein is probably the best and safest treatment for severe metabolic alkalemia.[583-585,587] Interestingly, some reports have also reported improved oxygenation following administration but this remains to be substantiated.[583,587] A central vein must be used because of the corrosive nature of this strong acid. Extravasation of HCl has been associated with severe soft tissue necrosis.[586] An estimation of the amount of hydrochloric acid to be initially administered can be calculated in the same way that the dose of bicarbonate was calculated in Equation 14-1.[584]

The solution should contain 100 mEq of HCl/L of NaCl. This solution is typically infused at a rate of 1 liter for 4 to 6 hours. Further therapy must be guided by arterial blood gas measurements after the initial dose.

Other acidifying agents (e.g., ammonium chloride or arginine monohydrochloride) may be used, but they require proper metabolism by the liver and may be associated with complications. Ammonium chloride should be avoided in patients with liver disease. Administration of arginine monohydrochloride may precipitate dangerous hyperkalemia.

High doses of acetazolamide may likewise be useful in helping to reverse metabolic alkalemia in the patient who can tolerate diuresis. Acetazolamide is particularly useful in patients with posthypercapnic metabolic alkalosis with normal volume status.[480] Nevertheless, it is not recommended for routine use because its administration is associated with increased renal excretion of water, sodium, and potassium, all of which are undesirable in metabolic alkalosis.

In addition, patients who are being mechanically ventilated may be hypoventilated during severe metabolic alkalemia in an effort to protect the pH (therapeutic compensation). This maneuver is only a stopgap, however, until other treatment can become effective.

In summary, acidifying agents may be indicated in severe metabolic alkalemia. Other forms of aggressive acid-base management (e.g., acetazolamide, hypoventilation) may also be appropriate. Some authors suggest that treatment for severe metabolic alkalosis should be reserved for only experts in acid-base management because indications for treatment are limited and therapy is potentially hazardous.[480] Probably most importantly, both moderate and severe metabolic alkalemia ultimately require potassium, chloride, and fluid maintenance.

Many cases of metabolic alkalosis can be prevented. This can be accomplished by maintaining a high index of suspicion in situations that are commonly associated with metabolic alkalosis (i.e., diuretic therapy, gastric drainage) and through prompt attention to fluid and electrolyte balance.

EXERCISES

Exercise 14-1 Factors Complicating Acid-Base Disturbances

Fill in the blanks or select the best answer.

1. State the two organ systems involved in the compensation of acid-base disturbances.

2. Indicate with an arrow whether the following blood gas parameters are typically above or below normal in severe COPD.
   $PaCO_2$ _____
   $[HCO_3]$ _____
   [BE] _____

3. The finding of metabolic alkalosis and a normal $PaCO_2$ on the blood gas report of a patient with severe COPD is likely to be the result of (bicarbonate treatment/compensation for previous hypercapnia).

4. It is not uncommon for (lactic acidosis/ketoacidosis) to complicate the blood gas finding in acute exacerbation of COPD.

5. The hallmark of acute exacerbation of COPD is the presence of a surprisingly normal (PaO_2/pH) despite severe hypercarbia.

Questions 6-8: Given the following blood gas:

pH	7.30
$PaCO_2$	75 mm Hg
[BE]	8 mEq/L
$[HCO_3]$	35 mEq/L
PaO_2	48 mm Hg

6. The patient most likely has (COPD/renal failure).

7. The patient should be treated initially with (low-flow O_2 therapy/mechanical ventilation).

8. The high bicarbonate is probably a result of (a primary metabolic problem/compensation).

9. Compensation for metabolic acidosis during mechanical ventilation may appear (more/less) complete than during spontaneous breathing.

10. Chronic renal failure most often presents with metabolic (acidosis/alkalosis).

Exercise 14-2   Mixed Acid-Base Disturbances

Fill in the blanks or select the best answer.

1. The coexistence of two primary acid-base disturbances is called a _____ acid-base disturbance.

2. The percentage of patients with simple acid-base disturbances that fall within the bands seen on the acid-base map is _____%.

3. When a patient's values fall within one of the bands on the acid-base map, it (does/does not) ensure that he or she has a single acid-base disturbance.

4. Given a patient with a simple, primary, acute respiratory acidemia resulting in a $PaCO_2$ of 70 mm Hg and pH of 7.22, state the approximate pH that results after maximal compensation.

5. Given a patient with a simple, primary, acute respiratory alkalosis resulting in a $PaCO_2$ of 20 mm Hg and a pH of 7.60, state the approximate pH that results after several days of compensation.

6. List the approximate $PaCO_2$ values that will accompany maximum compensation for simple, primary metabolic acidosis given the following pH values: 7.18, 7.30, and 7.22.

7. Compensation for respiratory acidosis usually leads to (hypochloremia/hyperchloremia).

8. Compensation for respiratory alkalosis usually leads to (hypochloremia/hyperchloremia).

9. The maximal compensatory response to metabolic acidosis may take up to 1 (hour/day).

10. State six situations that should alert the clinician to the likelihood of a mixed acid-base disturbance.

Exercise 14-3   Respiratory Acid-Base Treatment

Fill in the blanks or select the best answer.

1. State the two general directions or thrusts of therapeutic (treatment) interventions in acid-base disturbances.

2. The primary focus of treatment in acid-base disturbances is stabilization of the (pH/$PaCO_2$/[BE]).

3. *Ventilatory failure* is a term used to designate what primary acid-base disturbance?

4. In respiratory acidemia, the most sensitive indicator of the need for mechanical ventilation is the ($PaCO_2$/pH).

5. In general, mechanical ventilation should be considered in respiratory acidosis in the patient who does not have COPD when the pH falls below _____.

6. Before initiating mechanical ventilation in patients with COPD and with respiratory acidosis, it is wise to attempt _____ therapy.

7. List three variables that may be changed to alter $\dot{V}_A$ and correct respiratory acidemia or respiratory alkalemia during mechanical ventilation.

8. Acute, severe hypercapnia in patients with COPD should ideally be corrected (gradually/quickly).

Exercise 14-4 Treatment of Metabolic Acidosis

Fill in the blanks or select the best answer.

1. Primary metabolic acidosis with a pH of 7.23 generally (is/is not) treated with $NaHCO_3$.

2. Lactate and citrate, after passing through the _____, produce bicarbonate.

3. The drug most commonly used in the treatment of severe primary metabolic acidosis is _____.

4. In general, sodium bicarbonate may be indicated when the pH falls below _____ due to metabolic acidosis.

5. Bicarbonate administration may lead to plasma (hypokalemia/hyperkalemia).

6. A serious potential complication of bicarbonate therapy in neonates that is related to the hypertonicity of sodium bicarbonate is _____ hemorrhage.

7. If bicarbonate is administered to a patient who cannot alter alveolar ventilation, _____ may result.

8. Administration of sodium bicarbonate (has/has not) been associated with coma and decreased central nervous system function.

9. Two drugs purported to have advantages over sodium bicarbonate are _____ and _____.

10. Write the formula for estimating the dose of bicarbonate to be administered in metabolic acidemia.

11. Sodium bicarbonate (is/is not) indicated in metabolic acidosis associated with hyperkalemia or salicylate toxicity.

12. Sodium bicarbonate (is/is not) recommended for routine initial cardiac arrest management by the AHA.

13. During cardiopulmonary resuscitation, central venous PCO_2 may be (slightly/much) higher than arterial PCO_2.

14. The phenomenon of venous acidosis with arterial alkalosis has been called the _____.

15. The administration of $NaHCO_3$ results initially in a (fall/rise) in intracellular and cerebrospinal pH.

16. Calculate the dose of bicarbonate indicated for the treatment of metabolic acidemia when the [BE] is –20 mEq/L and the patient weighs 80 kg.

| Exercise 14-5 | **Treatment of Metabolic Alkalosis** |

Fill in the blanks or select the best answer.

1. State the three important elements in the treatment of mild-to-moderate metabolic alkalosis.

2. A drug that is useful in controlling the development of metabolic alkalosis secondary to gastric drainage by decreasing gastric secretion is _____.

3. A reasonable target of potassium replacement in metabolic alkalosis is a serum value above _____.

4. Potassium deficits must be replaced (slowly/quickly).

5. A useful diuretic that decreases blood bicarbonate level in metabolic alkalosis is _____.

6. Severe metabolic alkalemia is defined as a pH equal to or in excess of _____.

7. The treatment of choice in severe, sustained metabolic alkalemia is _____.

8. Dilute HCl should be administered through a (peripheral/central) vein.

9. The concentration of dilute HCl should be _____ mEq/L.

10. Metabolic alkalosis is (common/uncommon) in the hospital setting.

| Exercise 14-6 | **Internet Work** |

1. Go to the American Heart Association site and describe current recommendations for the use of sodium bicarbonate during cardiac arrest.

NBRC Challenge 14

Please select the best answer for the following multiple-choice questions.

1. An ICU patient with apparent hypovolemia has blood gases with electrolytes drawn. Results include: pH 7.53, $PaCO_2$ 50 mm Hg, [K] 3.1 mEq/L. Which of the following would be useful?
   A) Acetazolamide
   B) Mechanical ventilation
   C) Dilute HCl I.V.
   D) KCl I.V.
   E) Carbicarb
   (CSE-RRT EXAMINATION — NBRC MATRIX III,D,13)

2. An ICU patient with ARDS is being mechanically ventilated in the ICU in the control mode at 6 mL/Kg. Blood gases are drawn with the following results: pH 7.32, $PaCO_2$ 62 mm Hg, PaO_2 68 mm Hg. You are asked for recommendations regarding mechanical ventilation. You would recommend:
   A) increased tidal volume.
   B) increased respiratory rate.
   C) elimination of all mechanical deadspace.
   D) KCl I.V.
   E) leave the patient on the current settings.
   (CRT EXAMINATION — NBRC MATRIX III,E,3)

3. A patient with acute exacerbation of COPD is being treated with low-flow oxygen therapy but appears to be worsening with increased dyspnea and a mild increase in hypercapnia despite a PaO_2 of 62 mm Hg. pH has fallen slightly to 7.30.

   You would recommend:
   A) increased FIO_2.
   B) noninvasive positive pressure ventilation.
   C) mechanical ventilation.
   D) serum electrolytes.
   E) sodium bicarbonate I.V.
   (CRT EXAMINATION — NBRC MATRIX III,D,12,d)

4. Arterial blood gases drawn during a cardiac arrest show the following results: pH 7.45 and $PaCO_2$ 30 mm Hg. Based on these results, it is reasonable to assume that myocardial and tissue pH is:
   A) normal.
   B) most likely alkalotic.
   C) most likely acidotic.
   D) in need of HCl acid I.V.
   E) in need of sodium bicarbonate.
   (CSE-RRT EXAMINATION — NBRC MATRIX I,C,2,e)

5. Blood gases are drawn on a patient in ICU with the following results: pH 7.61 and $PaCO_2$ 55 mm Hg. Despite various attempts to correct acid-base status, it has remained essentially the same for the past 2 days and the physician is concerned about the potential for arrhythmias. At this time you might suggest:
   A) KCl I.V.
   B) NaCl I.V.
   C) $NaHCO_3$.
   D) dilute HCl acid I.V.
   E) Carbicarb therapy.
   (CSE-RRT EXAMINATION — NBRC MATRIX III,D,13)

Noninvasive Techniques and Case Studies

Pulse oximetry is arguably the most significant technological advance ever made in monitoring the well-being and safety of patients during anesthesia, recovery, and critical care.

J.W. Severinghaus and P.B. Astrup[588]

Monitors, of themselves, never improve patient outcome because they do not do anything. They provide information that must be interpreted. The decision to act (or not to act) must be made by a clinician.

Charles G. Durbin, Jr.[618]

Pulse oximetry and capnography are not replacements for arterial blood gas analysis, but rather serve as adjunctive monitoring tools.

J. Prouix[589]

Outline

INTRODUCTION

The assessment of blood oxygenation, carbon dioxide levels, and pH is crucial in the management of critically ill patients. Arterial blood gases remain the gold standard of evaluation in these areas. Nevertheless, acquisition of an arterial blood sample for analysis is an *invasive* procedure in which a foreign object (needle) penetrates the protective barrier of the skin and directly enters the bloodstream.

The use of invasive procedures is associated with an increased potential for complications, such as infection or trauma. In addition, invasive procedures generally cause increased discomfort and pain for the patient. Furthermore, invasive procedures are usually costly. Changes in governmental reimbursement policies have exerted considerable pressure on hospitals to use less expensive assessment techniques. Finally, acquired immunodeficiency syndrome has vastly increased our awareness regarding the potential hazards to health care workers in handling blood or blood products.

Emphasis and attention in recent years has been focused on the development of *noninvasive* techniques and methods for patient monitoring, treatment, and evaluation. The pulse oximeter is an example of a device developed for the noninvasive assessment of oxygenation. In view of the first quotation used at the beginning of this chapter, it is not surprising that pulse oximetry has caused a virtual revolution in the way that we approach the assessment of oxygenation.

Another trend has been the movement away from measurement devices and techniques toward monitoring devices and techniques. Measurement techniques, such as arterial blood gases, provide us with static information or data about a *single*, isolated point in time, a snapshot if you will. Often, these static measurements do not reflect the moment-to-moment changes in oxygenation and trends that occur within the body. Oxygenation is in reality a continuously changing, dynamic process.

Measurement techniques may be subdivided further into those that provide immediate *real-time* information, such as a pulmonary wedge pressure or an arterial blood pressure. Alternatively, measurements may provide us with delayed information about a single previous point in time. Unfortunately, this is the case with arterial blood gases.

Monitoring techniques such as pulse oximetry, on the other hand, are generally used *continuously*. Measurement techniques are used primarily to *evaluate* the patient during a specific point in time or during an acute cardiopulmonary crisis. Conversely, monitoring techniques are used more often in an ongoing fashion to indicate potentially harmful conditions for the patient. *Monitoring techniques* generally provide real-time information.

In this chapter, the traditional techniques of oximetry and CO-oximetry are reviewed and compared with noninvasive pulse oximetry. A brief review of transcutaneous gas measurement techniques is also included. Finally, capnometry and capnography are discussed. Throughout these discussions, the clinician should always keep in mind the quote by Charles Durbin at the beginning of this chapter. Monitors do not do anything, it is the clinician who must act and respond appropriately.

OXIMETRY

Historical Development

The technique of measuring the oxygen saturation of blood hemoglobin was described in 1932.[590] Use of the term *oximeter* to describe the particular measurement device, however, was not introduced until 10 years later in 1942.[591] Millikan (1906 to 1947) coined the term *oximeter* for the device that he invented to measure ear oxygen saturation.[591] At that time, Millikan was working on the problem of aviators losing consciousness while at high altitude during battle. He solved this problem by inventing a servo-controlled oxygen supply system attached to an ear oximeter.

Earlier, however, in 1860, invention of the spectroscope by Bunsen and Kirchhoff actually paved the way for the development of oximetry.[591] The spectroscope was a device that was used initially to measure the exact wavelengths of light emitted after introducing elements into the flame generated by a Bunsen burner.

Spectrophotometry

Qualitative Analysis

Interestingly, each substance studied with the spectroscope had its own unique light emission spectrum. Apparently, each substance absorbed and therefore emitted light of different wavelengths in its own unique manner much like each individual has his or her own distinct fingerprints. The particular pattern of light absorption/emission at sequential light wavelengths can be graphed, and this pattern is known as the *absorption spectrum* of that particular substance. The absorption spectra of some of the more common forms of hemoglobin that may be present in the body are shown in Figure 15-1. Measurement of the light spectrum of an unknown substance may thus serve as a useful technique for qualitative analysis.

Colorimetry

Early techniques for actually measuring light intensity over sequential light wavelengths were difficult. For this reason, *colorimetry*, a simplified measurement technique that did not actually require measurement of light intensity, was often used in qualitative analysis. Colorimetry was a methodology wherein the color of a known substance was compared with that of an unknown substance.[591] As such, colorimetry depended on visual acuity and perception and, consequently, was not highly exact. The current measurement technique of spectrophotometry is sometimes referred to incorrectly as a colorimetric method. This term is technically incorrect because color per se is not actually evaluated.

Photoelectric Effect

Discovery of the photoelectric effect and development of practical photoelectric cells (photo detectors) paved the way for spectrophotometry as it is used today. The *photoelectric effect* is the ability of light to release electrons from metals in proportion to the intensity of the light (Figure 15-2). A *photodetector* can use this principle to measure light intensity and to convert it into electrical energy.

In spectrophotometry, light is passed through a filter and is thus converted into a specific wavelength. This light is then passed through a cuvette that contains the substance being analyzed. The amount of light that passes through the cell is detected on the opposite side of the cuvette by a photo detector and is reflected on a meter (Figure 15-3). Thus, measurement of light emission at different wavelengths can be readily accomplished by using the technology

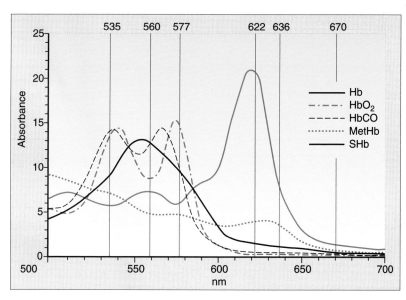

Figure 15-1. **Absorption spectra of common forms of hemoglobin.** Absorption spectra of oxyhemoglobin, deoxyhemoglobin, methemoglobin, carboxyhemoglobin, and sulfhemoglobin.

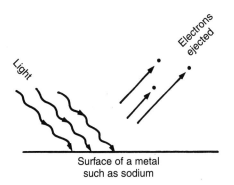

Figure 15-2.   Photoelectric effect. Light releases electrons from metals in proportion to the intensity of the light.

of spectrophotometry. The term *spectrophotometry* (spectro-photo-metry) is based on the measurement (-metry) of light (-photo-) spectrums (spectro-).

Quantitative Analysis

Interestingly, spectrophotometry can be used for quantitative analysis as well as for qualitative analysis; that is, the *amount* or concentration of a particular substance can also be evaluated by using the principles of spectrophotometry.

Lambert-Beer Law

Quantitative spectrophotometry is made possible by application of the Lambert-Beer law.

$$\log_{10} Io/Ix = kcd$$

Io = intensity of light incident on the specimen
Ix = intensity of the transmitted light

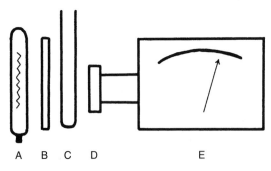

Figure 15-3.   Components of a spectrophotometer. A simplified diagram of a spectrophotometer. Components include (*A*) lamp, (*B*) filter, (*C*) cuvette, (*D*) photocell, and (*E*) meter.

k = a constant (characteristic of the substance and wavelength of the incident light)
c = concentration of the absorbing substance
d = pathlength in the absorbing medium (usually expressed in centimeters)

The Lambert-Beer law shows that light absorption of a substance depends not only on the substance per se but also on the concentration (c) of the substance present.

Optical Density

One of three things can happen to light as it enters a blood sample: (1) light may be absorbed by the solution; (2) it may be transmitted through the solution; or (3) it may be *reflected* from the solution.

During analysis of a substance, the ratio of light intensity incident on the substance (Io) is compared with the light intensity of the transmitted light (Ix). The ratio of Io/Ix is sometimes referred to as the *optical density*. Plotting out the optical density at various wavelengths leads to a graphic representation of the light absorption spectrum of a substance (see Fig. 15-1).

When *c* in the Lambert-Beer law is expressed in moles per liter, *k* is then referred to as the *molar extinction coefficient*.

Oximeters

An oximeter is an instrument that measures the amount of light transmitted through, or reflected from, a sample of blood at two or more specific wavelengths.[592] Thus, *oximetry* is a light measurement (photometric) technique that uses two or more specific wavelengths of the light spectrum to differentiate oxygenated from unoxygenated hemoglobin and to quantitate their relative concentrations. In other words, an oximeter is a dedicated *spectrophotometer* that is designed specifically to measure oxygen saturation (SO_2).

Transmission Oximetry

Because hemoglobin is a colored substance, it absorbs some of the light that is passed through a blood sample. Furthermore, according to the Lambert-Beer law, the amount of light absorbed at a particular wavelength (i.e., optical density) depends on the concentration of hemoglobin present.[591] Similarly, the amount of light *transmitted* through the blood sample at a given

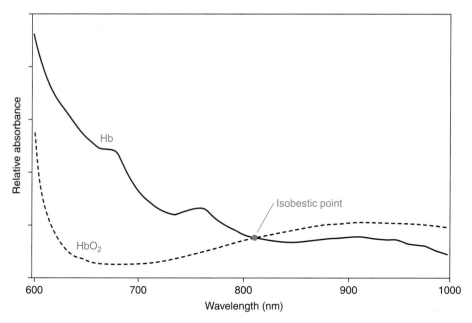

Figure 15-4.   **Light absorption spectra of oxygenated and deoxygenated hemoglobin.** At a wavelength of 805 nm, an isobestic point exists. At 650 nm, there is a large difference in absorption between oxyhemoglobin and deoxyhemoglobin.

wavelength is related inversely to the amount of light absorbed.

Each form of hemoglobin (e.g., HbO₂, Hb, HbCO, metHb) has its own unique absorption/transmission spectrum (see Fig. 15-1). The SaO₂ level can be measured because oxyhemoglobin and desaturated hemoglobin absorb light equally at some wavelengths, whereas they absorb light differently at other wavelengths. For example, at a wavelength of 805 nm in the near *infrared* region, oxyhemoglobin and desaturated hemoglobin have identical light absorption properties (Fig. 15-4).[593] When two substances absorb light equally at a given wavelength, an *isobestic* point is said to exist.[594]

On the other hand, at a wavelength of 650 nm in the *red* region of the spectrum, there is a large difference in light absorption properties between oxyhemoglobin and desaturated hemoglobin (see Fig. 15-4). The total hemoglobin can be determined at 805 nm and the amount of HbO₂ can be found at 650 nm. Thus, the difference in light absorption at these two wavelengths can be used to calculate SaO₂.

Hemolysis

Because the presence of cells in the blood tends to scatter light, measurements of SaO₂ by oximetry in the laboratory are made usually after breaking down the red blood cells (i.e., hemolysis). Typically, red blood cells are hemolyzed ultrasonically within the oximeter to make the sample more homogeneous and to increase the accuracy of the measurement. Transmission oximeters that use hemolyzed blood are generally accurate, stable, and precise.[595]

Backscatter Oximetry

As an alternative to transmission oximetry, one can measure the amount of light *reflected* at certain wavelengths and likewise determine the SaO₂ value. Each species of hemoglobin has its own unique reflection spectrum, just as each species has its own unique absorption spectrum.

Figure 15-5 illustrates the location of the major components used in transmission oximetry compared with backscatter (reflection) oximetry. Multiple (two) wavelength oximeters are shown in both examples that use red and infrared light sources. The major difference in

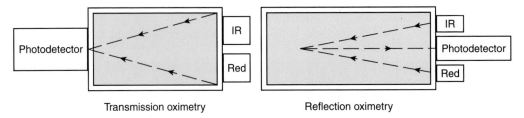

Figure 15-5.   **Location of major components of transmission and reflection oximeters.**

the two techniques is simply the location of the photodetector. In transmission oximetry, the photo detector is opposite the light source, whereas in reflection oximetry it is on the same side as the light source.

Functional Saturation

Regarding interpretation of data, it is important to understand two essential points when SaO_2 is measured using the two-wavelength method. First, when only two wavelengths are used, concentrations of abnormal forms of hemoglobin (e.g., HbCO, metHb) cannot be detected.[594] Second, the SaO_2 value measured in this way is the percentage of HbO_2 compared with the sum of HbO_2 and desaturated Hb only (however, HbCO and generally metHb will be picked up by the oximeter as HbO_2). Because this measurement does not include abnormal forms of hemoglobin, it is sometimes referred to as *functional* SaO_2.[594] Functional SaO_2 is the percentage of HbO_2 compared with the quantity of hemoglobin capable of carrying oxygen.

MetHb, HbCO, and sulfhemoglobin are incapable of carrying oxygen and are sometimes referred to as *dyshemoglobin species*. Dyshemoglobin species are not directly considered in the measurement of *functional* saturation via oximetry. Notwithstanding, the presence of significant dyshemoglobin species may lead to erroneous functional saturation.

CO-Oximetry

Functional SaO_2 is in contrast with the SaO_2 measurement resulting from use of a CO-oximeter (i.e., cuvette oximeter).[591] As the name implies, this instrument can measure HbCO% in addition to SaO_2. In addition, the percentage of methemoglobin is usually measured as well. With this instrument, major dyshemoglobin species are included in the determination of total hemoglobin and therefore the calculation of saturation.[596]

Thus, with this instrument, SaO_2 is the percentage of HbO_2 compared with *all* measured forms of hemoglobin (including dyshemoglobin species) in the arterial blood. SaO_2 measured in this way is sometimes referred to as *fractional* SaO_2 and may, at times, differ substantially from functional SaO_2.

The clinician should be aware that a potential error may occur when CO-oximetry is used in neonatal/premature infant SaO_2 assessment. Erroneously high HbCO% and erroneously low SaO_2 levels may be reported if substantial quantities of fetal hemoglobin are present. The error is introduced because the absorption properties of fetal oxyhemoglobin are similar to those of HbCO at the light wavelengths used.[597]

In review, the percentage of HbO_2 compared with the sum of desaturated hemoglobin and HbO_2 in arterial blood is called functional SaO_2, whereas the percentage of HbO_2 compared with *all* forms (including dyshemoglobin species) of hemoglobin in arterial blood is called fractional SaO_2. The presence of substantial quantities of fetal hemoglobin may distort HbCO% and SaO_2 readings obtained via CO-oximetry.

Ear Oximetry

Background

Unfortunately, conventional measurement of saturation via oximetry or CO-oximetry requires the acquisition of a blood sample. In other words, both of these measurements are *invasive*. Obviously, measurement of saturation noninvasively would be an attractive alternative.

As early as 1935, Matthes showed how transmission oximetry could be applied to the external ear.[598] Throughout the years, however, the major problem with noninvasive oximetry has been the inability to differentiate light absorption due to arterial blood from that due to all other blood and tissues in the light path. Two techniques were developed in an attempt to isolate arterial blood and to get a more accurate SaO_2 reading.

First, attempts were made to *arterialize* the ear by enhancing local perfusion. Arterialization could be accomplished by one or more of the following: heating the ear, applying a chemical vasodilator (e.g., nicotine cream),[599] or briskly rubbing the ear for about 15 seconds.

Second, a sensor was developed that incorporated a bladder that could be used to compress the earlobe and to render it bloodless. Thus, the optical properties of the bloodless ear could be compared with the optical properties of the perfused ear. This information could then be used to cancel out individual variations in skin pigmentation or ear characteristics.

Hewlett-Packard Ear Oximeter

In 1976, Hewlett-Packard incorporated these principles into the development of the model 47201A ear oximeter. This device used the aforementioned principles and measured light transmission at eight different equally spaced wavelengths from 650 to 1050 nm. Measurements at all eight wavelengths were incorporated into a complex formula that corrected for light absorption due to skin pigmentation and provided a measure of functional saturation. This clinical instrument was accurate over a saturation range of 65% to 100%.[600]

The original Hewlett-Packard ear oximeter was used widely in pulmonary function laboratories, cardiac catheterization laboratories, and physiologic research. Furthermore, the fact that ear oximetry could measure oxygen saturation under both stable and rapidly changing conditions rendered it a very useful diagnostic tool.[601] Simple ear oximetry has not, however, proved accurate enough to be used for determining the appropriate oxygen prescription for patients requiring supplemental oxygen during exercise.[602] Ear oximetry has never achieved prominence as a *clinical bedside* monitor because of its bulky nature and relatively high cost. The Hewlett-Packard ear oximeter is no longer

being manufactured.[603] Pulse oximeters are typically being used in its place.

PULSE OXIMETRY

Overview

The phenomenal growth and acceptance of pulse oximetry since the mid-1980s has made it the preeminent noninvasive monitor of oxygenation.

G.H. Hicks[628]

The simplicity and ready availability of *pulse oximetry* has literally revolutionized clinical oxygenation monitoring. Currently, blood oxygenation can easily be monitored *continuously* and *noninvasively* at the bedside or in the office or home. Application of this technology requires minimal technical skill and knowledge regarding the assembly, application, and maintenance of equipment. Pulse oximeters are typically calibrated at the factory and undergo a self-diagnostic check when powered up.[628] Furthermore, arterial blood gases with related risks, complications, and costs can often be avoided by using pulse oximetry.[289]

Indeed, pulse oximetry is currently a "standard of care" in the operating room and is probably soon to become a "standard of care" in critical care and other healthcare settings. It has already been referred to as a standard of care for nearly all patients in neonatal and pediatric intensive care.[628] No other medical device has achieved such widespread acceptance and implementation.[610]

A MEDLINE (National Library of Medicine) search of the term *pulse oximetry* in 2003 yielded more than 2300 citations,[628] and the list is growing rapidly. Furthermore, pulse oximetry has been demonstrated to be the single most important identifier of critical mishap events.[611] Capnography is second, with ECG a distant third. The value of pulse oximetry is such that it has often been referred to as a fifth vital sign.[612,628]

Diagnosis versus Monitoring

Historically, arterial blood gas assessment was commonly used for diagnostic purposes. On the other hand, arterial blood gases are limited in patient oxygenation monitoring because they represent a single, past moment in time. In contrast, pulse oximetry is much better suited for patient oxygenation monitoring than diagnosis.

The term *monitoring* is derived from the Latin word *monere*, which means "to warn." Although the accuracy of pulse oximetry may make it suspect in certain *diagnostic* applications, its value in *patient surveillance* is unquestionable. Pulse oximetry may help us identify potentially lethal oxygenation disturbances while we still have time to respond.

It has been estimated that more than one-third of patients are admitted to intensive care units primarily for the purpose of monitoring.[613,614] The essence of monitoring is continuous trending with concurrent alarms and signals of critical situations.

The true value of any alarm, however, relies on the ability of the clinician to recognize its significance and act upon it. He or she must be readily aware of clinical signs such as cyanosis or tachypnea, which are essential signs warning of impending distress. Indeed, the clinician remains the ultimate and most important patient monitor.

Conventional Underlying Technologies

Three technologies have been cleverly blended into the development of the pulse oximeter. *Photoelectric plethysmography* is used to determine the patient's pulse. *Spectrophotometry* is applied to determine the ratio of oxygenated to reduced hemoglobin. Finally, the development of *small light-emitting diodes* (LEDs) and *microprocessors* have made the production of pulse oximeters both feasible and relatively economical.

Historical Development

Although photoelectric plethysmography (to be described in the next section) and spectrophotometry have been available for decades, not until 1972 did the Japanese biochemical engineer Takuo Aoyagi[591] successfully combine these techniques in the development of the pulse oximeter. Also, the development of microprocessors and LEDs paved the way for *clinical* pulse oximetry by providing lightweight, stable light sources and bedside computerization of complex mathematical formulas. The Japanese firm Nihon Kohden developed Aoyagi's instrument and received a Japanese patent in 1974.[615]

By 1988, the number of companies that sold pulse oximeters under their own brand names increased to 29; 45 different oximeter models were available.[607] This relatively new technology had grown exponentially in just a few years. Furthermore, based on the expanding applications of pulse oximetry, it appears that this trend is likely to continue.

Photoelectric Plethysmography

A *plethysmograph* is a device for measuring and recording changes in volume of a part of the body or an organ. Photoelectric plethysmography, originally described in 1937,[604]

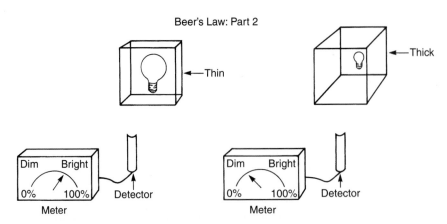

Figure 15-6.   **Thickness of the solution and light transmission.** All other things being equal, a red light appears dimmer as the thickness of the solution increases.

Photodetector   Light source

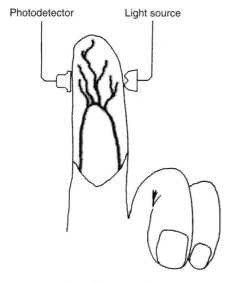

Figure 15-7.   Photoelectric plethysmography and pulse detection. The increased blood volume during systole results in decreased light transmission.

is a technology that makes use of light transmission properties to detect the changes from one moment to another in blood volume that occur in a finger or toe. These changes are presumably due to the pulsating arterial vascular bed. Thus, this technology may be used to detect the presence or magnitude of a pulse.[605]

As you may recall from the Lambert-Beer formula, the pathlength in an absorbing medium affects the amount of light absorption/transmission at a given wavelength. Simply, decreased light passes through the medium as the thickness (volume) increases (Fig. 15-6). If a vascular bed (e.g., finger) is positioned between a light source and a photo detector, pulsatile blood flow can be detected because the amount of light absorbed is in proportion to the volume of blood present (Fig. 15-7). The pulse oximetry sensors can be placed on a variety of sites as shown in Fig. 15-8.

The graphic representation of the pulse can also be displayed and is known as a *plethysmogram* (Fig. 15-9). Constant (static) light absorption occurs due to tissue and venous blood, whereas variable (dynamic) absorption occurs

Adult's or child's finger   Child's toe

Infant's or child's foot   Infant's hand

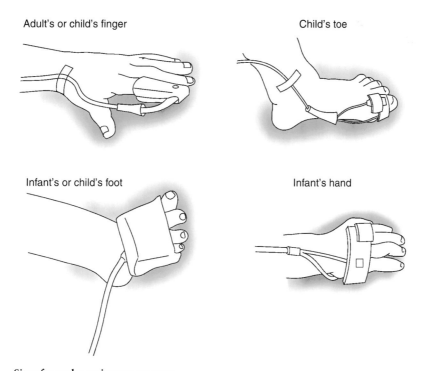

Figure 15-8.   **Sites for pulse oximetry sensors.**

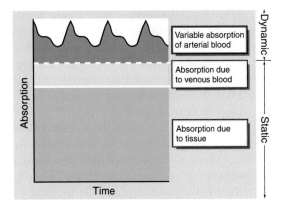

Figure 15-9. **Plethysmogram.** Pulse oximetry waveform illustrating static and dynamic absorption components.

due to pulsatile arterial blood. Photoelectric plethysmography has been used to monitor the hemodynamic status of patients after surgery. In general, when blood pressure or local blood flow is high, the pulse amplitude is high. Conversely, in the presence of vasoconstriction or hypotension, pulse amplitude decreases (Fig. 15-10). Changes in the plethysmogram may indicate the onset of hemodynamic problems and may suggest the need for prompt intervention. More important, detection of the pulse allows for the noninvasive determination of oxygen saturation.

In pulse oximetry, baseline absorption is the amount of light that is absorbed during diastole in the measured pulse cycle. The availability of the pulse allows light absorption due to tissue, bone, and venous blood to be canceled out. In addition, any ambient light that reaches the photo detector is likely canceled out. Thus, detection of the pulse and diastole allows us to zero out constant sources of interference and to calculate *baseline absorption*. Changes in light absorption during systole can therefore be presumed to be due to the addition of *pulsatile arterial blood* in the light path (see Fig. 15-9).[608]

Pulse/Circulation Dependency

In pulse oximetry, identification of the pulse facilitates comparison of the difference in light absorption in the two phases and thus isolates arterial blood from all other factors in the light path. Consequently, a measurable pulse is essential in the noninvasive assessment of oxygen saturation.

The mere functioning of a pulse oximeter, however, should not be interpreted as evidence of adequate perfusion or tissue oxygenation.[606] It is also wise to question pulse oximetry readings when the heart rate of the oximeter differs greatly from other indicators and measurements of heart rate. Newer pulse oximeter designs (e.g., signal extraction technology [SET]) actually calculate oxygen saturation as measured with pulse oximetry (SpO_2) through complex algorithms without first referencing the pulse rate.[629]

Two-Wavelength Methodology

The schematic illustration of two-wavelength transmission oximetry shown in Figure 15-5 is closely parallel to the structure and function of most pulse oximeters. On one side of the finger are two LEDs that transmit light alternately through the tissue to the photodetector (light detector) on the other side. Both the LEDs and the photodetector are aligned directly opposite each other and are encased within the probe. One LED emits light at a wavelength of 660 nm

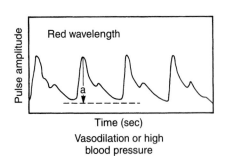

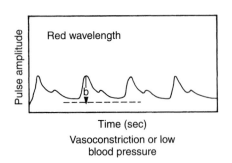

Figure 15-10. **Effects of hemodynamics on pulse amplitude.**

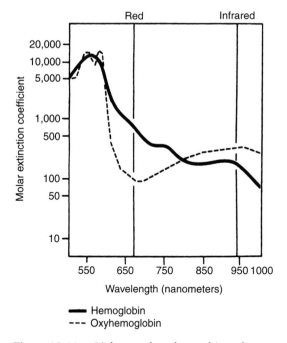

Figure 15-11.   **Light wavelengths used in pulse oximetry.** Light absorption characteristics of oxyhemoglobin and deoxyhemoglobin.

in the *red* range, whereas the other LED emits light at 940 nm in the *infrared* range.[608]

These two wavelengths are used because they facilitate differentiation of oxyhemoglobin from deoxygenated hemoglobin (Fig. 15-11) and calculation of saturation. At 660 nm in the red range, light absorption of deoxygenated hemoglobin is 10 times higher than light absorption by oxygenated hemoglobin. However, at a wavelength of 940 nm in the infrared range, light absorption by oxygenated hemoglobin is substantially higher than light absorption by deoxygenated hemoglobin. Thus, saturation can be computed through the ratio of light absorption changes (red/infrared) that occurs during systole (see Fig. 15-9; Fig. 15-12). The photodetector actually measures light during three modes: the red light mode, the infrared light mode, and when both lights are off.[616,630] The third mode (i.e., when both lights are out) helps insure that light (or noise) from any other source that may be reaching the detector is also canceled out.

Photodetectors may sample light as frequently as 480 times per second.[616] Although technology continues to improve, a reading should be attainable within at least 2 minutes.[617] The response time to actual arterial oxygenation changes also depends on the location of the probe.[630] Probes placed on the ear respond quickest whereas finger probes may take up to 12 seconds longer. Probes placed on the toes show an even greater lag time for response.

In summary, pulse oximeters are two-wavelength oximeters that measure light transmission both before and during a pulse by incorporating the principles of photoelectric plethysmography.[609] The difference in transmission at both wavelengths during a pulse provides a measure of blood oxygen saturation. If a pulse cannot be detected with traditional technology, oxygen saturation cannot be measured.

Technical Limitations

Accuracy

The accuracy of pulse oximeters in measuring exact saturation has been shown to be about ±4% as compared to blood oximetry measurements.[619,628] There is a general tendency to be less accurate (i.e., ± 6%[628]) as saturation falls particularly to less than 70%. The readings are

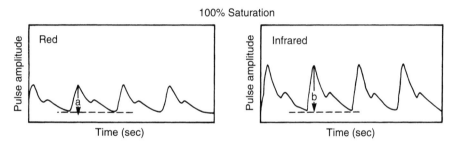

Figure 15-12.   **Calculation of saturation is based on the ratio of pulse amplitudes.** The ratio of pulse amplitude is defined as a/b = R.

most often falsely high at true low readings but some may actually be falsely lower.[620,621] This is not particularly surprising because different instruments use different pulse detection and SaO_2 calculation algorithms.[621] Furthermore, most of these algorithms were developed based on saturations of normal volunteers and therefore correlate better with high or normal saturations. One early study reported in 1991 found that only 10% of pulse oximetry readings in patients with poor perfusion were actually accurate to within ±4%,[631] but newer models and technology have improved accuracy substantially.

Some guidelines recommend comparing directly measured simultaneous saturations (i.e., CO-oximetry readings) with various pulse oximeter readings to get a baseline relationship.[622] These same guidelines also recommend periodic comparisons as the patient's condition changes. These comparisons would also help the clinician understand the standard biases of the specific devices being used. Notwithstanding, this is generally not practical or cost-effective. Most importantly, the clinician should understand that arterial blood gases are superior for diagnostic purposes whereas pulse oximetry is most beneficial as a *real-time monitoring device*.

Technical Error

Hemoglobin Variants

It is well known that high carboxyhemoglobin levels [HbCO] will falsely elevate SpO_2 readings. This is extremely important to remember since a high saturation reading in a patient with carboxyhemoglobinemia may lead to a false sense of security regarding oxygenation in the unsuspecting clinician. In any patient who is suspect for elevated HbCO (e.g., smoke inhalation, etc.), saturation should always be measured via arterial blood samples with CO-oximetry.

Interestingly, in one study of postoperative open-heart surgery patients, pulse oximetry seemed to cause slight elevations in readings as compared to saturations measured in the blood.[623] The authors suggested that perhaps slight elevations in HbCO secondary to hemolysis or infusion of stored blood may have been responsible for the elevated readings.

Methemoglobin may likewise alter pulse oximetry readings. The clinician should be mindful that nitrites, benzocaine (local anesthetic), or dapsone (antibiotic used in the treatment of malaria or *Pneumocystis carinii* infection) may cause serious methemoglobinemia. There is reasonable evidence to suggest that the readings tend to migrate toward 85% (see Chapter 7). Thus, lower than expected pulse oximetry readings would occur when true saturation exceeded 85% whereas higher readings would occur in severe methemoglobinemia. Like carboxyhemoglobinemia, the clinician should always be alert to the potential causes and possibility of methemoglobinemia especially when cyanosis is observed without substantial decreases in SpO_2. Like carboxyhemoglobinemia, sampling of blood via CO-oximetry is necessary for confirmation.

Surprisingly, fetal hemoglobin seems to behave very similar to adult hemoglobin despite its increased affinity for oxygen. Pulse oximetry seems to agree very well with directly measured arterial saturation in newborns despite high fetal hemoglobin levels (60% to 90%).

Dyes and Pigments

Vascular dyes administered during cardiac catheterization (i.e., methylene blue, indocyanine green, and indigo carmine) may similarly affect pulse oximetry readings. In particular, methylene blue, which is also used in the treatment of methemoglobinemia, may lead to a spurious *severe* decrease in SpO_2.[616]

Others have reported that brown, blue, and green nail polish may substantially affect readings and suggest routine removal.[616,619,632] If this problem is suspected, the probe can be placed on the lateral aspects of the digit instead of over the nail.[630,670]

Skin pigmentation may also be a factor as an SpO_2 less than 85% was shown to be less accurate in African Americans in some investigations.[619,627] Others have reported that skin pigmentation does not affect accuracy[628]; therefore, this remains controversial.

Finally, there has been some discussion regarding the impact of hyperbilirubinemia on pulse oximetry readings. AARC guidelines state the hyperbilirubinemia does not affect the accuracy of pulse oximetry readings.[622] This is most likely because the absorption peak of bilirubin is below that used in pulse oximetry. It is interesting to note, however, that the patients in some of these studies may also have had slight (i.e., 5% to 6%) elevations in HbCO secondary to heme metabolism.[618]

Optical Interference

Although this remains controversial, bright external ambient lights may impact oxygen saturation measured by pulse oximetry (SpO$_2$).[622] Typically, in the presence of optical interference (bright external lights), the pulse search alarm flashes and the digital display is blank. In one unusual anecdotal case that occurred in 1987 with an older model pulse oximeter, an ambient light in the operating room caused the SpO$_2$ display to remain at 100% even though the patient had cyanosis and was in distress.[624] This apparently occurred because the light had an unusual pulsatile quality, and the photodetector was sensing this quality as a pulse. As always, one cannot depend too heavily on any single technology as a replacement for a thorough clinical evaluation.

The potential for various forms of ambient light to affect pulse oximetry readings has been studied in more detail recently.[616] The findings of this study suggest that *ambient light has no significant effect on SpO$_2$* and that exposure to ambient light is clinically unimportant. In all likelihood, any light without a pulsatile quality should be automatically factored into baseline measurements and, therefore, should not affect readings.

Optical Shunting

Use of a sensor that is inappropriate for the patient or for the clinical setting may lead to *optical shunting*. This phenomenon occurs when part of the light emitted from the LED reaches the photo detector without passing through the finger. Optical shunting tends to bias the reading toward the 81% to 85% level.[625] Selecting the appropriate size of sensor and applying it correctly generally eliminates this problem. In particular, digit sensors should not be applied to fingers with long nails.[626]

Another potential type of optical interference is *optical cross-talk*. Optical cross-talk is a form of interference that may occur when multiple sensors are placed in proximity (e.g., two sensors on the same hand). Cross-talk error as well as other forms of optical shunting can easily be eliminated by covering each sensor with opaque material.

Decreased Perfusion

For years, low perfusion states have been recognized as a source of pulse oximeter malfunction or error.[622] Indeed, decreased perfusion and motion artifact (to be discussed in next section) have been cited as the two most common problems responsible for inaccurate SpO$_2$ readings.[628] A variety of factors may lead to decreased perfusion including decreased cardiac output, decreased arterial blood pressure, hypothermia, hypovolemia, or vasoactive drugs. Under vasoconstrictive conditions, the ear lobe appears to be the site least altered by compromised perfusion.[633]

When perfusion is insufficient, most monitors display a message indicating inadequate pulse signal or provide only intermittent readings. As stated earlier, most early pulse oximeters did not provide a measurement within ±4% of blood saturation measurements under conditions of decreased perfusion.[631] Early pulse oximeters amplified the pulse when it was weak. This, in turn, amplified the background noise which resulted in decreased accuracy.[628] Monitors are available that measure blood pressure and pulse oximetry independently and simultaneously.

Motion Artifact

Historically, motion of the probe (e.g., shivering) has likewise been a common source of error. Motion may cause decreased accuracy, loss of signal, desaturation alarms, or missed hypoxemic events. It was believed that erroneous signals could be reduced by synchronizing signals with electrocardiograph (ECG) signals. Notwithstanding, oximeters using ECG synchronization did not display increased accuracy.[634] Probably the best way to identify motion artifact is via pulse wave analysis (i.e., false or erratic pulse display), but this is also difficult and tedious. One method to minimize motion artifact was to attach the probe to an alternate site such as the ear or toe.[619]

It is not uncommon for hypoxemic patients to be agitated and move violently. Therefore, failure of the pulse oximeter to provide an accurate signal during motion could mean failure of the monitoring device when the patient is at greatest risk of hypoxia. Furthermore, motion artifact is probably the most common reason for abandoning the use of pulse oximeter monitoring.[636] Indeed, motion artifact may also cause both false-positive (false alarm) and false-negative (missed hypoxemic event) alarms.[637]

False Alarms

False alarms present a huge problem and obstacle particularly in intensive care. Nearly 90% of ICU alarms are false, while another 5% are true but irrelevant.[638] Furthermore, experienced nurses were unable to identify nearly 40% of critical alarms.[639] This may not be particularly surprising to anyone who has been subjected to the data overload present in critical care.

Pulse oximetry is especially prone to false alarms in the neonatal intensive care units. Approximately half of neonatal/pediatric alarms were due to pulse oximetry. Furthermore, 70% were false alarms and nearly 95% were considered clinically unimportant.[640]

Probably the most troubling issue related to false alarms is the impact on bedside clinicians, patients, and families. In addition to increased stress and inefficiencies, the numbing effect of alarm overload inevitably leads to a less than urgent response when true critical events occur. Furthermore, patients and families are subjected to additional stress and concern when alarms sound and especially when clinicians do not react expediently. In short, excessive false alarms subject everyone to unnecessary stress and strain in addition to the increased likelihood of true disaster. Any and all attempts to increase the accuracy and specificity of these monitors and alarms would certainly result in enhanced patient care. The new SET technology described subsequently in this chapter represents a welcome addition to current monitoring technology.

Other Sources of Error

Other factors that may affect readings include temperature variances above or below body temperature. These temperature changes can cause LEDs to shift their spectral outputs which, in turn, may cause additional errors of 1% to 4%.[628]

Furthermore, because different pulse oximeters use different algorithms and, in some cases, different technology, readings between different brands and models of pulse oximeters are likely to differ. When practical, it may be useful to get a concurrent blood saturation to serve as a baseline for future changes.

Hazards and Complications

Hazards or complications associated with the use of pulse oximeters are rare. Complications of a relatively minor nature have been reported occasionally in children. These complications include a localized skin burn due to a malfunctioning probe that heated to more than 70° C, skin erosion after a probe had been left on an ear of a 4-month-old infant for longer than 48 hours, and localized tanning of the skin.[705] Devices may overheat in the unusual event of cracking of the LED casing.[641] In general, pulse oximetry is a safe technology. A summary of some key points and issues detailed in the AARC Clinical Practice Guideline for Pulse Oximetry is shown in Box 15-1.[671]

Box 15-1	AARC Clinical Practice Guideline—Pulse Oximetry: Nuts & Bolts

Indications
  Prolonged continuous oxygen monitoring
  Spot-check of oxygenation
  Diagnosis of moderate to severe hypoxemia
    (Best to correlate with directly
    measured SaO_2)
Limitations
  No ventilation ($PaCO_2$) evaluation
  No acid-base pH evaluation
  Poor in detection of hyperoxemia
Potential Errors
  Motion artifact
  Dyshemoglobin species
  Intravascular dyes/pigments
  Ambient light
  Skin pigmentation
  Nail polish
  Degree of severe hypoxemia or hyperoxemia

Reference: AARC Clinical Practice Guideline: Pulse oximetry. Respir. Care, 36:1406–1409, 1991.

Advances in Technology

Signal Extraction Technology

SET is a term coined by Masimo Inc. describing new methods, algorithms, and probes used to (seemingly) more accurately determine SpO_2 during patient motion or decreased perfusion. SET was unveiled in 1998 and by 1999, there were many independent research studies claiming this technique to be more specific and sensitive than traditional pulse oximetry.[642]

Most importantly, SET functions better than conventional pulse oximeters during motion or poor perfusion,[628,645,646] the two most common technical limitations in pulse oximetry. In 2000, it was the only technology cleared by the US Food and Drug Administration to make claims regarding accuracy during motion or low perfusion.[642] Due to its rather unique approach to SpO_2 and pulse measurement, some key principles in its application will be discussed.

According to product literature,[629] the two keys to this new process for obtaining SpO_2 are the discrete saturation transform algorithm and the "low noise optical probe." The discrete saturation transform algorithm in conjunction with special adaptive filters allows for the identification of the SpO_2 without first referencing the pulse rate. This algorithm attempts to identify and ignore sources of pulse rate interference.[643,644]

The SET system also uses a special low noise optical probe (Fig. 15-13). Unlike conventional sensor design, the photo detector is recessed in a cavity to act like a shock absorber and minimize optical pathlength changes during motion.[629]

Studies have also demonstrated a substantial (7-fold or higher)[635,647] decrease in the number of false alarms while also purporting nearly 100% detection of true alarms with application of SET.[628,635,642,647,648]

Other New Methods

Other manufacturers and technologies have also been developed and some studies have purported their superiority to the SET technology.[649] Clearly, *all* current technology is improving as all new models outperform old models.[637] It is likely that the future will be even brighter than the remarkable past regarding pulse oximetry.

Despite some conflicting reports, at this point in time, there is a preponderance of evidence to support the superiority of the SET technology in reducing false alarms, particularly during motion and low perfusion states.

Most of these studies do not directly evaluate total cost. There have been reports of decreased sensor expense when using SET sensors[650]; however, to my knowledge, no clear comparisons of total cost. As times goes on, we will have to continue to monitor advances in this rapidly changing technology.

General Application

Usefulness

Pulse oximetry probably does offer a significant step at detecting hypoxemia while there's still something we can do about it.

C. Durbin (discussion)[618]

Pulse oximetry is, in all likelihood, our most valuable patient monitor. As described earlier, the pulse oximeter can be applied *noninvasively* and *continuously* to monitor oxygen saturation or more correctly desaturation. Handheld devices weighing as little as 1.3 oz without batteries[651] can be carried to the bedside for oxygenation assessment.

The true value of pulse oximetry is in surveillance and trending rather than for diagnosis, and it can be a valuable indicator of hypoxic crisis. Nevertheless, at times, pulse oximetry can also be a crude diagnostic index of benefit in the physician's office or the patient's home. In these scenarios, changes in the patient's SpO_2 following simple manipulations in patient position can sometimes aid in diagnosis.[652]

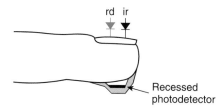

Figure 15-13. **Low noise optical probe.** Low noise optical probe design shows recessed photo detector.

In critical care, another potential application for pulse oximetry is its use in conjunction with continuous in vivo (within the body) measurement of oxygen saturation in the pulmonary artery by using a fiber-optic catheter. This *dual oximetry* can be used to monitor cardiac output *continuously* via the Fick equation.

Finally, when applied appropriately, pulse oximetry may result in cost savings. For example, the use of pulse oximetry instead of arterial blood gases during mechanical ventilation or oxygen therapy protocols can be cost-effective.

SpO$_2$ Targets

In most spontaneously breathing and mechanically ventilated patients, an SpO$_2$ of 92% to 94% is a reasonable goal for FIO$_2$ titration.[619] Some have suggested a slightly higher goal of 95% in African-American patients.[619] Similarly, a target of 93% may be best when prescribing oxygen during exercise for patients with COPD.[654]

In premature infants at risk of retinopathy of prematurity, one should keep the **high alarm** in the range of 92% to 95% or *lower* because this SpO$_2$ is on the flat portion of the oxyhemoglobin dissociation curve and the actual PaO$_2$ may be excessive.[628,618] Setting the alarm at 95% provides a 95% probability that the PaO$_2$ does not exceed 80 mm Hg; however, in this range, more than half of the alarms may be false.[655]

At high altitude (e.g., Denver), normal newborns to the first 4 months of life may have SpO$_2$s that are considerably low (i.e., as low as 80%); therefore, lower SpO$_2$s may be acceptable.[653] Finally, in the critically ill, it may be argued that SpO$_2$s as low as 75% to 80% may be less harmful than high alveolar pressures or excessive levels of positive end-expiratory pressure.[618] Precise targets for SpO$_2$ will remain an important issue to study for years to come.

Limitations

Despite its benefit, it is important to understand what pulse oximetry is not. First, the clinician must understand that pulse oximetry measures functional saturation and not fractional saturation. Secondly, it is essential to realize that pulse oximetry is only ±4% accurate and even less accurate when saturation is less than 70% to 80%. Therefore, the clinician should realize

that saturation is a much less sensitive indicator of blood oxygenation than PaO$_2$, especially when saturation is near or above 90% on the flat upper portion of the oxyhemoglobin curve.

Finally, one must always remember that pulse oximetry reveals absolutely nothing about ventilation, electrolyte changes, or acid-base balance. An arterial blood gas, despite its drawbacks concerning time and its invasive nature, provides the most complete picture of oxygenation and acid-base status.

Functional versus Fractional Saturation

Pulse oximetry will indeed be misleading in the patient with carboxyhemoglobinemia or methemoglobinemia. The clinician must always be cognizant of the fact that SpO$_2$ does not measure or indicate these conditions. Indeed, pulse oximetry will be normal and misleading in the presence of severe carboxyhemoglobinemia. Therefore, the clinician must maintain a high index of suspicion of these problems especially when the history of the patient suggests their presence (e.g., smoke inhalation). Most importantly, when cyanosis is present with normal SpO$_2$, these conditions should be ruled out through arterial blood sampling and CO-oximetry.

Accuracy of Pulse Oximetry

The accuracy of pulse oximetry in reflecting PaO$_2$ is not good on the flat upper portion of the oxyhemoglobin curve. In other words, if the SpO$_2$ is 92%, and given a ±4% accuracy, the actual PaO$_2$ could be anywhere from 55 to 80 mm Hg. If the SpO$_2$ were 97%, the PaO$_2$ might be anywhere from 65 to 500 mm Hg.

These relationships also assume a normal pH, which is unlikely in the critical care setting. It has been suggested by some that the limits of precision are more like ±5%, and that a reading of 95% could reflect a PaO$_2$ as low as 55 mm Hg and as high as 600 mm Hg.[618] Regardless of the exact ranges, the salient point is that a given pulse oximetry reading may be associated with a wide range of PaO$_2$.

When it is essential to know the actual PaO$_2$, such as during oxygenation of the premature infant (with concern of hyperoxemia and retinopathy of prematurity), pulse oximetry does not provide sufficient accuracy. Similarly, a pulse oximeter reading of 90% may be viewed as satisfactory when, in fact, it may represent clinically significant hypoxemia.

Similarly, pulse oximetry should be used very carefully in determining the need for chronic oxygen therapy in the home. First, use of only pulse oximetry could disqualify a significant number of patients truly in need of home oxygen therapy. Only 80% of patients with a resting PaO_2 of less than 55 mm Hg had a concomitant SpO_2 of less than 85%.[656] Thus, 20% of these patients would have been inappropriately denied home oxygen therapy based on pulse oximetry assessments alone. In addition, many patients could be deprived of necessary oxygen therapy or reimbursement perhaps based on HbCO artifact.

Another issue that has surfaced with the routine use of continuous pulse oximetry has been the identification of striking desaturation (<80%) in otherwise healthy, elderly postoperative patients.[657] Indeed, episodic severe hypoxemia may be normal in some patients and not associated with any adverse consequences. Please refer to the discussion on permissive hypoxemia in Chapter 10.

Ventilation and Acid-Base Balance

Again, the clinician must always keep in mind that pulse oximetry provides no information regarding the status of ventilation and acid-base balance. The subtle clues to developing and progressive acid-base disturbances are absent with pulse oximetry. Arterial blood gases are necessary when there is any question regarding these issues.

TRANSCUTANEOUS PO₂/PCO₂ MONITORING

Introduction

A relationship between blood PO_2 and skin PO_2 was shown in 1951.[658] In 1967, the PO_2 was measured on the skin surface by using a Clark electrode, and this measurement was correlated with PaO_2.[659] The PO_2 measured by using a modified Clark electrode applied directly to the skin is called transcutaneous PO_2 ($PtcO_2$). Most current transcutaneous monitors also measure $PtcCO_2$ concurrently.[619]

Transcutaneous PO_2 monitors are most often used in neonatal intensive care units owing to the thin skin layer in these patients and their special needs for oxygen monitoring. Transcutaneous PO_2 monitors are slightly more sensitive than pulse oximeters; however, they require a much greater degree of care and maintenance to ensure proper function. Improvements have been made in terms of ease of application and comfort, but other technical issues still complicate routine use.[669]

Anatomy of the Skin

The top three layers of the skin are important in the function of transcutaneous PO_2 monitors. The outermost layer (stratum corneum) is actually dead tissue, and it behaves functionally like a diffusion membrane (Fig. 15-14). The next layer is known as the *epidermis*. The epidermis does not contain blood vessels but consumes oxygen at a very high rate. The next layer of skin is called the *dermis*. The dermis consumes little oxygen in itself, but its capillaries provide the blood supply and oxygen for the epidermis as well.

Factors Determining PtcO₂

Arterial PO_2 represents the pressure of oxygen as blood enters the various tissues throughout the body. Obviously, the PO_2 normally falls as blood traverses the tissue capillaries because some oxygen is released to the tissues. The PO_2 does not fall as much in skin capillaries as in other capillaries because perfusion to the skin is far in excess of metabolic requirements. Furthermore, if perfusion is further increased due to heating the skin, capillary PO_2 begins to approach PaO_2. In fact, $PtcO_2$ may even exceed PaO_2 (measured at body temperature and pressure saturated [BTPS]) if it is measured at a higher temperature. If perfusion is diminished (e.g., in shock), capillary PO_2 is much lower than PaO_2 due to increased O_2 extraction by the cells. Conversely, $PtcCO_2$ will increase with decreased perfusion.

PO_2 decreases still more as the tissue distance increases from the capillary. The thicker the skin, the greater is the difference between capillary PO_2 and skin surface PO_2, which explains why $PtcO_2$ more nearly equals PaO_2 in newborns than in adults. Furthermore, the

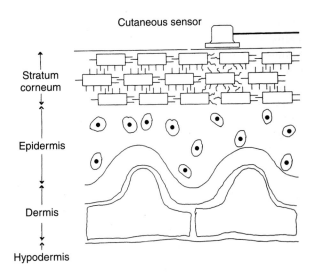

Figure 15-14. Skin layers and transcutaneous PO₂. The transcutaneous oxygen sensor detects oxygen that diffuses from the dermal capillary bed below the skin surface.

Cutaneous sensor

Stratum corneum

Epidermis

Dermis

Hypodermis

epidermis in preterms lacks a keratinized stratum corneum that is the main barrier to diffusion.[660] Therefore, $PtcO_2$ in the preterm will be higher than $PtcO_2$ in the term infant despite the same PaO_2 in both.[660]

All these factors help to explain why PO_2 tends to be lower on the skin surface compared with intra-arterial readings. Another important physical law must also be remembered, however, in understanding $PtcO_2$ as measured in the clinic. Gay-Lussac's law states that, given a constant gas volume, as temperature increases so does pressure. Transcutaneous PO_2 electrodes heat the skin to about 43.5° C. The direct physical effect of this heating is to increase PO_2 through stimulation of brownian movement of the gas molecules. Increasing the temperature from 37° to 44° C would have the direct physical effect of increasing a PO_2 of 100 to 140 mm Hg.[661] Of course, any local increase in temperature also tends to increase local metabolism. Nevertheless, this effect is less than the direct physical effects on the skin. Unlike oxygen, $PtcCO_2$ correlates well with $PaCO_2$ at body temperature.

Thus, one can see that the value for $PtcO_2$ depends on various factors. Most of these factors tend to make $PtcO_2$ lower than PaO_2, whereas the direct physical effect of an increase in temperature actually tends to make $PtcO_2$ higher. The actual $PtcO_2$ that is observed in a given patient, however, depends on the net interaction of all of these factors. In normal adults, $PtcO_2$ is generally about 20% less than PaO_2.[662] In infants, though, $PtcO_2$ is actually approximately 5% to 15% higher than PaO_2 because of the direct effects of the high temperature at the measurement site.[662]

PtcO₂–PaO₂ Agreement

Placement

Because function of the electrode depends greatly on the nature of the skin on which it is placed, the selection of an appropriate site is important to obtain $PtcO_2$ values that are approximate to PaO_2 values. Generally, one should choose a site where capillary pressure is high and vasoconstriction is usually minimal. The chest near the clavicles, the head, or the lateral sides of the abdomen are sites often used. The buttocks or inside upper thighs may also be used.

Some locations may show a very low $PtcO_2$ that fails to increase promptly when the microelectrode is applied. If this occurs, a different location should be tried. Placement of the electrode properly on the skin surface is also important. The electrode should be flat against the skin but should not indent or compress the skin.

The skin should be prepared by wetting it. Wet skin is more permeable than dry skin. Gels or glycerol are sometimes used and have the advantage of adhering to the skin better than water in some locations. Nevertheless, oxygen diffuses through the water more quickly than through gel.

Calibration

Transcutaneous PO_2 electrodes must be calibrated before being used. After initial application to the patient, $PtcO_2$ readings are low because the skin is cool. During the next 5 to 15 minutes as the skin warms, $PtcO_2$ increases and reaches a plateau.

Drift, or a change in the baseline with time, may also occur in these electrodes. Drift may be positive or negative and is usually approximately 1% to 5%. If the electrode is left in place for more than 6 hours, $PtcO_2$ usually decreases.[663] This problem can be discovered only by periodic recalibration. Transcutaneous PO_2 electrodes should be repositioned and calibrated every 2 to 6 hours, and more frequently in newborns.[630]

Response Time

The response time of the electrode depends on the age of the patient and more specifically on the skin thickness. In infants, the skin is thin and response time has been reported as 10 to 15 seconds.[662] In adults, the skin is thick and response time is 45 to 60 seconds.[662] In general, the older the individual, the longer is the response time. Other studies have shown response times that were considerably longer for oxygen (90% response took 5 minutes); however, CO_2 response times (90% response) occurred in one-third of this time.[669]

Perfusion and Drugs

Transcutaneous PO_2 does not agree well with PaO_2 when perfusion is poor. The lower the arterial pressure, the lower is the correlation between PaO_2 and $PtcO_2$. Similarly, shock and acidosis may decrease the correlation. Drugs and anesthetics that decrease the blood pressure or alter the distribution of perfusion may also disrupt the correlation.

Temperature

Even one degree of difference in the temperature at which skin PO_2 is measured can have a profound effect on the value obtained. When PO_2 is greater than 100 mm Hg, PO_2 increases 6 mm Hg/°C increase.[661] When PO_2 is less than 100 mm Hg, it increases 6%/°C increase.[661] The temperature of the $PtcO_2$ electrode should be set at 43.5° C.

The major complication associated with the application of transcutaneous PO_2 electrodes is burns to the skin. This complication can generally be avoided by rotating the electrode placement every 2 to 6 hours.[630]

Clinical Application

Transcutaneous PO_2/PCO_2 most often varies closely with arterial blood gases in infants and is a useful way to *continuously* monitor newborns and premature infants. In particular, transcutaneous PO_2 may be a sensitive indicator of hyperoxemia immediately following surfactant replacement therapy. Transcutaneous PO_2/PCO_2 may help guide application of special ventilator strategies such as high-frequency jet ventilation. They may also help to avoid infant stress and blood loss associated with excessive blood gas sampling. Finally, $PtcCO_2$ may assist in monitoring hypercapnia and the potential for increased intracranial perfusion and hemorrhage. Despite its numerous limitations, transcutaneous monitoring still seems to have a place in NICU monitoring.

Limitations

Despite its value, in some situations, transcutaneous gas measurement is still plagued with a host of limitations. Box 15-2 provides a brief summary of some of the key points from the AARC Clinical Practice Guideline related to Transcutaneous Blood Gas Monitoring for Neonatal/Pediatric Patients.[672] Furthermore, Box 15-3 likewise summarizes many of the overall limitations of transcutaneous monitoring. The clinician should always keep in mind that transcutaneous gas measurement is far from a direct process and many factors can disturb the delicate balance of measurement that ultimately is expected to accurately reflect arterial conditions.

Transcutaneous PO_2 versus Pulse Oximetry

Several early studies compared the clinical value of $PtcO_2$ with SpO_2 as measured via pulse oximetry.[664,665] The SpO_2 has been shown to be a more sensitive indicator of severe hypoxemia.[666,667] Furthermore, the response time of pulse oximetry is about five times faster than that for transcutaneous PO_2.

Box 15-2   AARC Clinical Practice Guidelines—Transcutaneous Blood Gas (O_2/CO_2) Monitoring for Neonatal and Pediatric Patients: Nuts & Bolts

Indications
   Continuous monitor of oxygenation and ventilation
   Quantify response to interventions (validate with ABGs initially and periodically)
Technical Limitations
   Labor intensive
   Prolonged stabilization time
   Oxygen electrode requires heating skin surface
   Calibration error potential
Clinical Limitations (i.e., decreased correlation with ABG)
   Hyperoxemia ($PaO_2 > 100$ mm Hg)
   Hypoperfusion and acidosis
   Electrode placement integrity
   Vasoactive drugs
   Skin injury or burns

Reference: AARC Clinical Practice Guideline: Transcutaneous blood gas monitoring for neonatal & pediatric patients. Respir. Care, 39:1176–1179, 1994.

From a practical standpoint, pulse oximetry offers several additional advantages when compared with transcutaneous PO_2 monitoring. Pulse oximetry requires no heating; therefore, there is essentially no risk of complication from burns. Conversely, the potential for burns is a major concern with $PtcO_2$ monitoring.

Transcutaneous PO_2 monitoring requires skin preparation, calibration of the electrode, technical warm-up time, and periodic rotation of the electrode site. Pulse oximetry, on the other hand, requires no skin preparation, no calibration, no warm-up, and no periodic movement of the probe. In the intensive monitoring of oxygenation in the adult, pulse oximetry is generally a superior technology.

The $PtcO_2$ is, however, a better index of hyperoxemia than SpO_2.[668] Because the saturation of oxygenated blood is relatively constant when PaO_2 is above 90 mm Hg, SpO_2 is not a sensitive indicator of hyperoxemia. Thus, $PtcO_2$ is the preferred index in infants at risk of retinopathy of prematurity secondary to excessive oxygenation.

CAPNOMETRY

Perhaps the most important thing to realize about $PetCO_2$ is that it is not $PaCO_2$.

D. Hess[673]

Introduction

Capnometry is the measurement of carbon dioxide (CO_2) in the exhaled gas. *Capnography* is the technique of displaying CO_2 measurements as waveforms (capnograms) throughout the respiratory cycle. Capnography is a "standard

---

Box 15-3   Limitations of Transcutaneous Monitoring

Frequent calibration required
Frequent position changes of electrode required
Relatively long equilibration time following electrode placement
Insufficient electrode temperature may adversely affect performance
Performance may be suboptimal over poorly perfused areas
$PtcO_2$ tends to underestimate PaO_2 and $PtcCO_2$ tends to overestimate of $PaCO_2$
Compromised hemodynamic status causes an underestimate of PaO_2 and an overestimate $PaCO_2$
Heated electrode may cause skin to blister
$PtcO_2$ may underestimate PaO_2 during hyperoxemia
Frequent membrane/electrolyte changes, and electrode maintenance required
Performance more reliable in neonates than adults (at least for $PtcO_2$)

From Hess, D.R., Kacmarek, R.M.: Essentials of Mechanical Ventilation, 2nd ed. New York, McGraw-Hill, 2002.

of care for general anesthesia."[704] The end-tidal CO_2, which is the maximum partial pressure of CO_2 exhaled during a tidal breath (just before the beginning of inspiration), is designated $PetCO_2$. Although technology associated with capnography continues to develop, clinical understanding of the meaning and limitations of this measurement lags behind.

Measurement Techniques

Carbon dioxide analyzers may use infrared, mass spectrometry, Raman spectra analysis, or a photoacoustic spectra technology.[674] The two methods most commonly employed are mass spectrometry and infrared analysis. Mass spectrometers are extremely precise instruments that can perform various functions including simultaneous measurement of several or all of the constituents of a gas mixture. They are accurate to within two decimal points within 0.1 second of the actual event. They are often used to monitor a large number of mechanical ventilators in the operating room. Nevertheless, mass spectrometers are labor-intensive, cumbersome, costly systems and are not practical in most critical care situations. Interestingly, the presence of Freon (used as a propellant in metered dose inhalers) may artificially increase CO_2 reading in mass spectrometers.[674]

Infrared Absorption Capnometers

Capnography is most often accomplished with free-standing infrared absorption capnometers. The infrared absorption technique is simpler and less expensive than mass spectrometry. Traditional response time is approximately

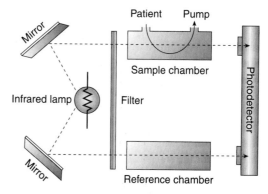

Figure 15-15. Schematic representation of a double-beam infrared capnometer.

0.25 seconds. Carbon dioxide has an absorption peak at 4250 nm. Nitrous oxide and water have absorption peaks close to this area. Thus, there is potential for the introduction of error with these substances; however, most analyzers have safeguards to minimize or prevent these technical errors. The units take advantage of the fact that CO_2 absorbs infrared radiation in proportion to its concentration (spectrophotometry). The accuracy of most capnometers is about ±12% or 4 mm Hg.[673]

Infrared analyzers may be double-beamed, positive-filter models (which include a reference chamber) as shown in Figure 15-15. In contrast, they may be single-beam, negative-filtered as shown in Figure 15-16. In both models, a spinning wheel (chopper), improves the accuracy of the sensor by periodically obstructing and opening the light channel(s). Older models required frequent calibration but some newer

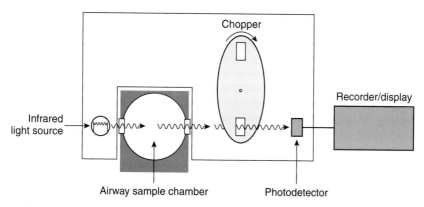

Figure 15-16. Single-beam infrared capnography. The basic components of a single-beam, negative-filter infrared carbon dioxide detector used in some mainstream sampling systems.

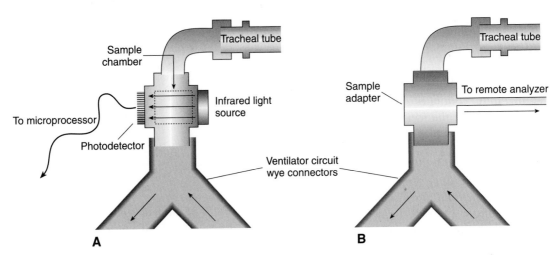

Figure 15-17.   **Mainstream vs. sidestream CO_2 sampling. A,** Mainstream CO_2 sampling. **B,** Sidestream CO_2 sampling.

models perform self-calibration, have no moving parts, and respond in approximately 100 milliseconds.[656]

Mainstream versus Sidestream Sampling

There are two general sampling techniques employed by the various capnometers: mainstream and sidestream analysis.

Mainstream Analyzers

Mainstream analyzers measure CO_2 directly in the airway (Fig. 15-17,A). Mainstream analyzers provide a very rapid, crisp, and accurate response. Early mainstream analyzers were criticized for their weight, fragile nature, or the addition of mechanical deadspace, however, newer designs have essentially eliminated these problems. The issue of water or sputum in the system contaminating readings, however, still remains. Most mainstream analyzers use a heating device to eliminate moisture accumulation. Mainstream designs are best suited for artificial airways.

Sidestream Analyzers

Sidestream analyzers aspirate the gas sample through a small bore tubing for analysis within a chamber (see Fig. 15-17,B). Sidestream analyzers can be used in the nonintubated patient by placement of the sampling tubing at the external nares or through a specially designed nasal cannula.[673]

 Unfortunately, mucus or moisture may be aspirated into the tubing along with exhaled gas, which will distort function and accuracy. Special water traps and foam barriers and, in some units, back-flushing systems have been designed to deal with this problem. In addition, aspiration flowrate must be set carefully (e.g., 150 mL/min) to avoid significant distortions in the waveform. At times, the continuous aspiration of gases causes some dampening or smoothing of CO_2 waveforms. In addition, if a leak is present in the system, PCO_2 readings decrease due to air dilution. Finally, sidestream analyzers usually have slower response times than do mainstream analyzers.[625]

Colorimetric CO_2 Analysis

Simple colorimetric techniques for evaluating the presence of CO_2 in exhaled gas have been available for many years. In 1916, Marriott described the use of a material that changed color in the presence of CO_2.[675] More recently, an end-tidal CO_2 detector has been described which is *purple* when CO_2 is less than 0.5%, then turns *tan* up to 2% CO_2, and finally becomes *yellow* when CO_2 exceeds 2%. The detector is said to be reliable and easy to use.[676] These devices are reliable and inexpensive and especially useful for detection of successful intubation.

Capnograms

Normal Capnogram

A normal single breath capnogram is shown in Figure 15-18. The partial pressure of expired CO_2 is plotted vertically against time on the

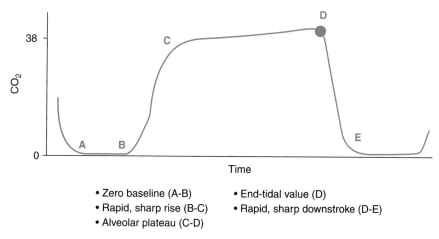

- Zero baseline (A-B)
- Rapid, sharp rise (B-C)
- Alveolar plateau (C-D)
- End-tidal value (D)
- Rapid, sharp downstroke (D-E)

Figure 15-18.   **Essentials of the normal capnographic waveform.**

horizontal axis. At the very onset of expiration, no CO_2 is observed because the first gas to leave the lungs comes from the anatomic deadspace (see Fig. 15-18,*A,B*). The anatomic deadspace is, of course, filled with fresh gas ($PCO_2 \cong 0$ mm Hg) from the previous inspiration.

As exhalation continues, some alveolar gas begins to be exhaled along with the anatomic deadspace, and an upward movement of the capnogram is observed. As the gas becomes proportionally more alveolar and less anatomic deadspace, there is a corresponding rise in the exhaled PCO_2 (see Fig. 15-18,*B,C*). Then, when essentially all of the gas being exhaled is coming from alveoli, an *alveolar plateau* (see Fig. 15-8, *C,D*) is observed.

Finally, when expiration is complete and inspiratory flow begins, CO_2 decreases quickly to zero (see Fig. 15-18,*D,E*). The PCO_2 level attained immediately before descent in the curve occurs is referred to as the *end-tidal partial pressure* of CO_2 (PetCO$_2$). This point is also shown in Figure 15-18,*D*.

Simultaneous capnograms produced by early model sidestream capnometer and a mainstream capnometer are shown in Figure 15-19. The smoothing of the waveform due to the old sidestream analyzer compared with the mainstream analyzer is readily apparent. Smoothing of the waveform occurs when the aspiration flow rate is too low. Newer sidestream analyzers eliminate this problem and demonstrate a waveform similar to that shown for the mainstream analyzer.

The clinician should also be aware that the graph paper may be run at a slow or fast speed. In the initial portion of the graphs in Figure 15-19, the paper is being run at a fast speed. Thus, fine details in the shape of the capnogram can be specifically analyzed. High-speed capnometry can often provide useful diagnostic information and fine detail of each breath.

The final portion of the graphs is being run at slow speed. Slow-speed capnography essentially provides a running monitor of the end-tidal CO_2 (PetCO$_2$) level. Some monitors display both slow and fast speed graphics. Slow-speed capnography is sometimes referred to as a CO_2 trend.

Abnormal Capnograms

The alveolar plateau will demonstrate an increased slope in the presence of ventilation-perfusion mismatch (e.g., COPD/ARDS).[680] Likewise, the alveolar plateau may flatten in a more normal manner following treatment of reversible ventilation-perfusion mismatch. Figure 15-20 illustrates capnographic improvement in a 2-year-old boy with severe croup following administration of racemic epinephrine.

The capnogram may also alert the clinician to rebreathing if the baseline continues to escalate as shown in Figure 15-21. Finally, the onset of patient spontaneous inspiration can be identified when sharply decreasing CO_2 is observed during the alveolar plateau. This phenomenon

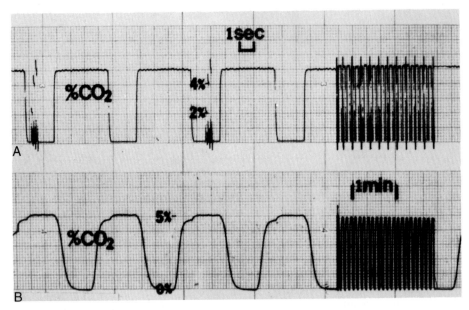

Figure 15-19. **Comparative tracings from mainstream and sidestream analyzers.** Simultaneous tracings from a mainstream analyzer (**A**) and a sidestream analyzer (**B**). The first portion of each graph represents fast-speed capnography, whereas the latter portion represents slow-speed capnography. Note the smoothing of the waveform with sidestream analysis during fast speed.

has been termed the "curare cleft" (Fig. 15-22) when observed in patients recovering from neuromuscular blockade.

Volumetric Capnograms

The partial pressure of carbon dioxide can be plotted against volume instead of time utilizing some recent technology (Fig. 15-23). The volumetric capnogram provides additional information regarding deadspace and CO_2 production heretofore not readily available at the bedside. Specifically, anatomical deadspace, alveolar deadspace, and CO_2 production per minute may be determined. This information can be particularly useful in evaluation of $PaCO_2$ changes during mechanical ventilation. It is also valuable when rapid increases in CO_2 production may indicate malignant hyperthermia in the operating room. Given stable metabolism and alveolar ventilation, flattening of phases II and III may indicate decreased pulmonary perfusion in volumetric capnography as shown in Figure 15-24.

Technology has also become recently available that allows for the volumetric capnogram in conjunction with partial rebreathing

to *noninvasively measure cardiac output.* A modified form of the Fick equation is used for this determination. This technique seems very promising as a method to determine the valuable cardiac output measurement without the need for invasive catheters.

PetCO₂ as an Indicator of PaCO₂

As described previously, the $PetCO_2$ represents the end-tidal pressure of carbon dioxide. In spontaneously breathing normal individuals, the $PetCO_2$ varies in concert with the $PaCO_2$. This fact, although true, is probably the origin of an abundance of confusion surrounding capnography. Only in the healthy spontaneously breathing individual does this fact hold true. Indeed, in sick individuals, the $PetCO_2$ and $PaCO_2$ are distinctly different entities that may, in fact, change in opposite directions. Although $PetCO_2$ is inviting as a simple, noninvasive, reflection of $PaCO_2$, it is not. Time and time again, this has been shown. Use of $PetCO_2$ as a predictor of $PaCO_2$ is deceiving and incorrect, and should be used with great caution for this purpose in mechanically ventilated patients.[619] Indeed, 73% of

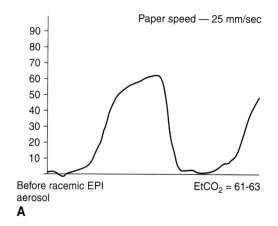
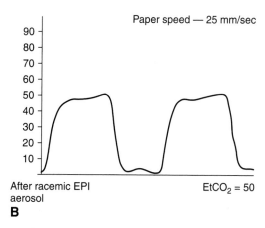

A   Before racemic EPI aerosol

B   After racemic EPI aerosol

Figure 15-20.   **Evaluating drug effectiveness with capnography.** Capnograms of 2-year-old boy with severe croup before (**A**) and after (**B**) administration of racemic epinephrine by aerosol.

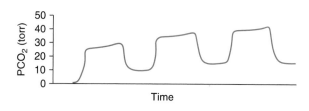

Figure 15-21.   **Capnogram produced with rebreathing.**

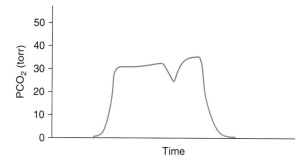

Figure 15-22.   **Capnogram produced with curare cleft.**

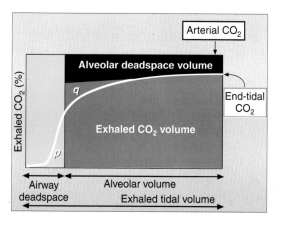

Figure 15-23.   **Volumetric capnogram.** Note that the area under the capnogram is carbon dioxide production. Also note that the volume-based capnogram allows determination of anatomic dead space, alveolar volume, and alveolar deadspace.

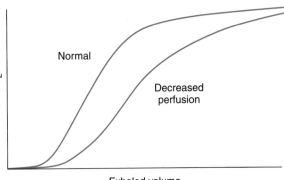

Figure 15-24. **Volumetric capnogram with decreased pulmonary perfusion.**

the variability in PetCO$_2$ has absolutely nothing to do with changes in PaCO$_2$.[677] Thus, more than half of the time it can be misleading if simply viewed, even as a trend monitor, in this manner.

There are two situations in which PetCO$_2$ may be considered to reflect PaCO$_2$. First is the patient with normal lungs, such as a patient being hyperventilated secondary to head trauma. Second, sudden substantial change in PetCO$_2$ has been shown to be of benefit in identifying mishaps.[678] This could be a ventilator disconnect or some other potentially catastrophic event.

Indeed, capnography has been identified as a valuable indicator of patient mishaps, second only to pulse oximetry, but more valuable than ECG tracings.[611]

Changes in PetCO$_2$ may be the result of changes in carbon dioxide production, alveolar ventilation, or equipment malfunctions. Potential causes of increased PetCO$_2$ are shown in Box 15-4. Causes of decreased PetCO$_2$ are shown in Box 15-5.

P(a–et)CO$_2$

If PaCO$_2$ and PetCO$_2$ are known, the gradient can be calculated. Normally, the gradient is less

---

Box 15-4 Causes of Increased PetCO$_2$
INCREASED CO$_2$ PRODUCTION AND DELIVERY TO THE LUNGS
Fever
Sepsis
Bicarbonate administration
Increased metabolic rate
Seizures
DECREASED ALVEOLAR VENTILATION
Respiratory center depression
Muscular paralysis
Hypoventilation
COPD
EQUIPMENT MALFUNCTION
Rebreathing
Exhausted CO$_2$ absorber
Leak in ventilator circuit

From Hess, D.: Capnometry and capnography: Technical aspects, physiological aspects, and clinical applications. Respir. Care, 35(6):562, June 1990.

Box 15-5 Causes of Decreased PetCO$_2$
DECREASED CO$_2$ PRODUCTION AND DELIVERY TO THE LUNGS
Hypothermia
Pulmonary hypoperfusion
Cardiac arrest
Pulmonary embolism
Hemorrhage
Hypotension
INCREASED ALVEOLAR VENTILATION
Hyperventilation
EQUIPMENT MALFUNCTION
Ventilator disconnect
Esophageal intubation
Complete airway obstruction
Poor sampling
Leak around endotracheal tube cuff

From Hess, D.: Capnometry and capnography: Technical aspects, physiological aspects, and clinical applications. Respir. Care, 35(6):562, June 1990.

than 5 mm Hg; however, it can be increased with deadspace disease such as pulmonary embolism or decreased cardiac output.[674] The presence of increased deadspace may also have some significance as a prognostic indicator in surgical patients, although further research is needed to confirm this.[681] Interestingly, $P(a-et)CO_2$ measured after forced exhalation seems to be best for evaluation of *acute* pulmonary embolism,[679] although this is not always practical in the clinic.

Occasionally, $PetCO_2$ may actually be higher than $PaCO_2$. The reasons for this are unclear but are most likely due to emptying of low $\dot{V}/\dot{Q}$ units with long time constants at the end of expiration.

Usefulness of PetCO_2

Verification of Intubation

As stated earlier, $PetCO_2$ is useful as a general indicator of $PaCO_2$ in the patient with normal lungs and has some value as a gross indicator of patient mishaps.

Monitoring of $PetCO_2$ via colorimetry is also clearly a valuable adjunct to assessing successful endotracheal intubation. Intubation of the esophagus is a serious problem that may occur during attempted intubation, during manipulation of the endotracheal tube, or during

movement of the patient's head. Assessment of $PetCO_2$ is the most reliable way to insure correct placement of an endotracheal tube.

Occasionally $PetCO_2$ may be high because of other reasons. Esophageal gas may be quite high in CO_2 following ingestion of carbonated beverages, or antacids. Nevertheless, the PCO_2 will decrease rapidly following 10 to 15 seconds of bag-resuscitator ventilation.

One must also keep in mind, however, that in the absence of circulation, as during cardiac arrest or very low perfusion states, $PetCO_2$ may be very low or absent. Notwithstanding, the American College of Emergency Physicians, as well as the International Guidelines for Emergency Cardiovascular Care recommend use of CO_2 detection to verify endotracheal tube placement.[674] Furthermore, new American Heart Association guidelines require secondary confirmation of proper tube placement in all patients by exhaled CO_2 immediately after intubation and during transport.[682] Colorimetric detectors are adequate for this purpose.[674]

PetCO_2 during Cardiopulmonary Resuscitation

$PetCO_2$ appears to be useful in the evaluation of cardiopulmonary resuscitation (CPR). First, the $PetCO_2$ increases with restoration of artificial circulation and correlates with

---

ON CALL | CASE 15-1 *ABGs and Critical Thinking*

You are the only person available to care for this patient. You must assess the patient/situation and act accordingly.

A 26-year-old woman is being mechanically ventilated following cranial surgery. She is being intentionally hyperventilated via mechanical ventilation to minimize intracranial pressure. She is also being monitored continuously via capnometry.

ARTERIAL BLOOD GASES

SaO_2	98%
pH	7.54
$PaCO_2$	27 mm Hg
PaO_2	94 mm Hg
$[HCO_3]$	23 mEq/L
FIO_2	0.40
$PetCO_2$	21 mm Hg

Suddenly, her $PetCO_2$ increases to 35 mm Hg.

ASSESSMENT

Abnormalities: List abnormal data and other noteworthy information. Classify ABG.

Explanation: List possible diseases, pathology, or other situations that may have led to this patient's condition.

Evaluation: Suggest additional data that would be useful in helping understand the situation or in making a diagnosis.

INTERVENTION

Importance: Prioritize concern(s) of treatment in order of urgency and/or seriousness as you see the overall situation.

Objective: Specifically state the measurable or observable outcomes you would like treatment to accomplish.

Action: Describe your specific plan of action.

ON CALL | CASE 15-2 *ABGs and Critical Thinking*

You are the only person available to care for this patient. You must assess the patient/situation and act accordingly.

A 64-year-old man is being mechanically ventilated in the surgical intensive care unit following heart surgery.

ARTERIAL BLOOD GASES

SaO_2	95%
pH	7.36
$PaCO_2$	37 mm Hg
PaO_2	74 mm Hg
$[HCO_3]$	22 mEq/L
FIO_2	0.50
$PetCO_2$	27 mm Hg

The patient appears uncomfortable and short of breath and a later ABG reveals a $PaCO_2$ of 50 mm Hg. Nevertheless, the $PetCO_2$ continues to read at approximately 27 mm Hg.

ASSESSMENT

Abnormalities: List abnormal data and other noteworthy information. Classify ABG.

Explanation: List possible diseases, pathology, or other situations that may have led to this patient's condition.

Evaluation: Suggest additional data that would be useful in helping understand the situation or in making a diagnosis.

INTERVENTION

Importance: Prioritize concern(s) of treatment in order of urgency and/or seriousness as you see the overall situation.

Objective: Specifically state the measurable or observable outcomes you would like treatment to accomplish.

Action: Describe your specific plan of action.

cardiac output and coronary perfusion pressure.[683,684,686] Perhaps most important, an abrupt increase (within 30 seconds) in $PetCO_2$ may be the earliest sign indicating that *spontaneous* circulation has been restored in the patient being resuscitated.[689] Thus, the $PetCO_2$ may be a very useful quantitative indicator of pulmonary perfusion and cardiac output during cardiac arrest.[689] Higher $PetCO_2$s were likewise observed when fatigued rescuers were relieved by fresh rescuers.[687] In addition, higher $PetCO_2$s were observed during successful resuscitation of animals than during unsuccessful resuscitation.[685] Likewise, $PetCO_2$ may be useful in identifying patients who were likely to be successfully resuscitated as those with a $PetCO_2$ of 15 mm Hg were more likely to be successfully resuscitated than those with a $PetCO_2$ of 7 mm Hg.[688] Administration of bicarbonate during CPR may negate the usefulness of $PetCO_2$ as an indicator of blood flow during CPR because it will artifactually increase carbon dioxide levels.

Summary

Clearly, colorimetric CO_2 analysis is useful to help verify endotracheal intubation. $PetCO_2$ also appears beneficial in tracking cardiac output (i.e., pulmonary perfusion) and response to

cardiopulmonary resuscitation. Capnography is a beneficial way to evaluate $PaCO_2$ in the patient with normal lungs. In addition, capnography and $PetCO_2$ are useful as indicators of patient mishaps.

$(PaCO_2 - PetCO_2)$ or the slope of the capnogram may be beneficial in many other situations to evaluate deadspace, equipment malfunctions, and response to therapy and ventilation-perfusion mismatch. Its benefit in assessing for pulmonary embolus and optimal positive end-expiratory pressure is less convincing. Likewise, its benefit in infants and children needs additional verification.[673] Most importantly, it should not be assumed to reflect $PaCO_2$ in most mechanically ventilated patients. Its use in this manner is misleading and dangerous.

Volumetric CO_2 analysis is useful for evaluating carbon dioxide production from metabolism and alveolar deadspace changes. Its use as a method to noninvasively monitor cardiac output is very promising and likely to expand.

Box 15-6 reviews key points from the AARC Clinical Practice Guideline regarding use of capnography during mechanical ventilation.[674] Notably, at this time, capnography is not held to the quality assurance standards imposed on invasive tests such as arterial blood gas analysis.

Box 15-6	AARC Clinical Practice Guidelines—Capnography/Capnometry during Mechanical Ventilation, 2003 Revision and Update: Nuts & Bolts

Indications: Conventional Capnometry/Capnography
  Verification endotracheal intubation
  Monitoring V/Q especially VD/VT
    Slope phase III capnograph
    $PaCO_2 - PetCO_2$ trends
    Assessment pulmonary embolus
Indications Volumetric Capnometry
  Assess CO_2 production per minute
  Assess alveolar deadspace
Clinical Limitations
  $PetCO_2$ is not a replacement for $PaCO_2$
Technical Error
  Oxygen, water, or nitrous oxide in light path
  Carbonated beverages or antacids in stomach
  Leaks in ventilator circuitry

Reference: AARC Clinical Practice Guideline. Capnography/capnometry during mechanical ventilation. (2003 update). Respir. Care, 48:534–539, 2003.

EXERCISES

Exercise 15-1 Basic Principles of Oximetry

Fill in the blanks or select the best answer.

1. The *gold standard* test in the evaluation of acid-base balance and oxygenation is _____.

2. (Monitoring/Measurement) techniques provide the clinician with static information about a single point in time.

3. Measurement of the light spectrum of an unknown substance is a useful method of (quantitative/qualitative) analysis.

4. The ability of light to release electrons from metals in proportion to the intensity of the light is known as the _____.

5. Quantitative spectrophotometry is made possible through application of the_____ law.

6. The ratio of light intensity at a given wavelength incident on a substance compared with the intensity of light transmitted through the substance is called its_____.

7. An instrument that measures the amount of light transmitted through (or reflected from) a sample of blood at two or more specific wavelengths to assess O_2 levels is called an _____.

8. An oximeter is a dedicated _____ specifically designed to measure SaO_2.

9. When two substances have identical light absorption properties at a given wavelength, an _____ point is said to exist.

10. In reflection oximetry, the photo detector is on the (same/opposite) side of the blood sample as the light source.

11. Transmission oximeters are more accurate if (hemolyzed/nonhemolyzed) blood is used.

12. When using two wavelength oximetry, abnormal forms of hemoglobin, such as methemoglobin, (are/are not) identified.

13. State the four hemoglobin species that are usually measured by a CO-oximeter.

14. SaO_2 measured via CO-oximetry is sometimes called (fractional/functional) saturation.

15. The _____ ear oximeter measured light at eight different wavelengths.

Exercise 15-2 Pulse Oximetry

Fill in the blanks or select the best answer.

1. Blood oxygen saturation can be monitored continuously and noninvasively at the bedside with the technology of _____.

2. A device for measuring and recording change in the volume of a part of the body or an organ is called a _____.

3. Photoelectric plethysmography is used in pulse oximeters to measure the _____.

4. In pulse oximetry, baseline absorption is the amount of light absorbed during (systole/diastole) of the heart cycle.

5. Pulse oximeters are generally (accurate/inaccurate) when large amounts of fetal hemoglobin are present.

6. Pulse oximeters use _____ wavelengths of light.

7. Pulse oximeters use light from what two light ranges?

8. When part of the light being emitted by a pulse oximeter reaches the photo detector by passing around rather than passing through the finger, _____ is said to exist.

9. Pulse oximetry (does/does not) measure carboxyhemoglobin levels.

10. Continuous simultaneous measurement of saturation through a fiber-optic pulmonary artery catheter and a pulse oximeter is called _____.

Exercise 15-3 Transcutaneous PO_2/PCO_2

Fill in the blanks or select the best answer.

1. The symbol for transcutaneous PO_2 is _____.

2. Transcutaneous PO_2 monitors require (more/less) maintenance and care than do pulse oximeters.

3. The $PtcCO_2$ electrode requires (more/less) skin heating than the $PtcO_2$ electrode.

4. State the three layers of the skin from the outermost layer inward.

5. The epidermis consumes oxygen at a (high/low) rate and contains (many/no) blood vessels.

6. Transcutaneous PO_2 electrodes heat the skin to approximately _____° C.

7. In the normal adult, $PtcO_2$ is approximately 20% (greater/less) than PaO_2.

8. In the normal infant, $PtcO_2$ is approximately 5% to 15% (higher/lower) than PaO_2.

9. (Wetting/Drying) the skin increases permeability.

10. Transcutaneous PO_2 electrodes (do/do not) require a warm-up period and calibration.

11. The major complication associated with $PtcO_2$ is skin _____.

12. It is usually recommended that electrode placement be rotated every _____ hours.

13. Transcutaneous PO_2 closely varies with PaO_2 in (adults/infants).

14. Between SpO_2 and $PtcO_2$, the better index of hyperoxemia is _____.

15. Which of the following is the most sensitive indicator of severe hypoxemia: SpO_2, $PtcO_2$.

Exercise 15-4 Capnometry Technique

Fill in the blanks or select the best answer.

1. The technique of displaying CO_2 measurements as waveforms throughout the respiratory cycle is called _____.

2. State the two most common types of machines that can be used to perform capnography.

3. (Mass spectrometers/Infrared capnometers) are often used to monitor a large number of mechanically ventilated patients simultaneously in the operating room.

4. Carbon dioxide absorbs (red/infrared) radiation in proportion to its concentration.

5. Radiation beams in infrared CO_2 analyzers are interrupted periodically by devices called _____ in order to increase accuracy and prevent electronic drift.

6. State the two general types of infrared CO_2 analyzers that are available depending on their actual measurement site.

7. (Sidestream/Mainstream) analyzers aspirate the gas into the sample chamber.

8. Mainstream designs are best suited for (artificial airways/spontaneously breathing patients).

9. Sidestream analyzers traditionally have (slower/faster) response times than do mainstream analyzers.

10. Problems with secretions and moisture are diminished with (sidestream/mainstream) CO_2 analyzers.

Exercise 15-5 Capnograms

Fill in the blanks or select the best answer.

1. The CO_2 concentration of the gas exhaled at the beginning of expiration is (high/almost zero).

2. The flat upper portion of the single breath capnogram is called the (anatomic deadspace/alveolar plateau).

3. Smoothing of the CO_2 waveform may occur with the (sidestream/mainstream) analyzer.

4. (Fast/Slow) speed capnography is essentially just a running monitor of end-tidal CO_2.

5. $PetCO_2$ (is/is not) a reliable indicator of $PaCO_2$ in most mechanically ventilated patients.

6. After ingestion of a carbonated beverage, $PetCO_2$ may be falsely (low/elevated) when evaluating the patient for correct placement of the endotracheal tube.

7. After a pulmonary embolus, one would expect $PetCO_2$ to (rise/fall).

8. At the onset of cardiac arrest, $PetCO_2$ (falls/rises).

9. An abrupt (rise/fall) in $PetCO_2$ may be the first sign of the restoration of spontaneous circulation after resuscitation for cardiac arrest.

10. A relatively large slope of the alveolar plateau is indicative of a/an (obstructive/restrictive) lung problem.

11. Volumetric CO_2 analysis is useful for evaluating (carbon dioxide production/$PaCO_2$).

12. Volumetric CO_2 analysis with a partial rebreathing technique may be useful for noninvasively monitoring (RQ/cardiac output).

Exercise 15-6 **Internet Work**

1. Search the web for noninvasive measurement of cardiac output and report on its validity compared to measurement of cardiac output by thermal dilution and the Fick method.

NBRC Challenge 15

Please select the best answer for the following multiple-choice questions.

1. A patient with arrhythmias experiences a sudden, substantial decrease in cardiac output. One would expect the following monitor change:
   A) increased $PetCO_2$.
   B) decreased $PetCO_2$.
   C) increased $PtcO_2$.
   D) increased metHb%.
   E) increased HbCO%.
   (CRT EXAMINATION — NBRC MATRIX I,B,10,a)

2. A surgical patient is on mechanical ventilation and is also being monitored with capnography. There is a sudden decrease in $PetCO_2$ without a change in $PaCO_2$; and there is a strong suspicion that the patient has recently had a pulmonary embolus. What is a logical cause for the decreased $PetCO_2$?
   A) The patient is hypoventilating.
   B) The patient is hyperventilating.
   C) The patient has increased shunting.
   D) The patient has increased deadspace.
   E) There is a likely ventilator disconnect.
   (RRT EXAMINATION — NBRC MATRIX I,B,10,a)

3. A premature newborn patient has recently been treated with surfactant therapy. The monitor that would likely be most important in follow-up is:
   A) $PtcO_2$.
   B) $PtcCO_2$.
   C) pulse oximetry.
   D) conventional capnography.
   E) volumetric capnography.
   (RRT EXAMINATION — NBRC MATRIX I,B,9,a)

4. Following administration of benzocaine before a bronchoscopy, a patient appears very cyanotic. At this point, you would recommend patient evaluation via:
   A) $PtcO_2$.
   B) $PtcCO_2$.
   C) pulse oximetry.
   D) conventional capnography.
   E) CO-oximetry.
   (CSE EXAMINATION — NBRC MATRIX I,C,2,e)

5. In order to maximize safety and prevent patient mishaps, rank the following monitors in order of their usefulness:
   I) ECG
   II) Pulse oximetry
   III) Capnography
   A) I, II, III
   B) I, III, II
   C) II, I, III
   D) II, III, I
   E) III, II, I
   (CSE EXAMINATION — NBRC MATRIX I,C,1,a)

Chapter
16
Arterial Blood Gas Case Studies

Outline

Case 1 NARCOTIC OVERDOSE

A 25-year-old man residing at sea level is brought to the emergency department after a narcotic overdose and possible aspiration. He is placed on a pulse oximeter, and arterial blood gases are drawn.

Arterial Blood Gases

FIO_2	0.21
pH	7.45
$PaCO_2$	36 mm Hg
$[HCO_3]$	23 mEq/L
PaO_2	145 mm Hg

Vital Signs

Pulse	55/min
Blood pressure (BP)	100/60
Temperature	37° C
Respiration rate (RR)	8/min

Pulse Oximetry

SpO_2	80%

1A Questions

1. Is the pulse oximeter reading congruent with the PaO_2?
2. Which of the two readings must be wrong?
3. (Air in the sample/Venous sampling) could explain these results.

Repeat blood gases are as follows:

Arterial Blood Gases

FIO_2	0.21
pH	7.21
$PaCO_2$	64 mm Hg
$[HCO_3^-]$	24 mEq/L
PaO_2	48 mm Hg

Vital Signs

Pulse	55/min
BP	100/60
Temperature	37° C
RR	8/min

Pulse Oximetry

SpO_2	80%

1B Questions

1. Classify the arterial blood gas.
2. What are the four common causes of hypoxemia in hospitalized patients?
3. Hypoventilation (is/is not) a cause of hypoxemia in this patient.
4. What index can be used to differentiate *simple hypoventilation* from *hypoventilation* in conjunction *with increased physiologic shunting?*
5. Write the clinical form of the alveolar air equation while breathing room air.

6. What is this patient's $P(A-a)O_2$ on room air?
7. This patient (does/does not) have abnormal increased physiologic shunting.
8. Treatment of this patient's acid-base status may require (sodium bicarbonate/mechanical ventilation).

Case 2 UNEXPLAINED ACIDEMIA

A 46-year-old woman who is comatose and has an unknown history is admitted to the emergency department. Arterial blood gases and laboratory data are as follows:

Arterial Blood Gases

FIO_2	0.21
pH	7.22
$PaCO_2$	25 mm Hg
$[HCO_3]$	10 mEq/L
PaO_2	96 mm Hg
SaO_2	96%

Vital Signs

Pulse	118/min
BP	170/110
Temperature	37° C
RR	18/min

Plasma Electrolytes

Na^+	137 mEq/L
CO_2	12 mEq/L
Cl^-	104 mEq/L
K^+	5.5 mEq/L

Bloodwork

Glucose	110 mg/dL
Creatinine	11 mg/dL
BUN	130 mg/dL
Lactate	12 mg/dL

2 Questions

1. Classify the arterial blood gas.
2. The anion gap is (high/low/normal).
3. The patient (appears/does not appear) to be hypoxic.
4. The lactate is (normal/increased).
5. The glucose is (normal/increased).
6. The creatinine is (normal/increased).
7. The BUN is (normal/increased).
8. The $[K^+]$ is (normal/increased).

9. What is the cause of the metabolic acidosis?
10. The hypocapnia appears to be (compensatory/a primary acid-base problem).

Case 3 GASTROINTESTINAL DISTURBANCE

A woman is admitted to the hospital with salmonella enteritis and a history of severe diarrhea for about 10 days before admission. Vital signs, blood gases, and electrolytes taken at admission are shown below:

Arterial Blood Gases

FIO_2	0.21
pH	7.15
$PaCO_2$	15 mm Hg
$[HCO_3]$	5 mEq/L
PaO_2	96 mm Hg
SaO_2	93%

Vital Signs

Pulse	112/min
BP	100/70
Temperature	37° C
RR	24/min

Plasma Electrolytes

Na^+	134 mEq/L
CO_2	7 mEq/L
Cl^-	113 mEq/L
K^+	3.2 mEq/L

3 Questions

1. Classify the arterial blood gas.
2. The anion gap is (high/low/normal).
3. The plasma chloride is (high/low/normal).
4. What is the cause of the metabolic acidosis?
5. The plasma $[K^+]$ is (high/low/normal).
6. What is the likely cause of the potassium disturbance?
7. The diuretic (Lasix/acetazolamide) could cause an acid-base disturbance similar to this, but the acidemia is usually less severe.
8. (Azotemic renal failure/Renal tubular acidosis) may cause a normal anion gap metabolic acidosis.

Case 4 STATUS ASTHMATICUS

A 17-year-old boy with a history of asthma has been continuously short of breath for approximately 2 days. He enters the hospital wheezing and with air hunger. Arterial blood gases and vital signs are as follows:

Arterial Blood Gases

FIO_2	0.21
pH	7.35
$PaCO_2$	22 mm Hg
$[HCO_3]$	12 mEq/L
PaO_2	41 mm Hg
SaO_2	77%

Vital Signs

Pulse	132/min
BP	150/90
Temperature	37° C
RR	28/min

4A Questions

1. Classify the blood gas according to the basic rules for blood gas classification discussed in Chapter 2.
2. Are there any signs to suggest that this is a mixed acid-base disturbance?
3. Do these values fall under the band on the acid-base map for simple metabolic acidosis? (See acid-base map in Chapter 14.)
4. Reclassify the acid-base status.
5. What is the cause of the respiratory alkalosis?
6. What is the probable cause of the metabolic acidosis?
7. What therapy is indicated?
8. Is it important to administer a low concentration of oxygen to this patient?
9. What could explain the elevated blood pressure, pulse, and RR in this patient?

Oxygen therapy and aerosol therapy with bronchodilators are administered, and the following blood gases are obtained about 3 hours later:

Arterial Blood Gases

FIO_2	0.5
pH	7.47
$PaCO_2$	24 mm Hg
$[HCO_3]$	16 mEq/L
PaO_2	55 mm Hg
SaO_2	92%

Vital Signs

Pulse	120/min
BP	140/90
Temperature	37° C
RR	22/min

4B Questions

1. Classify the arterial blood gas.
2. Lactate (can/cannot) be quickly metabolized in the presence of adequate oxygen.
3. The low bicarbonate concentration at this point is most likely due to (compensation/lactic acidosis).
4. The current values (do/do not) fall within the band for simple respiratory alkalosis on the acid-base map.

The patient's wheezing continued to be severe for the next 48 hours. He looked very tired at this point, and arterial blood gases were as follows:

Arterial Blood Gases

FIO_2	0.5
pH	7.32
$PaCO_2$	35 mm Hg
$[HCO_3]$	17 mEq/L
PaO_2	52 mm Hg
SaO_2	83%

Vital Signs

Pulse	135/min
BP	150/100
Temperature	37° C
RR	18/min (wheezing is less audible)

4C Questions

1. Classify the arterial blood gas.
2. It (can/cannot) be assumed that the patient has almost completely recovered.
3. The decreased wheezing (is/is not) clearly a positive sign.

The next day, the patient appears to be more comfortable and under much less stress. Arterial blood gases are as follows:

Arterial Blood Gases

FIO_2	0.28
pH	7.32
$PaCO_2$	40 mm Hg
$[HCO_3]$	20 mEq/L
PaO_2	90 mm Hg
SaO_2	96%

Vital Signs

Pulse	90/min
BP	120/80
Temperature	37° C
RR	14/min

4D Questions

1. Classify the arterial blood gas.
2. What is the most likely cause of the metabolic acidemia at this time?

Case 5   ACUTE RESPIRATORY ACIDEMIA

A 34-year-old man involved in an automobile accident arrives in the emergency department with severe head trauma. Arterial blood gases, vital signs, and pulse oximetry readings are as follows:

Arterial Blood Gases

FIO_2	0.21
pH	7.10
$PaCO_2$	95 mm Hg
[BE]	−5 mEq/L
$[HCO_3]$	29 mEq/L
PaO_2	60 mm Hg

Vital Signs

Pulse	60/min
BP	100/50
Temperature	37° C
RR	12/min

Pulse Oximetry

SpO_2	78%

5 Questions

1. What is the normal SaO_2 at a PaO_2 of 60 mm Hg?
2. Why is the SpO_2 only 78% in this patient despite a PaO_2 of 60 mm Hg?

3. Do these blood gas values fall in the band for acute respiratory acidosis on the acid-base map?
4. Does the plasma bicarbonate concentration of 29 mEq/L represent renal compensation?
5. Is it possible for a blood gas to be correct when the base excess of the blood is decreased and the actual bicarbonate is increased?
6. How much will the plasma bicarbonate increase acutely for every 10-mm Hg increase in $PaCO_2$ due to the hydrolysis effect?
7. What supportive treatment is indicated for this patient's acid-base status?

Case 6   NASOGASTRIC SUCTION

A nasogastric tube was placed in a 32-year-old woman with intestinal obstruction. For several days, large amounts of fluid were suctioned from the nasogastric tube. Arterial blood gases and electrolytes were as follows:

Arterial Blood Gases

FIO_2	0.21
pH	7.53
$PaCO_2$	49 mm Hg
$[HCO_3]$	39 mEq/L
PaO_2	92 mm Hg
SaO_2	98%

Vital Signs

Pulse	105/min
BP	110/70
Temperature	37° C
RR	18/min

Plasma Electrolytes

Na^+	142 mEq/L
CO_2	42 mEq/L
Cl^-	86 mEq/L
K^+	3.2 mEq/L

6 Questions

1. Classify the arterial blood gas.

2. Do the values fall within the band on the acid-base map for simple metabolic alkalosis?
3. What is the cause of the metabolic alkalosis?
4. Metabolic alkalosis is usually associated with (hyperchloremia/hypochloremia).
5. Hypokalemia (is/is not) common with a loss of gastric fluid.
6. Loss of body fluids (is/is not) an important aspect of this type of metabolic alkalosis.
7. What is the appropriate treatment for this type of metabolic alkalosis?

Case 7   UNEXPLAINED ALKALEMIA

A 28-year-old woman in her eighth month of pregnancy is admitted to the hospital after having severe vomiting for several days. Arterial blood gases, vital signs, and electrolytes are as follows:

Arterial Blood Gases

FIO_2	0.21
pH	7.58
$PaCO_2$	31 mm Hg
$[HCO_3]$	28 mEq/L
PaO_2	65 mm Hg
SaO_2	96%

Vital Signs

Pulse	110/min
BP	130/80
Temperature	37° C
RR	18/min

Plasma Electrolytes

Na^+	130 mEq/L
CO_2	32 mEq/L
Cl^-	86 mEq/L
K^+	3.1 mEq/L

7 Questions

1. Classify the arterial blood gas.
2. What is the likely cause of the metabolic alkalosis?
3. What is the likely cause of the respiratory alkalosis?
4. What mechanisms are responsible for hyperventilation during late pregnancy?

Case 8   OXYGENATION DISTURBANCE

A 4-month-old infant is admitted to the emergency department with cyanosis and mild cardiopulmonary distress. The family was from a rural area, and the infant had been receiving formula prepared with water taken from a well. Arterial blood gases, before the infant was given oxygen, were drawn and the blood specimen was noted to be dark. The blood gas results, pulse oximetry readings, and vital signs were as follows:

Arterial Blood Gases

FIO_2	0.21
pH	7.30
$PaCO_2$	28 mm Hg
[BE]	−12 mEq/L
PaO_2	105 mm Hg

Vital Signs

Pulse	140/min
BP	140/100
Temperature	37° C
RR	40/min

Pulse Oximetry

SpO_2	94%

8A Questions

1. Does the pulse oximeter reading and PaO_2 concur with the clinical picture of cyanosis and the appearance of a dark blood sample?
2. Should another blood gas sample be drawn?

The child is then placed on oxygen and repeat arterial blood gases are drawn. Surprisingly, when a small amount of the sample accidentally escapes from the syringe, the blood appears rusty brown or chocolate in color. Blood gas results and vital signs are as follows:

Arterial Blood Gases

FIO_2	0.5
pH	7.28
$PaCO_2$	28 mm Hg
$[HCO_3]$	13 mEq/L
PaO_2	240 mm Hg

Vital Signs

Pulse	140/min
BP	130/90
Temperature	37° C
RR	38/min

Pulse Oximetry

SpO_2	90%

8B Questions

1. What is the predicted normal PaO_2 on FIO_2 of 0.5?
2. Does the infant appear to have abnormal shunting?
3. Could the cyanosis and metabolic acidosis be due to hypoxia?
4. What type of oxygenation disturbance could be associated with cyanosis despite a normal PaO_2 and rust-colored blood on exposure of the blood to air?
5. Is there normally any methemoglobin present in the blood?
6. What is the normal percentage of methemoglobin in the blood?
7. Are infants more likely to have this particular disorder?
8. How can the level of methemoglobin be reduced?
9. Why is the pulse oximeter reading in the normal range?
10. Methemoglobin is (oxygenated/oxidized).
11. The definitive diagnosis would be made via (CO-oximetry, electrolytes)?

Case 9   DIABETIC PATIENT

A 32-year-old woman with a history of diabetes mellitus is admitted to the hospital with lethargy and confusion. Current arterial blood gases, laboratory data, and vital signs are shown below:

Arterial Blood Gases

FIO_2	0.21
pH	7.04
$PaCO_2$	15 mm Hg
$[HCO_3]$	10 mEq/L
PaO_2	125 mm Hg
SaO_2	95%

Vital Signs

Pulse	118/min
BP	90/50
Temperature	37° C
RR	32/min

Plasma Electrolytes

Na^+	136 mEq/L
CO_2	7 mEq/L
Cl^-	95 mEq/L
K^+	6.3 mEq/L

Bloodwork

Glucose	750 mg/dL
Acetoacetic acid	250 mg/dL
Blood urea nitrogen (BUN)	38 mg/dL
Lactate	30 mg/dL

9A Questions

1. Classify the arterial blood gas.
2. Why is the PaO_2 greater than 100 mm Hg on room air?
3. What is the maximum PaO_2 that can be achieved during hyperventilation while breathing room air?
4. This is a (high/normal) anion gap metabolic acidosis.
5. The primary cause of the metabolic acidosis is (lactic acidosis/ketoacidosis).
6. It is (expected/unexpected) to have some accumulation of lactic acid during ketoacidosis.
7. State the two ketoacids.
8. The concentration of acetoacetic acid is (normal/high).
9. Severe (hyperglycemia/hypoglycemia) is common during diabetic ketoacidosis and causes (polyuria/oliguria).
10. Hyperkalemia is (unexpected/expected) in ketoacidosis.
11. Dehydration is (common/uncommon) in ketoacidosis. Explain this.
12. The deep, rapid, breathing pattern observed in ketoacidosis is called _____ breathing.
13. Due to hypovolemia in ketoacidosis, blood pressure is frequently (high/low), and BUN is frequently (decreased/increased).

14. Ketosis and ketoacidosis are a result of increased (carbohydrate/protein/fat) metabolism.
15. The fruity odor often present on the breath during ketoacidosis is a result of (acetone/urea).
16. Sodium bicarbonate treatment (is/is not) recommended for this patient.

Follow-up

The patient was treated with bicarbonate, insulin, and fluids. Blood gases and electrolytes were drawn 6 hours later and were as follows:

Arterial Blood Gases

FIO_2	0.21
pH	7.54
$PaCO_2$	32 mm Hg
[BE]	4 mEq/L
PaO_2	97 mm Hg
SaO_2	98%

Plasma Electrolytes

Na^+	136 mEq/L
CO_2	33 mEq/L
Cl^-	90 mEq/L
K^+	3.1 mEq/L

9B Questions

1. Classify the arterial blood gas.
2. What mechanisms may be responsible for the metabolic alkalosis?
3. What mechanism is most likely responsible for the continued hyperventilation?

Case 10 ACUTE EXACERBATION OF CHRONIC OBSTRUCTIVE PULMONARY DISEASE

A 62-year-old (60 kg) man with a history of chronic bronchitis is examined in the emergency department for shortness of breath and expectoration of large amounts of yellow sputum. The following blood gases, vital signs, bloodwork, and electrolytes were drawn in the emergency department:

Arterial Blood Gases

FIO_2	0.21
pH	7.23
$PaCO_2$	80 mm Hg
$[HCO_3]$	34 mEq/L
PaO_2	39 mm Hg
SaO_2	52%

Vital Signs

Pulse	130/min
BP	130/110
Temperature	38.5° C
RR	35/min

Bloodwork

White blood cell [WBC]	17,000 mm^3
[Hb]	17 g%
Hct	51%

Plasma Electrolytes

Na^+	139 mEq/L
CO_2	36 mEq/L
Cl^-	89 mEq/L
K^+	4.1 mEq/L

10A Questions

1. Classify the arterial blood gas.
2. In general, what first-line supportive treatment is usually indicated when a normal patient presents with acute severe respiratory acidosis and hypoxemia?
3. Is intubation and mechanical ventilation indicated in this patient? Why? What special form of mechanical ventilation might be useful?
4. What is the most important priority in the treatment of this patient's blood gas? What treatment is indicated for supportive therapy?
5. What is the target PaO_2 in the clinical management of COPD associated with chronic hypercapnia?
6. In an acute exacerbation of COPD, how much does the PaO_2 usually increase for a 1% increase in inspired oxygen concentration?
7. What FIO_2 should be administered to this patient?
8. Is the plasma $[HCO_3]$ in the laboratory normal range?
9. Why is the plasma $[HCO_3]$ elevated in this patient? Is this an acute process?
10. Is the plasma $[HCO_3]$ consistent with the total CO_2 finding on the electrolyte report?

11. Is the chloride normal in this patient? Explain.
12. Are the values for [Hb] and Hct normal? Explain.
13. Is the WBC count normal? Explain.
14. Is the temperature normal?
15. Are the pulse and blood pressure readings within normal limits? Explain.

The patient was treated with low-flow oxygen therapy and aerosol bronchodilators. Nevertheless, his condition did not improve. He showed progressive hypercapnia, acidemia, and a diminished level of consciousness. The patient was therefore intubated and was placed on mechanical ventilation. Approximately 1 hour after the initiation of mechanical ventilation, the patient manifested seizures and arrhythmias. Arterial blood gases were drawn:

Arterial Blood Gases

FIO_2	0.4
pH	7.68
$PaCO_2$	35 mm Hg
$[HCO_3]$	40 mEq/L
PaO_2	120 mm Hg
SaO_2	99%

10B Questions

1. Classify the arterial blood gas.
2. What is the probable cause of the metabolic alkalosis?
3. What is a possible reason for the seizures and arrhythmias?
4. The $PaCO_2$ should be lowered (rapidly/slowly) via mechanical ventilation in acute exacerbation of COPD.
5. The target $PaCO_2$ during mechanical ventilation of this patient is approximately (40 mm Hg/50 mm Hg or higher).
6. This patient's response to oxygen therapy was (poor/good).
7. The response to oxygen therapy suggests (absolute/relative) shunting.

Case 11   MITRAL VALVE REPLACEMENT

A 53-year-old man is admitted to the hospital for mitral valve replacement. While awaiting surgery, he becomes disoriented. Arterial blood gases are drawn:

Arterial Blood Gases

FIO_2	0.21
pH	7.20
$PaCO_2$	22 mm Hg
[BE]	−18 mEq/L
PaO_2	82 mm Hg
SaO_2	92%

Vital Signs

Pulse	141/min
BP	75/P*
Temperature	37° C
RR	24/min

(P* = diastolic BP cannot be measured.)

Bloodwork

Hct	44%
[WBC]	9000 mm³

Plasma Electrolytes

Na^+	140 mEq/L
CO_2	11 mEq/L
Cl^-	108 mEq/L
K^+	5.1 mEq/L

11A Questions

1. The patient appears to have gone into (lactic acidosis/ketoacidosis).
2. The patient is most likely in (hypovolemic/septic/cardiogenic) shock.
3. The anion gap is (normal/decreased/increased).
4. Hypoxia (can/cannot) be present without hypoxemia.
5. Classify the blood gas.
6. Is the degree of compensation typical for a simple metabolic acidosis?

The patient is stabilized and later goes to the operating room. After surgery, the patient is put on a mechanical ventilator and the following arterial blood gases, vital signs, laboratory data, and hemodynamic data are obtained:

Arterial Blood Gases

FIO_2	1.0
pH	7.42

PaCO$_2$	32 mm Hg
[BE]	–4 mEq/L
PaO$_2$	240 mm Hg
SaO$_2$	99%

Vital Signs

Pulse	110/min
BP	130/80
Temperature	37° C
RR	12/min

Bloodwork

Hct	22%
[Hb]	5 g%
[WBC]	14,000 mm^3

Plasma Electrolytes

Na$^+$	140 mEq/L
CO$_2$	12 mEq/L
Cl$^-$	105 mEq/L
K$^+$	5.3 mEq/L

Hemodynamic Profile

Central venous pressure (CVP)	7 mm Hg
Pulmonary artery pressure (PAP)	28/12 mm Hg
Pulmonary wedge pressure (PWP)	9 mm Hg
Cardiac output (CO)	4.8 L/min
S$\bar{v}$O$_2$	60%
P$\bar{v}$O$_2$	32 mm Hg

11B Questions

1. Classify the arterial blood gas.
2. The mixed venous oxygen values are (less/greater) than normal.
3. What is the major problem in tissue oxygenation at this time?
4. This patient is presently (well/poorly) oxygenated.
5. What treatment does this patient need to improve oxygenation?
6. What is the likely cause of the respiratory alkalosis?
7. At this time, the metabolic acidosis is most likely (primary/compensatory).
8. The FIO$_2$ should be (reduced/left as is).

The patient was given many units of blood and the [Hb] was stabilized. The following

day, arterial blood gases and vital signs were as follows:

Arterial Blood Gases

FIO$_2$	0.5
pH	7.57
PaCO$_2$	32 mm Hg
[BE]	6 mEq/L
PaO$_2$	90 mm Hg
SaO$_2$	98%

Vital Signs

Pulse	110/min
BP	130/80
Temperature	37° C
RR	12/min

11C Questions

1. Classify the arterial blood gas.
2. What is the probable cause of the metabolic alkalosis?
3. The oxyhemoglobin curve in this patient is likely shifted to the (left/right).

Case 12   PATIENT WITH BURNS

A 28-year-old man is trapped in a fire in the hospital laundry room and has an inhalation injury and burns over 35% of his body. As oxygen is being initiated in the emergency department, he is placed on a pulse oximeter and arterial blood gases are drawn. Blood gases, electrolytes, pulse oximetry, and vital signs show the following:

Arterial Blood Gases

FIO$_2$	0.21
pH	7.29
PaCO$_2$	28 mm Hg
[BE]	–12 mEq/L
PaO$_2$	72 mm Hg
SaO$_2$	(calculated) 95%

Vital Signs

Pulse	118/min
BP	130/90
Temperature	38° C
RR	32/min

Pulse Oximetry

SpO$_2$	94%

Plasma Electrolytes

Na^+	136 mEq/L
CO_2	16 mEq/L
Cl^-	102 mEq/L
K^+	4.6 mEq/L

12A Questions

1. Is the PaO_2 a value that is usually considered clinically acceptable?
2. Is the calculated SaO_2 in the acceptable range?
3. Is the SpO_2 acceptable?
4. Classify the patient's blood gas.
5. The anion gap is (high/low/normal).
6. Is there any reason to believe that this patient is hypoxic?
7. What measurement device would provide a true measurement of fractional oxygen saturation?
8. The oxygen saturation as measured via pulse oximetry represents (functional/fractional) saturation.
9. Carboxyhemoglobin is read as (oxygenated/desaturated) hemoglobin via pulse oximetry.
10. The metabolic acidosis on the admission blood gas is most likely a result of (HbCO/decreased PaO_2).

The HbCO% is measured via a CO-oximeter and is 40%. Therefore, FIO_2 1.0 is administered to the patient. A pulmonary artery catheter is inserted because the fluid balance is an important aspect of severe burn management. Three hours later, arterial and mixed venous blood gases are drawn, and pulmonary hemodynamics are measured:

Arterial Blood Gases

FIO_2	1.0
pH	7.23
$PaCO_2$	25 mm Hg
[BE]	−16 mEq/L
PaO_2	68 mm Hg
SaO_2	88%

Vital Signs

Pulse	135/min
BP	75/P*
Temperature	38° C
RR	35/min

(P* = diastolic BP cannot be measured.)

CO-oximetry

HbCO%	12%

Bloodwork

Hct	52%
[WBC]	14,000 mm^3
Lactate	6 mM/L

Plasma Electrolytes

Na^+	128 mEq/L
CO_2	12 mEq/L
Cl^-	98 mEq/L
K^+	5.8 mEq/L

Hemodynamic Profile

CVP	1 mm Hg
PAP	20/8 mm Hg
PWP	4 mm Hg
CO	2.8 L/min
$S\bar{v}O_2$	54%
$P\bar{v}O_2$	30 mm Hg

12B Questions

1. Tissue hypoxia and lactic acidosis (do/do not) appear to be present in the follow-up patient data.
2. The lactic acidosis (is/is not) due to HbCO on this blood gas. Explain.
3. The half-life of HbCO on FIO_2 1.0 is approximately (1/5) hour(s).
4. The type of hypoxia that seems to be present is (hypoxemic/circulatory/anemic/histotoxic) hypoxia.
5. This patient appears to be in (cardiogenic/hypovolemic) shock.
6. The Hct is usually (low/high) in the first few hours after severe burns.
7. Why is the [K^+] increased?
8. The $S\bar{v}O_2$ and $P\bar{v}O_2$ are (normal/increased/decreased).
9. The FIO_2/PaO_2 relationship suggests (absolute/relative) shunting.
10. $\dot{V}CO_2$ in burn patients is often (increased/decreased).

After progressive hypoxemia and hypercapnia, 4 days later he is on a mechanical ventilator and 15 cm H_2O positive end-expiratory pressure (PEEP). Blood gas and hemodynamic data are as follows:

Arterial Blood Gases

FIO_2	0.8
pH	7.34
$PaCO_2$	38 mm Hg
[BE]	−5 mEq/L
PaO_2	58 mm Hg
SaO_2	88%

Mechanical Ventilation

PEEP	15 cm H_2O

Hemodynamic Profile

CVP	8 mm Hg
PAP	32/12 mm Hg
PWP	12 mm Hg
CO	3.7 L/min
$S\bar{v}O_2$	60%
$P\bar{v}O_2$	30 mm Hg

12C Questions

1. Is the absolute capillary shunting at this point due to congestive heart failure?
2. This patient most likely has (a pulmonary emboli/acute respiratory distress syndrome [ARDS]).
3. The $P\bar{v}O_2$ suggests that tissue oxygenation is (good/less than optimal).

After an increase in PEEP to 20 cm H_2O, the following blood gas and hemodynamic data are obtained:

Arterial Blood Gas

FIO_2	0.8
pH	7.35
$PaCO_2$	36 mm Hg
[BE]	−5 mEq/L
PaO_2	77 mm Hg
SaO_2	91%

Mechanical Ventilation

PEEP	20 cm H_2O

Hemodynamic Profile

CVP	16 mm Hg
PAP	35/14 mm Hg
PWP	14 mm Hg
CO	3 L/min
$S\bar{v}O_2$	50%
$P\bar{v}O_2$	25 mm Hg

12D Questions

1. Did the PaO_2 and SaO_2 improve with the higher level of PEEP?
2. At this point PEEP should be (increased/left as is/decreased).

Case 13 CHRONIC OBSTRUCTIVE PULMONARY DISEASE AND CONGESTIVE HEART FAILURE

This patient is a 53-year-old woman with emphysema and congestive heart failure. She is on a chronic regime of digitalis, Lasix, and steroids. She presents to the emergency department with weakness and shortness of breath. The following blood gases, vital signs, blood-work, and electrolytes were reported in the emergency department:

Arterial Blood Gases

FIO_2	0.21
pH	7.43
$PaCO_2$	78 mm Hg
[HCO_3]	50 mEq/L
PaO_2	51 mm Hg
SaO_2	88%

Vital Signs

Pulse	126/min
BP	110/80
Temperature	37° C
RR	26/min

Bloodwork

WBC	8000 mm^3
[Hb]	16 g%
Hct	48%

Plasma Electrolytes

Na^+	142 mEq/L
CO_2	51 mEq/L
Cl^-	80 mEq/L
K^+	2.6 mEq/L

13A Questions

1. Classify the arterial blood gas based on the simple principles of classification that are described in Chapter 2.
2. State any conditions that are present that might alert the clinician to the potential that a mixed disturbance exists.

3. Is the plasma [HCO_3] consistent with the total CO_2 reported on the electrolyte report?
4. Is the patient receiving any drugs that could cause metabolic alkalosis? If so, name them.
5. Are there any electrolyte abnormalities that could contribute to metabolic alkalosis in this patient? Explain.
6. Is it possible that congestive heart failure (disease itself) can cause metabolic alkalosis? Explain.
7. What drugs that this patient is receiving could lead to hypokalemia?
8. How should the metabolic alkalosis be treated in this patient?
9. Is oxygen therapy indicated? If so, what is the target PaO_2?
10. What FIO_2 is indicated?
11. What could explain the weakness in this patient?

Because of cardiac arrhythmias and this patient's marginal cardiovascular status, she was admitted to the hospital. A pulmonary artery catheter was inserted to evaluate more accurately her cardiac function and fluid status. Hemodynamic findings and mixed venous oxygenation values are shown below:

Hemodynamic Profile and Mixed Venous Oxygenation

CVP	15 mm Hg
PAP	45/25 mm Hg
PWP	9 mm Hg
$S\bar{v}O_2$	74%
$P\bar{v}O_2$	38 mm Hg
CO	5.4 L/min

13B Questions

1. Does the pulmonary wedge pressure indicate left-sided heart failure?
2. Is the CVP pressure normal?
3. The pulmonary vascular resistance appears to be (normal/above normal/ below normal) in this patient.
4. Increased pulmonary vascular resistance is common in chronic obstructive pulmonary disease (COPD) because of (low alveolar PO_2/alkalemia).

5. Pulmonary artery diastolic pressure is sometimes used as a substitute for PWP. Is this practice acceptable in this patient if the wedge balloon malfunctions?

Case 14 PULMONARY EDEMA

This 50-year-old patient was recently transferred to the intensive care unit from the emergency department after progressive cardiopulmonary distress that culminated in a cardiac arrest. The patient is presently intubated and receiving mechanical ventilation. Current arterial blood gases, laboratory data, and vital signs are shown below:

Arterial Blood Gases

FIO_2	0.7
pH	7.20
$PaCO_2$	50 mm Hg
[BE]	−9 mEq/L
PaO_2	64 mm Hg
SaO_2	85%

Vital Signs

Pulse	100/min
BP	70/P
Temperature	37° C
RR	20/min

Bloodwork

WBC	11,000 mm^3
BUN	25 mg/dL
Glucose	120 mg/dL
Lactate	75 mg/dL

Plasma Electrolytes

Na^+	140 mEq/L
CO_2	15 mEq/L
Cl^-	105 mEq/L
K^+	5.4 mEq/L

14A Questions

1. Classify the PaO_2.
2. Is mild hypoxemia associated with hypoxia in normal individuals?
3. The PaO_2 is a direct measure of (combined/dissolved) oxygen.
4. What percentage of arterial blood oxygen is usually in the dissolved state?

5. The PaO_2 provides (no/some indirect) information about the amount of combined oxygen.

6. The relationship between PaO_2 and SaO_2 is expressed in the (shunt equation/oxyhemoglobin dissociation curve).

7. The normal SaO_2 expected at a PaO_2 of approximately 60 mm Hg is _____ %.

8. As seen in this patient, an SaO_2 of only 85% with a PaO_2 of 64 mm Hg means that oxyhemoglobin affinity is (increased/decreased/normal).

9. In this patient, the oxyhemoglobin curve is shifted to the (left/right).

10. What could explain the change in oxyhemoglobin affinity in this patient?

11. Does this patient appear to have adequate tissue oxygenation?

12. What vital sign information may suggest that this patient has tissue hypoxia?

13. Classify this patient's acid-base status based on the blood gas report.

14. What underlying cause is probably responsible for the respiratory acidosis?

15. The first step in determining the cause of a metabolic acidosis is to calculate the _____ .

16. This patient's anion gap is _____.

17. This anion gap suggests (increased fixed acids/decreased bases) in the blood.

18. State four general causes of increased fixed acids.

19. What is the most likely cause of metabolic acidosis in this patient?

20. Is the lactate level normal?

21. What is the most likely explanation for why the potassium concentration has increased?

22. What are the four general mechanisms of hypoxemia in the acute care setting?

23. What is the normal PaO_2 when breathing FIO_2 of 0.7?

24. This patient (must/does not) have increased shunting.

25. This patient has predominantly (absolute/relative) shunting because the response to oxygen therapy is (good/poor).

26. State at least three common cardio-pulmonary disorders that can cause increased absolute shunting.

27. State the two major categories of pulmonary edema.

Invasive Monitoring

The patient's chest radiograph showed diffuse lung infiltrates consistent with cardiogenic pulmonary edema or ARDS. A pulmonary artery catheter was inserted, and the following readings were obtained:

Hemodynamic Profile and Mixed Venous Oxygenation

CVP	10 mm Hg
PAP	50/20 mm Hg
PWP	22 mm Hg
$S\bar{v}O_2$	40%
$P\bar{v}O_2$	28 mm Hg
CO	2.4 L/min

14B Questions

1. What is the most important hemodynamic index to differentiate cardiogenic pulmonary edema from noncardiogenic pulmonary edema?

2. (Left-sided heart failure/ARDS) is responsible for the pulmonary edema in this patient at this time.

3. Is the CVP usually high in left-sided heart failure?

4. Why is the CVP not excessively high in this patient?

5. What type of supportive pulmonary treatment is often effective in the treatment of absolute pulmonary shunting disorders?

6. Is PEEP contraindicated in this patient because of the low blood pressure?

7. Should this patient's feet be elevated because his blood pressure is low?

8. What type of drug can be given to this patient to decrease blood volume?

9. What drug is usually indicated to improve cardiac contractility and function in congestive heart failure?

10. The mixed venous oxygenation values are (low/high/normal) and suggest that the patient (is/is not) hypoxic.

The patient was managed aggressively with digitalis, diuretics, and fluid restriction. The next day, blood gases, hemodynamic measurements, and electrolytes were as follows:

Arterial Blood Gases

FIO_2	0.5
pH	7.54
$PaCO_2$	39 mm Hg
[BE]	−9 mEq/L
PaO_2	74 mm Hg
SaO_2	95%

Vital Signs

Pulse	110/min
BP	75/P
Temperature	37° C
RR	25/min

Plasma Electrolytes

Na^+	135 mEq/L
CO_2	30 mEq/L
Cl^-	90 mEq/L
K^+	2.5 mEq/L

Hemodynamic Profile

CVP	2 mm Hg
PAP	20/8 mm Hg
PWP	7 mm Hg
CO	3.1 L/min

14C Questions

1. Classify the blood gas.
2. Classify the blood gas based on the new base excess (see answer to question 1).
3. What factors may contribute to the metabolic alkalosis at this time?
4. Is this patient still in shock?
5. Should it be assumed that the patient is still in cardiogenic shock?
6. At this point in time the patient may benefit from being in the (sitting/supine) position.
7. What acid-base/electrolyte factors would contraindicate weaning the patient from the mechanical ventilator at this time?

ANSWERS TO ARTERIAL BLOOD GAS CASE STUDIES

CASE 1A

1. A saturation of 80% does not make sense with a PaO_2 of 145 mm Hg.

Both of these measurements cannot be correct.
2. The PaO_2 cannot be correct. A PaO_2 of 145 mm Hg cannot be achieved by breathing room air. Furthermore, the patient's vital signs are not congruent with the blood gas report.
3. Air in the sample could explain these results because it would increase the PaO_2 and decrease the $PaCO_2$.

CASE 1B

1. Uncompensated respiratory acidosis with moderate hypoxemia.
2. Hypoventilation, relative shunting, absolute shunting, diffusion defect.
3. Hypoventilation is present ($PaCO_2$ of 64 mm Hg), which is responsible, at least in part, for the hypoxemia.
4. The $P(A-a)O_2$ on room air can be used to make this differentiation. When the $P(A-a)O_2$ is less than 20 mm Hg, simple hypoventilation is the cause; however, when the value exceeds 20 mm Hg, increased physiologic shunting is also present.
5. $PAO_2 = (PB-PH_2O) \times 0.21 - 1.2 (PaCO_2)$.
6. $P(A-a)O_2 = 25$ mm Hg.
7. Does have increased physiologic shunting, which may be due to pulmonary aspiration.
8. Mechanical ventilation.

CASE 2

1. Partially compensated metabolic acidosis with normoxemia.
2. The anion gap is high (i.e., $A^- = 21$ mEq/L). $Na - (TCO_2 + Cl) = A^-$ (normal 12–14 mEq/L)
3. There is no evidence to support hypoxia.
4. The lactate concentration is in the normal range (<18 mg/dL). Note that the units are mg/dL. Normal values are much lower in mM/L or mEq/L.
5. The glucose concentration is normal (normal fasting glucose, 70 to 150 mg/dL).
6. The creatinine is greatly increased (normal < 1.5 mg/dL).

7. The BUN is greatly increased (normal < 23 mg/dL).
8. The [K+] is increased (normal < 5 mEq/L).
9. The metabolic acidosis is due to *azotemic renal failure*.
10. The hypocapnia appears to be compensatory; it is consistent with expected compensation because the $PaCO_2$ (25 mm Hg) approximates the last two digits of the pH (0.22). Furthermore, these values fall within the band for simple metabolic acidosis on the acid-base map.

CASE 3

1. Partially compensated metabolic acidosis with normoxemia.
2. The anion gap is normal (14 mEq/L).
3. The plasma chloride concentration is high (hyperchloremia). It is normally at a concentration of about 103 mEq/L.
4. The probable cause of the hyperchloremic (normal anion gap) acidosis in this patient is the history of *severe diarrhea*.
5. The potassium concentration is low (<3.5 mEq/L).
6. Potassium is lost secondary to GI fluid loss dehydration with the diarrhea.
7. Acetazolamide (Diamox) can cause hyperchloremic metabolic acidosis because it is a carbonic anhydrase inhibitor.
8. Renal tubular acidosis leads to normal anion gap metabolic acidosis.

CASE 4A

1. Compensated metabolic acidosis with severe hypoxemia.
2. Yes, the presence of *excessive (i.e., complete) compensation* suggests a mixed acid-base disturbance. In addition, the *history of asthma* and the presence of *severe hypoxemia* should be considered in the acid-base evaluation.
3. No, therefore we can be virtually sure that a mixed acid-base disturbance is present.
4. Mixed respiratory alkalosis and metabolic acidosis (two primary acid-base problems).
5. The severe hypoxemia is responsible for part, if not all, of the hyperventilation. Perhaps the restrictive component of the asthma may also contribute to the hyperventilation.
6. The most likely explanation for the metabolic acidosis is lactic acidosis as a consequence of severe hypoxemia and tissue hypoxia.
7. The most important treatment at this time is oxygen therapy to relieve the severe hypoxemia.
8. Recent evidence suggests it is best to first attempt low-flow (concentration) oxygen during acute exacerbation.[700] Nevertheless, higher FIO_2 may be required and it is imperative to correct the apparent lactic acidosis.
9. The increased blood pressure, heart rate, and respiratory rate are all normal physiologic responses to severe hypoxemia. These effects may be mediated via the peripheral chemoreceptors.

CASE 4B

1. Partially compensated respiratory alkalosis with moderate hypoxemia. The clinician should keep in mind that a mixed disturbance may still be present.
2. Lactate can be metabolized quickly by the liver in the presence of adequate oxygen. This may explain some improvement in [HCO_3].
3. Compensation alone may explain these results but lactic acidosis is also common in severe asthma. A lactate measurement would aid in diagnosis.
4. The current values fall within the band for chronic respiratory alkalosis.

CASE 4C

1. Uncompensated metabolic acidosis with moderate hypoxemia.
2. It cannot be assumed that the patient is better. He may have reached the point of exhaustion and may be headed toward ventilatory failure. The continued worsening of vital signs and PaO_2 are highly suggestive of this common phenomenon in status asthmaticus. The patient should be watched closely to determine if mechanical ventilation is required.

3. Is not. Decreased and inaudible wheezing may indicate decreased air flow and patient deterioration.

CASE 4D

1. Uncompensated metabolic acidosis with normoxemia.
2. Eucapnic ventilation after hypocapnia; the bicarbonate was low earlier owing to a compensatory mechanism. Now that the respiratory alkalosis has been corrected, the low bicarbonate appears as a primary metabolic acidosis. Nevertheless, other potential causes of primary metabolic acidosis should be considered and ruled out.

CASE 5

1. The SaO_2 at a PaO_2 of 60 mm Hg is normally 90%.
2. The oxyhemoglobin curve has shifted to the right owing to acidemia and hypercapnia.
3. Yes.
4. No, the increased bicarbonate is simply a result of the acute hypercapnia and the effect of hydrolysis (see Chapter 5).
5. Yes, in acute hypercapnia the *base excess of the blood* gives falsely low values due to in vivo/in vitro effects, and the actual bicarbonate reads falsely high owing to the hydrolysis effect (see Chapter 5).
6. The plasma $[HCO_3]$ increases approximately 1 mEq/L for every 10 mm Hg increase in PCO_2 acutely.
7. Intubation and mechanical ventilation is indicated. Hyperventilation may be indicated to decrease ICP.

CASE 6

1. Partially compensated metabolic alkalosis with normoxemia.
2. Yes.
3. Loss of excessive gastric secretions.
4. Hypochloremia.
5. Hypokalemia is common.
6. Loss of fluids is important (see Chapter 13).
7. Appropriate treatment must include replacement of fluids, chloride, and potassium.

CASE 7

1. Mixed respiratory and metabolic alkalosis with mild hypoxemia.
2. Severe vomiting can cause metabolic alkalosis.
3. Respiratory alkalosis is common in the third trimester of pregnancy.
4. Hyperventilation is common in the third trimester of pregnancy owing to: (1) mechanical difficulty (i.e., upward displacement of the diaphragm), and (2) progesterone stimulates ventilation.

CASE 8A

1. No, cyanosis and a sample of dark blood (suggesting poor oxygenation and possible methemoglobinemia) are incongruent with the PaO_2 and pulse oximeter readings (suggesting good oxygenation).
2. Yes, a repeat blood gas would be appropriate because of the incongruencies. It should also be analyzed via CO-oximetry.

CASE 8B

1. (Four to five × the percentage of oxygen inspired) $5 \times 50 = 250$ mm Hg.
2. No, 240 mm Hg is within the expected range.
3. Yes, the cyanosis suggests an oxygenation disturbance; however, an explanation of why this would occur must be sought. Remember, hypoxia can exist without hypoxemia.
4. Methemoglobinemia.
5. Yes.
6. (<1%–1.5%).
7. Yes, infants younger than 6 months of age are particularly vulnerable to methemoglobinemia, especially when exposed to water from a well, because it contains nitrates.
8. Administration of methylene blue accelerates the reduction of methemoglobin.
9. A pulse oximeter cannot detect methemoglobin but in its presence SpO_2 migrates toward 85%.
10. Oxidized.
11. CO-oximetry.

CASE 9A

1. Partially compensated metabolic acidosis with hyperoxemia.
2. Hyperventilation on room air can cause hyperoxemia (i.e., PaO_2 > 100 mm Hg).
3. The maximum PaO_2 that can be achieved during hyperventilation by breathing room air is approximately 130 mm Hg.
4. This is a very high anion gap metabolic acidosis (A^- = 34 mEq/L).
5. Ketoacidosis.
6. Some buildup of lactic acid is expected during ketoacidosis.
7. Acetoacetic acid and beta-hydroxybutyric acid.
8. The concentration of acetoacetic acid is high (normal < 10 mg/dL).
9. *Hyperglycemia* is seen in diabetic ketoacidosis because the glucose cannot enter the cells in the absence of insulin. Hyperglycemia also causes hyperosmolar diuresis (*polyuria* secondary to the high osmotic pressure).
10. Hyperkalemia is expected owing to intracellular/extracellular hydrogen ion–potassium exchanges. In addition, the general tissue breakdown that occurs in ketoacidosis releases intracellular potassium to the plasma.
11. Dehydration is common in diabetic keto-acidosis due to polyuria and vomiting.
12. Kussmaul's breathing.
13. Blood pressure is frequently *low*, and BUN is slightly increased.
14. Fat metabolism.
15. Acetone.
16. Sodium bicarbonate treatment is recommended because the pH is less than 7.10 and, most importantly, because the potassium is substantially elevated.

CASE 9B

1. Mixed respiratory and metabolic alkalosis with normoxemia.
2. Factors that may contribute to metabolic alkalosis include overcorrection with $NaHCO_3$, the conversion of ketones into bicarbonate by the liver, and hypokalemia.
3. Persistent hyperventilation is common after metabolic acidosis, probably secondary to CSF acidosis.

CASE 10A

1. Partially compensated respiratory acidosis with severe hypoxemia.
2. Intubation and mechanical ventilation.
3. No, because this patient has COPD. Intubation and mechanical ventilation should be avoided in these patients if at all possible, and low-flow oxygen therapy has worked well in many cases. Bronchial hygiene is also a very important part of therapy. Noninvasive positive pressure ventilation has also been shown to be effective.
4. Increasing the PaO_2 is the utmost priority. Low-flow oxygen therapy is indicated.
5. 60 mm Hg.
6. As a crude rule of thumb, in acute exacerbation of COPD, PaO_2 typically increases 3 mm Hg/0.01 FIO_2 increase (see Chapter 10).
7. The FIO_2 should be 0.28. (This is based on an expected 3-mm Hg increase/0.01 FIO_2 increase and a target PaO_2 of 60 mm Hg.) Pulse oximetry should be used to titrate therapy to 90% SpO_2.
8. No. Normal plasma bicarbonate is 24 ± 2 mEq/L. The plasma [HCO_3] is elevated in this patient.
9. The plasma [HCO_3] probably increased as a compensatory mechanism for the chronic respiratory acidosis and because of the hypercapnia and hydrolysis. In fact, if lactic acidosis is also present (a distinct possibility with a PaO_2 of 39 mm Hg), the plasma [HCO_3] may actually be lower than this patient's chronic normal baseline level.
10. Yes. The total CO_2 and [HCO_3] should be very close, and they are. It is also common for the TCO_2 to be slightly higher because it is measured in venous blood.
11. No. The patient has hypochloremia. This finding is expected in chronic respiratory acidosis. When the bicarbonate anion increases as a compensatory mechanism, the chloride anion decreases to maintain electroneutrality (see Chapter 12).

12. No. They are both elevated. The finding of secondary polycythemia is common in COPD, especially in chronic bronchitis. This is a compensatory mechanism to increase oxygen transport in the presence of hypoxemia.

13. No. The WBC count is elevated (normal < 10,000 cells/mm^3). This finding and the finding of yellow sputum suggest a bacterial infection/pneumonia.

14. The temperature is elevated, which is also consistent with infection or pneumonia.

15. The pulse and blood pressure are both slightly elevated. Again, this is the normal response to hypoxemia.

CASE 10B

1. Uncompensated metabolic alkalosis with hyperoxemia; however, it is known that the patient has COPD and is being mechanically ventilated. Therefore, these factors must be kept in mind.

2. The metabolic alkalosis is most likely due to eucapnic ventilation posthypercapnia. In other words, the patient is being ventilated at a lower $PaCO_2$ than is his normal chronic value. Therefore, the bicarbonate that was retained as compensation for both the acute and chronic respiratory acidosis now appears as a primary metabolic alkalosis.

3. Severe metabolic alkalemia may cause these effects. The CSF may be even more alkalotic than the blood because the CSF has less buffering capacity. Furthermore, seizures have been reported after the rapid reversal of hypercapnia in exacerbation of COPD.

4. Slowly.

5. 50 mm Hg or higher because this is probably near this patient's normal chronic baseline.

6. Good response to oxygen therapy (i.e., PaO_2 of 120 mm Hg on FIO_2 of 0.4).

7. Relative shunting, which is typical in COPD and $\dot{V}/\dot{Q}$ mismatch.

CASE 11A

1. Lactic acidosis is likely with a BP of 75/P.

2. Cardiogenic shock is likely based on the patient's cardiovascular history.

3. Anion gap increased ($A^- = 23$ mEq/L). (Normal 12–14 mEq/L)

4. Hypoxia can be present without hypoxemia.

5. Partially compensated metabolic acidosis with normoxemia.

6. Yes, the last two digits of the pH approximate the $PaCO_2$, and the values fall within the band for simple metabolic acidosis on the acid-base map.

CASE 11B

1. Completely compensated respiratory alkalosis with hyperoxemia.

2. The mixed venous oxygen values are less than normal. Normal $P\bar{v}O_2$ is greater than 35 mm Hg and normal $S\bar{v}O_2$ is greater than 75%. This suggests hypoxia.

3. Severe anemia ([Hb] 5 g%).

4. Poorly oxygenated due to the severe anemia despite a normal PaO_2 and cardiac output.

5. Blood transfusion.

6. Overzealous mechanical ventilation (or perhaps the mechanical ventilator is exaggerating the respiratory compensatory response to a primary metabolic acidosis).

7. Primary, based on the severe anemia and probable lactic acidosis.

8. The FIO_2 should probably be left as is until the severe anemia is treated; it should then be reduced because of the hyperoxemia.

CASE 11C

1. Combined respiratory and metabolic alkalosis with normoxemia.

2. The blood transfusions (citrate preservative) may be completely or partially responsible for the delayed metabolic alkalosis (see Chapter 13).

3. The curve would be shifted to the left because of the decreased [H$^+$] (alkalemia) and hypocapnia. Stored blood transfusions may also shift the curve to the left because of decreased DPG. However, DPG levels are usually back to normal 24 hours after transfusion.

CASE 12A

1. Yes. A PaO_2 of 72 mm Hg, although mildly hypoxemic, is usually considered to be clinically acceptable.
2. Yes. An SaO_2 of 95% is acceptable. Nevertheless, use of a calculated SaO_2, especially in a patient with burns, is not reliable.
3. The saturation reading on the pulse oximeter (SpO_2) is also acceptable. Here again, however, this reading is not reliable in the patient with burns and smoke inhalation.
4. Partially compensated metabolic acidosis with mild hypoxemia.
5. The A^- is high (18 mEq/L).
6. Yes. Carboxyhemoglobinemia is common after smoke inhalation, and metabolic acidosis may suggest lactic acidosis.
7. A CO-oximeter could measure fractional saturation as well as HbCO%.
8. Oxygen saturation measured by pulse oximetry represents functional saturation. Functional saturation does not reflect abnormal Hb species such as metHb or HbCO.
9. HbCO will be read as oxygenated Hb via pulse oximetry.
10. HbCO is most likely to be responsible for the metabolic acidosis on the blood gas when the patient was admitted to the hospital.

CASE 12B

1. Lactic acidosis is apparently still present and is shown by a high anion gap acidosis and increased lactate (normal < 2 mM/L). The low mixed venous oxygen values also suggest tissue hypoxia.
2. The current lactic acidosis is not due to HbCO because it has fallen from 40% to 12%. The hypoxia appears to be due to a low cardiac output (i.e., BP 75/P) and CO 2.8 L/min.
3. The half-life of HbCO on FIO_2 of 1.0 is approximately 1 hour. While the patient is breathing room air, the half-life of HbCO is 5 hours.
4. Circulatory hypoxia because the cardiac output is only 2.8 L/min and BP is very low.

5. The patient appears to be in hypovolemic shock, which is shown by the low CVP and low sodium. Furthermore, it is well known that sodium and fluids generally move to the extravascular space after severe burns. Cardiogenic shock is not present, which is substantiated by the low PWP.
6. The Hct is usually high in the first few hours after severe burns because of hemoconcentration secondary to the loss of intravascular fluid to the extravascular space.
7. The potassium concentration is usually elevated in burns due to the destruction of cells and to the release of intracellular potassium into the plasma. Also, the exchange of intracellular potassium ions for hydrogen ions in acidemia increases the serum potassium.
8. $S\bar{v}O_2$ and $P\bar{v}O_2$ are decreased and, because of the relatively normal PaO_2, this is highly suggestive of hypoxia of circulatory origin.
9. Absolute shunting. Oxygenation ratio <1.0.
10. CO_2 production is often increased in burn patients.

CASE 12C

1. No. Congestive heart failure would be associated with a high pulmonary wedge pressure (e.g., PWP > 18 mm Hg).
2. ARDS is common after severe burns with inhalation injury and is characterized by severe hypoxemia despite increased FIO_2.
3. Less than optimal.

CASE 12D

1. The PaO_2 and SaO_2 are both improved.
2. The PEEP should be decreased. Although the PaO_2 and SaO_2 have improved, the mixed venous oxygen indices and the cardiac output have deteriorated. The gains in reversing the pulmonary shunt are offset by an apparent decrease in cardiac output. Often these cases are further clouded as peripheral shunting in sepsis leads to higher mixed venous oxygen indices. This may occur despite patient deterioration.

CASE 13A

1. Compensated metabolic alkalosis with moderate hypoxemia.
2. Long-standing pulmonary disease (i.e., COPD) and excessive compensation (more than 50% compensation). Also, the administration of Lasix and steroids and the presence of serum hypokalemia.
3. Yes. The $[HCO_3]$ and total CO_2 are very close.
4. Yes. Both Lasix and, to a lesser extent, steroids can cause metabolic alkalosis.
5. Yes. Hypokalemia and hypochloremia may lead to metabolic alkalosis.
6. Yes. Poor renal perfusion may lead to secondary hyperaldosteronism.
7. Lasix, and to a lesser extent steroids, may cause hypokalemia.
8. Potassium replacement is indicated perhaps in the form of KCl. Fluids should not be administered because of the CHF. Perhaps the diuretic acetazolamide would help to counteract the metabolic acidosis while still providing some diuresis.
9. Yes. Oxygen therapy is indicated to try to achieve a target PaO_2 of 60 mm Hg.
10. The FIO_2 indicated is 0.24 (i.e., assume 3-mm Hg increase in $PaO_2/0.01$ FIO_2 increase in acute exacerbation of COPD). Oxygen should be titrated to SpO_2 90%.
11. Hypokalemia causes muscular weakness and, if severe, may cause hypoventilation.

CASE 13B

1. No. A PWP of 9 mm Hg is normal.
2. No. The CVP pressure is elevated (normal < 10 mm Hg).
3. Above normal as indicated by a normal PWP and an increased PAP.
4. Low alveolar PO_2.
5. No. The use of pulmonary artery diastolic pressure in place of wedge pressure is *acceptable only when the pulmonary vascular resistance is normal*, which is not the case here.

CASE 14A

1. Mild hypoxemia.
2. No. Oxygen content is still good at a PaO_2 greater than 60 mm Hg.
3. Dissolved oxygen.
4. 1% to 2% of CaO_2 is in the dissolved state.
5. Some indirect.
6. Oxyhemoglobin dissociation curve.
7. 90% SaO_2 at a PaO_2 of 60 mm Hg.
8. Decreased.
9. Shifted to the right.
10. The increased $PaCO_2$ and the increased hydrogen ion concentration (i.e., decreased pH) both shift the curve to the right.
11. No; cardiovascular status is poor (low B/P).
12. BP of 70/P is indicative of shock and severely compromised cardio-vascular function (i.e., circulatory hypoxia).
13. Mixed respiratory and metabolic acidosis.
14. Extreme ventilation-perfusion mismatch (suggested by the severe shunt) or exhaustion (suggested by the history) is likely to be responsible for the respiratory acidosis. Alternatively, cerebral hypoxia associated with the cardiac arrest may be causing a neurologic deficit or inadequate mechanical ventilation may be a factor (see Chapter 13).
15. Anion gap.
16. $A^- = 20$ mEq/L.
17. Increased fixed acids in the blood are suggested by the high anion gap.
18. Toxins, azotemic renal failure, lactic acidosis, ketoacidosis.
19. Lactic acidosis secondary to circulatory hypoxia.
20. No. Normal lactate is only up to 18 mg/dL.
21. Acidemia often causes plasma hyperkalemia owing to an intracellular-extracellular exchange of K^+ for H^+. Although plasma hyperkalemia is not always seen in organic acidosis, it is still fairly common.
22. Hypoventilation, absolute shunting, relative shunting, diffusion defects.
23. Normal PaO_2 is approximately $4-5 \times$ percent inspired oxygen. Thus, 280–350 mm Hg.
24. The patient must have increased shunting (oxygenation ratio <1.0).

25. The patient has predominantly absolute shunting because the response to oxygen therapy is poor.
26. Pneumonia, atelectasis, pulmonary edema, etc.
27. Cardiogenic (congestive heart failure) and noncardiogenic pulmonary edema (ARDS).

CASE 14B

1. Pulmonary wedge pressure (PWP).
2. Left-sided heart failure is responsible for the pulmonary edema, which is indicated by a wedge pressure of 22 mm Hg (normal <12 mm Hg).
3. Yes. This is how left-sided heart failure was usually monitored before the routine availability of pulmonary artery catheters.
4. The CVP does not *always* closely parallel the pulmonary wedge pressure, which is one of the important reasons why pulmonary artery catheters are more accurate than CVP lines.
5. PEEP therapy and ARDS/net protocol.
6. No. Although PEEP should always be applied carefully when the cardiac output or BP is low. Nevertheless, PEEP may actually improve the cardiac output in left-sided heart failure by decreasing venous return and by easing the workload on the heart. Furthermore, PEEP has been shown to be effective in the treatment of cardiogenic pulmonary edema.
7. Definitely not! This would increase the venous return to a heart that is already failing. Patients in acute congestive heart failure are best placed in the sitting position. This position helps to decrease venous return, to minimize heart strain, and perhaps to improve cardiac output. It is important to understand the origin of hypotension before determining optimal positioning for the patient. *In hypovolemic shock, the feet should be elevated. The sitting position is more appropriate for cardiogenic shock.*
8. Diuretics (e.g., Lasix).
9. Digitalis.
10. The mixed venous oxygenation indices are low and suggest hypoxia.

CASE 14C

1. This blood gas is not internally consistent and is therefore not possible. It is impossible to have alkalemia without either a respiratory or metabolic alkalosis. In this case, a transcribing error occurred. The base excess should have been 9 mEq/L.
2. Uncompensated metabolic alkalosis with mild hypoxemia.
3. Factors that may contribute to the metabolic alkalosis in this patient include diuretic therapy, hypokalemia, hypochloremia, and hyperaldosteronism secondary to poor renal perfusion.
4. Yes. The patient is still in shock, which is shown by the BP 75/P.
5. No. The wedge pressure is too low for cardiogenic shock. The low CVP and other hemodynamic pressures suggest hypovolemic shock, probably as a result of the aggressive diuresis and fluid restriction.
6. The patient may benefit from being placed in the supine position, which would enhance venous return. Nevertheless, this should be approached cautiously in the patient with CHF.
7. There are two areas that need to be corrected before weaning the patient: (1) metabolic alkalosis that causes hypoventilation as a compensatory mechanism must be reversed, and (2) the hypokalemia that causes muscle weakness must be corrected. Potassium chloride would correct the hypokalemia and hypochloremia.

References

1. National Committee for Clinical Laboratory Standards (NCCLS): Blood Gas and pH Analysis and Related Measurements; Approved Guideline. NCCLS document C46-A [ISBN 1-56238-444-9]. NCCLS, 940 West Valley Road, Suite 1400, Wayne, PA 19807-1898, 2001.

2. Filley, G. F.: Acid-Base and Blood Gas Regulation. Philadelphia, Lea & Febiger, 1971.

3. U.S. Dept. of Commerce, National Bureau of Standards, Public 450: Blood pH, Gases, and Electrolytes. Washington, DC, U.S. Dept. of Commerce, 1977.

4. Severinghaus, J. W.: Interpreting acid-base balance (Letter). Respir. Care, 27:1414–1415, 1982.

5. Bunker, J. P.: The great transatlantic acid-base debate. Anesthesiology, 26:591–593, 1965.

6. National Committee for Clinical Laboratory Standards: Blood Gas Pre-Analytical Considerations: Specimen Collection, Calibration, and Controls (proposed guideline). NCCLS publication C27–P. Villanova, PA, N.C.C.L.S., 1985.

7. Andrews, J. L., Jr., Copeland, B. E., Salah, A. M., et al: Arterial blood gas standards for healthy young non-smoking subjects. Am. J. Clin. Pathol., 75:773–780, 1981.

8. Weisberg, H. F.: Water, electrolytes, acid-base and oxygen. In Davidsohn, I., and Henry, J. B. (eds): Clinical Diagnosis and Management by Laboratory Methods, 17th ed. Philadelphia, W.B. Saunders, 1984.

9. Minty, B. D., and Nunn, H. F.: Regional quality control survey of blood-gas analysis. Ann. Clin. Biol. Chem., 14:245–253, 1977.

10. Shapiro, B. A., Peruzzi, W.T., Kozelowski-Templin, R.: Clinical Application of Blood Gases, 5th ed. St. Louis, Mosby-Year Book, 1994.

11. Sorbini, C. A., Grassi, V., Solinas, E., et al: Arterial oxygen tension in relation to age in normal subjects. Respiration, 25:3–13, 1968.

12. Mellemgaard, K.: The alveolar-arterial oxygen difference: Its size and components in normal man. Acta Physiol. Scand., 67:10–20, 1966.

13. Campion, E. W.: A retreat from SI units. N. Engl. J. Med., 327:49, 1992.

14. National Committee for Clinical Laboratory Standards (NCCLS): Percutaneous Collection of Arterial Blood for Laboratory Analysis–Second Edition: Approved Standard. NCCLS document H11–A2 (ISBN 1-56238-130-X). NCCLS, 771 E. Lancaster Avenue, Villanova, PA 19085, 1992.

15. Sampling for Arterial Blood Gas Analysis. AARC Clinical Practice Guideline. Respir. Care, 37:913–917, 1992.

16. American Lung Association of Pennsylvania PTS: Clinical Pulmonary Function Testing Manual of Uniform Lab Procedures. Harrisburg, PA, ALA/PTS, 1981.

17. Texas Department of Health: Recommendations for management of HIV infection and acquired immunodeficiency syndrome. Tex. Prev. Dis. News, 48(11), 1988.

18. Erslev, A. J., and Gabzuda, T. G.: Pathophysiology of Blood, 3rd ed. Philadelphia, W.B. Saunders, 1985.

19. Centers for Disease Control. Update: Universal precautions for prevention of transmission of human immunodeficiency virus, hepatitis B virus, and other bloodborne pathogens in health care settings. MMWR, 37:377–388, 1988.

20. Department of Labor, Occupational Safety and Health Administration: Occupational exposure to bloodborne pathogens. 29 CFRR Part 1910. 1030 Federal Register, December 6, 1991.

21. Mathews, P. J.: The validity of PaO_2 values 3, 6, and 9 minutes after an FIO_2 change in mechanically ventilated heart-surgery patients. Respir. Care, 32:1029–1034, 1987.

22. Howe, J. P., Alpert, J. S., Rickman, F. D., et al: Return of arterial PO_2 values to baseline after supplemental oxygen in patients with cardiac disease. Chest, 67:256–258, 1975.

23. Hess, D., Good, C., Didyoung, R., et al: The validity of assessing arterial blood gases 10 minutes after an FIO_2 change in mechanically ventilated patients without chronic pulmonary disease. Respir. Care, 30:1037–1041, 1985.

24. Sherter, C. B., Jabbour, S. M., Kounat, D. M., and Snider, G. I.: Prolonged rate of decay of arterial PO_2 following oxygen breathing in chronic airways obstruction. Chest, 67:259–261, 1975.

25. Woolf, C. R.: Arterial blood gas levels after oxygen therapy (Letter). Chest, 69:808–809, 1976.

26. Giner, J., Casan, P., Belda, J., et al: Pain during arterial puncture. Chest, 110:1443–1445, 1996.

27. National Committee for Clinical Laboratory Standards: Additives to Blood Collection Devices: Heparin (proposed standard). N.C.C.L.S. publication H24–P. Villanova, PA, 5(13), 1985.

28. Hansen, J. E. , and Simmons, D. H.: A systematic error in the determination of blood PCO_2. Am. Rev. Respir. Dis., 115:1061–1063, 1977.

29. Morgan, E., Baidwan, B., Petty, T., and Zwillich, C.: The effect of arterial puncture on steady state blood gas tensions (Abstract). Am. Rev. Respir. Dis., 119:152, 1979.

30. Petty, T. L.: Practical Pulmonary Function Tests. Philadelphia, Lea & Febiger, 1975.

31. Guenter, C. A., and Welch, M. H.: Pulmonary Medicine, 2nd ed. Philadelphia, J.B. Lippincott, 1982.

32. ACCP-National Heart, Lung and Blood Institute. National Conference on O_2 Therapy. Respir. Care, 29:922–935, 1984.

33. Dorland's Illustrated Medical Dictionary, 28th ed. Philadelphia, W.B. Saunders, 1994.

34. Liss, H. P., Payne, C. B.: Stability of blood gases in ice and at room temperature. Chest, 103:1120–1122, 1993.

35. Petty, T. L., Bigelow, B., and Levine, B. E.: The simplicity and safety of arterial puncture. J.A.M.A., 195: 181–182, 1966.

36. Sackner, M. A., Avery, W. G., and Sokolowski, J.: Arterial puncture by nurses. Chest, 59:97–98, 1971.

37. Mortensen, J. D.: Clinical sequelae from arterial needle puncture, cannulation, and incision. Circulation, 35: 1118–1123, 1967.

38. Allen, E. V.: Thromboangitis obliterans: Methods of diagnosis of chronic occlusive arterial lesions distal to the wrist with illustrative cases. Am. J. Med. Sci., 178:237–244, 1929.

39. Bedford, R. F.: Radial arterial function following percutaneous cannulation with 18- and 20-gauge catheters. Anesthesiol., 47:37–39, 1977.

40. Scanlan, C. L.: Analysis and monitoring of gas exchange. In Scanlan, C. L., Wilkins, R. L., Stoller, J. K. (eds): Egan's Fundamentals of Respiratory Care, 7th ed. St. Louis, C.V. Mosby, 1999, pp. 337–369.

41. Watson, M. A.: Median nerve damage from brachial artery puncture: A case study. Respir. Care, 40(11): 1141–1143, 1995.

42. Berger, A.: Brachial artery puncture: The need for caution. J. Fam. Pract., 28(6):720–721, 1989.

43. McCready, R. A., Hyde, G. L., Bivins B. A., et al: Brachial arterial puncture: A definite risk to the hand. South. Med. J., 77:786–789, 1984.

44. Plunkett, P. F.: Blood gas interpretation. In Barnes, T. A. (ed): Respiratory Care Practice. Chicago, Year Book, pp. 611–618, 1994.

45. Grombeck, C., and Miller, E. L.: Nonphysician placement of arterial catheters. Chest, 104:1716–1717, 1993.

46. Felkner, D.: A protocol for teaching and maintaining arterial puncture skills among respiratory therapists. Respir. Care, 18:700–705, 1973.

47. Horovitz, J. H., and Luterman, A.: Postoperative monitoring following critical trauma. Heart Lung, 4:269–278, 1975.

48. Cannon, B. W., and Meshier, W. T.: Extremity amputation following radial artery cannulation in a patient with hyperlipoproteinemia type V. Anesthesiology, 56:222–223, 1982.

49. Gurman, G. M., and Kriemerman, S.: Cannulation of big arteries in critically ill patients. Crit. Care Med., 13:217–220, 1985.

50. Falor, W. H., Hansel, J. R., and Williams, G. B.: Gangrene of the hand: A complication of radial artery cannulation. Am. Trauma, 16:713–716, 1976.

51. Marshall, G. M., Edelstein, G., and Hirshman, C. A.: Median nerve compression following radial artery puncture. Anesth. Analg., 59:953–954, 1980.

52. Slogoff, S., Keats, A. S., and Arlund, C.: On the safety of radial artery cannulation. Anesthesiology, 59:42–47, 1983.

53. Davis, F. M., and Stewart, J. M.: Radial artery cannulation. Br. J. Anaesth., 52:41–47, 1980.

54. Evans, P. J. D., and Kerr, J. H.: Arterial occlusion after cannulation. B.M.J., 3:197–199, 1985.

55. Band, J. D., and Maki, D. G.: Infections caused by arterial catheters used for hemodynamic monitoring. Am. J. Med., 67:735–741, 1979.

56. Gardner, R. M., Schwartz, R., Wong, H. C., and Burke, J. P.: Percutaneous indwelling radial-artery catheters for monitoring cardiovascular function. N. Engl. J. Med., 290:1227–1231, 1974.

57. Smoller, B. R., Kruskall, M. S.: Phlebotomy for diagnostic laboratory tests in adults. N. Engl. J. Med., 314:1233–1235, 1986.

58. Eyester, E., Bernene, J.: Nosocomial anemia. J.A.M.A., 223:73–74, 1973.

59. Henry, M. L., Garner, W. L., Fabri, P. J.: Iatrogenic anemia. Am. J. Surg., 151:362–363, 1986.

60. Lewis, L. L., Harrington, G. R., Stoltzfus, D. P.: The effect of arterial lines on blood-drawing practices and costs in intensive care units. Chest, 108:216–219, 1995.

61. Silver, M. J., Yue-Han, L., Gragg, L. A., et al: Reduction of blood loss from diagnostic sampling in critically ill patients using a blood-conserving system. Chest, 104:1711–1715, 1993.

62. Spiegel, J. S., Shapiro, M. F., Berman, B., et al: Changing physician test ordering in a university hospital: An intervention of physician participation, explicit criteria, and feedback. Arch. Intern. Med., 149:549–553, 1989.

63. Griner, P. F., and Glaser, R. J.: Misuse of laboratory tests and diagnostic procedures. N. Engl. J. Med., 307:1336–1339, 1982.

64. Critical Care in the United States: Coordinating Intensive Care Resources for Positive Cost-effective Patient Outcomes. Anaheim, CA, Society of Critical Care Medicine, 1992, 18.

65. Blood Gas Analysis and Hemoximetry: 2001 Revision and Update. AARC Clinical Practice Guideline. Respir. Care, 45:498-505, 2001.

66. Capillary Blood Gas Sampling for Neonatal & Pediatric Patients. AARC Clinical Practice Guideline. Respir. Care, 39:1180–1183, 1994.

67. McLain, B. I., Evans, J., Dear, P. F. R.: Comparison of capillary and arterial blood gas measurements in neonates. Arch. Dis. Child., 63:743–747, 1988.

68. Goldsmith, J. P., and Karotkin, E. H.: Assisted Ventilation of the Neonate, 3rd ed. Philadelphia, W.B. Saunders, 1996.

69. Gregory, G. A.: Respiratory Failure in the Child: Clinics in Critical Care Medicine. New York, Churchill Livingstone, 1981.

70. Tenholder, M.E.: The pendulum and the arterial line (Editorial). Chest, 104:1650–1651, 1993.

71. The Future of Blood Gases: Analysis & Monitoring. J. Resp. Care Practitioners, Dec/Jan 1993.

72. Goodwin, N. M., and Schreiber, M. T.: Effects of anticoagulants on acid-base and blood gas estimations. Crit. Care Med., 7:473–474, 1979.

73. Bageant, R. A.: Variations in arterial blood gas measurements due to sampling techniques. Respir. Care, 20:565–570, 1975.

74. Scanlan, C. L.: Physical principles in respiratory care. In Scanlan, C. L., Wilkins, R. L., Stoller, J. K. (eds): Egan's Fundamentals of Respiratory Care, 7th ed. St. Louis, C.V. Mosby, 1999, pp. 337–369.

75. Rennie, D.: High science, present and future. N. Engl. J. Med., 301:1343–1344, 1979.

76. Mueller, R. G., and Lang, G. E.: Blood gas analysis: Effect of air bubbles in syringe and delay in estimation (Letter). B.M.J., 285:1659–1660, 1982.

77. Biswas, C. K., Ramos, J. M., Agroyannis, B., and Kerr, D. N. S.: Blood gas analysis: Effect of air bubbles in syringe and delay in estimation. B.M.J., 284:923–927, 1982.

78. Ishikawa, S., Fornier, A., Borst, C., and Segal, M. S.: The effects of air bubbles and time delay on blood gas analysis. Ann. Allergy, 33:72–77, 1974.

79. Madiedo, G., Sciacca, R., and Hause, L.: Air bubbles and temperature effect on blood gas analysis. J. Clin. Pathol., 33:864–867, 1980.

80. Doty, D. B., and Moseley, R. V.: Reliable sampling of arterial blood. Surg. Gynecol. Obstet., 130:701–703, 1970.

81. Comroe, J. H.: Physiology of Respiration, 2nd ed. Chicago, Year Book, 1977.

82. National Committee for Clinical Laboratory Standards: Additives to Blood Collection Devices: Heparin (proposed standard). N.C.C.L.S. publication H24–P. Villanova, PA, 5(13), 1985.

83. Fan, L. E., Dellinger, K. T., Mills, A. L., et al: Potential errors in neonatal blood gas measurements. J. Pediatr., 97:650–653, 1980.

84. Hutchison, A. S., Ralson, S. H., Dryburgh, F. J., et al: Too much heparin: Possible source of error in blood gas analysis. B.M.J., 287:1131–1132, 1983.

85. Gauver, P., Friendman, J., and Imrey, P.: Effects of syringe and filling volume on analysis of blood pH, oxygen tension and carbon dioxide tension. Respir. Care, 25:558–563, 1980.

86. Turton, M.: Heparin solution as a source of error in blood gas determinations (Letter). Clin. Chem., 29: 1562–1563, 1983.

87. Clausen, J. L., and Zarins, L. P.: Pulmonary Function Testing Guidelines and Controversies. New York, Academic Press, 1982.

88. Adams, A. P., and Hahn, C. E. W.: Principles and Practice of Blood Gas Analysis. London, Franklin Scientific Products, 1979.

89. Fox, M. J., Brody, J. S., and Weintraub, L. R.: Leukocyte larceny: A cause of spurious hypoxemia. Am. J. Med., 67:742–746, 1979.

90. Robin, E. D.: Pathophysiology of hypoxia. Semin. Respir. Med., 3:112–127, 1981.

91. Shohat, M., Schonfeld, T., Zaizoz, R., et al: Determination of blood gases in children with extreme leukocytosis. Crit. Care Med., 16:787–788, 1988.

92. Severinghaus, J. W.: Blood gas concentrations. In Fenn, W. O., Rahn, H. (eds): Handbook of Physiology, Vol. 2. Washington, D.C., Am. Phys. Soc., 1965.

93. Walton, J. R., and Shapiro, B. A.: Value and application of temperature compensated blood gas data (Response to question). Respir. Care, 25:260–261, 1980.

94. Gilles, B., Ward, J. J., and Helmholz, Jr., H. F.: Clinical blood-gas data should be temperature-compensated. Respir. Care, 25:523, 1980.

95. Hansen, J. E., and Sue, D. Y.: Should blood gas measurements be corrected for the patient's temperature? (Letter). N. Engl. J. Med., 303:341, 1980.

96. Porter, T.: Value and application of temperature-compensated blood gas data. Respir. Care, 25:260, 1980.

97. Blume, P.: Blood gas measurements (Letter). Am. J. Pathol., 70:440–441, 1978.

98. Ashwood, E. R., Kost, G., and Kenny, M.: Temperature correction of blood-gas and pH measurements. Clin. Chem., 29:1877–1885, 1983.

99. Shapiro, B. A.: Temperature correction of blood gas values. Respir. Care Clin. North Am., 1:69–76, 1995.

100. Hess, C. E., Nichols, A. B., Hunt, W. B., Suratt, P. M.: Pseudohypoxemia secondary to leukemia and thrombocytosis. N. Engl. J. Med., 301:361–363, 1979.

101. Lyon, M. E., Fine, J. S., Henderson, P. J., Lyon, A. W.: D-phenylalanyl-L-prolyl-L-arginine chloromethyl ketone (PPACK): Alternative anticoagulant to heparin salts for blood gas and electrolyte specimens. Clin. Chem., 41:1038–1041, 1995.

102. Sachs, C., Rabovine, P., Chaneac, M., Kindermans, C., et al: Preanalytical errors in ionized calcium measurements induced by the use of liquid heparin. Ann. Clin. Biochem., 28:167–173, 1991.

103. Toffaletti, J.: Use of novel preparations of heparin to eliminate interference in ionized calcium measurements: Have all the problems been solved? (Editorial) Clin. Chem., 40:508–509, 1994.

104. Burnett, R. W., Covington, A. K., Fogh-Anderson, N. K., Ulpmann, W. R., et al: International Federation of Clinical Chemistry (IFCC). Scientific Division. Committee on pH, Blood Gases and Electrolytes. Approved IFCC recommendations on whole blood sampling, transport and storage for simultaneous determination of pH, blood gases and electrolytes. Eur. J. Clin. Chem. Clin. Biochem., 33:247–253, 1995.

105. Bunch, D.: AARC Videoconference Highlights RT Patient Assessment Skills. AARC Times, June 1999.

106. Lyons, J. H., Jr., and Moore, F. D.: Posttraumatic alkalosis: Incidence and pathophysiology of alkalosis in surgery. Surgery, 60:93, 1966.

107. National Committee for Clinical Laboratory Standards (NCCLS). Procedures for the Collection of Arterial Blood Specimens; Approved Standard–Third Edition. NCCLS document H11-A3 [ISBN 1-56238-374-4], 1999.

108. Levin, K. P., Hanusa, B. H., Rotondi, A. Singer, D. E., et al: Arterial blood gas and pulse oximetry in initial management of patients with community-acquired pneumonia. J. Gen. Intern. Med., 9:590, 2001.

109. Pennycook, A.: Are blood tests of value in the primary assessment and resuscitation of patients in the A&E department? Postgrad. Med. J., 832:81, 1995.

110. Cadden, K., Norman, E., Booth, J.: Use of ABG in trauma for early recognition of acidosis and hypoxemia (Abstract). Respir. Care, 46:1106, 2001.

111. Prause, G., Ratzenhofer-Komenda, B., Offner, A., Lauda, P., et al: Prehospital point of care testing of blood gases and electrolytes—An evaluation of IRMA. Crit Care (Lond.), 2:79, 1997.

112. Gokel, Y., Paydas, S., Koswoglu, Z., Alpaslan, N., et al: Comparison of blood gas and acid-base measurements in arterial and venous blood samples with

uremic and diabetic ketoacidosis in the emergency room. Am. J. Nephrol., 20:319, 2000.

113. Kaplan, D. E., Levine, S. M.: A critical reappraisal of the Allen test. Osler Med. J., 6: Feb. 2000.

114. Lanni, H. A., Smith, S. G.: Allen's test: Fact or myth? (Letter). Respir. Care, 46:274, 2001.

115. Hosokawa, K., Hata, Y., Yano, K., Kazunori, M., et al: Results of the Allen test on 2,940 arms. Ann. Plast. Surg., 24:149, 1990.

116. Smeenk, F. W., Janssen, J. D., Arends, B. J., van den Bosch, J. A., et al: Effects of four different methods of sampling arterial blood and gas storage time on gas tensions and shunt calculation in the 100% oxygen test. Eur. Respir. J., 4:910–913, 1997.

117. Lin, J. C., Strauss, R. G., Johnson, K. J., Zimmerman, M. B., et al: Phlebotomy overdraw in the neonatal intensive care nursery. Pediatrics, 106:E19, 2000.

118. Ejrup, B., Fischer, B., Wright, I. S.: Clinical evaluation of blood flow to the hand. The false-positive Allen test. Circulation, 33:778, 1966.

119. Spence, A. S.: Respiratory Monitoring in Intensive Care. New York, Churchill Livingstone, 1982.

120. Jensen, T. J.: Introduction to Medical Physics. Philadelphia, J.B. Lippincott, 1960.

121. Abramson, J. F.: Blood Gas Electrodes: A Self-instructional Multimedia Learning Series. Denver, Multi-Media Pubs, 1984.

122. Bennington, J. L.: Saunders Dictionary and Encyclopedia of Laboratory Medicine and Technology. Philadelphia, W.B. Saunders, 1984.

123. Adams, A. P., and Hahn, C. E. W.: Principles and Practice of Blood Gas Analysis. London, Franklin Scientific Products, 1979.

124. Burton, G. C., and Hodgkin, J. E. (eds): Respiratory Care, 2nd ed. Philadelphia, J.B. Lippincott, 1984.

125. Severinghaus, J. W., and Bradley, B. A.: Blood Gas Electrodes or What the Instructions Didn't Say. Copenhagen, Denmark, Radiometer A/S, 1971.

126. Burki, N. K.: Arterial blood gas measurement (Editorial). Chest, 88:3–4, 1985.

127. Itano, M.: CAP blood gas survey—1981 and 1982. Am. J. Clin. Pathol., 80:554–562, 1983.

128. Ehrmeyer, S. S., Laessig, R. H., and Garber, C. C.: Monthly inter-laboratory pH and blood gas survey. Am. J. Clin. Pathol., 81:224–229, 1984.

129. Winckers, E. K. A., Teunissen, A. H., Van den Camp, R. A. M., and Maas, A. J. H.: A comparative study of the electrode systems of three pH and blood gas apparatus. J. Clin. Chem. Clin. Biochem., 16:175–185, 1978.

130. Elser, R. C.: Quality control of blood gas analysis: A review. Respir. Care, 31:807–816, 1986.

131. Brinklov, M. M., Anderson, P. K., Stoke, D. B., and Hole, P.: Inaccuracy of oxygen electrode systems (Letter). Anesthesiology, 51:368–369, 1979.

132. Willis, N., and Latto, P.: Misunderstandings of telephoned blood-gas reports. Clin. Chem., 30:1262, 1983.

133. Blackburn, J. P.: What's new in blood gas analysis? Br. J. Anaesth., 50:51–62, 1978.

134. Tashman, L. J., and Lamborn, K. R.: The Ways and Means of Statistics. New York, Harcourt Brace Jovanovich, 1979.

135. General Diagnostics. Quality Assurance Manual; Blood Gas Analyzer. Morris Plains, NJ, General Diagnostics.

136. Moran, R. F.: Assessment of quality control of blood gas/pH analyzer performance. Respir. Care, 26: 538–546, 1981.

137. Abramson, J., Verkaik, G., Poltl, K., and Mohler, J. R.: Evaluation and comparison of commercial blood gas quality controls and tonometry. Respir. Care, 25:441–447, 1980.

138. Hall, J. R., and Shapiro, B. A.: Acute care/blood gas laboratories: Profile of current operations. Crit. Care Med., 12:530–533, 1984.

139. Miller, W. W., Gehrich, J. L., Hansmann, D. R., and Yafuso, M.: Continuous in vivo monitoring of blood gases. Lab. Med., 19:629–635, 1988.

140. Kontron Medical Intravascular PO_2 Monitor Module 636, Operating Manual, 1983.

141. American Bentley Laboratories, Irvine, CA 92714.

142. Peruzzi, W. T., Shapiro, B. A.: Blood gas monitors. Respir. Care Clin. North Am., 1:143–156, 1995.

143. Roupie, E. E., Brochard, L., Lemaire, F. J.: Clinical evaluation of a continuous intra-arterial blood gas system in critically ill patients. Intens. Care Med., 22: 1162–1168, 1996.

144. Oropello, J. M., Manasia, A., Hannon, E., Leibowitz, A., Benjamin, E.: Continuous fiberoptic arterial and venous blood gas monitoring in hemorrhagic shock. Chest, 109:1049–1055, 1996.

145. Abraham, E., Gallagher, T. J., Fink, S.: Clinical evaluation of a multiparameter intra-arterial blood gas sensor. Intensive Care Med., 22:507–513, 1996.

146. Machutte, C. K.: On-line arterial blood gas analysis with optodes: Current status. Clin. Biochem., 31: 119–130, 1998.

147. Kilger, E., Briegel, J., Schelling, G., Polasek, J., et al: Long-term evaluation of a continuous intra-arterial blood gas monitoring system in patients with severe respiratory failure. Transfusion Med., 22:98–104, 1995.

148. Kendall, J., Reeves, B., Clancy, M.: Point of care testing: Randomized controlled trial of clinical outcome. B.M.J., 316(7137):1052–1057, 1998.

149. Murthy, J. N.: Evaluation of i-STAT portable clinical analyzer in a neonatal and pediatric intensive care unit. Clin. Biochem., 30:385–389, 1997.

150. Schneider, J., Dudziak, R., Westphal, K., Vetterman, J.: The i-STAT analyzer. A new, hand-held device for the bedside determination of hematocrit, blood gases, and electrolytes. Anesthetist, 46:704–714, 1997.

151. Green, M.: Successful alternatives to alternate site testing. Use of a pneumatic tube system to the central laboratory. Arch. Pathol. Lab. Med., 119:943–947, 1995.

152. Gilbert, H. C., Vendor, J. S.: Arterial blood gas monitoring. Crit. Care Clin., 11:233–248, 1995.

153. Miller, C. C., Miller, M. K., Marlow, N.: Effects of lithium heparin concentration on whole blood analytes measured on a multichannel blood gas/electrode system. Respir. Care, 37(11):1250–1255, 1992.

154. Toffaletti, J., Ernst, P., Hunt, P., Abrams, B.: Dry electrolyte-balanced heparinized syringes evaluated for determining ionized calcium and other electrolytes in whole blood. Clin. Chem., 37:1730–1733, 1991.

155. West, J. B.: Ventilation/Blood Flow and Gas Exchange, 3rd ed. Oxford, London, Blackwell Scientific Pubs., 1977.

156. Heironimus, T. W., and Bageant, R. A.: Mechanical Artificial Ventilation, 3rd ed. Springfield, IL, Charles C. Thomas, 1977.

157. Vincent, J. L., Lignian, H., Gillet, J. B., et al: Increase in PaO_2 following intravenous administration of propanolol in acutely hypoxemic patients. Chest, 88:558–562, 1985.

158. Wagner, W. W.: Pulmonary circulatory control through hypoxic vasoconstriction. Semin. Respir. Med., 7:124–135, 1985.

159. Hales, C. A.: The site and mechanism of oxygen sensing for the pulmonary vessels. Chest, 88:234S–240S, 1985.

160. Staub, N. C.: Site of hypoxic pulmonary vasoconstriction. Chest, 88:240S–245S, 1985.

161. Buist, A. S.: The Measurement of Closing Volume. ATS slide-tape program, item 6051.

162. Mausell, A., Bryan, C., and Levison, H.: Airway closure in children. J. Appl. Physiol., 33:711–714, 1972.

163. Brooks, J. M., and Barber, M. O.: Changes in closing volume measurement after isoproterenol. Am. Rev. Respir. Dis., 109:198, 1974.

164. Rehder, K., Sessler, A. D., and Marsh, H. M.: General anesthesia and the lung (state of the art). Am. Rev. Respir. Dis., 112:541–559, 1975.

165. Damman, J. F., and McAslan, T. C.: PEEP: Its use in young patients with apparently normal lungs. Crit. Care Med., 7:14–19, 1979.

166. Scanlan, C. L., Wilkins, R. L., Stoller, J. K. (eds): Egan's Fundamentals of Respiratory Care, 7th ed. St. Louis, C.V. Mosby, 1999, pp. 337–369.

167. Stoneham, M. D., Saville, G. M., Wilson, I. H: Knowledge about pulse oximetry among medical and nursing staff. Lancet, 344:1339–1342, 1994.

168. Hess, D.: Detection and monitoring of hypoxemia and oxygen therapy. Respir. Care, 45:65–83, 2000.

169. Hess, D., Agarwal, N. N.: Variability of blood gases, pulse oximeter saturation, and end-tidal carbon dioxide pressure in stable, mechanically ventilated trauma patients. J. Clin. Monit., 8:111–115, 1992.

170. Demers, R. R., and Saklad, M.: Fundamentals of blood gas interpretation. Respir. Care, 18:153–159, 1973.

171. Ayres, S. M.: Equations, nomograms, and understanding acid-base abnormalities. Respir. Care, 19:280–284, 1971.

172. Mellor, L. D., and Innanen, V. T.: A source of error in determination of blood gases. Clin. Chem., 29(Pt. 1): 395, 1983.

173. Guyton, A. C.: Textbook of Medical Physiology, 9th ed. Philadelphia, W.B. Saunders, 1996.

174. Christensen, H. N.: Body Fluids and the Acid-Base Balance. Philadelphia, W.B. Saunders, 1964.

175. A.C.C.P.–A.T.S. Joint Committee on Pulmonary Nomenclature: Pulmonary terms and symbols. Chest, 67:583–593, 1975.

176. Kraut, J. A., Madias, N. E.: Approach to patients with acid-base disorders. Respir. Care, 46:392–403, 2001.

177. Adrogu'e, H. E., Adrogue'e, H. J.: Acid-base physiology. Respir. Care, 46:328–341, 2001.

178. Van Slyke, D. D., and Cullen, G. E.: Studies of acidosis. J. Biol. Chem., 30:289–346, 1917.

179. Van Slyke, D. D.: Studies of acidosis. J. Biol. Chem., 48:153–176, 1921.

180. Narins, R. G., and Emmett, M.: Simple and mixed acid-base disorders: A practical approach. Medicine (Baltimore), 59:161–187, 1980.

181. Armstrong, B. W., and Mohler, J. G.: The in-vivo CO_2 titration curve (Letter). Lancet, 1:759–761, 1966.

182. Simmons, D. H.: Evaluation of acid-base status. Basics of R. D., American Thoracic Society, 2(3):1974.

183. Winters, R. W., and Dell, R. B.: Acid-Base Physiology in Medicine. Boston, Little, Brown, 1982.

184. Mulhausen, R. O.: The affinity of hemoglobin for oxygen (Editorial). Circulation, XLII:195–197, 1970.

185. Slonim, N. B., and Hamilton, L. H.: Respiratory Physiology, 5th ed. St. Louis, C.V. Mosby, 1987.

186. Klocke, R. A.: Oxygen transport and 2,3-diphosphoglycerate. Chest, 62(Suppl. 2):79s–85s, 1972.

187. Benesch, R., and Benesch, R. E.: The effect of organic phosphates from the human erythrocyte on the allosteric properties of hemoglobin. Biochem. Biophys. Res. Commun., 26:162–167, 1967.

188. Chauntin, A., and Curnish, R. R.: Effect of organic and inorganic phosphates on the oxygen equilibrium of human erythrocytes. Arch. Biochem. Biophys., 121:96–102, 1967.

189. Bunn, H. F., and Jandl, J. H.: Control of hemoglobin function within the red cell. N. Engl. J. Med., 282: 1414–1421, 1970.

190. Edwards, M. J., and Cannon, B.: Normal levels of 2,3-DPG in red cells despite severe hypoxemia of chronic lung disease. Chest, 61:25s–26s, 1972.

191. Bunn, H. F., May, M. H., Kocholaty, W. F., et al: Hemoglobin function in stored blood. J. Clin. Invest., 8:311–321, 1969.

192. Duhm, J., Deuticke, B., and Gerlach, E.: Complete restoration of oxygen transport function and 2,3-DPG concentration in stored blood. Transfusion, 11:147–151, 1971.

193. Valtis, D. J., and Kennedy, A. C.: Defective gas transport function of stored red blood cells. Lancet, 1:119–125, 1954.

194. Hess, D.: Detection and monitoring of hypoxemia and oxygen therapy. Respir. Care, 45:65–83, 2000.

195. Kales, S. N., Feldman, J., Pepper, L., Fish, S. S., et al: Carboxyhemoglobin levels in patients with cocaine-related chest pain. Chest 106:147–150, 1994.

196. Haponik, E. F.: Smoke inhalation injury: Some priorities for respiratory care professionals. Respir. Care, 37:609–629, 1992.

197. Simmons, M.: Personal correspondence.

198. Poulton, T. J.: Carboxyhemoglobin levels in banked blood (Letter). Chest, 87:498–499, 1985.

199. Myers, R. A., Britten, J. S.: Are arterial blood gases of value in treatment decisions for carbon monoxide poisoning? Crit. Care Med., 17:139–142, 1989.

200. Norkool, D. M., and Kirkpatrick, J. N.: Treatment of acute carbon monoxide poisoning with hyperbaric oxygen: A review of 115 cases. Ann. Emerg. Med., 14:1168–1171, 1985.

201. Aronow, W. S., and O'Donohue, W. J.: Carboxy-hemoglobin levels in banked blood (Letter/response). Chest, 87:498–499, 1985.

202. Kindall, E. P.: Carbon monoxide poisoning treated with hyperbaric oxygen. Respir. Ther., 5:29–33, 1975.

203. Huff, J. S., Kardon, E.: Carbon monoxide toxicity in a man working outdoors with a gasoline-powered hydraulic machine. N. Engl. J. Med. 320:1564, 1989.

204. McGrath, R. B., Perry, S. M.: The production of methemoglobin by amyl nitrite: A case report. Respir. Care, 27:959–962, 1982.

205. Pierce, J. M. T., Nielsen, M. S.: Acute acquired methaemoglobinemia after amyl nitrite poisoning. B.M.J., 298:1566, 1989.

206. Perlson, R. M.: Blood gas corner #11. Respir. Care, 30:127–128, 1985.

207. Townes, P. L., Geertsma, M. A., White, M. R.: Benzocaine induced methemoglobinemia. Am. J. Dis. Child., 131:697–698, 1977.

208. Delwood, L., O'Flaherty, D., Prejean, E. J., Giesecke, A. H.: Methemoglobinemia and its effect on pulse oximetry. Crit. Care Med., 19:988, 1991.

209. Collins, J. F.: Methemoglobinemia as a complication of 20% benzocaine spray for endoscopy. Gastroenterology, 98:211–213, 1990.

210. Spielman, F. J., Anderson, J. A., Terry, W. C.: Benzocaine induced methemoglobinemia during general anesthesia. J. Oral Max. Surg., 42:740–743, 1984.

211. Ferree, S. M.: Blood gas corner #14: Cyanosis with hyperoxemia. Respir. Care, 31:827–828, 1986.

212. Anderson, S. T., Hajduczek, J., Barker, S. J.: Benzocaine-induced methemoglobinemia in an adult: Accuracy of pulse oximetry with methemoglobinemia. Anesth. Analg., 67:1099–1101, 1988.

213. Barker, S. J., Tremper, K. K., Hyatt, B. S., Zaccari, J.: Effects of methemoglobinemia on pulse oximetry and venous oximetry. Anesthesiology, 67:A171, 1987.

214. O'Connor, J. M.: Cyanosis and sulfhemoglobinemia: A case report. Respir. Care, 37:1346, 1992.

215. Benumof, J. L.: Anesthesia & Uncommon Diseases, 4th ed. St. Louis, Mosby Year Book, 1998.

216. Platt, O. S.: Easing the suffering caused by sickle cell disease. N. Engl. J. Med., 330:783–784, 1994.

217. Platt, O. S., Guinan, E. C.: Bone marrow transplantation in sickle cell anemia—The dilema of choice. N. Engl. J. Med., 335:426–427, 1996.

218. Rodger, G. P., Dover, G. J., Uyesaka, N., et al: Augmentation of erythropoietin of the fetal-hemoglobin response to hydroxyurea in sickle cell disease. N. Engl. J. Med., 328:73–80, 1993.

219. Platt, O. S., Brambilla, D. J., Rosse, W. F., et al: Mortality in sickle cell disease: Life expectancy and risk factors for early death. N. Engl. J. Med., 330:1639–1644, 1994.

220. Cohen, A. R.: Sickle cell disease—New treatments, new questions (Editorial). N. Engl. J. Med., 339:42–44, 1998.

221. Charache, S., Scott, J. C., Charache, P.: Acute chest syndrome in adults with sickle cell anemia. Arch. Intern. Med., 139:67–69, 1979.

222. Erslev, A.: Erythropoietin coming of age. N. Engl. J. Med., 316:101–103, 1987.

223. Erslev, A. J.: Erythropoietin. N. Engl. J. Med., 324:1339–1344, 1991.

224. Steinberg, M. H.: Erythropoietin for anemia of renal failure in sickle cell disease (Letter). N. Engl. J. Med., 324:1369–1370, 1991.

225. Maier, R. F., Obladen, M., Scigalla, P., et al: The effect of Epoetin (recombinant human erythropoetin) on the need for transfusion in very-low birth weight infants. N. Engl. J. Med., 330:1173–1178, 1994.

226. Blood transfusions in the critically ill patient: Questions, concerns, and alternatives. Medscape, 8/29/00.

227. Adamson, J. W.: Recombinant erythropoietin to improve athletic performance. N. Engl. J. Med., 324:698, 1991.

228. Bihari, D., Smithies, M., Gimson, A., and Tinker, J.: The effects of vasodilation with prostacyclin on oxygen delivery and uptake in critically ill patients. N. Engl. J. Med., 317:397–403, 1987.

229. Astrand, P. O., Rodahl, K.: Textbook of Work Physiology, 3rd ed. New York, McGraw Hill, 1986.

230. Aronow, W. S., and O'Donohue, W. J.: Carboxy-hemoglobin levels in banked blood (Letter/response). Chest, 87:498–499, 1985.

231. Strang, L. B.: Neonatal Respiration: Physiological and Clinical Studies. Oxford, Blackwell Scientific Publications, 1977.

232. Delivoria-Papadopoulos, M., Roncevic, N. P., and Oski, F. A.: Postnatal changes in oxygen transport of term, premature, and sick infants: The role of red cell 2,3 diphosphoglycerate and adult haemoglobin. Pediatr. Res., 5:235, 1971.

233. Erslev, A. J., and Gabzuda, T. G.: Pathophysiology of Blood. Philadelphia, W.B. Saunders, 1975.

234. Giulian, G. G., Gilbert, E. F., and Moss, R. I.: Elevated fetal hemoglobin levels in sudden infant death syndrome. N. Engl. J. Med., 316:1122–1126, 1987.

235. Perlson, R. M.: Blood gas corner #11. Respir. Care, 30:127–128, 1985.

236. Methemoglobinemia-sleuthing for a new cause. N. Engl. J. Med., 314:776–778, 1986.

237. Jobsis, F. F.: Oxidative metabolism at low PO_2. Fed. Proc., 31:1404–1413, 1972.

238. Fisher, A. B., and Dodia, C.: Lung as a model for evaluation of critical intracellular PO_2 and PCO_2. Am. J. Physiol., 241:E47–E50, 1981.

239. Lowenthal, D. T., and Pollock, M. P.: Cardiac response to exercise in health and disease. Sem. Resp. Med., 14:91–105, 1993.

240. Campbell, R. S., Branson, R. D., and Hurst, J. M.: Blood gas corner #27—Nonventilatory cause of hypercapnia during weaning. Respir. Care, 35:1001–1002, 1990.

241. (NCCLS): Blood Gas and pH Analysis and Related Measurements; Approved Guideline. NCCLS document C46-A. NCCLS, 940 West Valley Rd., Suite 1400, Wayne, PA 19087-1898, 2001.

242. Cerveri, I., Zoia, M. C., Fanfulla, L., et al: Reference values of arterial oxygen tension in the middle-aged and elderly. Am. J. Crit. Care Med., 152:934–941, 1995.

243. Wagner, P. D.: Interpretation of arterial blood gases (Editorial). Chest, 77:131–132, 1980.

244. Dantzker, D. R.: The influence of cardiovascular function on gas exchange. Clin. Chest Med., 4:140–159, 1983.

245. Phillips, B. A., McConnell, J. W., and Smith, M. D.: The effects of hypoxemia on cardiac output: A dose-response curve. Chest, 93:471–475, 1988.

246. Giovannini, I., Boldrini, G., Sganga, G., et al: Quantification of the determinants of arterial hypoxemia in critically ill patients. Crit. Care Med., 11:644–645, 1983.

247. Covelli, H. D., Nessan, V. J., and Tuttle, W. K.: Oxygen derived variables in acute respiratory failure. Crit. Care Med., 11:646–649, 1983.

248. Zetterstrom, H.: Assessment of the efficiency of pulmonary oxygenation: The choice of oxygenation index. Acta Anaesthesiol. Scand., 32:579–584, 1988.

249. Dganit, S., Maxwell, C., Hess, D., and Shefet, D. A.: A comparison of five common equations used to calculate QS/QT (Abstract). Respir. Care, 31: 943–944, 1986.

250. Harrison, R. A., Davison, R., Shapiro, B. A., and Meyers, S. N.: Reassessment of the assumed A-V oxygen content difference in the shunt calculation. Anesth. Analg., 54:198–202, 1975.

251. Hess, D., Maxwell, C., and Shefet, D.: Determination of intrapulmonary shunt comparison of an estimated shunt equation and a modified equation with the classic equation. Respir. Care, 32:268–273, 1987.

252. Cane, R. D., Shapiro, B. A., Templin, R., and Walther, K.: Unreliability of oxygen tension-based indices in reflecting intrapulmonary shunting in critically ill patients. Crit. Care Med., 16:1243–1245, 1988.

253. Granger, W. M.: Evaluating the oxygen-tension based indices of venous admixture. Respir. Care, 41: 607–610, 1996.

254. Harris, E. A., Kenyon, A. M., Nisbet, H. D., et al: The normal alveolar-arterial oxygen tension gradient in man. Clin. Sci. Mol. Med., 46:89–104, 1974.

255. Wasserman, K.: Summing $PaCO_2$ and PaO_2: A simple expedient for determining alveolar-arterial PO_2 difference (Letter). Am. Rev. Respir. Dis. 113:707, 1976.

256. Damman, J. F., and McAslan, T. C.: PEEP: Its use in young patients with apparently normal lungs. Crit. Care Med., 7:14–19, 1979.

257. Ward, R., Tolas, A., Benveniste, R., et al: Effect of posture on normal arterial blood gas tensions in the aged. Geriatrics, 21:139–143, 1966.

258. Martin, L.: Abbreviating the alveolar gas equation: An argument for simplicity. Respir. Care, 30:964–968, 1985.

259. Johnston, W. E., Vinten-Johansen, J., Strickland, R. A., and Bowton, D. L.: Comparison of two formulas to calculate alveolar oxygen tension in canine oleic acid pulmonary edema. Crit. Care Med., 17:176–179, 1989.

260. Cinel, D., Markwell, K., Lee, R., and Szidon, P.: Variability of the respiratory gas exchange ratio during arterial puncture. Am. Rev. Resp. Dis., 143:217–219, 1991.

261. Gilbert, R., and Keighley, J. F.: The arterial/alveolar oxygen tension ratio: An index of gas exchange applicable to varying inspired oxygen concentrations. Am. Rev. Respir. Dis., 109:142–145, 1974.

262. Gilbert, R., Auchincloss, J. H., Kuppinger, M., and Thomas, M. V.: Stability of the arterial/alveolar oxygen partial pressure ratio: Effects of low ventilation/perfusion regions. Crit. Care Med., 7:267–272, 1979.

263. Cohen, A., Taeusch, H. W., Jr., and Stanton, C.: Usefulness of the arterial/alveolar oxygen tension ratio in the care of infants with respiratory distress syndrome. Respir. Care, 28:169–173, 1983.

264. Gross, R., and Israel, R. H.: Graphic approach for prediction of arterial oxygen tension at different concentrations of inspired oxygen. Chest, 79:311–315, 1981.

265. Viale, J. P., Carlisle, J. P., Annat, G., et al: Arterial-alveolar oxygen partial pressure ratio: A theoretical reappraisal. Crit. Care Med., 14:153–154, 1986.

266. Robinson, N. B., Weaver, L. J., Carrico, C. H., and Hudson, L. D.: Evaluation of pulmonary dysfunction in the critically ill (Abstract). Am. Rev. Respir. Dis., 123(Suppl.):92, 1981.

267. Modell, J. H., Graves, S. A., and Ketover, A.: Clinical course of 91 consecutive near-drowning victims. Chest, 70:231–238, 1976.

268. Craig, K. C., Pierson, D. J., and Carrico, C. J.: The clinical application of PEEP in ARDS. Respir. Care, 30:184–201, 1985.

269. Lecky, J. H., and Ominsky, A. J.: Postoperative respiratory management. Chest, 62:50S–57S, 1972.

270. Dean, J. M., Wetzel, R., Gioia, F. R., and Rogers, M. C.: Use of oxygen derived variables for estimation of pulmonary shunt in critically ill children (Abstract). Crit. Care Med., 12:280, 1984.

271. Hess, D., and Maxwell, C.: Which is the best index of oxygenation—$P(A-a)O_2$, PaO_2/PAO_2, or PaO_2/FIO_2 (Editorial)? Respir. Care, 30:961–963, 1985.

272. Wallfisch, H. K., Tonnessen, A. S., and Huber, P.: Respiratory indices compared to venous admixture (Abstract). Crit. Care Med., 9:147, 1981.

273. Dean, J. M., Wetzel, R. C., and Rogers, M. C.: Arterial blood gas derived variables as estimates of intrapulmonary shunt in critically ill children. Crit. Care Med., 13:1029–1033, 1985.

274. Gross, R., and Israel, R. H.: Graphic approach for prediction of arterial oxygen tension at different concentrations of inspired oxygen. Chest, 79:311–315, 1981.

275. Peris, L. V., Boix, J. H., Salom, J. V., et al: Clinical use of the arterial/alveolar oxygen tension ratio. Crit. Care Med., 11:888–891, 1983.

276. Prys-Roberts, C., Kelman, G. R., Greenbaum, R., et al: Hemodynamics and alveolar-arterial PO_2 differences

at varying $PaCO_2$ in anesthetized man. J. Appl. Physiol., 25:80–87, 1968.

277. Owen-Thomas, J. B., Meade, F., and Jones, R. S.: Assessment of arterial blood gas tensions, inspired oxygen therapy and shunts (Abstract). Br. J. Anaesth., 43:1195, 1971.

278. Breivik, H., Grenvik, A., Millen, E., and Safar, P.: Normalizing low arterial CO_2 tension during mechanical ventilation. Chest, 63:525–531, 1973.

279. Burki, N. K.: Arterial blood gas measurement (Editorial). Chest, 88:3–4, 1985.

280. Schachter, E. N., Littner, M. R., Luddy, P., and Beck, G. J.: Monitoring of oxygen delivery systems in clinical practice. Crit. Care Med., 8:405–409, 1980.

281. Friedman, S. A., Weber, B., Briscoe, W. A., et al: Oxygen therapy: Evaluation of various air entraining masks. J.A.M.A., 228:474–478, 1974.

282. McCarthy, K., and Stoller, J.K.: Possible underestimation of shunt fraction in the hepatopulmonary syndrome. Respir. Care, 44:1486–1488, 1999.

283. Snider, G. L.: Interpretation of the arterial oxygen and carbon dioxide partial pressures: A simplified approach for bedside use. Chest, 63:801–806, 1973.

284. Klocke, R. A.: Interpretation of Blood Gases. New York, ATS Learning Resources Slide Tape Series, 1975.

285. Beall, C. E., Braun, H. A., and Cheney, F. W.: Physiological Bases for Respiratory Care. Missoula, MT, Mountain Press Pub., 1974.

286. Klocke, R. A.: Interpretation of Blood Gases. New York, ATS Learning Resources Slide Tape Series, 1975.

287. Harris, E. A., Kenyon, A. M., Nisbet, H. D., et al: The normal alveolar-arterial oxygen tension gradient in man. Clin. Sci. Mol. Med., 46:89–104, 1974.

288. West, J. B.: Ventilation/Blood Flow and Gas Exchange, 3rd ed. Oxford, London, Blackwell Scientific, 1977.

289. Glauser, L. G., Polatty, R. C., and Sessler, C. N.: Worsening oxygenation in the mechanically ventilated patient: Causes, mechanisms, and early detection (State of the art). Am. Rev. Respir. Dis., 138:458–465, 1988.

290. Bonner, R. A. J., Ralph, D. D.: Blood gas corner #15. Respir. Care, 31:1148–1150, 1986.

291. Cadranel, J. L., Millerson, B. J., Cadranel, J. F., et al: Severe hypoxemia-associated intrapulmonary shunt in a patient with chronic liver disease: Improvement after medical treatment. Am. Rev. Resp. Dis., 146:526–527, 1992.

292. Kocabas, A., Ozbek, S., and Colakogiu, S.: Arterial hypoxemia in patients with cirrhosis (Abstract). Chest, 103:167S, 1993.

293. Kramer, M. R., Springer, C., Berkman, N., et al: Rehabilitation of hypoxemic patients with COPD at low altitude at the Dead Sea, the lowest place on earth. Chest, 113:571–575, 1998.

294. Ashbaugh, D. G., Bigelow, D. B., Petty, T. L., Levine, B. E.: Acute respiratory distress in adults. Lancet, 2:319–323, 1967.

295. Dillard, T. A., Rosenberg, A. P., and Berg, B. W.: Hypoxemia during altitude exposure. Chest, 103:422–425, 1993.

296. Berg, B. W., Dillard, T. A., Rajagopal, K. R., and Mehm, W. J.: Oxygen supplementation during air travel in patients with chronic obstructive lung disease. Chest, 101:638–641, 1992.

297. Campbell, E. J. M.: The J. Burns Amberson Lecture—The management of acute respiratory failure in chronic bronchitis and emphysema. Am. Rev. Respir. Dis., 96:626–639, 1967.

298. American College of Chest Physicians—National Heart, Lung and Blood Institute: National conference on O_2 therapy. Respir. Care, 29:922–935, 1984.

299. Koo, K. W., Say, D. S., and Snider, G. L.: Arterial blood gases and pH during sleep in COPD. Am. J. Med., 58:663–670, 1975.

300. Warrel, D. A., Edwards, R. H. T., Godfrey, S. M. B., and Jones, N. L.: Effect of controlled blood gases in acute respiratory failure. B.M.J., 2:452–455, 1970.

301. Phillips, B. A., McConnell, J. W., and Smith, M. D.: The effects of hypoxemia on cardiac output: A dose response curve. Chest, 93:471–475, 1993.

302. Oxygen Therapy for Adults in the Acute Care Facility—2002 Revision and Update. AARC Clinical Practice Guideline. Respir. Care, 47:717–720, 2002.

303. Farias, E. M.: Partial- vs. Nonrebreathing Masks (Letter). Respir. Care, 39:154, 1994.

304. Selection of an Oxygen Delivery Device for Neonatal and Pediatric Patients. AARC Clinical Practice Guideline. Respir Care, 41:637–646, 1996.

305. Hess, D. R., and Kacmarek, R. M.: Essentials of Mechanical Ventilation, 2nd ed. New York, McGraw-Hill, 2002.

306. Smith, J. P., Stone, R. W., and Muschenheim, C.: Acute respiratory failure in chronic lung disease. Am. Rev. Respir. Dis., 97:791–803, 1968.

307. Hunt, W. B., Jr.: Low flow oxygen in respiratory failure treatment. Cont. Ed.: Feb. 1984.

308. Soto, F. J., and Varkey, B.: Evidence-based approach to acute exacerbations of COPD. Curr. Opin. Pulmon. Med., 9:117–124, 2003.

309. Schiff, M. M., and Massaro, D.: Effect of O_2 administration by a Venturi apparatus on arterial blood gas values in patients with respiratory failure. N. Engl. J. Med., 277:950–953, 1967.

310. Eldridge, F., and Gherman, C.: Studies of oxygen administration in respiratory failure. Ann. Intern. Med., 68:569–578, 1968.

311. Lejeune, P., Mols, P., Naeje, R., et al: Acute hemodynamic effects of controlled oxygen therapy in decompensated chronic obstructive pulmonary disease. Crit. Care Med., 12:1032–1035, 1984.

312. Kilburn, K. H.: Neurologic manifestations of respiratory failure. Arch. Intern. Med., 116:409–415, 1965.

313. Snider, G. L., and Maldonado, D.: Arterial blood gases in acutely ill patients. J.A.M.A., 204:133–136, 1968.

314. Craig, K. C., Pierson, D. J., and Carrico, C. J.: The clinical application of PEEP in the ARDS. Respir. Care, 30:184–201, 1985.

315. Dunlevy, C. L., and Tyl, S. E.: The effect of oral versus nasal breathing on oxygen concentrations received from nasal cannulas. Respir. Care, 37:357–360, 1992.

316. Carroll, G. C., and Rothenberg, D. M.: Carbon dioxide narcosis: Pathological or "pathillogical"? (Editorial) Chest, 102:986–987, 1992.

317. Block, E. R., and Ryerson, G. G.: Safe use of O_2 therapy (Pt. I). Respir. Ther., (Jan/Feb) 13:17–21, 1983.

318. Singer, M. M., Wright, F., Stanly, L. K., et al: O_2 toxicity in man. N. Engl. J. Med., 283:1473–1478, 1970.

319. Saussine, M., Colson, P., Alauzen, M., et al: Postoperative acute respiratory distress syndrome: A complication of amiodarone associated with 100 per cent oxygen ventilation (Letter). Chest, 102:980–981, 1992.

320. Rawles, J. M., and Kenmore, A. C. F.: Controlled trial of oxygen in uncomplicated myocardial infarction. B.M.J., 1:1121–1123, 1976.

321. Sweetwood, H. M.: Oxygen administration in the coronary care unit. Heart Lung, 3:102–107, 1974.

322. Martin, G. S.: Experts discuss ventilation strategies for improving outcomes in ALI/ARDS. 98th International Conference of the ATS. Medscape, 2002.

323. Brower, R. G., Matthay, M. A., Morris, A., et al: Ventilation with lower tidal volumes as compared with traditional tidal volumes for acute lung injury and the acute respiratory distress syndrome. N. Engl. J. Med., 342:1301–1308, 2000.

324. Shapiro, B. A., Cane, R. D., Harrison, R. A., and Steiner, M. C.: Changes in intrapulmonary shunting with administration of 100% oxygen. Chest, 77:138–141, 1980.

325. Barach, A. L., Marin, J., and Eckman, M.: Positive pressure respiration and its application in the treatment of acute pulmonary edema. Arch. Intern. Med., 12:754–795, 1938.

326. A.C.C.P.–A.T.S. Joint Committee on Pulmonary Nomenclature: Pulmonary terms and symbols. Chest, 67:583–593, 1975.

327. Spearman, C. B.: PEEP: Terminology and technical aspects of PEEP devices and systems. Respir. Care, 33:434–443, 1988.

328. Felton, C. R., Montenegro, H. D., and Saidel, G. M.: Inspiratory flow effects on mechanically ventilated patients: Lung volume inhomogeneity and arterial oxygenation. Intensive Care Med., 10:281–286, 1984.

329. Connors, A. F., McCaffree, D. R., and Gray, B. A.: Effect of inspiratory flowrate on gas exchange during mechanical ventilation. Am,. Rev. Respir. Dis., 124:537–543, 1981.

330. Scott, L. R., Benson, M. S., and Pierson, D. J.: Effect of inspiratory flowrate and circuit compressible volume on auto-PEEP during mechanical ventilation. Respir. Care, 31:1075–1082, 1986.

331. Hess, D.: The use of PEEP in clinical settings other than acute lung injury. Respir. Care, 33:581–595, 1988.

332. Hess, D.: The use of PEEP in clinical settings other than acute lung injury. Respir. Care, 33:581–595, 1988.

333. Dark, D. S., Pingleton, S. K., and Kerby, G. R.: Hypercapnia during weaning: A complication of nutritional support. Chest, 88:141–143, 1985.

334. Pare, P. D., Warriner, B., Baile, E. M., and Hogg, J. C.: Redistribution of pulmonary extra-vascular water

with PEEP in canine pulmonary edema. Am. Rev. Respir. Dis., 127:590–593, 1983.

335. Craig, K. C., Pierson, D. J., and Carrico, C. J.: The clinical application of PEEP in the ARDS. Respir. Care, 30:184–201, 1985.

336. Sugerman, H. J., Rogers, R. M., and Miller, L. D.: PEEP: Indications and physiological considerations. Chest, 62:s86–s93, 1972.

337. Venus, B., Cohen, L. E., and Smith, R. A.: Hemodynamics and intrathoracic pressure transmission during controlled mechanical ventilation and PEEP in normal and low compliant lungs. Crit. Care Med., 16:686–690, 1988.

338. Johnson, B., et al: Pressure-volume curve and compliance in acute lung injury. Am. J. Respir. Crit. Care Med., 159:1172–1179, 1999.

339. Carlon, G. C., Cole, R., Jr., Klein, R., et al: Criteria for selective PEEP and independent synchronized ventilation of each lung. Chest, 74:501–507, 1978.

340. Powner, J. D., Eross, B., and Grenvik, A.: Differential lung ventilation with PEEP in the treatment of unilateral pneumonia. Crit. Care Med., 5:170–172, 1977.

341. Pearce, L., Lilly, K., and Baigelman, W.: Effects of PEEP on intracranial pressure. Respir. Care, 26:754–756, 1981.

342. Demling, R. H., Staub, N. C., and Edmonds, L. H.: Effect of end-expiratory airway pressure on accumulation of extravascular lung water. J. Appl. Physiol., 38:907–912, 1975.

343. Benson, M. S., and Pierson, D. J.: Auto-PEEP during mechanical ventilation of adults. Respir. Care, 33:557–568, 1988.

344. Brown, D. G., and Pierson, D. J.: Auto-PEEP is common in mechanically ventilated patients: A study of incidence, severity, and detection. Respir. Care, 31:1069–1074, 1986.

345. Simbruner, G.: Inadvertent PEEP in mechanically ventilated newborn infants: Detection and effect on lung mechanics and gas exchange. J. Pediatr., 108:589–595, 1986.

346. PEEP: Intentional and Inadvertent (teleconference). Rancho Mirage, CA, Annenberg Center for Health Sciences, 1989.

347. Man-Lim, C., Jung, H., Kah, Y., et al: Effect of alveolar recruitment maneuver in early acute respiratory distress syndrome according to antiderecruitment strategy, etiological category of diffuse lung injury, and body position of the patient. Crit. Care Med., Feb. 27, 2003.

348. Reinhart, K., Bloos, F., Konig, F., et al: Reversible decrease in oxygen consumption by hyperoxia. Chest, 99:690–694, 1991.

349. Zapol, W. M., Falke, K. J., Hurford, W. E., and Roberts, J. D.: Inhaling nitric oxide: A selective pulmonary vasodilator and bronchodilator. Chest, 105:87S–91S, 1994.

350. Rossaint, R., Falke, K. J., Lopez, F., et al: Inhaled nitric oxide for the Adult Respiratory Distress Syndrome. N. Engl. J. Med., 328:399–405, 1993.

351. Craig, D. B., Wahba, W. M., Don, H. F., et al: "Closing volume" and its relationship to gas exchange

in seated and supine positions. J. Appl. Physiol., 31:717–721, 1971.

352. Norton, L. C., and Confort, C. G.: The effects of body position on oxygenation. Heart Lung, 14:45–52, 1985.

353. Langer, M., Mascheroni, D., Marcolin, R., and Gattinoni, L.: The prone position in ARDS patients. Chest, 94:103–107, 1988.

354. Stokes, D. C., Wohl, M. E. B., Khaw, K. T., and Strieder, D. J.: Postural hypoxemia in cystic fibrosis. Chest, 87:785–789, 1985.

355. Minh, V. D., Chun, D., Fairshter, R. D., et al: Supine change in arterial oxygenation in patients with chronic obstructive pulmonary disease. Am. Rev. Respir. Dis., 133:820–824, 1986.

356. Zack, M. B., Pontoppidan, H., and Kazemi, H.: The effect of lateral positions on gas exchange in pulmonary disease. Am. Rev. Respir. Dis., 110:49–55, 1974.

357. Neagley, S. R., and Zwillich, C. W.: The effect of positional changes on oxygenation in patients with pleural effusions. Chest, 88:714–717, 1985.

358. Rivara, D., Artucio, H., Aocos, J., and Hiriart, C.: Positional hypoxemia during artificial ventilation. Crit. Care Med., 12:436–438, 1984.

359. Davies, H., Kitchman, R., Gordon, I., and Helms, P.: Regional ventilation in infancy. N. Engl. J. Med., 313:1626–1628, 1985.

360. Chang, S. C., Chang, H. I., Shiao, G. M., and Perng, R. P.: Effect of body position on gas exchange in patients with unilateral central airway lesions. Chest 103:787–791, 1993.

361. Badr, M. S., and Grossman, J. E.: Positional changes in gas exchange after unilateral pulmonary embolism. Chest, 98:1514–1516, 1990.

362. Fraser, C.G.: Biological Variation: From Principle to Practice. Washington, DC, AACC Press, 2001.

363. Masoro, E. J., and Seigel, P. D.: Acid-Base Regulation: Its Physiology, Pathophysiology and Interpretation of Blood-Gas Analysis, 2nd ed. Philadelphia, W.B. Saunders, 1977.

364. Cohen, J. J., Kassirer, J. P. (eds.): Acid/Base. Boston, Little, Brown, 1982.

365. Bowen, F. W., Jr., and Williams, J. L.: The use and abuse of bicarbonate in neonatal acid-base derangements. Respir. Care, 23:465–475, 1978.

366. Daughaday, W. H.: Hydrogen ion metabolism in metabolic acidosis. Arch. Intern. Med., 107:63, 1961.

367. Simmons, D. H.: Evaluation of Acid-Base Status. Basics of R. D., vol. 2. Broadway, NY, American Thoracic Society, 1974.

368. Rooth, G.: Acid-Base and Electrolyte Balance. Chicago, Year Book, 1974.

369. Pierce, N. F., Fedson, D. S., Brigham, K. L., et al: The ventilatory response to acute base deficit in humans. Ann. Intern. Med., 72:633–640, 1970.

370. Statement on acid-base terminology. Report of the ad hoc committee on New York Academy of Sciences Conference. Anesthesiology, 27:7–12, 1966.

371. Okrent, D. G., and Kruse, J. A.: Metabolic acidosis in severe acute asthma; Acid-base nomenclature (Response to a letter). Crit. Care Med., 16:1255–1258, 1988.

372. Mosby's Nursing & Allied Health Dictionary. Philadelphia, W.B. Saunders, 2002.

373. Scanlan, C. L., Wilkins, R. L., and Stoller, J. K.: Egan's Fundamentals of Respiratory Therapy, 7th ed. St. Louis, C. V. Mosby, 1999.

374. Winters, R. W., and Dell, R. B.: Acid-Base Physiology in Medicine. Boston, Little, Brown, 1982.

375. Kruse, J. A.: Metabolic acidosis in severe acute asthma; Acid-base nomenclature. Crit. Care Med., 16:1255–1258, 1988.

376. Haldane, J. S.: Symptoms, causes, and prevention of anoxemia. B.M.J., 2:65, July 19, 1919.

377. Dantzker, D. R.: Oxygen transport and utilization. Respir. Care, 33:874–880, 1980.

378. West, J. B.: Everest—The testing place. Chest, 89:625–626, 1986.

379. Gray, F. D., and Horner, G. J.: Survival following extreme hypoxemia. J.A.M.A., 211:1815–1817, 1970.

380. James, T., Robin, E. D., Burke, C. M., et al: Impact of profound reductions of PaO_2 on O_2 transport and utilization in congenital heart disease. Chest, 87:293–302, 1985.

381. Thorson, S. H., Marini, J. S., Pierson, D. J., and Hudson, L. D.: Arterial blood gas variability in an ICU setting (Abstract). Am. Rev. Respir. Dis., 119:176, 1979.

382. American College of Chest Physicians—National Heart, Lung and Blood Institute: National conference on O_2 therapy. Respir. Care, 29:922–935, 1984.

383. Payne, J. B., and Severinghaus, J. W.: Pulse Oximetry. New York, Springer-Verlag, 1986.

384. Dennis, R. C., and Valeri, C. R.: Measuring per cent oxygen saturation of Hb, per cent carboxyhemoglobin and methemoglobin, and concentrations of total Hb and oxygen in blood of man, dog, and baboon. Clin. Chem., 26:1304–1308, 1980.

385. Barker, S. J., and Tremper, K. K.: The effect of carbon monoxide inhalation on pulse oximetry and the transcutaneous PO_2. Anesthesiology, 66:677–679, 1987.

386. Devalois, B., Strat, R., and Feiss, P.: Pulse oximeter: Clinical assessment in the recovery room (Abstract). Ann. Fr. Anesth. Reanim., 6:361–363, 1987.

387. Kim, J. M., Arakawa, K., Benson, K. T., and Fox, D. K.: Pulse oximetry and circulatory kinetics associated with pulse volume amplitude measured by photoelectric plethysmography. Anesth. Analg., 12:1333–1339, 1985.

388. Davidshohn, E., and Henry, J. B. (eds): Clinical Diagnosis by Laboratory Methods, 15th ed. Philadelphia, W.B. Saunders, 1974.

389. Pittiglio, D. H., and Sacher, R. A.: Clinical Hematology and Fundamentals of Hemostasis. Philadelphia, F.A. Davis, 1987.

390. Wallerstein, R. O.: Role of the laboratory in the diagnosis of anemia. J.A.M.A., 236:490–497, 1976.

391. Woodson, R. D., Willis, R. E., and Lenfant, C.: Effect of acute and established anemia on O_2 transport at rest, submaximal and maximal work. J. Appl. Physiol., 44:36–43, 1978.

392. Finch, C. A., and Lenfant, C. M.: O_2 transport in man. N. Engl. J. Med., 286:407–415, 1972.

393. Klein, H. G.: Blood transfusions and athletics. N. Engl. J. Med., 312:854–856, 1985.

394. Bryan-Brown, C. W.: Blood flow to organs: Parameters for function and survival in critical illness. Crit. Care Med., 16:170–178, 1988.

395. Czer, L. S. C., and Shoemaker, W. C.: Optimal hematocrit value in critically ill postoperative patients. Surg. Gynecol. Obstet., 147:363–368, 1978.

396. Skinner, N. S., Jr.: Blood flow regulation as a factor in regulation of tissue O_2 delivery. 14th Annual Aspen Conference on Research in Emphysema. Chest, 61:13s–14s, 1972.

397. Lough, M. D., Chatburn, R., and Schrock, W. A.: Handbook on Respiratory Care. Chicago, Year Book Medical, 1980.

398. Zschoche, D. A.: Mosby's Comprehensive Review of Critical Care, 2nd ed. St. Louis, C.V. Mosby, 1981.

399. Armstrong, P. W., and Baigrie, R. S.: Hemodynamic Monitoring in the Critically Ill. Philadelphia, Harper & Row, 1980.

400. Davidshohn, E., and Henry, J. B. (eds): Clinical Diagnosis by Laboratory Methods, 15th ed. Philadelphia, W.B. Saunders, 1974.

401. Weil, M. H., and Afifi, A. A.: Experimental and clinical studies on lactate and pyruvate as indicators of the severity of shock. Circulation, 41:989–1001, 1970.

402. Cady, L. D., Weil, M. H., Afifi, A. A., et al: Quantitation of severity of critical illness with special reference to blood lactate. Crit. Care Med., 1:75–80, 1973.

403. Kruse, J. A., Mehta, K. C., and Carlson, R. W.: Definition of clinically significant lactic acidosis (Abstract). Chest, 92:100s, 1987.

404. Flenley, D.C.: Oxygen transport in chronic ventilatory failure. In Payne, J. P., and Hill, D. W. (eds): Oxygen Measurements in Biology and Medicine. Boston, Butterworths, 1975.

405. Dantzker, D. R., and Gutierrez, G.: The assessment of tissue oxygenation. Respir. Care, 30:456–462, 1985.

406. Heironomus, T. W., and Bageant, R. A.: Mechanical Artificial Ventilation, 3rd ed. Springfield, IL, Charles C. Thomas, 1977.

407. Berry, M. N.: The liver and lactic acidosis. Proc. Roy. Soc. Med., 60:1260, 1967.

408. Braden, G. L., Johnston, S. S., Germain, M. J., et al: Lactic acidosis associated with the therapy of acute bronchospasm (Letter). N. Engl. J. Med., 313:890, 1985.

409. Relman, A. S.: Lactic acidosis and a possible new treatment (Editorial). N. Engl. J. Med., 298:564–566, 1978.

410. Dantzker, D. R.: Oxygen transport and utilization. Respir. Care, 33:874–880, 1980.

411. Astiz, M. E., Rackow, E. C., Kaufman, B., et al: Relationship of oxygen delivery and mixed venous oxygenation to lactic acidosis in patients with sepsis and acute myocardial infarction. Crit. Care Med., 16:655–658, 1988.

412. Collaborative Group on Intracellular Monitoring: Intracellular monitoring of experimental respiratory failure. Am. Rev. Respir. Dis., 138:484–487, 1988.

413. Davidson, L. J., and Brown, S.: Continuous SvO_2 monitoring: A tool for analyzing hemodynamic status. Heart Lung, 15:287–291, 1986.

414. Metcalfe, J.: Introduction: O_2 transport. 14th Annual Aspen Conference on Research on Emphysema. Chest, 61:12s–13s, 1972.

415. Mithoefer, J. C., Holford, F. D., and Keighley, J. F. H.: The effect of oxygen administration on mixed venous oxygenation in chronic obstructive pulmonary disease. Chest, 66:122–132, 1974.

416. Demers, R. R., Irwin, R. S., and Braman, S. S.: Criteria for optimum PEEP. Respir. Care, 22:596–601, 1977.

417. Shenaq, S. A., Casar, G., Chelly, J. E., et al: Continuous monitoring of mixed venous oxygen saturation during aortic surgery. Chest, 92:796–799, 1987.

418. Vaughn, S., and Puri, V. K.: Cardiac output changes and continuous mixed venous oxygen saturation measurement in the critically ill. Crit. Care Med., 16:495–498, 1988.

419. Dantzker, D. R.: Peripheral oxygen delivery and use. Semin. Respir. Med., 9(Suppl.):25–28, 1986.

420. Rashkin, M. C., Bosken, C., and Baughman, R. P.: Oxygen delivery in critically ill patients. Chest, 87:580–584, 1985.

421. Astiz, M. E., Rackow, E. C., Falk, J. L., et al: Oxygen delivery and consumption in patients with hyperdynamic septic shock. Crit. Care Med., 15:26–28, 1987.

422. Danek, S. J., Lynch, J. P., Weg, J. G., and Dantzker, D. R.: The dependence of oxygen uptake on oxygen delivery in adult respiratory distress syndrome. Am. Rev. Respir. Dis., 122:387–395, 1980.

423. Bihari, D., Gimson, A. E. S., Waterson, M., and Williams, R.: Tissue hypoxia during fulminant hepatic failure. Crit. Care Med., 13:1034–1038, 1985.

424. Mohsenifar, Z., Amin, D., Jasper, A. C., et al: Dependence of oxygen consumption on oxygen delivery in patients with chronic congestive heart failure. Chest, 92:447–450, 1987.

425. Brent, B. N., Matthay, R. A., Mahler, D. A., et al: Relationship between oxygen uptake and oxygen transport in stable patients with chronic obstructive pulmonary disease. Am. Rev. Respir. Dis., 129: 682–686, 1984.

426. Mohsenifar, Z., Jasper, A. C., and Koerner, S. K.: Relationship between oxygen uptake and oxygen delivery in patients with pulmonary hypertension. Am. Rev. Respir. Dis., 138:69–73, 1988.

427. Dorinsky, P. M., Costello, J. L., and Gadek, J. E.: Relationships of oxygen uptake and oxygen delivery in respiratory failure not due to ARDS. Chest, 93:1013–1019, 1988.

428. Bihari, D., Smithies, M., Gimson, A., and Tinker, J.: The effects of vasodilation with prostacyclin on oxygen delivery and uptake in critically ill patients. N. Engl. J. Med., 317:397–403, 1987.

429. Siegel, J. H., Cerra, F. B., Coleman, B., et al: Physiological and metabolic correlations in human sepsis. Surgery, 86:163–172, 1979.

430. Vincent, J. L., Roman, A., and Kahn, R. J.: Oxygen uptake/supply dependency: The dobutamine test (Abstract). Chest, 94:7s, 1988.

431. Shoemaker, W. C., Appel, P. L., and Kram, H. B.: Tissue oxygen debt as a determinant of lethal and nonlethal postoperative organ failure. Crit. Care Med., 16:1117–1120, 1988.

432. Groeneveld, A. B., Bronsveld, W., and Thijs, L. G.: Hemodynamic determinants of mortality in human septic shock. Surgery, 99:140–153, 1986.

433. Noble, W. H., and Kay, J. C.: Effect of continuous positive-pressure ventilation and oxygenation after pulmonary microemboli in dogs. Crit. Care Med., 13:412–416, 1985.

434. Walsh, J. M., Vanderwarf, C., Hoscheit, D., and Fahey, P. J.: Unsuspected hemodynamic alterations during endotracheal suctioning. Chest, 95:162–165, 1989.

435. Shively, M.: Effect of position change on mixed venous oxygen saturation in coronary artery bypass surgery patients. Heart Lung, 17:51–59, 1988.

436. Robin, E.D.: Part IV. Pathophysiology of hypoxia: Protocol 1. Semin. Resp. Med., 3:112–117, 1981.

437. Dantzker, D. R.: Tissue oxygen delivery. In Dantzker, D. R., MacIntyre, N. R., Bakow, E. D. (eds): Comprehensive Respiratory Care. Philadelphia, W.B. Saunders, 1995.

438. Marinella, M. A.: "Tomatophagia" and iron deficiency anemia (Letter). N. Engl. J. Med., 341:60–61, 1999.

439. Oski, F. A.: Iron deficiency in infancy and childhood. N. Engl. J. Med., 329:190–193, 1993.

440. Platt, O. S., Thorington, B. D., Brambilla, D. J., et al: Pain in sickle cell disease. N. Engl. J. Med., 325:11–16, 1991.

441. Perrine, S. P., Ginder, G. D., Faller, D. V., et al: A short-term trial of butyrate to stimulate fetal-globin-gene expression in the beta-globulin disorder. N. Engl. J. Med., 328:81–86, 1993.

442. Walker, R. H.: Transfusion risks. Am. J. Clin. Pathol., 88:374–378, 1987.

443. Pilla, M. A.: Blood transfusion in critical care (Letter). N. Engl. J. Med., 341:123, 1999.

444. Herbert, P. C., Wells, G., Blajchman, M. A., et al: A multicenter, randomized, controlled clinical trial of transfusion requirements in critical care. N. Engl. J. Med., 340:409–417, 1999.

445. Haryadi, D. G., Orr, J. A., Dipl-Ing, D. G., and McJames, B. S.: Evaluation of a partial CO_2 rebreathing Fick technique for measurement of cardiac output. Anesthesiology, 89:A536, 1998.

446. Gloe, D.: Common reactions to transfusions. Heart Lung, 20:506–514, 1991.

447. Bochner, B. S., and Lightenstein, L. M.: Anaphylaxis. N. Engl. J. Med., 324:1785–1790, 1991.

448. Shoemaker, W. C., Appel, P. L., and Kram, H. B.: Role of oxygen debt in the development of organ failure sepsis, and death in high-risk surgical patients. Chest, 102:208–215, 1992.

449. Tuchschmidt, J., Fried, J., Astiz, M., and Rackow, E.: Elevation of cardiac output and oxygen delivery improves outcome in septic shock. Chest, 102:216–220, 1992.

450. Chiolero, R., Mavrocordatos, P., Bracco, D., et al: Oxygen consumption by the Fick method: Methodologic factors. Am. J. Resp. Crit. Care Med., 149:1118–1122, 1994.

451. Phang, P. T., Cunningham, K. F., Ronco, J. J., et al: Mathematical coupling explains dependence of oxygen consumption on oxygen delivery in ARDS. Am. J. Respir. Crit. Care Med., 150:318–323, 1994.

452. Ronco, J. J., Fenwick, J. C., Wiggs, B. R., et al: Oxygen consumption is independent of increases in oxygen delivery by dobutamine in septic patients who have normal or increased lactate. Am. Rev. Resp. Dis., 147:25–31, 1993.

453. Corwin, H. L., Parsonnet, K. C., Gettinger, A.: RBC transfusion in the ICU: Is there a reason? Chest 108:767–770, 1995.

454. Krafft, P., Steltzer, H., Heismayer, M., Klimscha, W., and Hammerle, A.F.: Mixed venous oxygen saturation in critically ill septic shock patients. Chest, 103:900–906, 1993.

455. Attewell, J. V., Lidsky, J. M., Chandler, J. M., et al: Interstitial pH decreases postoperatively despite stability of oxygen transport variables in open-heart patients (Abstract). Chest, 102:135S, 1992.

456. Landow, L., Phillips, D. A., Heard, S. O., et al: Gastric tonometry and venous oximetry in cardiac surgery patients. Crit. Care Med., 19:1226, 1991.

457. Poole, J. W., Sammartano, R. J., and Boley, S. J.: The use of tonometry in the early diagnosis of mesenteric ischemia. Curr. Surg., 21:25, 1987.

458. Doglio, G. R., Pusajo, J. F., Egurrola, M. A., et al: Gastric mucosal pH as a prognostic index of mortality in critically ill patients. Crit. Care Med., 19: 1037–1039, 1991.

459. Ramage, J. E.: Hemodynamic and gas exchange monitoring. In Hess, D. R., et al. (eds): Respiratory Care: Principles and Practice. Philadelphia, W.B. Saunders, 2002.

460. Kulig, K.: Cyanide antidotes and fire toxicology. N. Engl. J. Med., 325:1801–1802, 1991.

461. Baud, F. J., Barriot, P., Toffis, V., et al: Elevated blood cyanide concentrations in victims of smoke inhalation. N. Engl. J. Med., 325:1761–1766, 1991.

462. Rooth, G.: Acid-Base and Electrolyte Balance. Chicago, Year Book, 1974.

463. Sassoon, C. S. H., Hassell, K. T., and Mahutte, C. K.: Hyperoxic-induced hypercapnia in stable chronic obstructive pulmonary disease. Am. Rev. Respir. Dis., 135:907–911, 1987.

464. Luft, U. C., Mostyn, E. M., Loepky, J. A., and Venters, M. D.: Contribution of the Haldane effect to the rise of arterial PCO_2 in hypoxic patients breathing oxygen. Crit. Care Med., 9:32–37, 1981.

465. Christensen, H. N.: Body Fluids and the Acid-Base Balance. Philadelphia, W.B. Saunders, 1964.

466. Frazier, H. S., and Yager, H.: The clinical use of diuretics (Pt. I). N. Engl. J. Med., 288:246–249, 1973.

467. Frazier, H. S., and Yager, H.: The clinical use of diuretics (Pt. II). N. Engl. J. Med., 288:455–457, 1973.

468. Coe, F. L.: Metabolic alkalosis. J.A.M.A., 238:2288–2290, 1977.

469. Sonneblick, M., Friedlander, Y., and Rosin, A. J.: Diuretic-induced severe hyponatremia. Chest, 103:601–606, 1993.

470. Burnell, J. M., Villamil, M. F., Myeno, B. T., and Scribner, B. H.: The effect in humans of extracellular pH change on the relationship between serum potassium concentration and intracellular potassium. J. Clin. Invest., 35:935–939, 1956.

471. Fulop, M.: Serum potassium in lactic acidosis and ketoacidosis. N. Engl. J. Med., 300:1087–1089, 1979.

472. Orringer, C. E., Eustace, J. C., Wunsch, C. D., and Gardner, L. B.: Natural history of lactic acidosis after grand mal seizures: A model for the study of an anion gap acidosis not associated with hyperkalemia. N. Engl. J. Med., 297:796–799, 1977.

473. Oster, J. R., Perez, G. O., and Vaamonde, C. A.: Relationship between blood pH and potassium and phosphorous during acute metabolic acidosis. Am. J. Physiol., 235:F345–351, 1978.

474. Narins, R. G., Jones, E. R., Stom, M. C., et al: Diagnostic strategies in disorders of fluid, electrolyte and acid-base homeostasis. Am. J. Med., 72:496–519, 1982.

475. Stewart, P. A.: How to Understand Acid-Base. New York, Elsevier, 1981.

476. Swenson, E. R.: The strong ion difference approach: Can a strong case be made for its use in acid-base analysis? (Editorial). Respir. Care, 44:26–27, 1999.

477. Morfei, J.: Stewart's strong ion difference approach to acid-base analysis. Respir. Care, 44:45–52, 1999.

478. Vera, Z., Janzen, D., Desai, J.: Acute hypokalemia and inducibility of ventricular tachyarrhythmia in a nonischemic canine model. Chest, 100:1414–1420, 1991.

479. Molfino, N. A., Nannini, L. J., Martelli, A. N., and Slutsky, A. S.: Respiratory arrest in near-fatal asthma. N. Engl. J. Med., 324:285–288, 1991.

480. Khanna, A., and Kurtzman, N. A.: Metabolic alkalosis. Respir. Care, 46:354–365, 2001.

481. Figge, J., et al: Anion gap and hypoalbuminemia. Crit. Care Med., 26:1807–1810, 1998.

482. Thomas, C. L.: Taber's Cyclopedic Medical Dictionary, 16th ed. Philadelphia, F.A. Davis, 1989.

483. Cohen, J. J., and Kassirer, J. P. (eds.): Acid/Base. Boston, Little, Brown, 1982.

484. Swenson, E. R.: Metabolic acidosis. Respir. Care, 46:342–353, 2001.

485. Epstein, S. E., and Singh, N.: Respiratory acidosis. Respir. Care, 46:366–383, 2001.

486. Eldridge, F., and Gherman, C.: Studies of oxygen administration in respiratory failure. Ann. Intern. Med., 68:569–578, 1968.

487. Schiff, M. M., and Massaro, D.: Effect of O_2 administration by a Venturi apparatus on arterial blood gas values in patients with respiratory failure. N. Engl. J. Med., 277:950–953, 1967.

488. Hunt, W. B., Jr.: Low flow oxygen in respiratory failure treatment. Cont. Ed., Feb. 1984.

489. Lejeune, P., Mols, P., Naeje, R., et al: Acute hemodynamic effects of controlled oxygen therapy in decompensated chronic obstructive pulmonary disease. Crit. Care Med., 12:1032–1035, 1984.

490. Sassoon, C. S. H., Hassell, K. T., and Mahutte, C. K.: Hyperoxic-induced hypercapnia in stable chronic obstructive pulmonary disease. Am. Rev. Respir. Dis., 135:907–911, 1987.

491. American College of Chest Physicians—National Heart, Lung and Blood Institute: National conference on O_2 therapy. Respir. Care, 29:922–935, 1984.

492. Weil, J. V., McCullough, R. E., Kline, J. S., and Sodal, B. S.: Diminished ventilatory response to hypoxia and hypercapnia after morphine in normal man. N. Engl. J. Med., 292:1103, 1975.

493. Driver, A. G., and LeBrun, M.: Iatrogenic malnutrition in patients receiving ventilatory support. J.A.M.A., 244:2195–2196, 1980.

494. Covelli, H. D., Black, J. W., Olsen, M. S., and Beekman, J. F.: Respiratory failure precipitated by high carbohydrate loads. Ann. Intern. Med., 95:579–581, 1981.

495. Herve, P., Simonneau, G., Girard, P., et al: Hypercapnic acidosis induced by nutrition in mechanically ventilated patients: Glucose versus fat. Crit. Care Med., 13:537–540, 1985.

496. Sage, J. I., Van Uitert, R. L., and Duffy, T. E.: Simultaneous measurement of cerebral blood flow and unidirectional movement of substances across the blood-brain barrier: Theory, method and application to leucine. J. Neurochem., 36:1731–1738, 1981.

497. Clivati, A., Ciofetti, M., Cavestri, R., and Longhini, E.: Cerebral vascular responsiveness in chronic hypercapnia. Chest, 102:135–138, 1992.

498. Tuxen, D. V.: Permissive hypercapnic ventilation. Am. J. Respir. Crit. Care Med., 150:870–874, 1994.

499. Begin, P., and Grassino, A.: Inspiratory muscle dysfunction and chronic hypercapnia in chronic obstructive pulmonary disease. Am. Rev. Respir. Dis., 143:905–912, 1991.

500. Rochester, D. F.: Respiratory muscle weakness, pattern of breathing, and CO_2 retention in COPD. Am. Rev. Respir. Dis., 143:901–903, 1991.

501. Vitacca, M., Foglio, K., Scalvini, S., et al: Time course of pulmonary function before admission into ICU. Chest, 102:1737–1741, 1992.

502. Lasky, T., Terracciano, G. J., Magder, L., et al: The Guillain-Barré syndrome and the 1992–1993 and 1993–1994 influenza vaccines. N. Engl. J. Med., 339:1797–1802, 1998.

503. Drachman, D. B.: Myasthenia gravis. N. Engl. J. Med., 330:1797–1810, 1994.

504. Larach, M. G.: Malignant hyperthermia: The respiratory care practitioner's critical role. Respir. Care, 35:949–951, 1990.

505. Vakharia, N., and Hall, R.: Malignant hyperthermia: A review of current concepts. Respir. Care, 35:977–986, 1990.

506. Dietch, E. A.: The management of burns. N. Engl. J. Med., 323:1249–1254, 1990.

507. Talpers, S. S., Romberger, D. J., Bucnce, S. B., and Pingleton, S. K.: Nutritionally associated increased carbon dioxide production. Chest, 102:551–555, 1992.

508. Foster, G. T., Vaziri, N. D., and Sassoon, S. H.: Respiratory alkalosis. Respir. Care, 46:384–391, 2001.

509. Hudson, L. D., Hurlow, R. S., Craig, K. C., et al: Does intermittent mandatory ventilation correct respiratory alkalosis in patients receiving assisted mechanical ventilation? Am. Rev. Respir. Dis., 132:1071–1075, 1985.

510. Contreras, G., Guiterrez, M., Beroiza, T., et al: Ventilatory drive and respiratory muscle function in pregnancy. Am. Rev. Resp. Dis., 144:837–841, 1991.

511. Gardner, W. M.: The pathophysiology of hyperventilation disorders. Chest, 109:516–534, 1996.

512. Saisch, S. G. N., Wessely, S., and Gardner, W. N.: Patients with acute hyperventilation presenting to an inner-city emergency department. Chest, 110:953–957, 1996.

513. Poison Pearls and Perils: A Bulletin from the National Capital Poison Center. Vol. 1, no. 4, 1995.

514. Jacobsen, D.: New treatment for ethylene glycol poisoning (Editorial). N. Engl. J. Med., 340:879–881, 1999.

515. Narins, R. G., and Emmett, M.: Simple and mixed acid-base disorders: A practical approach. Medicine (Baltimore), 59:161–187, 1980.

516. Goldberger, E.: A Primer of Water, Electrolyte and Acid-Base Syndromes, 5th ed. Philadelphia, Lea & Febiger, 1974.

517. Sutheimer, C., Bost, R., Sunshine, I., et al: Volatiles by deadspace chromatography. In Sunshine, I., and Jatlow, P. (eds): Methodology for Analytical Toxicology, vol. 2. Boca Raton, FL, CRC Press, 1982, pp. 1–9.

518. Foster, D. W., and McGarry, J. D.: The metabolic derangements and treatment of diabetic ketoacidosis. N. Engl. J. Med., 309:159–169, 1983.

519. Schade, D. S., and Eaton, P.: Differential diagnosis and therapy of hyperketonemic state. J.A.M.A., 241:2064–2065, 1979.

520. Fischman, C. M., and Oster, J. R.: Toxic effects of toluene: A new cause of high anion gap acidosis. J.A.M.A., 241:1713–1715, 1979.

521. Narins, R. G., Jones, E. R., Stom, M. C., et al: Diagnostic strategies in disorders of fluid, electrolyte and acid-base homeostasis. Am. J. Med., 72:496–519, 1982.

523. Goldberger, E.: A Primer of Water, Electrolyte and Acid-Base Syndromes, 5th ed. Philadelphia, Lea & Febiger, 1974.

524. Orringer, C. E., Eustace, J. C., Wunsch, C. D., and Gardner, L. B.: Natural history of lactic acidosis after grand mal seizure. N. Engl. J. Med., 297:796–799, 1977.

525. Tietz, N. W.: Fundamentals of Clinical Chemistry, 3rd ed. Philadelphia, W.B. Saunders, 1987, p. 659.

526. Relman, A. S.: Lactic acidosis and a possible new treatment (Editorial). N. Engl. J. Med., 298:564–566, 1978.

527. Heinig, R. E., Clarke, E. F., and Waterhouse, C.: Lactic acidosis and liver disease. Arch. Intern. Med., 13:1229–1232, 1979.

528. Miller, P. D., Heinig, R. E., and Waterhouse, C.: Treatment of alcoholic acidosis. Arch. Intern. Med., 38:67–72, 1978.

529. Cohen, J. J., Kassirer, J. P. (eds.): Acid/Base. Boston, Little, Brown, 1982.

530. Okrent, D. G., Tessler, S., Twersky, R. A., and Tashkin, D. P.: Metabolic acidosis not due to lactic acidosis in patients with severe acute asthma. Crit. Care Med., 15:1098–1101, 1987.

531. Hodgkin, J. E., Soeprono, F. F., and Chan, D. M.: Incidence of metabolic alkalemia in hospitalized patients. Crit. Care Med., 8:725–728, 1980.

532. Lyons, J. H., Jr., and Moore, F. D.: Posttraumatic alkalosis: Incidence and pathophysiology of alkalosis in surgery. Surgery, 60:93, 1966.

533. Coe, F. L.: Metabolic alkalosis. J.A.M.A., 238:2288–2290, 1977.

534. Madias, N. E., Ayus, J. C., and Adrogue, H. J.: Increased anion gap in metabolic alkalosis. N. Engl. J. Med., 300:1421–1423, 1979.

535. Driscoll, D. F., Bistrian, B. R., Jenkins, R. L., et al: Development of metabolic alkalosis after massive transfusion during orthotopic liver transplantation. Crit. Care Med., 15:905–908, 1987.

536. Sheldon, G. F.: Blood from bag through patient. Emerg. Med., 12:36–38, 1980.

537. Winters, R. W., and Dell, R. B.: Acid-Base Physiology in Medicine. Boston, Little, Brown, 1982.

538. Gallagher, T. J.: Metabolic alkalosis complicating weaning from mechanical ventilation. South. Med. J., 72:786–787, 1979.

539. Riccio, J. F., and Irani, F. A.: Posthypercapnic metabolic alkalosis: Common and neglected cause. South. Med. J., 72:7, 1979.

540. Kraut, J. A., and Madias, N. E.: Approach to patients with acid-base disorders. Respir. Care, 46:392–403, 2001.

541. Rahman, A. R., McDevitt, D. G., Struthers, A. D., and Lipworth, B.J.: The effects of enalapril and spironolactone on terbutaline-induced hypokalemia. Chest, 102:91–95, 1992.

542. Farese, R. V., Biglieri, E. G., Schackleton, C. H. L., et al: Licorice-induced hypermineralocorticoidism. N. Engl. J. Med., 325:1223–1227, 1991.

543. Campbell, E. J. M.: The J. Burns Amberson Lecture—The management of acute respiratory failure in chronic bronchitis and emphysema. Am. Rev. Respir. Dis., 96:626–639, 1967.

544. Smith, J. P., Stone, R. W., and Muschenheim, C.: Acute respiratory failure in chronic lung disease. Am. Rev. Respir. Dis., 97:791–803, 1968.

545. Rooth, G.: Acid-Base and Electrolyte Balance. Chicago, Year Book, 1974.

546. Pierce, N. F., Fedson, D. S., Brigham, K. L., et al: The ventilatory response to acute base deficit in humans. Ann. Intern. Med., 72:633–640, 1970.

547. Javaheri, S., and Kazemi, H.: Metabolic alkalosis and hypoventilation in humans. Am. Rev. Respir. Dis., 136:1011–1016, 1987.

548. Bradstetter, R. D., Tamarin, F. M., Washington, D., et al: Occult mucous airway obstruction in diabetic ketoacidosis. Chest, 91:575–578, 1987.

549. van Ypersele de Strihou, C., Brasseur, L., and DeConnick, J.: The carbon dioxide response curve for chronic hypercapnia in man. N. Engl. J. Med., 275:117–130, 1966.

550. Rodriguez, J. L., Askanazi, J., Weissman, C., et al: Ventilatory and metabolic effects of glucose infusions. Chest, 88:512–518, 1985.

551. Pierson, D. J.: Indications for mechanical ventilation in acute respiratory failure. Respir. Care, 28: 570–576, 1983

552. Hunt, W. B.: Low flow oxygen in respiratory failure treatment. Cont. Ed., February 1984.

553. Smith, J. P., Stone, R. W., and Muschenheim, C.: Acute respiratory failure in chronic lung disease. Am. Rev. Respir. Dis., 97:791–803, 1968.

554. Warrel, D. A., Edwards, R. H. T., Godfrey, S., and Jones, N. L.: Effects of controlled oxygen therapy on arterial blood gases in acute respiratory failure. B.M.J., 2:452–455, 1970.

555. Cooper, C. B.: Life expectancy in severe COPD (Editorial). Chest, 105:335–336, 1994.

556. Hill, N. S.: Noninvasive ventilation: Does it work, for whom, and how? (Editorial). Am. Rev. Resp. Dis., 147:1050–1055, 1993.

557. Leger. P., Bedicam, J. M., Cornette, A., et al: Nasal intermittent positive pressure ventilation. Chest, 105:100–105, 1994.

558. Wysocki, M., Tric, L., Wolff, M. A., et al: Noninvasive pressure support ventilation in patients with acute respiratory failure. Chest, 103:907–913, 1993.

559. Lum, L. C.: The syndrome of habitual chronic hyperventilation. Rec. Adv. Psychosom. Med., 3:196–229, 1976.

560. Rotherman, E. B., Jr., Safar, P., and Robin, E. D.: CNS disorder during mechanical ventilation in chronic pulmonary disease. J.A.M.A., 189:993–996, 1964.

561. Bendixen, H. H.: Rational ventilator modes for respiratory failure. Crit. Care Med., 2:225–227, 1974.

562. Hubmayer, R. D., Gay, P. C., and Tayyab, M.: Respiratory system mechanics in ventilated patients: Techniques and indications. Mayo Clin. Proc., 62:358–368, 1987.

563. De Guire, S., Gevirtz, R., Kawahara, Y., et al: Hyperventilation syndrome and the assessment of treatment for functional cardiac symptoms. Am. J. Cardiol., 70:673–677, 1992.

564. Kilburn, K. H.: Shock, seizures and coma with alkalosis during mechanical ventilation. Ann. Intern. Med., 65:977–984, 1966.

565. Kelly, B. J., and Luce, J. M.: Current concepts in cerebral protection. Chest, 103:1246–1254, 1993.

566. Kette, F., Weil, M. H., and Gazmuri, R. J.: Buffer solutions may compromise cardiac resuscitation by reducing the coronary perfusion pressure. Concepts Emerg. Crit. Care, 266:2121–2126, 1991.

567. Weil, M. H., Rackow, E. C., Trevino, R., et al: Difference in acid base state between venous and arterial blood during cardiopulmonary resuscitation. N. Engl. J. Med., 315:153–156, 1986.

568. Relman, A. S.: Blood gases: Arterial or venous? N. Engl. J. Med., 315:188–189, 1986.

569. Weil, M. H., Grundler, W., Yamaguchi, M., et al: Arterial blood gases fail to reflect acid-base status during cardiopulmonary resuscitation: A preliminary report. Crit. Care Med., 13:884–885, 1985.

570. Niemann, J. T., and Rosborough, J. P.: Effects of acidemia and sodium bicarbonate therapy in advanced cardiac life support. Ann. Emerg. Med., 13:781–784, 1984.

571. Grundler, W., Weil, M. H., Rackow, E. C., et al: Selective acidosis in venous blood during human cardiopulmonary resuscitation: A preliminary report. Crit. Care Med., 13:886–887, 1985.

572. Bowen, F. W., Jr., and Williams, J. L.: The use and abuse of bicarbonate in neonatal acid-base derangements. Respir. Care, 23:465–475, 1978.

573. Wiklund, L., and Sahlin, K.: Induction and treatment of metabolic acidosis: A study of pH changes in porcine and skeletal muscle and cerebrospinal fluid. Crit. Care Med., 13:109–113, 1985.

574. Kette, F., Weil, M. H., Plant, M., Gazmuri, R. J., and Rackow, E. C.: Buffer agents do not reverse intramyocardial acidosis during cardiac resuscitation. Circulation, 81:1660–1666, 1990.

575. Weisfeldt, M. L.: Sodium bicarbonate and CPR (Editorial). J.A.M.A., 266:2129–2130, 1991.

576. Rhee, K. H., Torro, L. O., McDonald, G. G., Nunally, R. L., and Levin, D. L.: Carbicarb, sodium bicarbonate, and sodium chloride in hypoxic lactic acidosis. Chest, 104:913–918, 1993.

577. Lyons, J. H., Jr., and Moore, F. D.: Posttraumatic alkalosis: Incidence and pathophysiology of alkalosis in surgery. Surgery, 60:93, 1966.

578. Bustamante, E. A., and Levy, H.: Severe alkalemia, hyponatremia, and diabetic ketoacidosis in an alcoholic man. Chest, 110:273–275, 1996.

579. Wilson, R. F., Gibson, D., Percinel, A. K., et al: Severe alkalosis in critically ill surgical patients. Arch. Surg., 105:97, 1972.

580. Weisberg, H. F.: Water, electrolytes, acid-base and oxygen. In Davidsohn, I., and Henry, J. B. (eds): Clinical Diagnosis by Laboratory Methods, 15th ed. Philadelphia, W.B. Saunders, 1974.

581. Marik, P. E., Hons, D. A., Kussman, B. D., Lipman, J., and Kraus, P.: Acetazolamide in the treatment of metabolic alkalosis in critically ill patients. Heart Lung, 20:455–458, 1991.

582. Cohen, J. J.: Physiology of metabolic alkalosis. In Schwartz, A. B., Lyons, H. (eds): Acid-Base and Electrolyte Balance. New York, Grune & Stratton, 1977.

583. Brimioulle, S., Berre, J., Dufaye, P., Vincent, J. L., et al: Hydrochloric acid infusion for treatment of metabolic alkalosis associated with respiratory acidosis. Crit. Care Med., 17:232–236, 1989.

584. Warren, S. E., Swerdlin, A. R. H., and Steinberg, S. M.: Treatment of alkalosis with ammonium chloride: A case report. Clin. Pharmacol. Ther., 25:624–627, 1979.

585. Wagner, C. W., Nesbit, R. R., Jr., and Mansberger, A. R., Jr.: Treatment of metabolic alkalosis with intravenous HCl. South. Med. J., 72:1241–1245, 1979.

586. Jankauskas, S. J., Gursel, E. T. I., and Antonenko, D. R.: Chest wall necrosis secondary to hydrochloric acid use in the treatment of metabolic alkalosis. Crit. Care Med., 17:963, 1989.

587. Brimioulle, S., Vincent, J. L., Dufaye, P., et al: Hydrochloric acid infusion for treatment of metabolic alkalosis: Effects on acid-base balance and oxygenation. Crit. Care Med., 13:738–742, 1985.

588. Severinghaus, J. W.: Interpreting acid-base balance (letter). Respir. Care, 27:1414–1415, 1982.

589. Prouix, J.: Respiratory monitoring: Arterial blood gas analysis, pulse oximetry, and end-tidal carbon dioxide analysis. Clin. Tech. Small Animal Pract., 14:227–230, 1999.

590. Neuman, M. R.: Pulse Oximetry: Physical Principles, Technical Realization and Present Limitations. New York, Plenum Press, 1986.

591. Severinghaus, J. W., and Astrup, P. B.: History of blood gas analysis. VI: Oximetry. J. Clin. Monit., 2:270–288, 1986.

592. Cole, P. V.: Bench analysis of blood gases. *In* Spence, A. A. (ed): Respiratory Monitoring in Intensive Care. New York, Churchill Livingstone, 1982.

593. Adams, A. P., and Hahn, C. E. W.: Principles and Practice of Blood Gas Analysis. London, Franklin Scientific Products, 1979.

594. Payne, J. B., and Severinghaus, J. W.: Pulse Oximetry. New York, Springer-Verlag, 1986.

595. Cole, P. V.: Bench analysis of blood gases. *In* Spence, A. A. (ed): Respiratory Monitoring in Intensive Care. New York, Churchill Livingstone, 1982.

596. Dennis, R. C., and Valeri, C. R.: Measuring per cent oxygen saturation of Hb, per cent carboxyhemoglobin and methemoglobin, and concentrations of total Hb and oxygen in blood of man, dog, and baboon. Clin. Chem., 26:1304–1308, 1980.

597. Zwart, A., Buursma, A., Oeseburg, B., et al: Determination of Hb derivatives with the IL 282 CO-oximeter as compared with a manual spectrophotometric five-wavelength method. Clin. Chem., 27:1903–1907, 1981.

598. Neuman, M. R.: Pulse Oximetry: Physical Principles, Technical Realization and Present Limitations. New York, Plenum Press, 1986.

599. Burki, N. K., and Albert, R. K.: Noninvasive monitoring of arterial blood gases: A report of the ACCP section on respiratory pathophysiology. Chest, 83:666–670, 1983.

600. ACCP–National Heart, Lung and Blood Institute. National Conference on O_2 Therapy. Respir. Care, 29:922–935, 1984.

601. Wanger, J., and Zeballos, R. J.: PFT Corner no. 7— Ear oximetry in the clinical laboratory. Respir. Care, 29:161–162, 1984.

602. Bland, D. K., and Anholm, J. D.: Arterial oxygen saturation during exercise: Erroneous results with ear oximetry (Abstract). Am. Rev. Respir. Dis., 137:150, 1988.

603. Cahan, C., Decker, M., Arnold, J., et al: Agreement between non-invasive oximetry values for oxygen saturation (Abstract). Am. Rev. Respir. Dis., 137:451, 1988.

604. Hertzman, A. B., and Spealman, C. R.: Observation on the finger volume pulse recorded photo-electrically. Am. J. Physiol., 119:334–335, 1937.

605. Altemeyer, K. H., Mayer, J., Berg-Seiter, S., and F'osel, T.: Pulse oximetry as a continuous, noninvasive monitoring procedure: Comparison of 2 instruments. Anesthetist, 35:43–45, 1986.

606. Lawson, D., Norley, L., Korben, G., et al: Blood flow limits and pulse oximeter signal detection. Anesthesiology, 67:599–603, 1987.

607. Berlin, S. L., Branson, P. S., Capps, J. S., et al: Pulse oximetry: A technology that needs direction (Editorial). Respir. Care, 33:243–244, 1988.

608. Costarino, A. T., Davis, D. A., and Keon, T. P.: Falsely normal saturation reading with the pulse oximeter. Anesthesiology, 67:830–831, 1987.

609. Mihm, F. G., and Halperin, B. D.: Noninvasive detection of profound arterial desaturation using a pulse oximetry device. Anesthesiology, 62:85–87, 1985.

610. Wahr, J. A., Tremper, K. K., and Diab, M.: Pulse oximetry. Respir. Care Clin. North Am., 1:77–105, 1995.

611. Tinker J. H., Dull, D. L., Caplan, R. A., Ward, R. J., and Cheney, F. W.: Role of monitoring devices in prevention of anesthetic mishaps: A closed claim analysis. Anesthesiology, 71:541–546, 1989.

612. Neff, T. A.: Routine oximetry: A fifth vital sign? (Editorial) Chest, 94:227, 1988.

613. Henning, R. J., McGlish, D., Daly, B., et al: Clinical resource utilization of ICU patients: Implications for organization of intensive care. Crit. Care Med., 15:264–269, 1987.

614. Sdivack, D.: The high cost of acute health care: A review of escalating costs and limitations of such exposure in intensive care units. Am. Rev. Resp. Dis., 137:1007–1111, 1987.

615. Severinghaus, J. W., Honda, Y.: History of blood gas analysis. VII. Pulse oximetry. J. Clin. Monit., 3:135–138, 1987.

616. Fluck, R. R., Schroeder, C., Franil, G., Kropf, B., and Engbertson, B.: Does ambient light affect the accuracy of pulse oximetry? Respir. Care, 48:677–680, 2003.

617. The Pulse Oximeter Guide. AARC Times, 13:29–35, 1989.

618. Welsch, J. P., DeCesare, R. and Hess, D.: Pulse oximetry: Instrumentation and clinical applications (and discussion). Respir. Care, 35:584–601, 1990.

619. Hess, D. R., and Kacmarek, R. M.: Essentials of Mechanical Ventilation, 2nd ed. New York, McGraw-Hill, 2002.

620. Sidi, A., Rush, W., Gravenstein, N., et al: Pulse oximetry fails to accurately detect low levels of arterial hemoglobin oxygen saturation in dogs. J. Clin. Monit., 3:257–262, 1987.

621. Hannhart, B., Michalski, H., Delorme, N., Chapparo, G., and Polu, J.: Reliability of six pulse oximeters in chronic pulmonary disease. Chest, 99:842–846, 1991.

622. Pulse Oximetry. AARC Clinical Practice Guidelines. Respir. Care, 36:1406–1409, 1991.

623. Palve, H., and Vuori, A.: Pulse oximetry during low cardiac output and hypothermia states immediately after open-heart surgery. Crit. Care Med., 17:66–69, 1989.

624. Costarino, A. T., Davis, D. A., and Keon, T. P.: Falsely normal saturation reading with the pulse oximeter. Anesthesiology, 67:830–831, 1987.

625. Harris, K. H.: Noninvasive monitoring of gas exchange. Respir. Care, 32:544–557, 1987.

626. Nellcor Troubleshooting Guide for Optical Interference. Hayward, CA, Nellcor Inc., 1987.

627. Zeballos, J., and Weisman, I. M.: Reliability of noninvasive oximetry in black subjects during exercise and hypoxia. Am. Rev. Resp. Dis., 144:1240–1244, 1991.

628. Hicks, G. H.: Blood gas and acid-base measurement. In Dantzker, D. R., MacIntyre, N. R., and Bakow, E. D. (eds): Comprehensive Respiratory Care. Philadelphia, W.B. Saunders, 1995.

629. Signal Extraction Technology. Masimo Corporation. Irvine, CA. Available at: www.masimo.com. Product literature 2001.

630. Cairo, J. M.: Blood gas monitoring. In Cairo, J. M., and Pilbeam, S. P. (eds): Mosby's Respiratory Care Equipment. St. Louis, Mosby, 2004.

631. Clayton, D., Webb, R. K., Ralston, A. C., et al: A comparison of the performance of 20 pulse oximeters under conditions of poor perfusion. Anesthesia, 46:3–10, 1991.

632. Cote, C. J., Goldstein, E. A., Fuchsman, W. H., et al: The effect of nail polish on pulse oximetry. Anesth. Analg., 67:683–686, 1988.

633. Evans, M. L., and Geddes, L. A.: An assessment of blood vessel vasoactivity using photoplethysmography. Med. Instrum., 22:29–32, 1988.

634. Severinghaus, J. W., Naifeh, K. H., and Koh, S. O.: Errors in 14 pulse oximeters during profound hypoxemia. J. Clin. Monit., 5:72–81, 1989.

635. Blonshine, S.: Technology advances: pulse oximetry. AARC Times, p. 45, 1999.

636. Moller, J. T., Pederson, T., Rasmussen, L. S., et al: Randomized evaluation of pulse oximetry in 20,802 patients: I. Anesthesiology, 78:436–444, 1993.

637. Barker, S. J.: "Motion-resistant" pulse oximetry: A comparison of new and old models. Anesth. Analg., 95:967–972, 2002.

638. Tsein, C. L., and Fackler, J. C.: Poor prognosis for existing monitors in the intensive care unit. Crit. Care Med., 25:614–619, 1997.

639. Cropp, A. J., Woods, L. A., Raney, D., and Bredle, D. L.: Name that tone: The proliferation of alarms in the intensive care unit. Chest, 105:1217–1220, 1994.

640. Lawless, S. T.: Crying wolf: False alarms in pediatric intensive care unit. Crit. Care Med., 22:981–985, 1994.

641. Thermal injury due to pulse oximeter probes. Aust. Patient Saf. Found. (APSF) News, 2:4, 1988.

642. Medical Strategic Planning (MSP) Industry Alert, 2:1, 2000.

643. Goldman, J. M., Petterson, M. T., Kopotic, R. J., and Barker, S. J.: Masimo signal extraction pulse oximetry. J. Clin. Monit. Comput., 16:475–483, 2000.

644. Next generation pulse oximetry: Focusing on Masimo signal extraction technology. Health Devices, 29:349–370, 2000.

645. Elfadel, I. M, Weber, W. M., and Barker, S. J.: Motion-resistant pulse oximetry. J. Clin. Monit., 11:262, 1995.

646. Goldstein, M. R., Liberman, R. I., Taschuk, R. D., Thomas, A., and Vogt, J. F.: Pulse oximetry in transport of poorly perfused babies. Pediatrics, 102:818, 1988.

647. Poets, C. F., Urschitz, M. S., and Bohnhorst, B.: Pulse oximetry in the neonatal intensive care unit (NICU): Detection of hyperoxemia and false alarm rates. Anesth. Analg., 94(Suppl. 1):S41–S43, 2002.

648. Miyaska, K.: Pulse oximetry in the management of children in the PICU. Anesth. Analg., 94:967–972, 2002.

649. Barcelona, S. L., Roth, A. G., and Cote, C. J.: Comparison of four pulse oximeters on pediatric patients during anesthesia and the initial phases of recovery: Does the new generation offer an advantage? (Abstract). Am. Soc. Anesthesiol. Available at: www.Asa-abstracts.com. Accessed Feb. 18, 2003.

650. Holmes, A., Vogt, J., Gangitano, E., Stephenson, C., and Liberman, R.: Useful life of pulse oximeter sensors in a NICU. Respir. Care, 43:860, 1998.

651. Onyx Model 9500 Finger Pulse Oximeter Product Literature. Nonin Medical, Plymouth, MN, 2000.

652. Guy, H. J.: Pulse oximetry. J. Resp. Care Pract., 89, 1997.

653. Niermeyer, S., Shaffer, E. M., Thilo, E., Corbin, C., and Moore, L. G.: Arterial oxygenation and pulmonary artery arterial pressure in healthy neonates and infants at high altitude. J. Pediatr., 123:767–772, 1993.

654. Carone, M., Patessio, A. Appendi, L., et al: Comparison of invasive and noninvasive saturation monitoring in prescribing oxygen during exercise in COPD patients. Eur. Resp., 10:446–451, 1997.

655. Bohnhorst, B., Peter, C. S., and Poets, C. F.: Detection of hyperoxemia in neonates: Data from three new pulse oximeters. Arch. Dis. Child Fetal Neonatal Educ., 87:F217–F219, 2002.

656. Ramage, J. E.: Hemodynamic and gas exchange monitoring. In Hess, D. R., et al, (eds): Respiratory Care: Principles and Practice. Philadelphia, W.B. Saunders, 2002.

657. Rosenberg, J., Rasmussen, V., von Jenssen, F., Ullstad, T., and Kehlet, H.: Late postoperative episodic and constant hypoxemia and associated ECG abnormalities. Br. J. Anesth., 65:684–691, 1990.

658. Baumberger, J. P., and Goodfriend, R. B.: Determination of arterial oxygen tension in man by equilibration through intact skin. Fed. Proc. Fed. Am. Soc. Exp. Biol., 10:10–16, 1951.

659. Evans, N. T. S., and Naylor, P. R. D.: The systemic oxygen supply to the surface of human skin. Respir. Physiol., 3:21–26, 1967.

660. Vyas, H., Helms, P., and Cheriyan, G.: Transcutaneous oxygen monitoring beyond the neonatal period. Crit. Care Med., 16:844–847, 1988.

661. Severinghaus, J. W.: Transcutaneous blood gas analysis (the 1981 Donald F Egan Lecture). Respir. Care, 27:152–159, 1982.

662. Spence, A. S.: Respiratory Monitoring in Intensive Care. New York, Churchill Livingstone, 1982.

663. Burki, N. K., and Albert, R. K.: Noninvasive monitoring of arterial blood gases: A report of the ACCP section on respiratory pathophysiology. Chest, 83:666–670, 1983.

664. Viitanen, A., Salemper'a, M., and Heinonen, J.: Noninvasive monitoring of oxygenation during one-lung ventilation: A comparison of transcutaneous oxygen tension and pulse oximetry. J. Clin. Monit., 2:90–95, 1987.

665. Jennis, M. S., and Peabody, J. L.: Pulse oximetry: An alternative method for the assessment of oxygenation in newborn infants. Pediatrics, 4:524–528, 1987.

666. Lafeber, H. N., Fetter, W. P., and van der Weil, A. R.: Pulse oximetry and transcutaneous oxygen tension in hypoxemic neonates and infants with bronchopulmonary dysplasia. Adv. Exp. Med. Biol., 220:181–186, 1987.

667. Bossi, E., Meister, B., and Pfenninger, J.: Comparison between transcutaneous PO_2 and pulse oximetry for monitoring O_2 treatment in newborns. Adv. Exp. Med. Biol., 220:171–176, 1987.

668. Baeckert, P., Bucher, H. U., Fallenstein, F., et al: Is pulse oximetry reliable in detecting hyperoxemia in the neonate? Adv. Exp. Med. Biol., 220:165–169, 1987.

669. Kesten, S., Chapman, K. R., and ReBuck, A. S.: Response characteristics of a dual transcutaneous oxygen/carbon dioxide monitoring system. Chest, 99:1211–1215, 1991.

670. Chan, M. M.: What is the effect of fingernail polish on pulse oximetry? Chest, 123:2163–2164, 2003.

671. AARC Clinical Practice Guideline: Pulse oximetry. Respir. Care, 36:1406–1409, 1991.

672. AARC Clinical Practice Guideline: Transcutaneous blood gas monitoring for neonatal & pediatric patient. Respir. Care, 39:1176–1179, 1994.

673. Hess, D.: Capnometry and capnography: Technical aspects, physiological aspects, and clinical applications. Respir. Care, 35:557–576, 1990.

674. AARC Clinical Practice Guideline. Capnography/capnometry during mechanical ventilation (2003 update). Respir. Care, 48:534–539, 2003.

675. Marriott, W. M.: The determination of alveolar carbon dioxide by a simple method. J.A.M.A., 66:1594–1596, 1916.

676. AARC Bulletin. Adult Critical Care Section. Sept. 1992.

677. Graybeal, J. M., and Russell, G. B.: Capnometry in the surgical ICU: A meta-analysis of the arterial and end-tidal carbon dioxide difference. PS News Literary Award, 1992. Also presented at the AARC Open Forum, 1991, Atlanta, GA.

678. Kumar, A., Bithal, P., Chouhan, R. S., and Sinha, P. K.: Should one rely on capnometry when a capnogram is not seen? J. Neurosurg. Anesthesiol., 14:153–156, 2002.

679. Hatle, L., and Rokseth, R.: The arterial to end-expiratory carbon dioxide gradient in acute pulmonary embolism and other cardiopulmonary diseases. Chest, 66:352–357, 1974.

680. Graybeal, J. M.: Capnography–A key to understanding physiology (Editorial). Respir. Care, 42:200–201, 1997.

681. Domsky, M., Wilson, R. F., and Heins, J.: Intraoperative end-tidal carbon dioxide values and derived calculations correlated with outcome: Prognosis and capnography. Crit. Care Med., 23:1497–1503, 1995.

682. Bhende, M. S., and La Covey, D. C.: End-tidal carbon dioxide monitoring in the prehospital setting. Prehosp. Emerg. Care, 5:208–213, 2001.

683. Weil, M. H., Bisera, J. Trevino, R. P., and Rackow, E. C.: Cardiac output and end-tidal carbon dioxide. Crit. Care Med., 13:907–909, 1985.

684. Trevino, R. P., Bisera, J., Weil, M. H., Rackow, E. C., et al: End-tidal CO_2 as a guide to successful cardiopulmonary resuscitation: A preliminary report. Crit. Care Med., 13:910–911, 1985.

685. Sanders, A. B., Ewy, G. A., Bragg, S. Atlas, M., et al: Expired PCO_2 as a prognostic indicator of successful resuscitation from cardiac arrest. Ann. Emerg. Med., 14:948–952, 1985.

686. Garnett, A. R., Ornato, J. P., Gonzalez Johnson, B.: End-tidal carbon dioxide monitoring during cardiopulmonary resuscitation. J.A.M.A., 257:512–515, 1987.

687. Kalenda, Z.: The capnogram as a guide to the efficacy of cardiac massage. Resuscitation, S6:259–263, 1978.

688. Sanders, A. B., Kern, K. B., Otto, C. W., Milander, M. M., et al: End-tidal carbon dioxide monitoring during cardiopulmonary resuscitation: A prognostic indicator for survival. J.A.M.A., 262:1347–1351, 1989.

689. Falk, J. L., Rackow, E. C., and Weil, M. H.: End-tidal carbon dioxide concentration during cardiopulmonary resuscitation. N. Engl. J. Med., 318:607–611, 1988.

690. National Committee for Clinical Laboratory Standards: Blood Gas Pre-analytical Considerations: Specimen Collection, Calibration, and Controls (Proposed guideline). NCCLS publication C27—P. Villanova, PA, N.C.C.L.S., 1985.

691. National Committee for Clinical Laboratory Standards: Procedure for the Collection of Diagnostic Blood Specimens by Venipuncture (Approved Standard), 4th ed. NCCLS document H3-A4. Wayne, PA, NCCLS, 1998.

692. Nocturnal Oxygen Therapy Trial Group: Continuous or nocturnal oxygen therapy in hypoxemic chronic obstructive lung disease: A clinical trial. Ann. Intern. Med., 93:391–398, 1980.

693. Report of the Medical Research Council Working Party: Long term domiciliary oxygen therapy in

chronic hypoxic cor pulmonale complicating chronic bronchitis and emphysema. Lancet, 1:681–685, 1981.

694. Code of Federal Regulations, Title 14 CFR, Part 25.841. Washington, DC, US Government Printing Office, 1986.

695. Gong, H. J.: Air travel and oxygen therapy in cardiopulmonary patients. Chest, 101:1104–1113, 1992.

696. Downs, J. B.: Has oxygen administration delayed appropriate respiratory care? Fallacies regarding oxygen therapy (2002 Donald F. Egan Scientific Lecture). Respir. Care, 48:611–620, 2003.

697. DeWitt, A. L.: Routine ABGs can carry big risk too. ADVANCE for Respiratory Care Practitioners. Aug. 12, 1996, p 4.

698. Fairas, E. M., et al: Delivery of high inspired oxygen by face mask. J. Crit. Care, 6:119–124, 1991.

699. ACCP-NLHBI: Report of national conference on oxygen therapy. Arch. Intern. Med., 144:1645–1655, 1984.

700. Rodrigo, G. J., et al: 100% oxygen can be harmful to asthmatics. Chest, 124:1312–1317, 2003.

701. Pierson, D. J.: The future of respiratory care. Respir. Care, 46:705–718, 2001.

702. Lyght, C. E.: The Merck Manual, 11th ed. West Point, PA, Merck, Sharpe and Dohme, 1966.

703. Cummins, R. O. (ed.): Textbook of Advanced Cardiac Life Support. American Heart Association, 1994.

704. Eichorn, J. H., Cooper, J. B., Cullen, D. J., et al: Standards of patient monitoring during anesthesia at Harvard Medical School. J.A.M.A., 256:1017–1020, 1986.

705. Miyasaka, K., and Ohata, J.: Burn, erosion, and sun tan with the use of pulse oximetry in infants. Anesthesiology, 67:1008–1009, 1987.

Answers

CHAPTER 1

ON-CALL CASE 1-1 ABGs and Critical Thinking

Assessment

Abnormalities:

Blood gases were not drawn during a steady state.
Only a few minutes elapsed since O_2 was placed on the patient.
ABGs should not be drawn for 30 minutes as a general rule.
A repeat sample should be drawn.
Repeat sample on room air.

Assessment

Abnormalities:

Normal pH
↓ $PaCO_2$ (hypocapnia)
↓ PaO_2
↓ $[HCO_3]$

Explanation:

One must keep in mind that blood gas values are different in Denver than they would be at sea level (i.e., PaO_2 will be lower due to high altitude). See Chapter 2.

One should also note that the patient is 70 years old. The lower normal limit of PaO_2 in the elderly is approximately 75 mm Hg at sea level.

One should also remember that it is common for normal females to have slightly lower $PaCO_2$ values than males. When $PaCO_2$ is low for a prolonged period, the bicarbonate will tend to decrease as explained in Chapter 2.

It appears that the blood gas is generally normal for a female of 70 years old in Denver, CO.

Evaluation:

Additional useful information would be a patient history and physical examination, including vital signs.

ON-CALL CASE 1-2 ABGs and Critical Thinking

Assessment

Abnormalities:

Normal blood gas oxygenation and acid-base status

↓ $PaCO_2$ (very mild)

Standard procedure for selecting the optimal site for drawing an arterial blood gas was not followed. The radial artery (preferably in the non-dominant hand) is the first artery of choice for arterial blood gas sampling. A modified Allen test should also be performed to ensure sufficient collateral circulation to the hand through the ulnar artery; this should be documented. The blood gas values reflect normal oxygenation and acid-base balance with the exception of mild hyperventilation (hypocarbia).

Explanation:

The pain and decreased mobility of the right hand could be a result of injury to the median nerve when attempting arterial puncture of the brachial artery (see Fig. 1-11). The course of the median nerve closely parallels that of the brachial artery. Cases have been described in which median nerve damage followed brachial artery puncture. Furthermore, selection of the brachial artery in the dominant hand as a first choice is somewhat controversial and could lead to undue harm and potential litigation (see Legal Issues in the section on Common Sample Sites). The mild hyperventilation may have been a result of pain, which accompanied the arterial puncture.

EXERCISES

EXERCISE 1-1 Blood Gas Values

1. pH   7.35–7.45
   $PaCO_2$ 35–45 mm Hg
   $[BE]$ 0 ± 2 mEq/L
   PaO_2 80–100 mm Hg
   $[HCO_3]$ 24 ± 2 mEq/L
   SaO_2 97%–98%
2. PaO_2
   SaO_2
3. $[HCO_3]$
   $[BE]$
4. False. Either of these metabolic indices alone is sufficient for interpretation provided that the metabolic index is completely understood.

5. 95%
6. Lower
7. Age PaO_2
   84 ± 10 mm Hg at age 58
   78 ± 10 mm Hg at age 72
   Formula $PaO_2 = 109 - (0.43 \times \text{age})$
8. 97% to 98%
9. 5
10. 90, 75
11. Kilopascal (kPa)
12. 13.3 kPa
13. 2
14. 7.5 mm Hg
15. 8 kPa = 60 mm Hg
16. Level off

EXERCISE 1-2 Arterial versus Venous Blood

1. Arteries are blood vessels that carry blood *away* from the heart. Veins are blood vessels that carry blood *to* the heart.
2. Arterial
3. Arterial
4. Localized tissue
5. Arterial pH

EXERCISE 1-3 Preparation for Arterial Sampling

1. Heparin
   Coumadin
   Aspirin
   Dipyridamole
   Streptokinase
2. Hemophilia
3. Steady state
4. 30 min
5. Should
6. 20 to 25 gauge
7. 25 gauge
8. Plastic
9. Lithium heparin (sodium heparin, 1000 U/mL was the previous standard and may still be used)
10. 1000 U/mL
11. 0.05 mL
12. Continue
13. Aseptic
14. Nosocomial
15. Optional

EXERCISE 1-4 Arterial Blood Sampling

1. Radial
   Brachial
   Femoral
2. Ulnar
   Axillary
   Dorsalis pedis
   Temporal
3. Thrombus (clot) formation with possible dislodgement
   Hemorrhage
   Infection
   Pain
   Arteriospasm
   Peripheral nerve damage
   Vasovagal response
4. Vasovagal
5. Modified Allen test
6. 5 to 15 sec
7. Median
8. Femoral
9. 30
10. 45
11. A *flashing pulsation* of blood upon entry into the vessel and *auto-filling* of the syringe with blood
12. 3–5 min
13. a. Readily available source for serial or emergency blood gases
    b. Accurate, continuous monitor of blood pressure
14. Closed
15. Non-dominant
16. Should not

NBRC Challenge 1

1. C) The modified Allen test evaluates radial artery collateral circulation and should be performed before radial *artery* puncture.
2. C) Inadvertent venous puncture is most common when attempting femoral artery puncture due to proximity of vein.
3. D) An arterial blood gas is the gold standard to evaluate the combination of oxygenation, acid-base, and ventilation.
4. E) Mild hypoxemia is common in the elderly and a PaO_2 of 75 mm Hg is the lower limit of normal at the age of 70.[242]
5. E) Low $PaCO_2$ values are common in young females.

(The multiple-choice questions given initially are less complex than those typically on NBRC exams because they are intended for the novice as an introduction to NBRC job-related format.)

CHAPTER 2

ON-CALL CASE 2-1 ABGs and Critical Thinking

Assessment

Abnormalities:
$\downarrow\downarrow$ pH
$\uparrow\uparrow$ $PaCO_2$
Normal $[HCO_3]$
Mild hypoxemia ($\downarrow PaO_2$)
$\downarrow SaO_2$
ABG classification: Uncompensated respiratory acidosis (acute ventilatory failure) with mild hypoxemia.

A young person with slow respiratory rate and comatose in the emergency department.

Explanation:
Unexplained acute respiratory acidosis in the emergency department and a very slow respiratory rate could likely be a narcotic or other drug overdose. Mild hypoxemia is likely secondary to hypoventilation.

Evaluation:
Patient history and physical might unveil the events that led up to the condition. A drug screen would also be useful.

Intervention

Importance:
First priority is to get ventilation at an acceptable level.

Because the patient is comatose, she is likely to have obtunded reflexes and is at risk for aspiration. Thus, the patient should be intubated and placed on mechanical ventilation to normalize $PaCO_2$.

ON-CALL CASE 2-2 ABGs and Critical Thinking

Assessment

Abnormalities:
$\downarrow$ pH
$\uparrow\uparrow$ $PaCO_2$

$\uparrow [HCO_3]$
Moderate hypoxemia (very near severe)
$\downarrow\downarrow PaO_2$
$\downarrow\downarrow SaO_2$
ABG classification: Partially compensated respiratory acidosis with moderate hypoxemia.

Barrel chest, smoking history, age, and pulmonary secretions all suggest chronic lung disease. The mild pH disturbance despite substantial hypercapnia also suggests some chronic compensation secondary to chronic respiratory acidosis.

Explanation:
This ABG would likely represent an acute exacerbation of chronic obstructive pulmonary disease (COPD).

Evaluation:
A chest radiograph could further clarify the presence of chronic lung disease. One might also evaluate the patient for the presence of an acute bacterial infection. Fever, increased white blood cell count (leukocytosis), and the presence of purulent secretions would help confirm this. Pulmonary function studies would also help confirm pulmonary disease and impairment.

Intervention

Importance:
First priority is to get oxygenation to an acceptable level while always keeping in mind that patients with COPD may hypoventilate in response to oxygen therapy (i.e., they are oxygen sensitive). Excessive oxygen therapy in these patients may be very dangerous and should be avoided unless absolutely necessary. It is common practice to try to get the PaO_2 to approximately 60 mm Hg by using low-flow oxygen. Low-flow oxygen is really low oxygen concentrations as administered by nasal cannula (e.g., 1–3 L/min) or Venti-masks. This is an important group of patients that we must recognize have chronic lung disease and in whom oxygen should be administered sparingly. Notwithstanding, oxygen must be administered in quantities sufficient to preclude hypoxia.

EXERCISES

EXERCISE 2-1 pH Assessment

1. pH
2. Extracellular
3. Overall
4. 6.80 to 7.80
5. Depressive
6. Alkalemia
7. Does not
8. Acidemia
9. Acidosis
10. Acid-base status
    Basic (primary) acid-base disturbance(s)
    Compensation assessment
11. pH
    $PaCO_2$
    $[HCO_3]$
    PaO_2
12. a. Acidosis
    b. Acidosis
    c. Alkalosis
    d. Normal pH
    e. Acidosis
    f. Alkalosis
    g. Alkalosis
    h. Normal pH
    i. Alkalosis

EXERCISE 2-2 Respiratory Acid-Base Status

1. Carbonic
2. $PaCO_2$
3. Hypercarbia
4. a. Respiratory alkalosis
    b. Normal $PaCO_2$
    c. Normal $PaCO_2$
    d. Respiratory alkalosis
    e. Respiratory acidosis
5. a. Decrease
    b. Decrease
    c. Increase
    d. Decrease
    e. Increase

EXERCISE 2-3 Metabolic Acid-Base Status

1. Metabolic
2. Nonrespiratory
3. Actual
4. 24 ± 2 mEq/L

5. a. Normal $[HCO_3]$
    b. Metabolic alkalosis
    c. Metabolic acidosis
6. a. Decrease
    b. Increase
    c. Decrease
7. $[HCO_3]$ and [BE]
8. 0 ± 2 mEq/L
9. Base deficit
10. a. Metabolic acidosis
    b. Metabolic alkalosis
    c. Metabolic alkalosis
    d. Metabolic acidosis
    e. Normal [BE]
    f. Metabolic alkalosis

EXERCISE 2-4 Compensation Assessment

1. Compensation
2. Respiratory
3. Renal
4. Hypocarbia
5. Acute
6. Partial
7. pH
8. Partially
9. Increased
10. a. Respiratory acidosis
    b. Respiratory acidosis
    c. Respiratory alkalosis
    d. Metabolic alkalosis
    e. Metabolic acidosis

EXERCISE 2-5 Acid-Base Classification

Set A

1. Uncompensated respiratory acidosis
2. Uncompensated metabolic alkalosis
3. Mixed (combined) respiratory and metabolic alkalosis
4. Mixed (combined) respiratory and metabolic acidosis
5. Uncompensated respiratory alkalosis
6. Uncompensated metabolic alkalosis
7. Mixed (combined) respiratory and metabolic alkalosis
8. Uncompensated metabolic acidosis
9. Uncompensated metabolic acidosis
10. Uncompensated respiratory acidosis

Set B
1. Compensated respiratory acidosis
2. Partially compensated respiratory acidosis
3. Partially compensated respiratory alkalosis
4. Normal acid-base status
5. Partially compensated metabolic acidosis
6. Uncompensated metabolic acidosis
7. Partially compensated respiratory alkalosis
8. Uncompensated metabolic alkalosis (PaCO$_2$ is still in the normal range)
9. Partially compensated metabolic alkalosis
10. Mixed (combined) respiratory and metabolic acidosis

EXERCISE 2-6 Alternative Terminology

1. Failure
2. Temporal
3. Acute
4. Respiratory
5. a. Chronic respiratory acidosis or chronic ventilatory failure
   b. Acute respiratory acidosis or acute ventilatory failure
   c. Acute respiratory alkalosis
   d. Uncompensated metabolic acidosis (remember that temporal adjectives are inappropriate for primary metabolic problems)
   e. Acute respiratory alkalosis
   f. Uncompensated metabolic alkalosis

EXERCISE 2-7 Oxygenation Assessment

1. PaO$_2$
2. 80 to 100 mm Hg
3. Normoxemia
4. Hypoxemia
5. Partial pressure
6. Hyperoxemia
7. Lower
8. Is not
9. 90%
10. Cardiovascular
11. Should
12. 4–5

EXERCISE 2-8 PaO$_2$ Classification Adults

1. Hyperoxemia
2. Severe hypoxemia
3. Moderate hypoxemia
4. Severe hypoxemia
5. Moderate hypoxemia
6. Hyperoxemia
7. Mild hypoxemia
8. Hyperoxemia
9. Normoxemia
10. Normoxemia

EXERCISE 2-9 Complete Blood Gas Classification

1. Partially compensated respiratory alkalosis with mild hypoxemia
2. Compensated metabolic alkalosis with severe hypoxemia
3. Uncompensated respiratory acidosis with moderate hypoxemia
4. Compensated respiratory alkalosis with hyperoxemia
5. Mixed (combined) alkalosis with moderate hypoxemia
6. Partially compensated metabolic alkalosis with mild hypoxemia
7. Normal acid-base status with hyperoxemia
8. Uncompensated metabolic alkalosis with moderate hypoxemia
9. Uncompensated metabolic alkalosis with normoxemia
10. Normal acid-base status with normoxemia

EXERCISE 2-10 Complete Blood Gas Classification Using [BE] as the Metabolic Index

1. Partially compensated metabolic acidosis with moderate hypoxemia
2. Mixed (combined) respiratory and metabolic alkalosis with severe hypoxemia
3. Uncompensated metabolic acidosis with hyperoxemia
4. Respiratory alkalosis and metabolic acidosis with normoxemia (perhaps this is complete compensation, but given only this information, one cannot be sure of the precise primary problem)
5. Mixed acidosis with mild hypoxemia
6. Uncompensated respiratory acidosis with normoxemia
7. Uncompensated respiratory alkalosis with mild hypoxemia
8. Partially compensated metabolic acidosis with severe hypoxemia

9. Compensated respiratory acidosis with moderate hypoxemia
10. Normal acid-base status with hyperoxemia

EXERCISE 2-11 Complete Blood Gas Classification: Additional Examples

Set A

1. Mixed acidosis with moderate hypoxemia
2. Uncompensated respiratory alkalosis with severe hypoxemia
3. Normal acid-base status with hyperoxemia
4. Partially compensated metabolic acidosis with normoxemia
5. Uncompensated respiratory acidosis with mild hypoxemia
6. Partially compensated respiratory acidosis with normoxemia
7. Mixed alkalosis with severe hypoxemia
8. Compensated metabolic acidosis with severe hypoxemia
9. Compensated metabolic alkalosis with normoxemia
10. Compensated respiratory acidosis with hyperoxemia

Set B

1. Uncompensated respiratory alkalosis with normoxemia
2. Partially compensated respiratory acidosis with severe hypoxemia
3. Mixed acidosis with moderate hypoxemia
4. Uncompensated respiratory alkalosis with hyperoxemia
5. Partially compensated metabolic acidosis with moderate hypoxemia
6. Mixed acidosis with mild hypoxemia
7. Normal acid-base status with hyperoxemia
8. Uncompensated metabolic alkalosis with moderate hypoxemia
9. Mixed alkalosis with normoxemia
10. Partially compensated respiratory acidosis with normoxemia

NBRC Challenge 2

1. A) Mechanical ventilation. Patient has uncompensated respiratory acidosis, which is also known as acute ventilatory failure. Treatment for ventilatory failure is to re-establish adequate ventilation.

2. C) Compensation for severe metabolic acidosis. The basic primary acid-base disturbance is metabolic and not respiratory. The respiratory hyperventilation is compensatory or a secondary acid-base disturbance. This situation is compatible with diabetic ketoacidosis and the deep breathing pattern (Kussmaul's breathing) that accompanies it. Therapy must be directed at the primary disturbance and not the body's compensatory mechanisms.

3. E) COPD. This is a classic blood gas for compensated respiratory acidosis or chronic ventilatory failure. COPD is likewise the classic cause of chronic ventilatory failure. The elevated bicarbonate and relatively normal pH are essential clues to this determination.

4. C) Oxygen mask. The most critical problem with this blood gas is the severe hypoxemia. Remember, it is wise to assume severe hypoxemia will result in hypoxia. Hypoxia is life-threatening and must be treated immediately and aggressively. An oxygen mask will deliver more oxygen faster than a nasal cannula; therefore, it is the treatment of choice. The uncompensated respiratory alkalosis is a normal response of the body to severe hypoxemia and will be corrected if PaO_2 returns to normal.

5. C) Primary respiratory acidosis and primary metabolic acidosis (mixed acidosis) and likely hypoxia secondary to severe hypoxemia. The tissue hypoxia appears to be causing lactic (metabolic) acidosis.

CHAPTER 3

ON-CALL CASE 3-1 ABGs and Critical Thinking

Assessment

Abnormalities:

↑ pH
↓$PaCO_2$
↑PaO_2

It is noteworthy that the sample contained froth.

Explanation:

A PaO_2 of 153 mm Hg on room air indicates a technical error. Samples with froth should be discarded because they obviously contain a substantial amount of air. The most pronounced effect of air contamination in a blood gas sample is a change in PaO_2. The maximum PaO_2 attainable with room air and hyperventilation is only approximately 130 mm Hg. The decrease in $PaCO_2$ and increase in pH could also be attributable to air contamination because the PCO_2 in room air is near zero and a low $PaCO_2$ would increase pH. A repeat blood gas sample is necessary to provide information about this patient's oxygenation and acid-base status. Treatment and intervention cannot be based on this obviously erroneous data.

ON-CALL CASE 3-2 ABGs and Critical Thinking

Assessment

Abnormalities:

$\downarrow\downarrow SaO_2$	$\uparrow$B/P
$\uparrow$ pH	$\uparrow$RR
$\downarrow PaCO_2$	$\uparrow$HR
$\uparrow\uparrow\uparrow PaO_2$	Fever
Normal [HCO_3]	$\downarrow\downarrow SpO_2$

Explanation:

It is noteworthy that an experienced clinician observed a flash of blood and auto-filling of the syringe. Although the PaO_2 is the same as normal mixed venous PO_2, other clinical information tends to confirm that this is an arterial sample. For example, the pulse oximeter also indicates hypoxemia and the presence of cyanosis suggests a problem with oxygenation. Cardiopulmonary stress is also apparent from the elevated vital signs and hypocarbia, which again is suggestive of an oxygenation disturbance. *A venous sample cannot be identified or confirmed by blood gas values alone.* Sick patients may indeed have arterial values that resemble normal venous values. Looking at the entire situation, data, and patient description, it appears that this is an arterial sample from a severely hypoxemic patient.

EXERCISES

EXERCISE 3-1 Basic Physics of Gases

1. Brownian movement
2. Pressure is defined as force per unit area.
3. Water vapor pressure
4. Barometer
5. 760 mm Hg
6. Decreased
7. Dalton's law states that the sum of the partial pressures in a mixture of gases is equal to the total pressure.
8. Kinetic
9. Will not
10. Will not
11. Fractional concentration of inspired oxygen in a dry gas phase
12. a. 150 mm Hg
    b. 137 mm Hg
    c. 340 mm Hg
    d. 232 mm Hg
    e. 483 mm Hg
13. Gay-Lussac's law states that if volume and mass remain fixed, the pressure exerted by a gas varies directly with the absolute temperature of the gas.
14. Body temperature and pressure saturated (37° C, 760 mm Hg, 47 mm Hg water vapor)
15. 150 mm Hg
16. Henry's law states that when a gas is exposed to a liquid, the partial pressure of a gas in a liquid phase equilibrates with the partial pressure of a gas in a gaseous phase.
17. *Charles' law*: Pressure is constant (remember that Charles' law is always the same pressure [acronym CLASP]).[98]
    Boyle's law: Temperature is constant (remember that Boyle's law is always the same temperature [acronym BLAST]).
    Gay-Lussac's law: Volume is constant.[98]
18. *a* (lowercase)
19. Humidification and external respiration
20. Absolute, potential

EXERCISE 3-2 Air in Blood Gas Samples

1. Are not
2. (c) Change in PaO_2
3. Is not
4. Duration of exposure
5. Greater than
6. a. Increased
   b. Increased
   c. Decreased
   d. Increased
   e. Decreased
7. Is not

8. 2
9. Decrease
10. Increase

EXERCISE 3-3 Venous Sampling or Admixture

1. Will
2. Discarded
3. Short
4. Does not necessarily mean
5. Is not
6. Pulmonary artery
7. $P\bar{v}O_2 = 40$ mm Hg
   $P\bar{v}CO_2 = 48$ mm Hg
   $S\bar{v}O_2 = 75\%$
8. Femoral

EXERCISE 3-4 Blood Gas Anticoagulation

1. Lithium heparin
   Sodium
2. 1000 U/mL
3. Decreased PCO_2
4. Is not
5. Dilution
6. Low (because of the dilution effect)
7. 2 mL
8. 1%
9. a. New syringe designs
   b. Use of dry, crystalline heparin

EXERCISE 3-5 Blood Gas Error Due to Metabolism

1. Does
2. PaO_2 decreases
   $PaCO_2$ increases
   pH decreases
3. 5 mm Hg
   0.05
4. High
5. Half
6. 10%
7. 30
8. 30
9. Is not
10. Leukocytes (white blood cells)
    Reticulocytes (immature red blood cells)
    Platelets
11. Leukocyte larceny
12. 2
13. Leukocytosis
14. More

EXERCISE 3-6 Temperature Effects on Blood Gases

1. High
2. 5
3. 0.03 (see Table 3-8)
4. 10%
5. Not be

EXERCISE 3-7 Summary of Potential Sampling Errors

Air in the blood sample
Venous sampling or admixture
Excessive or improper anticoagulant
Rate of metabolism
Temperature disparities between patient and machine (see Box 3-1)

EXERCISE 3-8 Blood Gas / Electrolyte Specimens

1. Will
2. Balanced
3. Mixing
4. PPACK
5. Elevate

NBRC Challenge 3

1. A) PaO_2. Because the increased leukocytes will consume oxygen from the sample more quickly than normal.
2. D) I & II only. The partial pressures of gases have the greatest effect with pH of the heparin also having some effect.
3. B) II & III. A bluish sample suggests possible venous blood as does failure of the syringe to auto-fill.
4. C) III only. Temperature correction is easily accomplished but generally not recommended for clinical application.
5. D) Electrolytes. Icing samples leads to hemolysis and elevated potassium and decreased ionized calcium.

CHAPTER 4

ON-CALL CASE 4-1 ABGs and Critical Thinking

Assessment

Abnormalities:

↓SaO_2
↓↓PaO_2

Patient is known to have thrombocytosis.
Pulse oximeter reading is inconsistent with ABG saturation.

Explanation:

The PaO_2 on the blood gas report may be surprisingly low due to the presence of thrombocytosis. Remember, very high white blood cell counts, platelet counts, or reticulocyte counts, could lead to excessive oxygen consumption from within the blood gas sample due to the high metabolism of these cells. This is the same phenomenon that occurs with leukemia and leukocyte larceny and could explain the low PaO_2 seen despite a very good pulse oximeter reading. The saturation on the blood gas report, which is a calculated value, is also low because it is *calculated* based on PaO_2.

Evaluation:

Additional useful information would be vital signs to determine if there are any other physiologic indications of hypoxemia. If an additional blood gas is drawn, it should be acquired in an iced, glass syringe and analyzed as quickly as possible after acquisition to minimize error due to continued metabolism. Analysis of saturation via CO-oximetry would also be useful to determine precise saturation.

ON-CALL CASE 4-2 ABGs and Critical Thinking

Assessment

Abnormalities:

↓ PaO_2
↓ SaO_2
↓ pH
Patient is severely febrile (41°C).
Blood gases have been temperature corrected.

Explanation:

The patient seems only mildly hypoxemic; however, the blood gases have been temperature-corrected and normal values are not known for this temperature. Blood gases should be interpreted at BTPS where normal values are known.

Evaluation:

Additional useful information would be blood gas values at normal body temperature.

At BTPS, the PaO_2 would actually be 48 mm Hg. Therefore, this patient is quite hypoxemic. Furthermore, the high temperature would lead to increased metabolism and oxygen need. Thus, the patient is in dire need of oxygen. This fact is somewhat obscured because blood gases are temperature-corrected and provides an example as to why temperature correction is not advocated and may be misleading.

Intervention

Importance:

Clearly, oxygen therapy is in dire need.

Objective:

Get (BTPS) PaO_2 to an acceptable level (e.g., 80–100 mm Hg) as a first priority. Secondary issues include bronchial hygiene needs, chest radiography, possibly sputum culture, and identification of the type of pneumonia present.

Action:

Place the patient on an oxygen mask.

Interpret all future blood gases at BTPS. If blood gas values are reported at a temperature other than BTPS, BTPS values should be recorded along with temperature-corrected values.

EXERCISES

EXERCISE 4-1 Basic Electrical Principles

1. Electricity
2. Cathode, anode
3. Electromotive
4. Volt
5. Potentiometer
6. Ampere
7. Ohm
8. Voltage = amp × ohm
9. Watts
10. Conductor

EXERCISE 4-2 Electrodes and Terminology

1. Electrochemical cell systems
2. An entire measuring system for one of the blood gases

3. Electrode terminal
4. Metal, glass
5. Half-cell
6. Working half-cells
   Reference half-cells
7. Working (or measuring)

EXERCISE 4-3 The PO_2 Electrode

1. Ammeter
2. Platinum
3. Silver chloride
4. Consumes
5. Polarographic
6. Clark
7. Polypropylene
8. Cuvette
9. Anode
10. Voltage

EXERCISE 4-4 The pH Electrode

1. Glass
2. Working
3. Is not
4. Potentiometric
5. Nernst equation
6. Silver chloride
7. Calomel
8. Mercury/mercurous chloride
9. Liquid junction
10. Calomel

EXERCISE 4-5 The PCO_2 Electrode

1. Does not
2. Teflon or silicone rubber
3. Bicarbonate
4. 2
5. Is not
6. Hydrolysis
7. Severinghaus
8. Voltage
9. 1
10. PO_2

EXERCISE 4-6 Quality Assurance/Preventive Maintenance

1. Clinical
2. Quality assurance
3. Analytical
4. 0.1
5. 1 to 3 min

EXERCISE 4-7 Quality Control and Statistics

1. Quality control
2. Proficiency testing
3. Mean
4. Standard deviation
5. 68%
6. 95%
7. PaO_2 = 5 mm Hg standard deviation
   $PaCO_2$ = 2.5 mm Hg standard deviation
8. Less
9. Coefficient of variation (CV)
10. Percent (%)

EXERCISE 4-8 Quality Control Charts—1

1. Controls, or control samples
2. 2 levels, 8 hours
3. Performance records
   Quality control charts
4. Levey-Jennings
5. Systematic error
6. Trending
7. Shifting
8. Random error
9. Dispersion
10. "In control"

EXERCISE 4-9 Quality Control Charts—2

1. Accuracy
2. Precision
3. Precision
4. Accuracy
5. Aging of the electrode or battery
   Protein contamination
6. 0.02 pH units
7. Alkaline
8. 1% to 2%
9. Results
10. Two

EXERCISE 4-10 Types of Controls

1. Do not
2. Do not
3. Tonometer
4. Time
5. An infectious risk
6. Emulsions
7. Emulsions
8. Commercially

9. PO_2
10. Fluorocarbon

EXERCISE 4-11 Continuous Blood Gas Monitoring

1. Measurement
2. Do not
3. In vivo
4. Clark
5. Must
6. Oxygen or carbon dioxide
7. Cardiac output
8. Gas Stat system
9. Wall
10. Ex vivo (on demand)

NBRC Challenge 4

1. A) The cathode should be cleaned and the membrane should be changed.
2. B) II and IV only. This is proficiency testing for external quality control and helps evaluate accuracy not precision.
3. B) Trending is a form of systematic error that may result from these conditions.
4. D) Precision
5. C) CIABG. Measurement of tissue wall PO_2 may occur with these devices.

CHAPTER 5

ON-CALL CASE 5-1 ABGs and Critical Thinking

Assessment

Abnormalities:

$\downarrow SaO_2$
$\uparrow pH$
$\uparrow PaCO_2$
$\downarrow\downarrow$ [BE]
$\downarrow PaO_2$

ABG classification: The blood gas cannot be classified because it is not internally consistent. It is not possible to have a high pH (alkalemia) when both a respiratory acidosis (increased $PaCO_2$) and metabolic acidosis (decreased [BE]) are present. There must be an error in the data reported. It is noteworthy that this was a telephone report, which could have resulted in a miscommunication of data.

Explanation:

The acid-base data cannot be explained because they are not internally consistent.

Evaluation:

The clinician should call the lab to double-check the laboratory results.

Intervention

Importance:

If internally consistent results are not available, a repeat sample is necessary. Therapeutic intervention should not occur until we are sure we have reliable data. The administration of bicarbonate (although commonplace years ago during cardiac arrest) is inappropriate for two reasons. First, and most important, one should never administer bicarbonate to a patient with a pH of 7.52. The pH should be the primary focus of acid-base treatment and not simply the [BE], [HCO$_3$], or $PaCO_2$. Second, one should never initiate treatment when acid-base data are not internally consistent. Upon calling the laboratory, it was found that the [BE] was actually + 11 mEq/L and there was an error in the telephone report. Administration of bicarbonate to this patient was totally inappropriate and could be life-threatening. Recognition of lack of internal consistency could have been life-saving.

ON-CALL CASE 5-2 ABGs and Critical Thinking

Assessment

Abnormalities:

$\downarrow\downarrow SaO_2$
$\downarrow\downarrow pH$
$\uparrow\uparrow PaCO_2$
$\uparrow$ [HCO$_3$]
$\downarrow$ [BE]
$\downarrow\downarrow PaO_2$

ABG classification: Uncompensated respiratory acidosis (acute ventilatory failure) with moderate hypoxemia. (Note this blood gas would have been classified as a partially compensated respiratory acidosis using the rules described in Chapter 2. See discussion, which follows under explanation.) Plasma bicarbonate is elevated whereas the base excess of the blood (another metabolic index) is decreased.

Explanation:
The data are consistent with a drug overdose and acute respiratory acidosis. The hypoxemia is likely a result of simple hypoventilation. The apparently conflicting messages regarding metabolic status provided by the bicarbonate and base excess simply represents flaws in these indices associated with hypercapnia. Again, the bicarbonate level is elevated due to hydrolysis in hypercapnia and the base excess of the blood is decreased due to in vitro–in vivo discrepancies. These values are normal for acute respiratory acidosis and do not represent renal compensation.

Evaluation:
A drug screen and history and physical examination are indicated.

Intervention

Importance:
Immediate intervention might include a narcotic antagonist. If this was not effective, intubation to ensure a patent and protected airway and mechanical ventilation to restore normal ventilation and acid-base balance would be indicated.

EXERCISES

EXERCISE 5-1 Gross Inconsistency

1. I
2. C
3. I
4. I
5. I
6. C
7. C
8. C
9. I
10. C

EXERCISE 5-2 Principles of Indirect Metabolic Assessment

1. Can
2. 0.10
3. 0.06
4. 7.60
5. 7.22
6. Normal
7. Acidosis
8. Alkalosis
9. Normal
10. Can

EXERCISE 5-3 Calculation of Expected pH

In Hypocarbia: Expected pH = 7.40 + (40 mm Hg − $PaCO_2$)0.01
In Hypercarbia: Expected pH = 7.40 − ($PaCO_2$ − 40 mm Hg)0.006

1. Expected pH = 7.40− (50 mm Hg − 40 mm Hg)0.006
   Expected pH = 7.40 − 0.06
   Expected pH = 7.34
2. Expected pH = 7.40− (60 mm Hg − 40 mm Hg)0.006
   Expected pH = 7.28
3. Expected pH = 7.40 + (40 mm Hg − $PaCO_2$)0.01
   Expected pH = 7.40 + (40 mm Hg − 25 mm Hg)0.01
   Expected pH = 7.40 + 0.15
   Expected pH = 7.55
4. Expected pH = 7.25
5. Expected pH = 7.60
6. Expected pH = 7.50
7. Expected pH = 7.22
8. Expected pH = 7.31
9. Expected pH = 7.58
10. Expected pH = 7.37

EXERCISE 5-4 Indirect Metabolic Assessment

Actual pH	Expected pH Relationship	Indirect Metabolic Status
Actual pH	= expected pH±0.03	Normal metabolic status
Actual pH	> expected pH + 0.03	Metabolic alkalosis
Actual pH	< expected pH − 0.03	Metabolic acidosis

	Actual pH	Expected pH	Indirect Metabolic Status
1.	7.34	= 7.34	Normal metabolic status
2.	7.30	= 7.28 + 0.02	Normal metabolic status

3.	7.52	$= 7.55 - 0.03$	Normal metabolic status
4.	7.15	< 7.25	Metabolic acidosis
5.	7.62	$= 7.60 + 0.02$	Normal metabolic status
6.	7.56	> 7.50	Metabolic alkalosis
7.	7.38	> 7.22	Metabolic alkalosis (probably compensatory)
8.	7.20	< 7.31	Metabolic acidosis
9.	7.48	< 7.58	Metabolic acidosis (probably compensatory)
10.	7.34	$= 7.37 - 0.03$	Normal metabolic status

EXERCISE 5-5 Accuracy Check by Comparing Direct and Indirect Metabolic Status

	Indirect Status	Direct Status	Consistency
1.	Normal	Normal	Consistent
2.	Normal	Alkalosis	Inconsistent
3.	Normal	Acidosis	Inconsistent
4.	Acidosis	Normal	Inconsistent
5.	Normal	Normal	Consistent
6.	Alkalosis	Alkalosis	Consistent
7.	Alkalosis	Normal	Inconsistent
8.	Acidosis	Acidosis	Consistent
9.	Acidosis	Normal	Inconsistent
10.	Normal	Alkalosis	Inconsistent

EXERCISE 5-6 The Rule of Eights in Accuracy Check

$(\text{Factor} \times PaCO_2) = \text{predicted bicarbonate}$

pH	Factor
7.60	8/8
7.50	6/8
7.40	5/8
7.30	4/8
7.20	2.5/8
7.10	2/8

	Predicted	Actual	Consistency
1.	30	28	C
2.	42	40	C
3.	22.5	29	I
4.	9	20	I
5.	15	25	I
6.	40	39	C
7.	10	9	C
8.	50	30	I
9.	19	19	C
10.	17.5	10	I

EXERCISE 5-7 pH – [H⁺] Conversion

pH
1. 7.35
2. 7.24
3. 7.48
4. 7.50
5. 7.32
6. Linear relationship does not hold true outside the range of 7.20 to 7.50 (30–60 nEq/L)
7. 7.20
8. 7.41
9. 7.52 (Again, remember that the linear relationship begins to deteriorate beyond 7.50; nevertheless, this is a reasonable estimate.)
10. 7.29

EXERCISE 5-8 Application of Modified Henderson's Equation

	pH	[H⁺] (nEq/L)	$PaCO_2$ (mm Hg)	[HCO₃] (mEq/L)
1.	7.32	48		
2.	7.43	37		
3.	7.47	33		
4.		60		20
5.	7.40	40		
6.		50	50	
7.	7.50	30		
8.	7.20		45	
9.	7.40			18
10.		52		18

EXERCISE 5-9 Calculation of [HCO₃] From Total CO₂

1. 36.2 mEq/L
2. 24.8 mEq/L
3. 16.5 mEq/L
4. 19.2 mEq/L
5. 20.0 mEq/L

EXERCISE 5-10 Metabolic Indices

1. CO_2 combining power
   Total CO_2
2. Does not
3. Does
4. 10 mm Hg
5. 5 mm Hg
6. Standard bicarbonate
7. Low
8. T_{40} standard bicarbonate
9. Whole blood buffer base ([BB])
10. Base excess ([BE]) or [BE] blood
11. Low

12. In vitro
13. [BE]ecf
14. [Hb] 5 g%
15. 0.10 units

NBRC Challenge 5

1. C) The blood gas should be checked and/ or run again. It is impossible to have a respiratory and metabolic acidosis and a high pH.
2. E) Increased plasma bicarbonate due to hydrolysis. The bicarbonate will go up roughly 1 mEq/L for each 10 mm Hg acute increase in $PaCO_2$. Therefore, this blood gas represents a simple acute respiratory acidosis with a bicarbonate elevation secondary to hydrolysis, not compensation.
3. D) The blood gas and pulse oximeter readings are incongruent. Saturation is very different from partial pressure. When SpO_2 is 90%, PaO_2 is typically about 60 mm Hg.
4. D) 7.55. The acute $PaCO_2$–pH relationship would apply. For every 1 mm Hg drop in $PaCO_2$, pH will acutely increase approximately 0.01 units.
5. D) The change in [BE] and [HCO_3] is due to hypercapnia. This blood gas shows how acute hypercapnia will affect bicarbonate and base excess of the blood in opposing directions.

CHAPTER 6

ON-CALL CASE 6-1 ABGs and Critical Thinking
Assessment
Abnormalities:

$\downarrow SaO_2$	$\uparrow$B/P
Normal pH	$\uparrow$HR
Normal $PaCO_2$	Normal temperature
$\downarrow\downarrow PaO_2$	$\uparrow$RR
Normal [HCO_3]	$\uparrow\uparrow \dot{V}$

ABG classification: Normal acid-base status with moderate hypoxemia. Large minute ventilation – $PaCO_2$ disparity suggests deadspace disease. In normal lungs, tripling the minute ventilation should result in a $PaCO_2$ of approximately 25 mm Hg.

Explanation:
Given postoperative leg surgery in an elderly individual, there should be a high index of suspicion for pulmonary emboli. The high minute ventilation – $PaCO_2$ disparity and the abrupt onset of shortness of breath are also typical of pulmonary embolus. Hemoptysis, chest pain, and hypoxemia are also frequent findings. Elevation in vital signs (increased HR/BP) is most likely secondary to moderate hypoxemia.

Evaluation:
Pulmonary angiography confirms the diagnosis. A lung perfusion scan is inconclusive because perfusion will tend to match ventilation in primary ventilatory disturbances.

Intervention
Importance:
First priority is to get oxygenation at an acceptable level.
 Anticoagulant or thrombolytic drug therapy should also be initiated.

ON-CALL CASE 6-2 ABGs and Critical Thinking
Assessment
Abnormalities:

$\downarrow SaO_2$	$\uparrow$B/P
$\uparrow$ pH	$\uparrow$HR
$\downarrow PaCO_2$	$\uparrow$Temperature
$\downarrow\downarrow PaO_2$	$\uparrow$RR
Normal [HCO_3]	

ABG classification: Uncompensated respiratory alkalosis with moderate hypoxemia.

Explanation:
Given postoperative abdominal status, patients may avoid deep breathing due to pain and anesthesia that may lead to atelectasis (collapsed alveoli) and pneumonia (lung infection). Elevated temperature (fever) and hypoxemia suggest pulmonary shunting, and we need to be concerned about progressive shunt producing disease (e.g., pneumonia/atelectasis) following surgery. Elevation in vital signs (increased HR/BP) and hyperventilation (low $PaCO_2$) are most likely secondary to moderate hypoxemia. Remember, when there is a problem with low blood oxygenation (hypoxemia), the circulatory system attempts to compensate

(increased HR/BP) and assure tissue oxygenation. Hyperventilation also ensues.

Evaluation:
Additional data: Chest radiograph, [WBC], sputum culture—to identify potential microbes, would all help to facilitate definitive diagnosis. White-out on chest radiograph and/or increased white blood cells (leukocytosis) confirms bacterial pneumonia.

Intervention
Importance:
First priority is to get oxygenation to an acceptable level.

If pneumonia and secretions are present, antibiotics and bronchial hygiene (secretion removal) are indicated. Most abnormal laboratory data will normalize if the root problem is corrected.

Objective:
The first goal is to get the PaO_2 and/or SpO_2 in an acceptable adult range.

Action:
Place the patient on a moderately high FIO_2 (e.g., 50% aerosol mask would also provide humidity to loosen secretions). Monitor with pulse oximetry to ensure saturation moves to an acceptable range. Encourage deep breathing with incentive spirometry.

EXERCISES

EXERCISE 6-1 Introduction to Oxygenation
1. Cardiopulmonary
2. The exchange of O_2 and CO_2 between the alveoli and the pulmonary capillaries
3. The quantitative movement of a sufficient volume of O_2 from the pulmonary capillaries to its cellular destination
4. The exchange of O_2 and CO_2 between the systemic capillaries and the body cells or tissue
5. Quantitative
6. O_2 loading
   O_2 transport
   O_2 unloading

7. More
8. Secondary polycythemia
9. Blood
10. Hypoxia
11. May be
12. May be

EXERCISE 6-2 External Respiration and Normal Pulmonary Perfusion
1. a. Adequate ventilation
   b. Adequate ventilation-perfusion match
   c. Adequate diffusion
2. $PaCO_2$
3. Partial pressure of O_2 (PO_2)
4. 60 mm Hg
5. Most
6. Absent
7. Is not
8. 2
9. 3
10. 1

EXERCISE 6-3 Normal Distribution of Ventilation
1. Compliance
   Resistance
2. Apices
3. More
4. $(+2 \text{ cm } H_2O) - (-8 \text{ cm } H_2O) =$
   $(+2 \text{ cm } H_2O + 8 \text{ cm } H_2O) = 10 \text{ cm } H_2O$
5. Larger
6. Compressive
7. Higher
8. Bases
9. Tidal volume
10. More

EXERCISE 6-4 Abnormal Pulmonary Perfusion
1. Compensatory
2. Generalized
3. Higher
4. a. Heart failure (decreased cardiac output)
   b. Positive pressure ventilation
5. The perfusion zones may shift downward if an increased pulmonary vascular resistance is associated with a weak or damaged heart that could not increase the force of contraction.

6. a. Acidemia
   b. Hypoxemia
7. Pulmonary fibrosis or COPD
8. PAO_2

EXERCISE 6-5 Abnormal Distribution of Ventilation

1. Will
2. Secretions
3. Airway resistance
4. Airway resistance
5. Gravity
6. Decrease
7. Obese
8. Smokers
9. Supine
10. 44 years of age
11. $PACO_2$

EXERCISE 6-6 Ventilation-Perfusion Matching

1. Cardiac minute output
2. Alveolar minute ventilation
3. 1/1
4. More
5. 0.8
6. 3
7. 0.6
8. 130 mm Hg
9. True capillary shunt
10. True alveolar deadspace

EXERCISE 6-7 Physiologic Deadspace

1. No
2. Higher
3. 200 mL
4. Low
5. Physiologic
6. 0.5
7. Mean
8. 0.2 to 0.4
9. Less than 0.6
10. Mechanical deadspace
11. Wasted
12. Increase
13. Will not
14. 30 mm Hg
15. Increased physiologic deadspace
16. Normal deadspace
17. Carbon dioxide (CO_2)

EXERCISE 6-8 Physiologic Shunting

1. Lower
2. Silent
3. Anatomic and capillary
4. 2%
5. Bronchial
   Pleural
   Thebesian
6. True (absolute)
   Relative
7. Absolute
8. (Any 2)
   Pneumonia
   Pulmonary edema
   Atelectasis
9. Approximately 1%
10. Hypoxemia

EXERCISE 6-9 Diffusion

1. Equilibration time, adequate surface area
2. Pulmonary capillary transit
3. 0.75 sec
4. 0.25 sec
5. Smaller
6. Faster
7. Graham's law
8. 1 μ
9. Decreased
10. 70 m^2

NBRC Challenge 6

1. D) Physiologic deadspace measurement will be increased in the presence of deadspace disease (e.g., decreased cardiac output, pulmonary embolus) or application of mechanical ventilation.
2. E) To calculate physiologic deadspace, mean exhaled gas must be collected in a Douglas bag and the average PCO_2 measured.
3. D) The Acute Respiratory Distress Syndrome and congenital heart defects (shunt-producing diseases) may lead to elevated pulmonary shunt fractions. Although a slight increase in the shunt may accompany pulmonary embolus, it is primarily a deadspace producing disease.
4. A) Tuberculosis is most often seen in the upper lung zones due to the high PO_2 levels in this area.

5. C) A decrease in PaO_2 during exercise suggests a problem with lung diffusion such as pulmonary fibrosis.

CHAPTER 7

ON-CALL CASE 7-1 ABGs and Critical Thinking

Assessment

Abnormalities:

↓ pH	↑ HR
Normal $PaCO_2$	↑ B/P
↓ $[HCO_3]$	↓↓ [Hb]
Normoxemia	↑ RR

ABG classification: Uncompensated metabolic acidosis with normoxemia.

The PaO_2 is only 94 mm Hg on FIO_2 of 0.60. Oxygenation ration 1.3. The [Hb] is one-third of normal.

Explanation:

The data are consistent with severe anemia and a substantial decrease in arterial oxygen content; probably secondary to bleeding following surgery. Despite the fact that oxygenation appears acceptable via the blood gases, the patient has severe anemic hypoxia, which needs to be corrected immediately. The concurrent metabolic acidosis suggests lactic acidosis secondary to hypoxia.

Evaluation:

Although the heart rate and blood pressure are slightly elevated, the patient should be evaluated for hypovolemia and bleeding. Auscultation and a chest radiograph would be indicated to evaluate the poor oxygenation ratio.

Intervention

Importance:

Immediate intervention would include a transfusion to ensure sufficient hemoglobin for carrying oxygen.

ON-CALL CASE 7-2 ABGs and Critical Thinking

Assessment

Abnormalities:

↓ pH	↑↑ HR
↓ $PaCO_2$	↑ RR
↓ $[HCO_3]$	↓↓ B/P
↓ PaO_2	

ABG classification: Uncompensated metabolic acidosis with mild hypoxemia. The patient appears to be in cardiopulmonary distress and shows signs and symptoms of shock (cold and clammy). The B/P is very low.

Explanation:

The data are consistent with shock and circulatory hypoxia. Again, despite the fact that oxygenation appears acceptable according to the blood gases, the patient has substantial circulatory hypoxia, which needs to be corrected immediately. The concurrent metabolic acidosis suggests lactic acidosis secondary to hypoxia.

Evaluation:

The source of the hypotension must be sought. It could be due to cardiac pump failure, hypovolemia, or systemic vasodilation.

Intervention

Importance:

Intervention depends on the nature of the cardiovascular disturbance but should aim to improve cardiovascular status and blood pressure.

EXERCISES

EXERCISE 7-1 Oxygen Transport

1. Dissolved oxygen
   Combined oxygen
2. 0.003 mL O_2/100 mL blood/mm Hg
3. Vol%
4. Decrease
5. Linear
6. Hemoglobin
7. Iron (Fe)
   Porphyrin
8. 4
9. SaO_2
10. Combined

EXERCISE 7-2 Oxyhemoglobin Dissociation Curve

1. PaO_2
2. Nonlinear

3. 26 mm Hg
   60 mm Hg
   250 mm Hg
4. Large
5. Small
6. Association
7. End
8. 97%–98%
9. 90%
10. Upper
    Lower

EXERCISE 7-3 Oxyhemoglobin Affinity

1. P_{50}
2. 26 mm Hg
3. PCO_2
   pH
   Temperature
   DPG
4. Right
   Decreased
5. Bohr
6. Detrimental
7. Unloading
8. Decrease
   Increase
9. 7.40
   40 mm Hg
10. Men

EXERCISE 7-4 2,3-Diphosphoglycerate

1. Decreases
2. Abundant
3. Unloading
4. Increase
5. Infusion of stored blood
6. Possible
7. 24 hours
8. Decreased
9. Sustained
10. Acid-citrate dextrose

EXERCISE 7-5 Oxygen Content

1. CaO_2
2. 0.3 vol%
   0.18 vol%
   1.2 vol%
3. 19.095 vol%
   14.472 vol%
   10.72 vol%

4. 12.81 vol%
   18.60 vol%
   9.34 vol%
5. 20 vol%
6. 40 mm Hg
   75%
7. 5.0 vol%
8. Fick
9. Increases
10. 250 mL/min

EXERCISE 7-6 Cyanosis

1. Cyanosis
2. Peripheral
3. Mucous membranes
4. 20% desaturated
5. Average 5 g% desaturated Hb in capillaries
6. 2 g%
7. Anemia
8. Polycythemia
9. (100% − 80% = 20% Hb desat in arterial blood)
   (100% − 60% = 40% Hb desat in venous blood)
   (20 g% × 0.2) + (20 g% × 0.4)/2
   (4 g%) + (8 g%)/2 = 6 g% Hb desat in capillaries
   Because the average amount of Hb desat in the capillaries of this patient is more than 5 g%, this patient appears cyanotic.
10. (100% − 80% = 20% Hb desat in arterial blood)
    (100% − 60% = 40% Hb desat in venous blood)
    (10 g% × 0.2) + (10 g% × 0.4)/2
    (2 g%) + (4 g%)/2 = 3 g% Hb desat in capillaries
    Because the average amount of Hb desat in the capillaries of this patient is less than 5 g%, this patient does not appear cyanotic.

EXERCISE 7-7 O_2 Transport/ HbCO/HbF

1. 15 mL O_2/min
2. 1000 mL O_2/min
3. 750.18 mL O_2/min
   499.95 mL O_2/min
   418.02 mL O_2/min
4. 245 times
5. Carboxyhemoglobin

6. HbCO is incapable of carrying O_2. HbCO shifts the oxyhemoglobin curve to the left.
7. 20 mm Hg
8. Greater
9. CO-oximeter
10. 80%

EXERCISE 7-8 Methemoglobinemia and Sickle Cell Disease

1. Methemoglobin
2. Methemoglobinemia
3. Methemoglobinemia
4. Methylene blue
5. Cyanosis
6. HbF
7. Chest pain
   Fever
   Leukocytosis
8. 85%
9. metHb
10. 10%

EXERCISE 7-9 Internal Respiration

1. Decreased O_2, decreased pH, increased temperature, increased CO_2
2. 11 vol% in the heart
   1 vol% in the skin
3. Mitochondria
4. 10%
5. 0.8
6. 1.0
7. 10
8. Krebs cycle
9. Lactic acid
10. Central
11. 1.3

NBRC Challenge 7

1. D) CO-oximetry. It is likely the patient has methemoglobinemia because it may be observed following administration of topical anesthetics and appears as abrupt cyanosis.
2. B) Methylene blue I.V.
3. E) II, III, and IV only. Hypercapnia and acidemia could cause this due to a right shift of the oxyhemoglobin curve. Alternatively, some forms of abnormal Hb species may also have decreased affinity for oxygen.

4. B) A low cardiac output is the classic cause of an increased arteriovenous difference.
5. E) Lipogenesis secondary to a high carbohydrate intake can result in an RQ as high as 1.3.

CHAPTER 8

ON-CALL CASE 8-1 ABGs and Critical Thinking

Assessment

Abnormalities:

$\downarrow\downarrow$ pH
$\uparrow$ $PaCO_2$
$\downarrow$ $[HCO_3]$
$\downarrow\downarrow$ PaO_2
$\downarrow\downarrow$ SaO_2

ABG classification: Mixed respiratory acidosis and metabolic acidosis with moderate hypoxemia.

Explanation:

Regarding acid-base, the metabolic acidosis is likely due to the renal failure described. The recent respiratory acidosis is most likely due to the administration of bicarbonate to a patient with controlled ventilation. Bicarbonate will produce CO_2 via the hydrolysis reaction that is normally excreted; however, this patient cannot increase alveolar ventilation; therefore, $PaCO_2$ rises. The worsening hypoxemia is probably secondary to the acute hypercapnia superimposed on the pulmonary shunting from the acute respiratory distress syndrome (ARDS).

No additional data are needed to confirm the interpretation.

Intervention

Importance:

An increase in alveolar ventilation would normalize the $PaCO_2$. This would improve acid-base balance as well as oxygenation. This is probably best done by increasing the respiratory rate while avoiding dangerous lung pressures in ARDS. If this could not be done without increasing lung pressures significantly, an alternative would be permissive hypercapnia. However, in this case, FIO_2 or positive end-expiratory pressure (PEEP) would have to be used to increase oxygenation and more bicarbonate may need to be administered if one wanted to keep the pH > 7.30.

ON-CALL CASE 8-2 ABGs and Critical Thinking

Assessment

Abnormalities:

$\uparrow\uparrow$ pH
$\downarrow\downarrow$ $PaCO_2$
Normal [HCO_3]
Normal oxygenation
ABG classification: Uncompensated respiratory alkalosis with normoxemia while breathing FIO_2 0.4.

Explanation:

Regarding acid-base balance, the mechanical deadspace did not increase $PaCO_2$ as intended but, in fact, $PaCO_2$ decreased. Mechanical deadspace is ineffective in the patient who simply increases alveolar ventilation on their own by either increasing rate or tidal volume.

Intervention

Importance:

The patient should have alveolar ventilation reduced.

Objective:

It would be desirable to get the pH below 7.50 and the $PaCO_2$ above 30 mm Hg.

Action:

The patient's tidal volume and/or rate should be reduced in order to decrease alveolar ventilation. Another alternative might be to sedate the patient.

EXERCISES

EXERCISE 8-1 Hydrogen Ions and pH

1. Is not
2. Negative log of the free [H^+]
3. 7.35 to 7.45
4. Inverse, logarithmic
5. 0.3
6. Acid
7. Base
8. Homeostasis
9. Lungs, kidneys

10. Acid
11. Lungs
12. Volatile
13. Carbonic acid (H_2CO_3)
14. Kidneys
15. Bicarbonate (HCO_3^-)

EXERCISE 8-2 Underlying Chemistry of H_2CO_3 Regulation

1. Does not
2. Closed
3. Left
4. Law of mass action
5. Left
6. $H_2O + CO_2 \xrightarrow{\longleftarrow} H_2CO_3 \xrightarrow{\longleftarrow} HCO_3 + H^+$
7. Direct, linear
8. $PaCO_2$
9. Increase
10. Acidic

EXERCISE 8-3 CO_2 Homeostasis

1. Metabolic rate
2. $\dot{V}CO_2$
3. Alveolar ventilation
4. $\dot{V}_A$
5. Massive burns, sepsis
6. Sodium bicarbonate ($NaHCO_3$)
7. Decreased
8. Tidal volume
9. $VT \times RR = \dot{V}$
10. Is not
11. $PaCO_2$
12. $\dot{V}_A = (VT - V_D) \times RR$
13. Inversely
14. Increase
15. Decreases

EXERCISE 8-4 CO_2 Transport

1. Dissolved CO_2
   Carbonic acid
   Bicarbonate
   Carbamino compounds
2. Higher
3. 0.03 mEq/L/mm Hg
4. 80 mm Hg $\times$ 0.03 mEq/L/mm Hg
   = 2.4 mEq/L
5. Is
6. Slow
7. Bicarbonate
8. Faster

9. Carbonic anhydrase
10. Hemoglobin
11. Chloride (Cl^-)
12. Hamburger
13. Erythrocytes
14. Carbamino compound
15. Carbamino-hemoglobin
16. Does not
17. Less
18. Haldane
19. 10%
20. 2%

EXERCISE 8-5 The Kidney and Acid-Base Balance

1. Excretion of fixed acids
   Regulation of blood [HCO_3]
2. Cannot
3. Protein
4. Lipid
5. Ketoacids
6. Lactic acid
7. 50 to 60
8. Hydrochloric acid (HCl)
9. Excrete and produce
10. [HCO_3]

EXERCISE 8-6 Basic Chemistry Related to Buffers

1. Base
2. Conjugate acid-base pair
3. HCO_3^-, Hb^-
4. Different
5. High
6. Greater
7. Weaker
8. Deoxygenated
9. Strong
10. Acid or a base
    Amphoteric

EXERCISE 8-7 Blood Buffer Systems

1. Do not
2. Weaker acids
3. Weak acid
   Salt of the conjugate base of the weak acid
4. Salt
5. Carbonic acid (H_2CO_3)
   Sodium bicarbonate ($NaHCO_3$)
6. Carbonic acid (H_2CO_3) and sodium chloride (NaCl)
7. $NaHCO_3 + H_2O$

8. Bicarbonate
   Inorganic phosphates
   Proteins
9. Quantity of the buffer
   pK of the weak acid in the buffer system
   Open versus closed buffer system
10. 50%
11. Open
12. 1
13. Bicarbonate
14. Hemoglobin
15. Isohydric principle

EXERCISE 8-8 Henderson-Hasselbalch Equation

1. Henderson's equation
2. p
3. pH = pKc + log [HCO_3]/[H_2CO_3]
4. 6.1
5. 24 mEq/L
6. 40 mm Hg × 0.03 mEq/L/mm Hg = 1.2 mEq/L
7. 20:1
8. 1.3
9. pH ≈ [HCO_3]/$PaCO_2$
10. Denominator
11. Ratio between the numerator and denominator
12. Compensation
13. 24 mEq/L/40 mm Hg

EXERCISE 8-9 Acid-Base Physiology and Terminology

1. Renal
2. Alkalosis
3. Acidosis
4. Metabolic
5. 48 to 72 hours
6. Rarely
7. a. Metabolic acidosis
   b. Respiratory acidosis
   c. Respiratory alkalosis
   d. Metabolic alkalosis
8. Primary
9. Laboratory or secondary
10. Hypobasemia

NBRC Challenge 8

1. C) I and II only. The patient appears to have COPD and chronic renal bicarbonate retention for compensation.

2. E) These results are consistent and expected. Venous bicarbonate should be higher due to CO_2 transport.
3. E) The pulmonary changes (hypoventilation and mild hypoxemia) suggest compensation for a metabolic alkalosis.
4. A) Increased CO_2 production is a common cause of CO_2 retention in burn patients.
5. C) Blood buffers respond immediately to protect the pH.

CHAPTER 9

ON-CALL CASE 9-1 ABGs and Critical Thinking

Assessment

Abnormalities:

↓↓ SaO_2
↓ pH
↓ $PaCO_2$
↓↓ PaO_2
↓↓ $[HCO_3]$

ABG classification: Partially compensated metabolic acidosis with moderate hypoxemia.

Explanation:

The respiratory alkalosis appears to be secondary to the acute hypoxemia. The patient had a substantial shunt earlier at 10:00 AM as evidenced by the $P(A-a)O_2$ and FIO_2/PaO_2 ratio. Because it was stated that the patient had pneumonia, this is the likely cause of the pulmonary shunt and hypoxemia. The acute onset of hypoxemia appears to be due to a decreased cardiac output as evidenced by the hypotension, arrhythmias, chest pain, and shortness of breath. In healthy individuals, a decrease in cardiac output would only have a minimal effect on PaO_2 because of the small percentage of shunted blood. In this individual, however, the decrease in cardiac output could have a substantial impact on PaO_2 because of the high shunt fraction, which was pre-existing.

Evaluation:

Additional data: Measurement of cardiac output and shunt fraction would be ideal if the patient had a Swan-Ganz catheter in place. Pulmonary wedge pressure and central venous pressure would also help guide fluid and drug therapy.

Intervention

Importance:

First priority would be to get oxygenation and cardiac output to an acceptable level. It would probably be wise to increase FIO_2 to maintain an SpO_2 of at least 90%. The next priority would be to evaluate cardiac output more specifically and maintain B/P through appropriate use of cardiotonics and fluids.

ON-CALL CASE 9-2 ABGs and Critical Thinking

Assessment

Abnormalities:

↓↓ SaO_2
↓↓ pH
↑ $PaCO_2$
↓ PaO_2
↓ $[HCO_3]$

ABG classification: Mixed respiratory and metabolic acidosis with mild hypoxemia.

Explanation:

The hypoxemia is due at least in part to hypoventilation. The hypoventilation is secondary to the drug overdose and depression of ventilatory drive with subsequent decrease in alveolar oxygen. Calculation of the $P(A-a)O_2$ on room air yields a value of 28 mm Hg. Because the normal $P(A-a)O_2$ is less than 20 mm Hg, this value suggests another factor contributing to the hypoxemia, specifically an increased physiologic shunt. The increased shunt could be a consequence of aspiration. Therefore, the likelihood of aspiration and additional gas exchange impairment is likely.

Evaluation:

Additional data: A chest radiograph would provide additional evidence of aspiration.

Intervention

Importance:

The first priority is to establish an airway and maintain sufficient alveolar ventilation. Therefore, if the hypoventilation could not be quickly reversed, the patient should be intubated and ventilated. Also, the patient should be observed for worsening hypoxemia and shunting as a result of the likely aspiration. Bronchial clearance maneuvers should be initiated as necessary.

EXERCISES

EXERCISE 9-1 Hypoxemia and the Role of Cardiac Output

1. Adequacy
   Efficiency
2. **H**ypoventilation
   Absolute shunting
   Relative shunting
   Diffusion defects
   (Note that these four common causes form the acronym HARD.)
3. Relative shunting
4. Always
5. Minimal
6. Lower
7. Fall
8. A large percentage of venous blood entering the arteries
9. Cannot
10. Increased

EXERCISE 9-2 Alveolar-Arterial O_2 Gradients

1. $P(A-a)O_2$
2. 10 mm Hg
   20 mm Hg
3. Ventilation-perfusion mismatch
4. Mean
5. $PAO_2 = PIO_2 - 1.2(PaCO_2)$
6. $PIO_2 = (PB - PH_2O) \times FIO_2$
7. 50
8. Absorption atelectasis
9. Increases
10. $PAO_2 = PIO_2 - PaCO_2$

EXERCISE 9-3 Oxygenation Ratios

1. More
2. 0.75
3. 0.3 to 1.0
4. 100 mm Hg
5. 400
6. Oxygenation
7. 2.0
8. Does not
9. PaO_2/PAO_2
10. Do

EXERCISE 9-4 Indices of Physiologic Shunting

1. Corrects
2. Classic
3. Mixed venous blood
4. Pulmonary artery catheter
5. $C(a-\bar{v})O_2$
6. $\dot{Q}sp/\dot{Q}T$
7. $P(A-a)O_2$
8. $P(A-a)O_2$
9. PaO_2/FIO_2 or the oxygenation ratio $(PaO_2/\%FIO_2)$
10. 20%

EXERCISE 9-5 Differential Diagnosis of Hypoxemia and Effects of Altitude on Hypoxemia

1. Multiple mechanisms
2. Hypoventilation
3. Poor
4. White-out
5. Edema
6. Decreased cardiac output
7. Hyperventilation
   Excessive oxygen therapy
8. Relative
9. 130 mm Hg
10. Bronchodilators
    Nitrides
11. Hemodialysis
12. Liver
13. Increase
14. 5000
15. 4

EXERCISE 9-6 The $P(A-a)O_2$ in Differential Diagnosis

$$PAO_2 = PIO_2 - 1.2(PaCO_2)$$

	$P(A-a)O_2$ (mm Hg)	Diagnosis
1.	38	Hypoventilation with increased physiologic shunting
2.	28	Hypoventilation with increased physiologic shunting
3.	10	Simple hypoventilation
4.	14	Simple hypoventilation
5.	25	Hypoventilation with increased physiologic shunting

6. Absolute shunting
7. Relative shunting
8. Absolute shunting
9. Relative shunting
10. Absolute shunting

NBRC Challenge 9

1. B) Pneumonia. The $P(A-a)O_2$ of 35 mm Hg on room air suggests increased physiological shunting. Pneumonia is the only shunt producing disease listed.
2. A) Hypoventilation. A normal $P(A-a)O_2$ indicates the patient has simple hypoventilation without shunting disease.
3. D) PaO_2. In the presence of a substantial shunt (e.g., 30%), a drop in cardiac output will decrease mixed venous PO_2 and will cause hypoxemia.
4. E) Decrease very slightly or not at all. Since the normal shunt fraction is so small, a decrease in cardiac output tends to have only very minimal effect on PaO_2.
5. A) Increase, increase. Since the PaO_2/PAO_2 is inversely proportional to shunting, both indices of shunting will increase when the ratio decreases.

CHAPTER 10

ON-CALL CASE 10-1 ABGs and Critical Thinking

Assessment

Abnormalities:

$\downarrow\downarrow$ SaO_2
$\downarrow$ pH
$\uparrow\uparrow$ $PaCO_2$
$\downarrow\downarrow\downarrow$ PaO_2
$\uparrow$ $[HCO_3]$

ABG classification: Partially compensated respiratory acidosis with severe hypoxemia.

Explanation:

The patient appears to be in acute exacerbation of COPD that is most likely secondary to the recent acute infection.

Evaluation:

Additional data: Chest radiography, vital signs, and blood work would help to evaluate for possible pneumonia. Elevated temperature and [WBC] and white-out on chest radiograph confirms bacterial infection. Sputum culture may be beneficial to determine the type of microbe involved.

Intervention

Importance:

The patient needs to be oxygenated first to preclude hypoxia. Bronchial hygiene with bronchodilators would be useful. Appropriate antibiotics would also be useful.

Objective:

The goal in oxygen therapy is to keep PaO_2 at 60 mm Hg and SaO_2 at 90% in acute exacerbation of COPD.

Action:

Mechanical ventilation should be avoided if at all possible in COPD because these patients are prone to other problems and are difficult to wean. Low concentration FIO_2 should be initiated at approximately FIO_2 0.28. This FIO_2 is most likely to result in an increase in PaO_2 of about 18 mm Hg, which is the appropriate target. This can be administered with 2 LPM nasal cannula or Ventimask. The patient should be watched for signs of further deterioration (decreasing pH, increasing $PaCO_2$, or progressive loss of consciousness) and/or deterioration of vital signs. Arterial blood gases should be drawn at least 30 minutes after initiation of therapy.

ON-CALL CASE 10-2 ABGs and Critical Thinking

Assessment

Abnormalities:

$\downarrow\downarrow$ SaO_2
$\downarrow\downarrow$ pH
$\uparrow$ $PaCO_2$
$\downarrow\downarrow$ PaO_2
$\downarrow$ $[HCO_3]$

ABG classification: Mixed respiratory and metabolic acidosis with moderate hypoxemia.

Explanation:

The patient appears to be in severe acute respiratory distress syndrome. The chest radiograph and pulmonary wedge pressure are consistent with this. The history of hypotension and sepsis also makes this patient a good candidate for acute respiratory distress syndrome. Finally, the oxygenation ratio less than 1 indicates severe pulmonary shunting. If the oxygenation ratio were greater than 2, the diagnosis would be acute lung injury.

Evaluation:

Additional data: Measurement of cardiac output and shunt fraction would reinforce the diagnosis because the patient apparently has a Swan-Ganz catheter in place.

Intervention

Importance:

The patient needs oxygen to prevent tissue hypoxia, positive end-expiratory pressure to address the true shunting (10–20 cm H_2O), and, finally, the ventilatory failure would ideally be corrected.

Objective:

Ideally, we can restore this patient to a normal $PaCO_2$ and ventilation. We can also ensure that oxygenation is adequate with a PaO_2 of at least 60 mm Hg, and SaO_2 greater than 90%. It would also be desirable to normalize the pulmonary shunt, though we do not want to exacerbate VILI or MODS.

Action:

The patient should be intubated and placed on mechanical ventilation using the ARDS/Net approach. This would include using a tidal volume goal of no more than 6 mL/kg ideal body weight, a maximal alveolar pressure of 30 cm H_2O, using permissive hypercapnia, if necessary, while maintaining a pH at least greater than 7.20. (Refer to the section in the chapter regarding ARDS/Net.)

EXERCISES

EXERCISE 10-1 Oxygen Therapy

1. Oxygen therapy
2. Severe
3. $PaO_2 < 60$ mm Hg
   $SaO_2 < 90\%$
4. Alveolar oxygen supply
5. Relative
6. High-flow
7. FIO_2 0.24
8. Higher
9. Low-flow
10. 0.40–0.70

EXERCISE 10-2 Hazards and Guidelines in Oxygen Therapy

1. *55*
2. 7.20
3. 60
4. FIO_2
   PaO_2
   Duration of exposure
5. 150 mm Hg
6. Pulse oximetry
7. Correction of hypoxia
8. COPD
9. 3
10. CO_2 narcosis

EXERCISE 10-3 General Treatment and Positioning in Oxygen-Loading Problems

1. Maintain an *adequate* PaO_2
   Minimize cardiopulmonary work
   Prevent or alleviate hypoxia
2. Oxygen therapy
   Body positioning
   PEEP/CPAP
   Mechanical ventilation
   Alveolar recruitment maneuvers
   Nitric oxide
3. Cardiac output may change
   Effects of airway closure
   Ventilation-perfusion relationships
4. Supine
5. Sitting
6. Sitting
7. Up
8. Down
9. Is not
10. Prone

EXERCISE 10-4 Oxygen Toxicity/ ALI/ARDS

1. Bleomycin
2. Amiodarone
3. Paraquat
4. 50 mm Hg
5. Acute Lung Injury and Acute Respiratory Distress Syndrome
6. Less
7. Heterogeneous
8. 30 cm H_2O
9. Volume induced lung injury
10. Multiple organ dysfunction syndrome
11. ARDS/Net

12. 6
13. Permissive hypercapnia
14. Decreased
15. 7.20

EXERCISE 10-5 PEEP/CPAP

1. ARDS
2. CPAP
3. PEEP
4. EPAP
5. Threshold
6. Continuous
7. 10–20
8. Is
9. Improves
10. Beneficial

EXERCISE 10-6 Complications of PEEP

1. Decreased cardiac output
   Pulmonary barotrauma
2. Hypovolemic
3. High
4. Above
5. Mean
6. Unilateral
7. Threshold
8. Decreased venous return
9. Increase
10. Differential

EXERCISE 10-7 Auto-PEEP

1. Auto-PEEP
2. COPD
3. High
4. Increases
5. Is not
6. Expiratory
7. Increasing
8. High
9. Decrease
10. Should not

NBRC Challenge 10

1. D) Nasal cannula 1 LPM. Because it is a patient with COPD, we administer low FIO_2. Because the target PaO_2 in COPD exacerbation is 60 mm Hg, and as a guideline, PaO_2 increases approximately 3 torr per 1% increase in FIO_2, a nasal cannula at 1 LPM should deliver FIO_2 of 0.24 and increase PaO_2 approximately 9 mm Hg.

2. C) I and II only. A tidal volume 6 mL/kg ideal body weight and a maximum alveolar pressure of 30 cm H_2O are consistent with ARDS/Net. PEEP is usually set between 10 and 20 cm H_2O.
3. A) PEEP. PEEP therapy is effective in cardiogenic pulmonary edema because it decreases preload and improves cardiac function.
4. D) II and III only. Prone positioning and nitric oxide therapy have been shown to improve $\dot{V}/\dot{Q}$ in ARDS.
5. C) Decrease PEEP to 5 cm H_2O. Current thinking (reference 305) is that once FIO_2 is decreased to 0.50, PEEP should be reduced to 5 cm H_2O. Decreasing FIO_2 to 0.40 and then extubation should then follow this action.

CHAPTER 11

ON-CALL CASE 11-1 ABGs and Critical Thinking

Assessment

Abnormalities:

Normal acid-base status (pH, $PaCO_2$, and $[HCO_3]$)

↓ PaO_2

↓↓ Oxygenation ratio (PaO_2/FIO_2)

↓↓ $P\bar{v}O_2$

ABG classification: Normal acid-base status with mild hypoxemia

Explanation:

The patient's pulmonary shunt seems slightly improved as evidenced by the PaO_2 increase with the increased PEEP on the same FIO_2. Nevertheless, the substantial decrease in $P\bar{v}O_2$ indicates that tissue oxygenation has deteriorated. This is most likely due to a decrease in cardiac output associated with the PEEP. PEEP is usually beneficial in cardiogenic pulmonary edema, however, it appears that 15 cm H_2O is too much in this patient.

Evaluation:

Evaluation of hemodynamic data (if a Swan-Ganz catheter or central venous pressure line is in place) would be useful. Perhaps the patient has become hypovolemic secondary to drug therapy such as Lasix.

Intervention

Importance:

The most important priority is tissue oxygenation.

Objective:

The $P\bar{v}O_2$ must be returned to the normal range of 35 to 45 mm Hg.

Action:

PEEP should be restored to the previous level.

ON-CALL CASE 11-2 ABGs and Critical Thinking

Assessment

Abnormalities:

$\downarrow$ pH
Normal $PaCO_2$
$\downarrow$ [HCO_3]
$\downarrow PaO_2$
$\downarrow SaO_2$
$\uparrow P\bar{v}O_2$
$\uparrow\uparrow$ Lactate
ABG classification: Uncompensated metabolic acidosis with mild hypoxemia.

Explanation:

The patient appears to be hypoxic as indicated by the lactic acidosis. Other indices of oxygenation (PaO_2, SaO_2, $P\bar{v}O_2$) all look acceptable, but sepsis is often characterized by a problem with internal respiration and systemic arterial-venous shunting or failure of the cells to accept oxygen.

Intervention

Importance:

The immediate concern is to minimize the apparent hypoxia and decrease the lactic acidosis.

Objective:

Because this patient may be suffering from pathologic oxygen supply dependency (see section on Covert Hypoxia), it would probably be wise to increase oxygen transport to see if this would improve the patient's overall oxygenation status (i.e., decrease lactate).

EXERCISES

EXERCISE 11-1 Hypoxic Assessment

1. **A**rterial oxygenation
   Blood Hemoglobin Concentration
   Circulatory Status
2. Hypoxia
3. Is not
4. Arterial oxygenation status
5. Usually
6. Is not
7. 60
8. Does not ensure
9. 55
10. Cardiovascular system

EXERCISE 11-2 SaO_2

1. Is not
2. Do not
3. Functional
4. Is not
5. Fractional
6. Fractional
7. Functional
8. Trending of
9. Are not
10. 2

EXERCISE 11-3 Laboratory Diagnosis of Anemia

1. Normal [RBC] 5 million/mm^3 ($\pm$ 700,000) in men
   Normal [RBC] 4.5 million/mm^3 ($\pm$ 500,000) in women
   Normal [Hb] is 15 g% in men
   Normal [Hb] is 13 to 14 g% in women
2. Anemia
3. Hematocrit
4. Anisocytosis
5. Macrocytosis
6. MCV
7. Poikilocytosis
8. Reticulocytes
9. 34 $\pm$ 2%
10. Hypochromia

EXERCISE 11-4 Types of Anemia and Treatment

1. Aplastic
2. Iron deficiency

3. Thalassemia
4. Erythropoietin, folic acid, vitamin B_{12}
5. Pernicious anemia
6. Folic acid deficiency
7. Increased cardiac output, increased DPG
8. 30%–45%
9. Hemolytic
10. Thalassemia

EXERCISE 11-5 Cardiovascular System/Shock

1. Cardiac minute output
2. C.O. or $\dot{Q}$
3. Cardiac index (C.I.)
4. Thermodilution, Fick equation
5. Is
6. Urine output, neurological status, blood pressure, pulse, capillary refill, cyanosis, warmth of extremities
7. Heart, blood volume, blood vessels
8. Shock
9. Vasoconstriction
10. Restlessness, anxiety, alteration of level of consciousness, cyanosis, decreased urine output, lactic acidosis, respiratory alkalosis, cold clammy extremities

EXERCISE 11-6 Types of Shock

1. C.O. = heart rate × stroke volume
2. Decreases
3. Increases, decreases
4. Cardiogenic shock
5. Hypovolemia
6. Low
7. Congestive heart failure
8. Hypovolemic shock
9. Septic
10. Anaphylactic

EXERCISE 11-7 Hemodynamic Monitoring

1. Right atrium
2. 2 to 10
3. Heart failure
4. Swan-Ganz catheter
5. 25/10
6. 5 to 12
7. Left-sided heart failure
8. ARDS
9. Diastolic

EXERCISE 11-8 Cardiovascular Treatment

1. Sitting
2. Feet up
3. Detrimental, beneficial
4. Chronotropic

EXERCISE 11-9 Lactate

1. Lactic
2. Lactate
3. 0.9–1.9 mM/L
4. 9
5. Correlates
6. Liver, quickly
7. Is not
8. 10:1
9. Increased
10. Is not

EXERCISE 11-10 Mixed Venous Oxygenation Indices

1. Swan-Ganz catheter (pulmonary artery catheter)
2. 75%
3. $S\bar{v}O_2$
4. 35 mm Hg
5. Both pulmonary and cardiovascular changes
6. Increased
7. Decreased
8. Normal PaO_2, low $P\bar{v}O_2$
9. High
10. Usually

EXERCISE 11-11 Oxygen Uptake/Utilization

1. Is not
2. Critical oxygen delivery point
3. 8 to 10
4. Unnecessary because the additional oxygen is not used
5. May be increased
6. Covert
7. Poor
8. Multiple organ dysfunction syndrome
9. Prostacyclin
10. Unchanged, may be increased
11. Pathologic

NBRC Challenge 11

1. C) Hypovolemic shock. The low hemodynamic pressures throughout (especially CVP) suggest low blood volume in the cardiopulmonary system.
2. C) Gastric tonometry. Gastric tonometry is a relatively new technique for evaluation of mucosal acidosis reflective of poor perfusion.
3. A) Cardiogenic shock. The high CVP and especially the high PWP is diagnostic of LHF.
4. A) Sitting. The sitting position is likely to minimize venous return, which is optimal in the failing heart.
5. E) III and IV only. An increased $C(a-\bar{v})O_2$ and a decreased SvO_2 both are suggestive of a decreased cardiac output.

CHAPTER 12

ON-CALL CASE 12-1 ABGs and Critical Thinking

Assessment

Abnormalities:

↑ pH	↑↑ CO_2
↑ $PaCO_2$	↓↓ K
↑↑ [HCO_3]	↓ Na
	↓ Cl

ABG classification: Partially compensated metabolic alkalosis with normoxemia.

Explanation:

The history of thiazide diuretics should alert one to the possibility of hyponatremia, fluid depletion, and hypokalemia. Symptoms associated with hypokalemia are present; namely, weakness, lethargy, and muscle cramps, and electrocardiography (ECG) demonstrates an inverted T wave and a prominent U wave. It appears to be a classic case of hypokalemia associated with chronic diuretic therapy.

Intervention

Importance:

To prevent dangerous arrhythmias, correct the potassium level as soon as possible. Administer potassium slowly to allow for movement into the intracellular space. The patient also appears to need some sodium and chloride.

Objective:

The goal is to restore potassium and the other electrolytes to the normal range.

ON-CALL CASE 12-2 ABGs and Critical Thinking

Assessment

Abnormalities:

↓↓ pH
↓↓ $PaCO_2$
↓↓ [HCO_3]

↓↓ CO_2 10 mEq/L
↑ K 5.2 mEq/L
↓ Albumin 3.2 g/dL

ABG classification: Partially compensated metabolic acidosis with normoxemia.

Explanation:

The patient appears to have a primary metabolic acidosis. The first step in evaluating a metabolic acidosis is to calculate the anion gap. The anion gap equals 16 mEq/L, which is near the upper limits of normal; however, the anion gap reads falsely low when hypoalbuminemia is present. Therefore, the anion gap should be higher by approximately 3 mEq/L. This anion gap is beyond the normal range for that level of albumin and indicates an increased fixed acid in the blood.

Evaluation:

Evaluate the patient to see if he or she ingested a toxin. Measurement of blood glucose helps to rule out diabetic ketoacidosis, and assessment of blood urea nitrogen and creatinine levels helps to rule out renal failure. Oxygenation should be suspected because of the history of anemia. The [Hb] should be checked. Furthermore, cardiovascular assessment and lactate measurement would help determine if lactic acidosis is present.

Intervention

Importance:

The most important priority is to determine the cause of the metabolic acidosis. If the pH falls below 7.20 (or hyperkalemia worsens), administration of sodium bicarbonate may be indicated. If serious anemia is present, blood transfusion may be indicated.

EXERCISES

EXERCISE 12-1 Regulation of Ventilation

1. Medulla
2. CSF
3. Gases, ions
4. Cheyne-Stokes respiration
5. Carotid, aortic
6. May stimulate the peripheral chemoreceptors:
   b) Hypoxemia
   c) Cyanide poisoning
   d) Hypercarbia ($PaCO_2$ 70 mm Hg)
   e) Cardiogenic shock
7. Peripheral
8. 60
9. Central
10. Depressed
11. Greater
12. Hypoxemia
13. Hypercarbia
14. Hypercarbia
15. J-receptor

EXERCISE 12-2 Renal Function

1. Cortex, medulla
2. Ureters
3. Nephron
4. Glomerulus
5. Afferent
6. Proximal convoluted tubule
7. Cannot
8. Oliguria
9. Secretion
10. Glomerular filtrate

EXERCISE 12-3 Body Fluids and Electrolytes

1. Intracellular
2. Intravascular
3. Serum
4. Interstitial
5. Non-electrolyte
6. Cations
7. Potassium
8. Sodium   142 mEq/L
   Potassium   4 mEq/L
   Calcium   5 mEq/L
   Magnesium   2 mEq/L
9. Sodium
10. Na^+

EXERCISE 12-4 Chemical Mechanisms of Sodium Reabsorption and the Renin-Angiotensin System

1. NaCl mechanism and the $NaHCO_3$ mechanism
2. Chloride (Cl^-)
3. Hydrogen (H^+) or potassium (K^+) ion
4. Is
5. Hydrolysis
6. In alkalemia, K^+ is secreted and H^+ is retained
7. Juxtaglomerular
8. Renin
9. Aldosterone
10. $NaHCO_3$

EXERCISE 12-5 Total Sodium Reabsorption and Diuretics

1. Proximal tubule
2. 80%
3. $NaHCO_3$
4. Reclaimed
5. Proximal
6. NaCl
7. Loop
8. Alkalosis, hypokalemia
9. Is
10. Acetazolamide

EXERCISE 12-6 Hyperaldosteronism, Urinary Buffers, and Potassium

1. Alkalosis
2. Increased H^+ excretion
   Hypokalemia
3. Secondary
4. Mineralocorticoid
5. Primary
6. Glucocorticoids
7. pH of 4.50
8. Bicarbonate
   Ammonia
   Phosphate
9. Increases
10. Intracellular

EXERCISE 12-7 Law of Electroneutrality, Anion Gap, and Stewart's Strong Ion Difference

1. Hypochloremia
2. Acidosis

3. $Na^- (TCO_2 + Cl) = A^-$
4. 12 to 14
5. Hyperchloremic metabolic acidosis
6. Increases
7. A^- 28 mEq/L; increased fixed acids
8. A^- 22 mEq/L; increased fixed acids
9. A^- 10 mEq/L; decreased base
10. A^- 15 mEq/L; decreased base
11. Decrease
12. Dependent
13. PCO_2, (SID), $[A_{TOT}]$

NBRC Challenge 12

1. C) Serum electrolytes. The recommended first step in the diagnosis of primary metabolic acidosis is to calculate the anion gap from the serum electrolyte report.
2. D) Holding the administration of KCl. The patient currently has a normal plasma potassium concentration.
3. B) Serum potassium. The ECG, especially in a patient with chronic renal failure, suggests hyperkalemia.
4. A) Albumin. Hypoalbuminemia will lower the anion gap and hyperalbuminemia will increase it. Hypoalbuminemia is a common condition in the critically ill.
5. C) Had lactic acidosis. Hypoxia is the most common cause of high anion gap lactic acidosis. The normalization of the anion gap following oxygen therapy is highly suggestive of hypoxic lactic acidosis.

CHAPTER 13

ON-CALL CASE 13-1 ABGs and Critical Thinking

Assessment

Abnormalities:

↑ PaO_2	↑ Salicylate level
↓↓ $PaCO_2$	↑↑ Anion gap (23 mEq/L)
↓↓ $[HCO_3]$	[K]

ABG classification: Compensated respiratory alkalosis with hyperoxemia. However, it is more likely that this represents mixed respiratory alkalosis and metabolic acidosis with hyperoxemia.

Explanation:
The blood gas and laboratory data are consistent with acute salicylate intoxication. The high anion gap suggests a metabolic acidosis, but the blood gas also appears to indicate a primary respiratory alkalosis. This is the classic picture of an adult with salicylate toxicity.

Evaluation:
Serial blood gas and salicylate levels should be measured because the patient may get progressively worse, especially if the aspirin was enteric coated. The enteric coating may slow absorption and delay serious symptoms. In a reported case, a patient was shown to have a salicylate level greater than 125 mg/dL 24 hours after presentation.[513]

Intervention

Importance:
Carefully monitor the patient for any signs of worsening toxicity. Initiate hemodialysis quickly following any signs of deterioration.

ON-CALL CASE 13-2 ABGs and Critical Thinking

Assessment

Abnormalities:
↓↓ PaO_2
↑ $PaCO_2$
↑↑ $[HCO_3]$ and Total CO_2
↓ Na
↓↓ K
↓↓ Cl

ABG classification: Partially compensated metabolic alkalosis with moderate hypoxemia.

Explanation:
The blood gas and electrolytes are consistent with severe dehydration secondary to vomiting.

Intervention

Importance:
The patient needs I.V. therapy, including sodium chloride to restore fluids. Potassium should likewise be administered slowly because abrupt increases to dangerous levels could precipitate arrhythmias. Oxygen therapy would be useful because the patient is hypoventilating at substantial levels to compensate for the metabolic alkalosis. If the pH does not respond to

fluid and potassium replacement, dilute HCl might be indicated for treatment of severe alkalemia.

EXERCISES

EXERCISE 13-1 Respiratory Acidosis

1. Accumulation
2. COPD
3. COPD
4. Should not
5. Are
6. Status asthmaticus
7. Vital capacity
8. Hypokalemia
9. Less
10. Increases
11. Quantity
12. An increased
13. Pickwickian
14. Ondine's
15. COPD
    O_2 excess in COPD
    Drugs
    Extreme ventilation-perfusion mismatch
    Exhaustion
    Neuromuscular disorders
    Iatrogenic respiratory acidosis
    Neurologic disorders
    Excessive CO_2 production
    (The acronym *code nine* may help when recalling these major causes.)

EXERCISE 13-2 Respiratory Alkalosis

1. Depleting
2. Hypoxemia
3. Hering-Breuer
4. J-receptor
5. Stimulate
6. Acidosis
7. Decreased
8. Respiratory alkalosis
9. Acidosis
10. Hypoxemia (moderate to severe)
    Overzealous mechanical ventilation
    Restrictive lung disorders
    Neurologic origin
    Shock/Decreased cardiac output
    (The acronym *horns* may help when recalling these major causes.)

EXERCISE 13-3 High Anion Gap Metabolic Acidosis: Toxins and Azotemic Renal Failure

1. Increase in fixed acids
2. Salicylate
3. Methanol (wood alcohol)
4. Ethylene glycol
5. Toluene
6. Azotemic renal failure
7. BUN and creatinine
8. Prerenal
9. Uremia
10. 4 mg/dL

EXERCISE 13-4 High Anion Gap Metabolic Acidosis: Lactic Acidosis and Ketoacidosis

1. Common
2. Hepatic
3. Acetoacetic acid
   Beta-hydroxybutyric acid
4. Acetone
5. Ketone
6. Starvation
   Alcoholic ketoacidosis
   Diabetes mellitus
7. Acetest
8. Mellitus, hyperglycemia
9. Insulin
10. Hyperglycemia
11. Dehydration
12. 500 mg/dL
13. Kussmaul's breathing
14. Glycosuria
15. Toxins
    Azotemic renal failure
    Lactic acidosis
    Ketoacidosis
    (The acronym *talk* may help when recalling these major causes.)

EXERCISE 13-5 Normal Anion Gap Metabolic Acidosis

1. Hyperchloremic
2. Kidneys
   Intestines
3. Renal tubular acidosis (RTA)
4. High
5. Enteric
6. Diarrhea
7. Acetazolamide

8. Children
9. High
10. Renal tubular acidosis
    Enteric drainage tubes
    Diarrhea
    Urinary diversion
    Carbonic anhydrase inhibitors
    Early renal disease
    Dilution acidosis
    Biliary or pancreatic fistulas
    Acidifying salts
    Sulfur, hydrogen sulfide, and drugs
    Eucapnic ventilation post-hypocapnia
    (The acronym *reduced base* may help
    when recalling these major causes.)

EXERCISE 13-6 Metabolic Alkalosis

1. Cannot
2. Intracellular
3. Gastric fluid loss
4. (HCO$_3^-$) anion
5. Bartter's
6. Acidosis, alkalosis
7. Primary hyperaldosteronism
8. Glucocorticoids
9. Alkalosis
10. Hypokalemia
    Ingestion of large amounts of alkali or licorice
    Gastric fluid loss
    Hyperaldosteronism secondary to non-adrenal factors
    Bicarbonate administration
    Adrenocortical hypersecretion
    Steroids
    Eucapnic ventilation post-hypercapnia
    (The acronym *high base* may help when
    recalling these major causes.)

NBRC Challenge 13

1. C) Diamox. A carbonic anhydrase inhibitor
   would tend to lower pH.
2. C) Tissues are likely acidotic. It has been
   shown that tissue pH and PCO$_2$ are most
   often acidotic and hypercapnic despite
   arterial hypocapnia during profound circulatory shock.
3. A) [Hb]. The high lactate and anion gap
   suggest hypoxia. Anemia is a potential
   cause of tissue hypoxia.

4. E) Discontinue the narcotic. Narcotics are
   known to depress ventilation in COPD and
   should be avoided.
5. D) I. I, II and III only. Blood glucose, BUN,
   and lactate all provide clues as to possible
   causes of high anion gap acidosis.

CHAPTER 14

ON-CALL CASE 14-1 ABGs and Critical Thinking

Assessment

Abnormalities:
↓ PaO$_2$ and SaO$_2$
↑↑ PaCO$_2$
↑↑ [HCO$_3$]
↓ K
↓↓ Cl
↑↑ Anion gap

ABG classification: On first impression, it
appears to be a compensated metabolic alkalosis; however, the degree of compensation seems
excessive and the history suggests primary respiratory acidosis. The best classification would be
a mixed respiratory acidosis and metabolic alkalosis. Plotting the data on an acid-base map is
also consistent with a mixed acid-base disorder.

Explanation:
The long-standing COPD has probably caused
the respiratory acidosis. Diuretics and steroids
often cause primary metabolic alkalosis and
this may be the reason for this. Hypokalemia is
also consistent with the effects of these drugs.
The high anion gap suggests that lactic acidosis is also present but is masqueraded by the
other acid-base disorders. This may actually be
termed a triple acid-base disorder.

Evaluation:
A lactate measurement may confirm the presence of lactic acid accumulation.

Intervention

Importance:
The patient probably requires careful rehydra-
tion and potassium replacement. Both should be
approached slowly to avoid hyperkalemia and
fluid overload especially considering the CHF.

If plasma lactic acidosis appears to be present, the patient should also receive oxygen therapy.

ON-CALL CASE 14-2 ABGs and Critical Thinking

Assessment

Abnormalities:
$\downarrow$ PaO_2 and SaO_2 (mild)
$\downarrow\downarrow$ pH
$\downarrow\downarrow$ $PaCO_2$
$\downarrow\downarrow$ $[HCO_3]$
$\uparrow\uparrow$ [K]
$\uparrow\uparrow$ Anion gap
ABG classification: Partially compensated metabolic acidosis with mild hypoxemia.

Explanation:
It appears that the patient has metabolic acidosis secondary to renal failure. The high anion gap is consistent with this diagnosis. The hyperkalemia, although common in metabolic acidosis, is also consistent with this. The hyperkalemia is also a matter of some concern because it may lead to serious complications.

Evaluation:
Measurement of blood urea nitrogen [BUN] and creatinine would facilitate the diagnosis of azotemic renal failure. These values are likely substantially elevated.

Intervention

Importance:
The foremost concern is to decrease the serum potassium to a safe level. A secondary goal might be to correct the metabolic acidosis.

Objective:
It is best to decrease the potassium below 6.0, preferably lower.

Action:
Sodium bicarbonate is useful in metabolic acidosis accompanied with hyperkalemia because alkalinization of the extracellular fluid would facilitate the movement of potassium back into the intracellular space. Despite the fact that the pH is above 7.10, sodium bicarbonate intravenously may be indicated to help lower the serum potassium. If hyperkalemia persists or worsens, dialysis will likely be necessary.

EXERCISES

EXERCISE 14-1 Factors Complicating Acid-Base Disturbances

1. Respiratory system
   Renal system
2. $PaCO_2$ increased
   $[HCO_3^-]$ increased
   [BE] increased
3. Compensation for previous hypercapnia
4. Lactic acidosis
5. pH
6. COPD
7. Low-flow O_2 therapy
8. Compensation
9. More
10. Acidosis

EXERCISE 14-2 Mixed Acid-Base Disturbances

1. Mixed
2. 95%
3. Does not
4. pH 7.31 after maximal compensation (50% return)
5. pH 7.50 after maximal compensation (50% return)
6. 18 mm Hg
   30 mm Hg
   22 mm Hg
7. Hypochloremia
8. Hyperchloremia
9. Day
10. Absence of compensation
    Long-standing renal or pulmonary disease
    Excessive compensation
    Respiratory assistance
    Temporal inconsistencies
    Settings conducive to mixed disturbances
    (Note that the acronym *alerts* may help when recalling these situations.)

EXERCISE 14-3 Respiratory Acid-Base Treatment

1. Supportive (palliative) treatment
   Corrective treatment

2. pH
3. Respiratory acidosis (acidemia)
4. pH
5. 7.25
6. Low FIO_2 (0.24 to 0.40) or noninvasive positive-pressure ventilation
7. Respiratory rate
   Tidal volume
   Mechanical deadspace
8. Gradually

EXERCISE 14-4 Treatment of Metabolic Acidosis

1. Is not
2. Liver
3. Sodium bicarbonate ($NaHCO_3$)
4. pH < 7.10
5. Hypokalemia
6. Intracranial
7. Hypercapnia (respiratory acidosis)
8. Has
9. THAM or Carbicarb
10. [BE] × 0.3 × weight in kg/2 = HCO_3^- dose
11. Is
12. Is not
13. Much
14. Venous paradox
15. Fall
16. [20] × 0.3 × 80 kg/2 = HCO_3^- dose
    480/2 = HCO_3^- dose = 240 mEq

EXERCISE 14-5 Treatment of Metabolic Alkalosis

1. Potassium, chloride, fluid volume replacement
2. Cimetidine or ranitidine
3. 3.5 mEq/L
4. Slowly
5. Acetazolamide (Diamox)
6. 7.55
7. Dilute hydrochloric acid
8. Central
9. 100 mEq/L
10. Common

NBRC Challenge 14

1. D) KCl I.V. Therapy for mild-to-moderate metabolic alkalosis typically includes KCl I.V., especially in the patient with hypokalemia.

The kidney cannot correct metabolic alkalosis in the absence of sufficient potassium.
2. E) Leave the patient on the current settings. This is classic permissive hypercapnia. The key in ARDS is to minimize alveolar pressures whereas mild-to-moderate hypercapnia is secondary and generally of minimal consequence.
3. B) Noninvasive positive-pressure ventilation is effective in the management of COPD and helps to avoid mechanical ventilation and intubation.
4. C) Most likely acidotic. Typically during cardiac arrest, there is a venous paradox and tissue pH remains acidotic despite arterial blood gases that manifest respiratory alkalosis.
5. D) Dilute HCl acid I.V. This is the treatment of choice for severe sustained metabolic alkalosis; however, an experienced intensivist should administer it carefully.

CHAPTER 15

ON-CALL CASE 15-1 ABGs and Critical Thinking
Assessment
Abnormalities:
Normal PaO_2 and SaO_2
↑ pH
↓ $PaCO_2$
Normal [HCO_3]
↓ $PetCO_2$ followed by an abrupt increase
ABG classification: Uncompensated respiratory alkalosis with normoxemia.

Explanation:
The patient is being intentionally hyperventilated to minimize intracranial pressure due to her head surgery. The original $PaCO_2$–$PetCO_2$ gradient is appropriately about 6 mm Hg, which is normal. This gradient is expected in a healthy young female with otherwise normal lungs.

Evaluation:
Although we need to be skeptical about $PetCO_2$ changes reflecting $PaCO_2$ changes in all patients, there is usually a good correlation between changes in $PetCO_2$ and $PaCO_2$ in this type of patient. Therefore, we should carefully

evaluate the ventilator circuit and obtain an arterial blood gas. If intracranial pressure is being monitored, it should also be checked to ensure it is not increasing.

Intervention

Importance:
The foremost concern is to decrease the carbon dioxide to a safe level.

Objective:
Restore $PaCO_2$ levels back to 25 to 30 mm Hg.

Action:
Ensure ventilator circuit is intact and make necessary changes to restore hyperventilation.

ON-CALL CASE 15-2 ABGs and Critical Thinking

Assessment

Abnormalities:
↓ PaO_2 (mild hypoxemia)
Normal pH
Normal $PaCO_2$
Normal $[HCO_3]$
↓ $PetCO_2$
ABG classification: Normal acid-base status with mild hypoxemia.

Explanation:
The patient is being appropriately ventilated via mechanical ventilation. The $PaCO_2$ to $PetCO_2$ gradient is slightly elevated (10 mm Hg). This could be due to a variety of reasons including $\dot{V}/\dot{Q}$ mismatch or increased deadspace. The increase in arterial $PaCO_2$ without a concurrent rise in $PetCO_2$ is not uncommon in mechanically ventilated patients. This could reflect an increase in deadspace or a variety of other things. Most importantly, the clinician must recognize that $PetCO_2$, although stable in this patient, does not adequately reflect $PaCO_2$ in most mechanically ventilated patients and should not be relied on as an indicator of $PaCO_2$. Assuming that $PaCO_2$ was unchanged in this patient would have left the hypercarbic problem unidentified. When in doubt, an arterial blood gas measurement should be obtained.

Evaluation:
The increased gradient may suggest the development of increased deadspace such as a pulmonary embolus but the results are inconclusive.

Intervention

Importance:
The foremost concern is to restore arterial $PaCO_2$ to an acceptable level.

Objective:
Restore $PaCO_2$ levels back to 35 to 45 mm Hg.

Action:
Ensure ventilator circuit is intact and make necessary changes to restore ventilation.

EXERCISES

EXERCISE 15-1 Basic Principles of Oximetry
1. Arterial blood gas analysis
2. Measurement
3. Qualitative
4. Photoelectric effect
5. Lambert-Beer
6. Optical density
7. Oximeter
8. Spectrophotometer
9. Isobestic
10. Same
11. Hemolyzed
12. Are not
13. Oxyhemoglobin
    Desaturated hemoglobin
    Carboxyhemoglobin
    Methemoglobin
14. Fractional
15. Hewlett-Packard

EXERCISE 15-2 Pulse Oximetry
1. Pulse oximetry
2. Plethysmograph
3. Pulse
4. Diastole
5. Accurate
6. 2
7. Red and infrared
8. Optical shunting
9. Does not
10. Dual oximetry

EXERCISE 15-3 Transcutaneous PO$_2$/PCO$_2$

1. PtcO$_2$
2. More
3. Less
4. Stratum corneum
   Epidermis
   Dermis
5. High, no
6. 43.5°C
7. Less
8. Higher
9. Wetting
10. Do
11. Burn
12. 2 to 6
13. Infants
14. PtcO$_2$
15. SpO$_2$

EXERCISE 15-4 Capnometry Technique

1. Capnography
2. Mass spectrometers
   Infrared absorption capnometers
3. Mass spectrometers
4. Infrared
5. Choppers
6. Sidestream
   Mainstream
7. Sidestream
8. Artificial airways
9. Slower
10. Mainstream

EXERCISE 15-5 Capnograms

1. Almost zero
2. Alveolar

3. Sidestream
4. Slow
5. Is not
6. Elevated
7. Fall
8. Falls
9. Rise
10. Obstructive
11. Carbon dioxide production
12. Cardiac output

NBRC Challenge 15

1. B) Decreased PetCO$_2$. Decreased perfusion of the lungs results in decreased carbon dioxide in the exhaled gas.
2. D) The patient has increased deadspace. Although the PaCO$_2$ to PetCO$_2$ is less than foolproof, an increasing gradient is consistent with increased alveolar deadspace such as might occur with a pulmonary embolus.
3. A) PtcO$_2$. The patient needs to be carefully monitored for progression into hyperoxemia. Transcutaneous measurement is best suited for this monitoring because it is most sensitive.
4. E) CO-oximetry. The most likely explanation is that methemoglobinemia has developed, which can be detected with CO-oximetry.
5. D) II, III, I. The best monitors for identifying patient mishaps are shown to be in rank order: pulse oximetry, capnography, and ECG.

Illustration Credits

Chapter 1

Figure 1-1, Modified from Croxton, F. E.: Elementary Statistics with Applications in Medicine. Mineola, Dover Publications, 1953;

Figure 1-2, From Thibodeau, G. A., and Patton, K. T.: Anatomy and Physiology, 5th ed. St. Louis, Mosby, 2003;

Figure 1-4, A, Redrawn from Marquest Medical Products, Inc., 1989; and *B,* From Retractable Technologies, Inc.;

Figure 1-5, From Jacob, S. W., and Francone, C. A.: Structure and Function in Man, 5th ed. Philadelphia, W.B. Saunders, 1982;

Figure 1-6, From Goldsmith, J. P., and Karotkin, E. H.: Assisted Ventilation of the Neonate, 3rd ed. Philadelphia, W.B. Saunders, 1996;

Figure 1-7, From Jacob, S. W., and Francone, C. A.: Structure and Function in Man, 5th ed. Philadelphia, W.B. Saunders, 1982;

Figure 1-8, From Goldsmith, J. P., and Karotkin, E. H.: Assisted Ventilation of the Neonate, 3rd ed. Philadelphia, W.B. Saunders, 1996;

Figure 1-9, From McMinn, R. M. H., Hutchings, R. T., Pegington, J., and Abrahams, P.H.: Color Atlas of Human Anatomy, 3rd ed. Mosby-Year Book Europe Limited, 1993;

Figure 1-10, From Jacob, S. W., and Francone, C. A.: Structure and Function in Man, 5th ed. Philadelphia, W.B. Saunders, 1982;

Figure 1-13, From Goss, C. M. (ed): Gray's Anatomy of the Human Body, 29th ed. Philadelphia, Lea & Febiger, 1973;

Figure 1-15, From Millar, S., Sampson, L. K., and Soukup, M. (eds): AACN Manual for Critical Care, 2nd ed. Philadelphia, W.B. Saunders, 1985;

Figure 1-20, From Goldsmith, J. P., and Karotkin, E. H.: Assisted Ventilation of the Neonate, 3rd ed. Philadelphia, W.B. Saunders, 1996.

Chapter 3

Figure 3-4, From Guyton, A. C.: Textbook of Medical Physiology, 9th ed. Philadelphia, W.B. Saunders, 1996;

Figure 3-5, Courtesy Radiometer, Inc.;

Figure 3-6, Courtesy Radiometer, Inc.;

Figure 3-7, From Miller, A.: Pulmonary Function Tests: A Guide for the Student and House Officer. Orlando, FL, Grune & Stratton, 1987.

Chapter 4

Figure 4-5, From Siggaard-Andersen, O.: The Acid-Base Status of the Blood, 4th ed. Baltimore, Lippincott Williams and Wilkins, 1974, Copyright 1963 by O. Siggaard-Andersen, Copenhagen, Denmark;

Figure 4-7, From Burtis, C. A., and Ashwood, E. R. (eds): Tietz: Fundamentals of Clinical Chemistry, 5th ed. Philadelphia, W.B. Saunders, 2001;

Figure 4-9, From Siggaard-Andersen, O.: The Acid-Base Status of the Blood, 4th ed. Baltimore, Lippincott Williams and Wilkins, 1974, Copyright 1963 by O. Siggaard-Andersen, Copenhagen, Denmark;

Figure 4-10, From Fraser, C. G.: Biological Variation: From Principles to Practice. Washington D.C., AACC Press, 2001;

Figure 4-11, From Burtis, C. A., and Ashwood, E. R. (eds): Tietz: Fundamentals of Clinical Chemistry, 5th ed. Philadelphia, W.B. Saunders, 2001;

Figure 4-12, From Burtis, C. A., and Ashwood, E. R. (eds): Tietz: Fundamentals of Clinical Chemistry, 5th ed. Philadelphia, W.B. Saunders, 2001;

Figure 4-13, From Henry J. B.: Clinical Diagnosis and Management by Laboratory Methods, 20th ed. Philadelphia, W.B. Saunders, 2001;

Figure 4-14, From Dantzker D. R., MacIntyre, N. R., and Bakow, E. D. (eds): Comprehensive Respiratory Care. Philadelphia, W.B. Saunders, 1995;

Figure 4-15, From Burtis, C. A., and Ashwood, E. R. (eds): Tietz: Fundamentals of Clinical Chemistry, 5th ed. Philadelphia, W.B. Saunders, 2001;

Figure 4-16, Adapted from Dantzker, D. R., MacIntyre, N. R., and Bakow, E. D. (eds): Comprehensive Respiratory Care. Philadelphia, W.B. Saunders, 1995;

Figure 4-17, Modified from Shapiro, B. A., Peruzzi, W. T., and Kozelowski-Templin, R.: Clinical Application of Blood Gases, 5th ed. St. Louis, Mosby, 1994;

Figure 4-18, Reference: Shapiro, B. A., Peruzzi, W. T., and Kozelowski-Templin, R.: Clinical Application of Blood Gases, 5th ed. St. Louis, Mosby, 1994.

Chapter 6

Figure 6-2, Adapted from Wandrup, J. H.: Assessment of Blood Oxygen Profiles in Critically Ill Patients, 16th Annual Respiratory Care Symposium, Pittsburgh. PA, February 29, 1996 [Radiometer America Inc., Ohio];

Figure 6-3, From Naclerio, E. A.: Chest Injuries. Orlando, FL, Grune & Stratton, 1971;

Figure 6-6, From West, J. B., Dollery, C. T., and Naimark, A.: Distribution of blood flow in isolated lung; relation to vascular and alveolar pressures. J. Appl. Physiol. 19:713, 1964;

Figure 6-7, From West, J. B., Dollery, C. T., and Naimark, A.: Distribution of blood flow in isolated lung; relation to vascular and alveolar pressures. J. Appl. Physiol. 19:713, 1964;

Figure 6-8, From Fraser, R. G., and Paré, J. A. P.: Diagnosis and Diseases of the Chest, vol. IV, 3rd ed. Philadelphia, W.B. Saunders, 1997;

Figure 6-11, From West, J. B.: Ventilation/Blood Flow and Gas Exchange, 3rd ed. Oxford, London, Blackwell Scientific Publications, 1977. [Data from Bryan, A. C., Bentivoglio, L. G., Beerel, F., Macleish, H., et al.: Factors affecting regional distribution of ventilation and perfusion in the lung. J. Appl. Physiol. 19:395–402, 1964.];

Figure 6-15, Modified from Lee, A. R., and Schumaker, P. T.: Respiratory Physiology: Basics and Applications. Philadelphia, W.B. Saunders, 1993;

Figure 6-16, From Cherniack, R. M.: Respiration in Health and Disease, 3rd ed. Philadelphia, W.B. Saunders, 1983;

Figure 6-17, From West, J. B.: Regional differences in gas exchange in the lung of erect man. J. Appl. Physiol. 17:893, 1962;

Figure 6-18, Modified from Alspach, A.: AACCN Instructors Resource Manual for the AACCN Core Curriculum for Critical Care Nurses. Philadelphia, W.B. Saunders, 1992;

Figure 6-19, Adapted from Burke, J. F.: Surgical Physiology. Philadelphia, W.B. Saunders, 1983;

Figure 6-20, Redrawn from Alspach, A.: AACCN Instructors Resource Manual for the AACCN Core Curriculum for Critical Care Nurses. Philadelphia, W.B. Saunders, 1992;

Figure 6-22, From Dantzker, D. R.: Gas exchange. In Montenegro. H. (ed): Chronic Obstructive Pulmonary Disease. New York, Churchill Livingstone, 1983;

Figure 6-23, From Cherniack, R. M.: Respiration in Health and Disease, 3rd ed. Philadelphia, W.B. Saunders, 1983;

Figure 6-24, From Comroe, J. H. Jr., et al.: The Lung. Chicago, Year Book Medical, 1962. Original illustration from Low, F. N.: Anat. Rec. 117:241, 1953, Reprinted by permission of Wiley-Liss, Inc., a subsidiary of John Wiley and Sons, Inc.

Chapter 7

Figure 7-1, Adapted from Wandrup, J. H.: Assessment of Blood Oxygen Profiles in Critically Ill Patients, 16th Annual Respiratory Care Symposium, Pittsburgh, PA, February 29, 1996 [Radiometer America Inc., Ohio];

Figure 7-4, From Henry, J. B.: Clinical Diagnosis and Management by Laboratory Methods, 20th ed. Philadelphia, W.B. Saunders, 2001;

Figure 7-5, From Schloo, B. L.: Normal development of the hematopoietic system. *In* Lake, C. L., and Moore, R. A. (eds): Blood: Hemostasis, Transfusion, and Alternatives in the Perioperative Period. New York, Raven Press, 1995;

Figure 7-6, From Wilson, S. F., and Thompson, J. M.: Mosby's Clinical Nursing Series: Respiratory Disorders. St. Louis, Mosby, 1990;

Figure 7-7, From Skalak, R., and Branemark, P. I.: Deformation of red blood cells in capillaries. Science, 164:717, 1969. Copyright 1969 by the American Association for the Advancement of Science;

Figure 7-8, From Oxygen Transport Physiology Slide Series. Hayward, CA, Nellcor Incorporated, 1987;

Figure 7-14, From Leff, A. R., and Schumaker, P. T.: Respiratory Physiology: Basics and Application. Philadelphia, W.B. Saunders, 1993;

Figure 7-15, Modified from Murray, J. F.: The Normal Lung. Philadelphia, W.B. Saunders, 1976;

Figure 7-18, From LeVeen, H. H., Ip, M., Ahmed, N., et al.: Lowering blood viscosity to overcome vascular resistance. Surg. Gynecol. Obstet. 150:139–149, 1980;

Figure 7-19, From Hinshaw, H. C., and Murray, J. F.: Diseases of the Chest. Philadelphia, W.B. Saunders, 1979, p 767;

Figure 7-20, From personal correspondence, Simmons, M.;

Figure 7-21, From Stamatoyannopoulos, G., Bellingham, A. J., Lenfant, C., and Finch, C. A.: Abnormal hemoglobins with high and low oxygen affinity, Annual Review of Medicine, vol. 22, 1971, Reprinted from Annual Reviews (www.annualreviews.org);

Figure 7-22, From Barker, S. J., Tremper, K. K., Hyatt, B. S., and Zaccari, J.: Effects of methemoglobinemia on pulse oximetry and mixed venous oximetry. Anesthesiology 67:A171, 1987;

Figure 7-23, Adapted from Platt, O. S.: Easing the suffering caused by sickle cell disease. N. Engl. J. Med. 330:783–784, 1994;

Figure 7-24, Courtesy of Ann Bell, MS, SH (ASCP), Professor of Clinical Laboratory Sciences, University of Tennessee, Memphis. *In* Rodak, B. F.: Hematology: Clinical Principles and Applications, 2nd ed. Philadelphia, W.B. Saunders, 2002;

Figure 7-25, Adapted from Wandrup, J.H.: Assessment of Blood Oxygen Profiles in Critically Ill Patients, 16th Annual Respiratory Care Symposium, Pittsburgh, PA, February 29, 1996 [Radiometer America Inc., Ohio];

Figure 7-26, Adapted from Comroe, J.: Physiology of Respiration, 2nd ed. Chicago, Year Book Medical, 1977.

Chapter 8

Figure 8-8, From Guyton, A. C.: Textbook of Medical Physiology, 10th ed. Philadelphia, W.B. Saunders, 2000;

Figure 8-10, From Jacob, S. W., and Francone, C. A.: Structure and Function in Man, 2nd ed. Philadelphia, W.B. Saunders, 1970.

Chapter 10

Figure 10-6, Modified from Hinshaw, H. C., and Murray, J. F.: Diseases of the Chest, 4th ed. Philadelphia, W.B. Saunders, 1980;

Figure 10-7, From Benumof, J. L.: Anesthesia for Thoracic Surgery, 2nd ed. Philadelphia, W.B. Saunders, 1995;

Figure 10-8, From Benumof, J. L.: Anesthesia for Thoracic Surgery, 2nd ed. Philadelphia. W.B. Saunders, 1995;

Figure 10-9, From Benumof, J. L.: Anesthesia for Thoracic Surgery, 2nd ed. Philadelphia, W.B. Saunders, 1995;

Figure 10-10, From Benumof, J. L.: Anesthesia for Thoracic Surgery, 2nd ed. Philadelphia, W.B. Saunders, 1995;

Figure 10-11, From O'Quin, R., and Marini, J. J.: Pulmonary artery occlusion pressure: Clinical physiology, measurement and interpretation. Am. Rev. Respir. Dis. 128:319–326, 1983.

Chapter 11

Figure 11-1, From LeVeen, H. H., Ip, M., Ahmed, N., et al.: Lowering blood viscosity to overcome vascular resistance. Surg. Gynecol. Obstet. 150:139–149. 1980 (now J Am Coll Surg);

Figure 11-2, From Rodak, B. F.: Hematology: Clinical Principles and Applications, 2nd ed. Philadelphia, W.B. Saunders, 2002;

Figure 11-3, From Rodak, B. F.: Hematology: Clinical Principles and Applications, 2nd ed. Philadelphia, W.B. Saunders, 2002;

Figure 11-4, From Rodak, B. F.: Hematology: Clinical Principles and Applications, 2nd ed. Philadelphia, W.B. Saunders, 2002;

Figure 11-5, From Rodak, B. F.: Hematology: Clinical Principles and Applications, 2nd ed. Philadelphia, W.B. Saunders, 2002;

Figure 11-6, Modified from Sabiston, D. C. Jr.: Sabiston's Textbook of Surgery, 16th ed. Philadelphia, W.B. Saunders, 2001;

Figure 11-7, Modified from Sabiston, D. C., Jr.: Sabiston's Textbook of Surgery, 16th ed. Philadelphia, W.B. Saunders, 2001;

Figure 11-8, Modified from Sabiston, D. C., Jr.: Sabiston's Textbook of Surgery, 16th ed. Philadelphia, W.B. Saunders, 2001;

Figure 11-9, Courtesy Baxter Healthcare Corp., Irvine, CA;

Figure 11-10, From Luce, J. M., Tyler, M. L., and Pierson, D. J.: Intensive Respiratory Care, 2nd ed. Philadelphia, W.B. Saunders, 1993;

Figure 11-11, Redrawn from Alspach, A.: AACCN Instructors Resource Manual for the AACCN Core Curriculum for Critical Care Nurses. Philadelphia, W.B. Saunders Company, 1992;

Figure 11-12, Redrawn from Alspach, A.: AACCN Instructors Resource Manual for the AACCN Core Curriculum for Critical Care Nurses. Philadelphia, W.B. Saunders, 1992.

Chapter 12

Figure 12-1, From Weinberger, S. E.: Principles of Pulmonary Medicine, 3rd ed. Philadelphia, W.B. Saunders, 2003;

Figure 12-2, From Weinberger, S. E.: Principles of Pulmonary Medicine, 3rd ed. Philadelphia, W.B. Saunders, 2003;

Figure 12-3, From Guyton, A. C.: Textbook of Medical Physiology, 10th ed. Philadelphia, W.B. Saunders, 2000;

Figure 12-4, From Guyton, A. C.: Textbook of Medical Physiology, 10th ed. Philadelphia, W.B. Saunders, 2000;

Figure 12-5, From Guyton, A. C.: Textbook of Medical Physiology, 10th ed. Philadelphia, W.B. Saunders, 2000;

Figure 12-6, Modified from Andreoli, T. E., Carpenter, C. C. J., Griggs, R. C., Loscalzo, J., and Cecil, R. L.: Cecil Essentials of Medicine, 5th ed. Philadelphia, W.B. Saunders, 2001;

Figure 12-7, From Guyton, A. C.: Textbook of Medical Physiology, 10th ed. Philadelphia, W.B. Saunders, 2000;

Figure 12-8, From McCance, K. L., and Heuther, S. E.: Pathophysiology: The Biologic Basis for Disease in Adults and Children, 2nd ed. St. Louis, Mosby, 1994;

Figure 12-9, Modified from Guyton, A. C.: Basic Human Physiology, 2nd ed. Philadelphia, W.B. Saunders, 1977;

Figure 12-10, Modified from Guyton, A. C.: Basic Human Physiology. 2nd ed. Philadelphia, W.B. Saunders, 1977;

Figure 12-11, Modified from Guyton, A. C.: Basic Human Physiology, 2nd ed. Philadelphia, W.B. Saunders. 1977;

Figure 12-12, Modified from Alspach, A.: AACCN Instructors Resource Manual for the AACCN Core Curriculum for Critical Care Nursing. Philadelphia, W.B. Saunders, 1992;

Figure 12-13, Modified from Guyton, A. C.: Basic Human Physiology, 2nd ed. Philadelphia, W.B. Saunders, 1977;

Figure 12-14, From Guyton, A. C.: Basic Human Physiology, 2nd ed. Philadelphia, W.B. Saunders, 1977;

Figure 12-15, From Guyton, A.C.: Basic Human Physiology, 2nd ed. Philadelphia, W.B. Saunders, 1977;

Figure 12-17, From Beeson, P. B., and McDermott, W.: Textbook of Medicine, vol. II, 14th ed. Philadelphia, W.B. Saunders, 1975.

Chapter 13

Figure 13-2, From Ropper, A. H.: ICU management of acute inflammatory-postinfectious polyneuropathy. *In* Ropper, A. H., and Kennedy, S. K., (eds): Neurological and Neurosurgical Intensive Care, 2nd ed. Rockville, MD, Aspen, 1988, pp 253–268;

Figure 13-3, Modified from Drachman, D. B.: Myasthenia gravis. N. Engl. J. Med. 330:1797–1810, 1994;

Figure 13-8, From Finberg, L., Kravath, R. E., and Fleischman, A. R.: Water and Electrolytes in Pediatrics. Philadelphia, W.B. Saunders, 1982.

Chapter 14

Figure 14-1, From Halsted, C. H., and Halsted, J. A.: The Laboratory in Clinical Medicine. Philadelphia, W.B. Saunders, 1981;

Figure 14-2, Modified from Halsted, C. H., and Halsted, J. A.: The Laboratory in Clinical Medicine. Philadelphia, W.B. Saunders, 1981.

Chapter 15

Figure 15-1, Modified from Radiometer Medical A/S. Blood Gas, Oximetry, and Electrolyte Systems Reference Manual. Copenhagen, 1996;

Figure 15-2, From Nave, C. R., and Nave, B. C.: Physics for the Health Sciences, 3rd ed. Philadelphia, W.B. Saunders, 1985, p 251;

Figure 15-3, From Davidsohn, I., and Bernard, J. H. (eds): Todd-Sanford Clinical Diagnosis by Laboratory Methods, 15th ed. Philadelphia, W.B. Saunders, 1974;

Figure 15-4, From Neuman, M. R.: Pulse Oximetry: Physical Principles, Technical Realization and Present Limitations. New York, Plenum Press, 1986;

Figure 15-5, From Neuman, M. R.: Pulse Oximetry: Physical Principles, Technical Realization and Present Limitations. New York, Plenum Press, 1986;

Figure 15-6, From Oxygen Transport Physiology Slide Series. Hayward, CA, Nellcor Incorporated, 1987;

Figure 15-7, From Brown, M., and Vender, J. S.: Noninvasive oxygen monitoring. *In* Vender, J. S. (ed): Critical Care Clinics: Intensive Care Monitoring, vol. 4. Philadelphia, W.B. Saunders, 1988, p 495;

Figure 15-8, From Ramage, J. E. Hemodynamic and gas exchange monitoring. *In* Hess, D. R., et al. (eds): Respiratory Care: Principles and Practice. Philadelphia, W.B. Saunders, 2002;

Figure 15-9, Modified from materials courtesy Novametrix Medical Systems, Wallingford, CT;

Figure 15-10, From Oxygen Transport Physiology Slide Series. Hayward, CA, Nellcor Incorporated, 1987;

Figure 15-11, From Brown, M., and Vender, J. S.: Noninvasive oxygen monitoring. *In* Vender, J. S. (ed): Critical Care Clinics: Intensive Care Monitoring, vol. 4. Philadelphia, W.B. Saunders, 1988;

Figure 15-12, From Oxygen Transport Physiology Slide Series. Hayward, CA, Nellcor Incorporated, 1987;

Figure 15-13, From Masimo Corporation product literature, Irvine, CA;

Figure 15-14, From, Brown, M., and Vender, J. S.: Noninvasive oxygen monitoring. *In* Vender, J. S. (ed): Intensive Care Monitoring, vol. 4. Philadelphia, W.B. Saunders. 1988;

Figure 15-15, From Scanlon, C. L.: Analysis and monitoring of gas exchange. *In* Scanlan, C. L., Wilkins, R. L., and Stoller, J. K. (eds): Egan's Fundamentals of Respiratory Care, 7th ed. St. Louis, Mosby, 1999;

Figure 15-16, From Hicks, G. H.: Blood gas and acid-base measurement. *In* Dantzker, D. R., MacIntyre, N. R., and Bakow, E. D. (eds): Comprehensive Respiratory Care. Philadelphia, W.B. Saunders, 1995;

Figure 15-17, From Scanlan, C. L.: Analysis and monitoring of gas exchange. *In* Scanlan, C. L., Wilkins, R. L., and Stoller, J. K. (eds): Egan's Fundamentals of Respiratory Care, 7th ed. St. Louis, Mosby, 1999;

Figure 15-18, From Capnography: A Quick Reference. Hayward, CA, © Nellcor Incorporated, 1988;

Figure 15-19, From Snyder, J. V., Elliot, J. L., and Grenvik, A.: Capnography. *In* Spence, A. A.: Clinics in Critical Care Medicine: Respiratory Monitoring in Intensive Care. Edinburgh, Churchill Livingstone, 1982;

Figure 15-20, From Nuzzo, P. E., and Anton, W. R.: Practical applications of capnography. Respir. Ther. Nov/Dec:12–17, 1986;

Figure 15-21, From Hess, D.: Capnometry and capnography: Technical aspects, physiological aspects, and clinical applications. Respir. Care 35(6):563, June 1990;

Figure 15-22, From Hess, D.: Capnometry and capnography: Technical aspects, physiological aspects, and clinical applications. Respir. Care 35(6):564, June 1990;

Figure 15-23, From Ramage, J. E.: Hemodynamic and gas exchange monitoring. *In* Hess, D. R., et al. (eds): Respiratory Care: Principles and Practice. Philadelphia, W.B. Saunders, 2002;

Figure 15-24, From Single Breath Carbon Dioxide (product literature). Novametrix Medical Systems, Inc.

Index

Note: Page numbers followed by f indicate figures; those followed by t indicate tables; and those followed by b indicate boxed material.